D0938328

Measuring Occupational Performance

SUPPORTING BEST PRACTICE IN OCCUPATIONAL THERAPY

SECOND EDITION

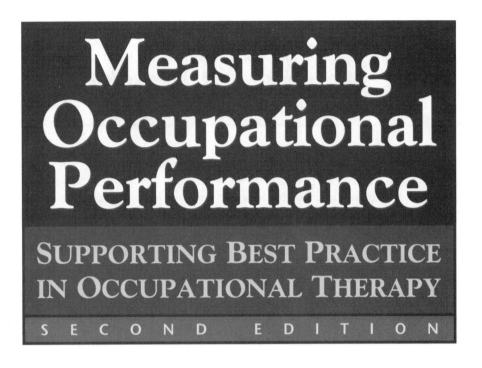

Measuring Occupational Performance

SUPPORTING BEST PRACTICE IN OCCUPATIONAL THERAPY

SECOND EDITION

MARY LAW, PhD, OT REG. (ONT.), FCAOT
McMaster University
Hamilton, Ontario, Canada

CAROLYN BAUM, PhD, OTR/C, FAOTA
Washington University School of Medicine
St. Louis, Missouri

WINNIE DUNN, PhD, OTR, FAOTA
University of Kansas Medical Center
Kansas City, Kansas

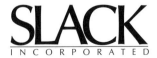
SLACK
INCORPORATED

An innovative information, education, and management company
6900 Grove Road • Thorofare, NJ 08086

Copyright © 2005 by SLACK Incorporated

ISBN 10: 1-55642-683-6

ISBN 13: 978-1-55642-683-4

The *Measuring Occupational Performance: Supporting Best Practice in Occupational Therapy, Second Edition Instructor's Manual* is also available from SLACK Incorporated. Don't miss this important companion to *Measuring Occupational Performance: Supporting Best Practice in Occupational Therapy, Second Edition*. To obtain the Instructor's Manual, please visit http://www.efacultylounge.com.

Library of Congress Cataloging-in-Publication Data

Measuring occupational performance : supporting best practice in occupational therapy / [edited by] Mary Law, Carolyn Baum, Winnie Dunn.-- 2nd ed.
    p. ; cm.
Rev. ed. of: Measuring occupational performance / Mary Law, Carolyn Baum, Winnie Dunn. c2001.
Includes bibliographical references and index.
ISBN-13: 978-1-55642-683-4 (pbk. : alk. paper)
ISBN-10: 1-55642-683-6 (pbk. : alk. paper)
1. Occupational therapy. 2. Outcome assessment (Medical care) 3. Occupational therapy--Decision making.
[DNLM: 1. Occupational Therapy--standards. 2. Outcome Assessment (Health Care) 3. Evidence-Based Medicine. WB 555 M484 2005] I. Law, Mary C. II. Baum, Carolyn Manville. III. Dunn, Winnie. IV. Law, Mary C. Measuring occupational performance.
RM735.L39 2005
615.8'515--dc22

2005010132

Printed in the United States of America

Published by: SLACK Incorporated
               6900 Grove Road
               Thorofare, NJ 08086 USA
               Telephone: 856-848-1000
               Fax: 856-853-5991
               www.slackbooks.com

Contact SLACK Incorporated for more information about other books in this field or about the availability of our books from distributors outside the United States.

DEDICATION

To all the persons and their families who have informed us about the importance of measurement.

CONTENTS

Dedication . . . . *v*

Acknowledgments . . . . *viii*

About the Editors . . . . *ix*

Contributing Authors . . . . *x*

Preface . . . . *xi*

Foreword . . . . *xii*

Section I: Foundations of Occupational Therapy Measurement Practice

Chapter 1   Measurement in Occupational Therapy 3
           Mary Law, PhD, OT Reg. (Ont.), FCAOT, and Carolyn Baum, PhD, OTR/C, FAOTA

Chapter 2:   Measurement Issues and Practices 21
           Winnie Dunn, PhD, OTR, FAOTA

Chapter 3:   Guiding Therapist Decisions About Measuring Outcomes in Occupational Therapy 33
           Mary Law, PhD, OT Reg. (Ont.), FCAOT; Gillian King, PhD; and Dianne Russell, MSc

Section II: Measurement in Occupational Therapy

Chapter 4:   Establishing the Integrity of Measurement Data: Identifying Impairments
           That Can Limit Occupational Performance and Threaten the Validity of Assessments 49
           Carolyn Baum, PhD, OTR/C, FAOTA; Monica Perlmutter, MA, OTR/L;
           and Winnie Dunn, PhD, OTR, FAOTA

Chapter 5:   Using Qualitative Measurement Methods to Understand Occupational Performance 65
           Mary Corcoran, PhD, OTR(L), FAOTA

Chapter 6:   Measuring Occupational Performance Using a Client-Centered Perspective 81
           Mary Ann McColl, PhD, OT Reg. (Ont.) and Nancy Pollock, MSc, OT Reg. (Ont.)

Chapter 7:   Occupational Performance: Measuring the Perspectives of Others 93
           Dorothy Edwards, PhD and Carolyn Baum, PhD, OTR/C, FAOTA

Chapter 8:   Measuring Participation 107
           Mary Law, PhD, OT Reg. (Ont.), FCAOT; Winnie Dunn, PhD, OTR, FAOTA;
           and Carolyn Baum, PhD, OTR/C, FAOTA

Chapter 9:   Measuring Play Performance 129
           Anita C. Bundy, ScD, OTR, FAOTA

Chapter 10: Measuring Work Performance From an Occupational Performance Perspective 151
           Sue Baptiste, MHSc, OT Reg. (Ont.), FCAOT; Susan Strong, MSc, OT Reg. (Ont.);
           and Brianna McGuire, MScOT, OT Reg. (Ont.)

Chapter 11: Measuring Occupational Performance in Basic Activities of Daily Living 179
           Lori Letts, PhD, OT Reg. (Ont.) and Jackie Bosch, MSc, OT Reg. (Ont.)

Chapter 12: Measuring Performance in Instrumental Activities of Daily Living 227
           Laura N. Gitlin, PhD

Chapter 13: Measuring Leisure Performance 249
           Kate Connolly, PhD, MPA; Mary Law, PhD, OT Reg. (Ont.), FCAOT;
           and Brianna MacGuire, MScOT, OT Reg. (Ont.)

Chapter 14: Measurement of Occupational Role 277
         Janice P. Burke, PhD, OTR/L, FAOTA and T. Brianna Lomba, OTS

Chapter 15: Occupational Balance: Measuring Time Use and Satisfaction Across Occupational
         Performance Areas 287
         Catherine Backman, PhD, OT(C)

Chapter 16: Measuring Community Integration and Social Support 301
         Mary Ann McColl, PhD, OT Reg. (Ont.)

Chapter 17: Measuring Environmental Factors 315
         Patricia Rigby, MHSc, OT Reg. (Ont.); Barbara Cooper, PhD; Lori Letts, MA, OT Reg. (Ont.);
         Debra Stewart, MSc, OT Reg. (Ont.); and Susan Strong, MSc, OT Reg. (Ont.)

Section III: Using Measurement in Practice

Chapter 18: Measuring Occupational Performance within a Sociocultural Context 347
         Pollie Price, PhD, OTR/L

Chapter 19: Using Information to Influence Policy 367
         Carolyn Baum, PhD, OTR/C, FAOTA; Sue Baptiste, MHSc, OT Reg. (Ont.), FCAOT;
         and Mary Law, PhD, OT Reg. (Ont.), FCAOT;

Chapter 20: Challenges and Strategies in Applying an Occupational Performance Measurement Approach 375
         Mary Law, PhD, OT Reg. (Ont.), FCAOT; Carolyn Baum, PhD, OTR/C, FAOTA;
         and Winnie Dunn, PhD, OTR, FAOTA

Appendices

Appendix A: List of Measures (Alphabetical) *383*
Appendix B: List of Measures by Occupational Performance Area *385*
Appendix C: List of Measures by Source/Author *387*
Appendix D: List of Measures Mapped to the International Classification of Functioning *390*
Appendix E: Outcome Measures Rating Forms and Guidelines *396*

Index *411*

ACKNOWLEDGMENTS

We are very grateful to all the authors who have shared their knowledge in the chapters of this book. Their ability to analyze measures and to synthesize that information in easy-to-use tables is outstanding. Thanks also to our colleagues at McMaster University, Washington University in St. Louis, and the University of Kansas Medical Center for your continuing support of our work.

Mary wishes to acknowledge the ongoing support that she receives from her family—thanks to Brian, Mike, Geoff, and Andy. Thanks to Brianna MacGuire who provided research assistant services for the second edition.

Carolyn would like to acknowledge the colleagues and subjects who have fostered her interest in measurement and particularly Charles Christiansen and Mary Law, who share unselfishly their knowledge and support.

Winnie would like to acknowledge Jeannie Rigby, Joan Delahunt, and Marguerite Green for their work preparing references and obtaining background material.

ABOUT THE EDITORS

Mary Law, PhD, OT Reg. (Ont.), FCAOT, is Professor and Associate Dean of Rehabilitation Science and Co-Director of CanChild Centre for Childhood Disability Research at McMaster University, Hamilton, Canada.

Carolyn Baum, PhD, OTR/C, FAOTA, is the Elias Michael Director and Assistant Professor of Occupational Therapy and Neurology at Washington University School of Medicine in St. Louis, MO.

Winnie Dunn, PhD, OTR, FAOTA, is Professor and Chair of the Department of Occupational Therapy Education at the University of Kansas, Kansas University Medical Center, Kansas City, KS.

Contributing Authors

Catherine Backman, PhD, OT(C) is Head, Division of Occupational Therapy in the School of Rehabilitation Sciences at the University of British Columbia, Vancouver, Canada.

Sue Baptiste, MHSc, OT Reg. (Ont.), FCAOT, is Chair of the Occupational Therapy Programme in the School of Rehabilitation Science at McMaster University, Hamilton, Canada.

Jackie Bosch, MSc, OT Reg. (Ont.), is a research fellow in the Canadian Cardiovascular Collaboration and Assistant Clinical Professor in the School of Rehabilitation Science at McMaster University, Hamilton, Canada.

Anita C. Bundy, ScD, OTR, FAOTA, is a professor in the Department of Occupational Therapy at Colorado State University in Fort Collins, CO.

Janice P. Burke, PhD, OTR/L, FAOTA, is Chair of Occupational Therapy in the College of Health Professions at Thomas Jefferson University in Philadelphia, PA.

Kate Connolly, MPA, is currently a PhD candidate in the School of Urban and Regional Planning and the Department of Recreation and Leisure Studies at the University of Waterloo, Waterloo, Canada.

Barbara Cooper, PhD is a professor in the School of Rehabilitation Science at McMaster University, Hamilton, Canada.

Mary Corcoran, PhD, OTR(L), FAOTA, is currently the Associate Department Chairman, Director of Research, Department of Health Care Sciences, School of Medicine and Health Sciences, The George Washington University, Washington, DC.

Dorothy Edwards, PhD, is a research assistant professor in Occupational Therapy and Neurology at Washington University School of Medicine, St. Louis, MO.

Laura N. Gitlin, PhD, is a professor in the Department of Occupational Therapy and Director, Community and Homecare Research Division in the College of Health Professions at Thomas Jefferson University, Philadelphia, PA. She is also Director of Research, Senior Health Institute in the Jefferson Health System.

Gillian King, PhD, is Research Program Manager at Thames Valley Children's Centre in London, an Investigator with the CanChild Centre for Childhood Disability Research and Assistant Clinical Professor in the School of Rehabilitation Science at McMaster University in Hamilton, Canada.

Lori Letts, MA, OT Reg. (Ont.), is Assistant Professor in the School of Rehabilitation Science, McMaster University, Hamilton, Canada.

T. Brianna Lomba, OTS is a graduate student in the master's degree program at Jefferson College of Health Professions, Thomas Jefferson University in Philadelphia, PA.

Brianna MacGuire, MScOT, OT Reg. (Ont.) is an occupational therapist with the Halton Infant Program, Halton Region, Canada.

Mary Ann McColl, PhD, OT Reg. (Ont.), is a professor of Rehabilitation Therapy and of Community Health and Epidemiology at Queen's University in Kingston, Canada.

Monica Perlmutter, MA, OTR/L, is an instructor in the Program in Occupational Therapy, Washington University School of Medicine, St. Louis, MO.

Nancy Pollock, MSc, OT Reg. (Ont.), is Associate Professor in the School of Rehabilitation Science and an Investigator in the CanChild Centre for Childhood Disability Research at McMaster University, Hamilton, Canada.

Pollie Price-Lackey, PhD (Cand.), OTR, is a doctoral candidate at the University of Southern California in the Department of Occupational Science and Occupational Therapy and is currently a Teaching Associate in the Department of Occupational Therapy at the University of Kansas Medical Center in Kansas City, KS.

Patricia Rigby, MHSc, OT Reg. (Ont.), is Assistant Professor in the Department of Occupational Therapy at the University of Toronto and Clinical Leader in Occupational Therapy at Bloorview MacMillan Children's Centre in Toronto, Canada.

Dianne Russell, MSc, is a research coordinator with the CanChild Centre for Childhood Disability Research and Assistant Professor in the School of Rehabilitation Science at McMaster University, Hamilton, Canada.

Debra Stewart, MSc, OT Reg. (Ont.), is Assistant Clinical Professor in the School of Rehabilitation Science and an Associate Member of the CanChild Centre for Childhood Disability Research at McMaster University, Hamilton, Canada.

Susan Strong, MSc, OT Reg (Ont.), is a research coordinator at the Work Function Research Unit, McMaster University and an occupational therapist at Hamilton Psychiatric Hospital, Hamilton, Canada.

PREFACE

The journey from the conceptualization of an idea for a book to its completion is often a long, meandering pathway. That is the case with this text. We initially conceived the idea for this book in conversations during the Can-Am Occupational Therapy Conference in Boston, 1994. All of us were enthusiastic about the idea of assembling knowledge about the measurement of occupational performance in occupational therapy practice. As you can imagine, the tasks of identifying the focus and content of the book and appropriate authors and writing have taken longer than expected. However, there has been a benefit from the time taken. Measurement in occupational therapy has become more sophisticated, and this is reflected in many assessments reviewed in this book.

It has been exciting and rewarding to work together on this text. There is no doubt that this book has been enriched from the collaboration between the three of us. From the many faxes and e-mails to the time that we spent together at conferences and over 2 days in St. Louis, our interactions have been stimulating and fun. This time to work together has been a wonderful opportunity.

It is our hope that student occupational therapists, occupational therapy practitioners, and occupational therapy educators will find the material in this book useful in their daily studies and practice. We welcome your comments and thoughts about the content and layout of the book.

Mary Law, Carolyn Baum, and Winnie Dunn

Foreword

In my foreword for the first edition of this book, I stated that global health care trends were becoming congruent with the core values and beliefs of occupational therapy. I am happy to report that now, several years later, these trends continue as health care policy and the prevalent health paradigm increasingly support our values and beliefs. Among these values and beliefs are that health is greater than or even different from the sum of the intact anatomical, physiological, and behavioral components of individuals; that client-centered experience of well-being is essential to health; and that health is inseparable from the social and physical environment of daily living.

These trends have been fueled by globalization, research findings, and evidence-based practice. As different cultures have come together and exchanged knowledge, practices, and artifacts of living, it has become clear that the traditional Western view of health as the absence of bodily pathology is only partially true, and therefore, only a partially effective model for improving health. A more bio-psycho-social-cultural view is required. Research findings generally have supported the need for a model of health in which mind, body, action, and situation are interactive and transactive. The rise of evidence-based practice has encouraged critical scholarship and the testing of deeply held assumptions by the various health care disciplines, creating and supporting the climate of change that underlies the emerging trends.

Although the trends in health care are promising, they have far to go. The new policies are not yet backed uniformly or consistently by economic and management systems that provide the infrastructure for the practices needed to implement these trends. Practitioners continue to hold disparate and non-convergent models of health, either because of lack of training relevant to the new trends or inability to accommodate to these trends because of the poor infrastructure. There is a need for leadership on how to do the health care represented in these trends: specifically, a need for the clear explication of healthy living, for the development of interventions to promote it, for the valid and trustworthy assessment of its achievement, and for the dissemination of this body of knowledge to clients, health care providers, managers, and policy makers.

Now, more than ever, occupational therapy has much to contribute to the path of health care. We are trained in mind-body health and its relationship with the meaning and importance of the routines of daily living; we are experts in the content, rhythms, and situations of living; and we have a philosophy of optimism and pragmatism that girds our intervention—a seeing of possibilities, and the roll-your-sleeves-up, hands-on doing of what needs to be done. Most importantly, we aim to see clients' lives through their eyes, to understand what is important from their point of view. Having this aim, even if its achievement is difficult, is essential to effective cross-ethnicity and cross-cultural therapeutic relationships, as well as to the development of high quality and globally relevant assessments, interventions, practice theory, and research.

However, in fulfilling our potential as leaders in health care, we occupational therapists also have much to learn. Only now are we recognizing that our "commonsense" approach to daily living is our primary strength, that, indeed, it is worthy of the intense critical scholarship, research, and theory development that we had seen previously as secondary to the doing of our work with clients, or as reserved for the more "basic science" disciplines. The editors of this text, Mary Law, Carolyn Baum, and Winnie Dunn, have been instrumental in naming the strengths of an occupational paradigm and giving a voice to the meaning of health from an occupational perspective. Among their many works, they have brought together the esteemed contributors to this book to explain how our core values and beliefs can be put into everyday practice in this changing environment.

What I stated in my foreword to the first edition bears repeating because it continues to be true in this second edition. The contributors to this book show how the manifestation of our values and beliefs in practice creates the best practice for our clients and supports the continued integration of these values and beliefs into the larger health care system. Their guidance is based specifically upon current research evidence about the importance and validity of measuring occupational performance. They summarize the measurement tools needed to assess client occupational performance, to provide the best intervention, and to document the effectiveness of that intervention. The tools are not merely a compilation of all that are available for measurement relevant to occupational therapy; rather, they are an elite group of tools carefully selected by the contributors through a process of rigorous theoretical, clinical, and scientific reasoning. As a result, the book is an essential reference manual for the evidence-based practitioner, the occupational performance researcher, and the health care policy consultant.

Although occupational therapy continues to develop as a profession, it has recently achieved a new level of rigor and expertise in its scholarship and research-based knowledge. Now, several years after the printing of the first edition, I believe that occupational therapists are ready to play major roles in defining the multi- and inter-disciplinary approach to health. The assessments in this book address health concepts and constructs that are at the intersections of the various disciplines, and they bridge the dichotomies that often differentiate the disciplines. These assessments connect mind to body, action to environment, and individual to community. They do so because this is how occupational therapists view health. Occupational therapists are ready to lead the way to a new and collaborative health care paradigm, using the voice of connection that exists within the assessment procedures of this book.

Linda Tickle-Degnen, PhD, OTR/L, FAOTA
Boston University
Boston, MA

SECTION I

FOUNDATIONS OF OCCUPATIONAL THERAPY MEASUREMENT PRACTICE

Occupational therapists work with persons, groups, and organizations that are experiencing difficulties in performing the occupations of life (i.e, self-care, work, voluntary activities, play, leisure). The desired outcome of occupational therapy services is optimal occupational performance, defined as the satisfactory experience of a person participating in everyday occupations. The World Health Organization (WHO) has recognized the importance of participation in occupations and its influence on health and well-being in their new International Classification of Functioning, Disability and Health (WHO, 2001). This book focuses on the measurement of occupational performance, providing readers with a guide to the application of measurement and introduction of tools to support best practice in occupational therapy.

What are the challenges that occupational therapists face as they pursue the measurement of occupational performance? Let's illustrate a few of them:

"I want to be able to evaluate the occupational performance outcomes of my clients, but the team I work with expects me to provide information about range of movement, strength, and endurance. They also want numbers."

"It would be easier to justify reimbursement for services if we had and used outcomes measures that provided evidence of the changes that we see in day-to-day activities in our clients. It's so hard to know where to start in using outcomes measures. How do we decide what it is we want to measure, and what are the best assessments to use?"

"I know that I should encourage my clients to identify the occupational performance issues for which they need occupational therapy services, but I just don't have enough time to allow them to do that. It's so much easier just to do our standard assessment of performance components (e.g., cognitive status, balance) and start therapy right away."

In writing this book, we hope to address these issues and help practitioners eliminate concerns that limit measurement practices in occupational therapy. We have identified five fundamental objectives for the book.

Mine the Gold

There is a wealth of information in the occupational therapy literature and the broad health and social sciences literature that can be used by the occupational therapy practitioner to support occupational therapy measurement practices. Using such information will enable occupational therapists to support their clinical observations and, indeed, will lend credibility to their day-to-day clinical observations. Occupations are complex, individualized, and essential for health and well-being. Evaluation of occupational performance, the outcomes of doing occupation, is enhanced by the development of a broad measurement perspective. The unique contribution of occupational therapy to the health care team will be recognized.

Become Systematic

Occupational therapists can use the information in this text to develop a consistent approach to measuring the outcomes of their practice. The reader is given a systematic guide to make decisions about measurement of occupational performance. This guide is provided to enable therapists and clients to knowledgeably identify outcomes of interest and select the most reliable and valid methods to assess these desired outcomes. Resources for the selection of assessments are provided to support therapists in selecting the best outcomes measures for their clinical situation. Measures are indexed by assessment area, chapter and title for ease of identification.

Use Evidence in Practice

Occupational therapists, as well as all other health care providers, strive to practice in a manner that is effective and efficient. Providing cost-effective, evidence-based health care is the goal of every health professional. One of the most important underpinnings of an evidence-based occupational therapy practice is the consistent use of outcomes measures to evaluate occupational therapy service. Information from the application of outcomes measurement enables therapists to make decisions about which programs are most effective, thus building evidence to support occupational therapy intervention. In this text, we provide information about the selection and application of outcomes measurement to support an evidence-based occupational therapy practice.

Make Occupational Therapy Contribution Explicit

Occupational therapy, as a profession, makes a unique contribution to health care through our focus on the occupations of everyday life. Through ongoing analysis of persons doing the occupations of their choice within different environments, occupational therapists identify factors that support or hinder performance and intervene to enable optimal performance. Mattingly and Fleming, in a study of the occupational therapy clinical reasoning process, stated that "what occupational therapists do looks simple, what they know is quite complex" (1994, p. 24). The consistent use of measurement enables occupational therapists to identify the unambiguous outcomes of effective occupational therapy services, thus clarifying the contribution of occupational therapy to the health and well-being of persons needing our services and to others on the health care team.

Engage in Occupation-Based, Client-Centered Practice

There is increasing research evidence to support the relationship between engagement in occupation and positive outcomes for a person's health and well-being (Clark, Corcoran & Gitlin, 1995; Law, Steinwender, & LeClair, 1998; Wilcock, 1998). Therapy to enable persons to do the occupations of their choice is most effective when delivered using a client-centered service delivery model (Law, 1998). Information in this text focuses on measurement of occupational performance from a client-centered perspective and can be used by therapists to support an occupation-based, client-centered practice.

This book is organized to be a tool for the student occupational therapist and the practicing therapist as they strive to organize and classify their occupational therapy experiences to best serve their clients. Section I of this text addresses the foundations of occupational therapy measurement practices. In Chapter 1, the theoretical foundations for an occupation-based, client-centered practice are outlined. Chapter 2 focuses on central concepts to understand regarding measurement, including the importance of considering the context of measurement. In Chapter 3, we present a decision-making framework to guide occupational therapists in the identification, selection, and use of best measurement practices.

1

MEASUREMENT IN OCCUPATIONAL THERAPY

Mary Law, PhD, OT Reg. (Ont.), FCAOT and Carolyn Baum, PhD, OTR/C, FAOTA

"Our conception of man is that of an organism that maintains and balances itself in the world of reality and actuality by being in active life and active use."

Adolph Meyer, 1922, p. 1

Occupational therapists work with individuals, groups, and organizations to enable them to participate in the occupations of everyday life. The goal for occupational therapy services is to enhance occupational performance (i.e., the doing and experience of occupation in order to satisfy life needs). Occupational therapists' unique contribution to society, therefore, is to enable clients to achieve their goals by helping them overcome problems that limit their occupational performance (Baum & Law, 1997). Occupational therapists enhance participation in occupations. To achieve this goal, our discipline must learn about the clients' physical, cognitive, neurobehavioral, and psychological capacities; their culture; their physical, social, and institutional environments; and the activities, tasks, and roles that the clients define as important. The process of providing occupational therapy is complex.

Within the health care arena, each discipline has a developed area of focus. For example, physicians' clinical practice and clinical research centers on patients' impairments, medical history, and physical exam; physical therapists' on their movement; dietitian's on their nutrition; and occupational therapists' on their occupational performance. Rogers (1982) describes medicine's efforts to limit the impact of disease as a contrast to occupational therapy's efforts in enabling the performance of work, play, or self-care "occupations." A critical point of Rogers

is that there are individuals who experience occupational performance problems that are not accompanied by disease (i.e., joblessness, behavior disorders, teen mothers, people living in times of war). The broad focus of occupational therapy on the "occupations of everyday life" makes it necessary to use measurement methods that are not dependent on a medical condition to determine the extent of the occupational performance dysfunction. Rogers argues convincingly that through the emphasis on disease and functional deficit, rather than occupational performance and competence, the biomedical influences on traditional health care have been a limiting factor in the development of occupational therapy (and its measurement methods).

There is a sizable population of persons with disabilities in the world. For example, about 45 million Americans, or one in six (Brandt & Pope, 1997), and one of seven Canadians over the age of 15 years, about 3.4 million people (Statistics Canada, 2002), have an impairment that limits their daily activities. Approximately one-third of these disabilities are severe enough that they limit participation in work and/or community life (Statistics Canada, 2002). Disability is a public health problem—it affects not only individuals with disabling conditions and their immediate families, but also society (Pope & Tarloff, 1991). There are even more persons who are experiencing limitations in occupational performance for other reasons such as poverty, social crises, or war. Measurement of the outcomes of occupational therapy practice in all these situations improves our ability to work together with clients, their families, and other groups in a client-centered occupational therapy practice.

In this chapter we will discuss the foundations of occupational therapy measurement practices, including the philosophical influences, sociocultural factors, central concepts for contemporary practice, interdisciplinary models that are consistent with our philosophy, and models for considering occupational performance in a best practice measurement process.

PHILOSOPHICAL INFLUENCES ON OCCUPATIONAL THERAPY

The values, beliefs, and principles of a discipline have a major influence on its identity and development and are known collectively as its philosophy. Throughout our history, occupational therapy's value of occupation and on performance of occupations have been central. There have been ongoing discussions of measurement, but until the past two decades, there was a lack of measures of occupational performance to support the profession's values and beliefs.

Adolph Meyer, a notable psychiatrist and neurobiologist who taught at Johns Hopkins University and was a proponent of occupational therapy during its early years, is widely credited with making an important contribution to the development of philosophy in the field. He also has had a major impact on measurement because he stated the first hypothesis of our discipline. In an address given at the fifth annual meeting of the National Society for the Promotion of Occupational Therapy in Baltimore, Maryland, in 1921, Meyer suggested that occupational therapy represents an important manifestation of human philosophy, namely, "the valuation of time and work" (1922, p. 6) and the role of performance and completion in bringing meaning to life.

Meyer stated that "man learns to organize time and he does it in terms of doing things" (p. 6), thus emphasizing his view of the importance of doing to achieving self-fulfillment. Meyer suggested that the view of mental illness as a problem of living rather than a structural, toxic, or constitutional disorder was an important characteristic of the field, and that occupational therapists could provide opportunities for the individual to work, to plan, to create, and to learn to use tools and materials. These opportunities, Meyer thought, would assist patients in gaining pleasure and pride in achievement. If we were to apply these concepts in today's practice, we would provide people an opportunity to use their minds in planning, organizing, sequencing, and carrying out a task (executive skills).

In summarizing Meyer's address, we can observe that he viewed the individual and health in a holistic rather than structural sense and believed that engagement in occupations, or doing, provided a sense of reality, achievement, and temporal organization. Meyer perceived occupational

therapy as providing opportunities for engagement that would contribute to learning and improving one's sense of fulfillment and self-esteem. In doing so, he was proclaiming occupational therapy's concern for quality of life and suggesting a clear relationship between the ability to perform daily occupations and one's life satisfaction.

Meyer's themes have been repeated in more recent contributions by scholars reflecting on the unique characteristics of the field. For example, Yerxa (1967), in her Eleanor Clarke Slagle address, emphasized the role of occupational therapy in providing opportunities for fulfillment in doing when she wrote:

In occupational therapy, the patient experiences the reality of his physical environment and his capacity to function within it. Our clinics may be chambers of horror for some individuals as they confront their physical disability for the first time by trying to do something, perhaps as simple as [eating]. Yet, if the individual is to function with self-actualization, he must discover both his limitations and his possibilities. We meet our responsibilities to the client when we provide opportunities to readjust his or her value system through the development of both new capacities and the ability to substitute for some lost capacities. We are like mirrors which can reflect, without the distortion of wish-fulfillment or self-deprecation, a true image of the client's potential. (p. 5)

Similarly, Fidler and Fidler (1978) emphasized the role of occupation, or doing, in gaining self-actualization, when they wrote:

The ability to adapt, to cope with the problems of everyday living, and to fulfill age-specific life roles requires a rich reservoir of experiences gathered from direct engagement with both human and non-human objects in one's environment. Doing is a process of investigating, trying out, and gaining evidence of one's capacities for experiencing, responding, managing, creating, and controlling. It is through such action with feedback from both non-human and human objects that an individual comes to know the potential and limitations of self and the environment and achieves a sense of competence and intrinsic worth. (p. 306)

Both Elizabeth Yerxa and the Fidlers reaffirmed Adolph Meyer's beliefs and values in the opportunities occupational therapy affords for self-actualization. They also emphasized the role of the therapist in assisting the individual to cope with problems of everyday living and to adapt to limitations that interfere with competent role performance.

Rogers (1982) declared that functional independence is not only the core concept of occupational therapy theory, but also the goal of the occupational therapy process. Noting that the requirements for independence are competence and autonomy, she suggested that autonomy is reflected in the ability to make choices and have control over the environment. The opportunities afforded within occupational therapy practice for developing competence and teaching strategies for exerting autonomy make it unique among the rehabilitation disciplines. To say we influence autonomy and independence, it is necessary to use a measurement strategy that demonstrates these effects.

Occupation has always been central to the practice of occupational therapy. Writers over the decades have given direction to that practice. A sampling of these writers is presented here to lay the context for the measurement of occupational performance.

- "[A human] is an organism that maintains and balances itself in the world of reality and actuality by being in active life and active use... It is the use that we make of ourselves that gives the ultimate stamp to our every organ" (Meyer, 1922, p.1).

- Reilly (1962) suggests that human beings need to produce, create, master, and improve their environment in order to achieve health and well-being.

- Fidler & Fidler (1963) conceptualized activity as a valuable vehicle to acquire, maintain, or redevelop skills necessary to fulfill occupational roles and provide satisfaction.

- Individuals who perceive that they have control over their environments and can address obstacles derive satisfaction from their occupational roles (Burke, 1977; Sharrott & Cooper-Fraps, 1986).

- Function results from a series of complex relationships among cognitive, psychological, sensory, neuromotor, and physiological capabilities as the individual interacts with his or her environment (Christiansen, 1991).

- Occupational dysfunction can be viewed as a "breakdown in habits that leads to physiological deterioration with the concomitant loss of ability to perform competently in daily life" (Kielhofner, 1992, p. 30).

- When occupational therapists present the opportunity for individuals to engage in activity, not only does the individual's functional status improve (Baum, 1995), but occupational therapy makes explicit its unique contribution to the enhancement of human function.

- "...purposeful and fulfilling occupations can provide individuals with sufficient exercise to maintain homeostasis, to keep body parts and neuronal physiology and mental capacities functioning at peak efficiency, and enable maintenance and development of satisfying and stimulating social relationships... If they are able, or encouraged to pursue this need, they will, apart from supplying sustenance for survival and safety, enhance their health" (Wilcock, 1993, p. 23).

- "Occupational therapy, at its best, is client-centered. The person receiving occupational therapy services leads the way in making decisions about the focus and nature of therapy intervention. The relationship between that person, his or her family, and the occupational therapist is a collaborative partnership whose goal is to enhance occupational performance, health, and well-being" (Law, 1998, Preface).

Bing (1991) proposed the following six enduring values. These values can serve as hypotheses for guiding intervention and measurement and challenging students and faculty into action to empirically test these core principles.

1. Engagement in occupation is of value because it provides opportunities for individuals to influence their well-being by gaining fulfillment in living.

   Question: Does participation in occupation provide opportunities for individuals to influence their well-being?

2. Through the experience of occupation (or doing), the individual is able to achieve mastery and competence by learning skills and strategies necessary for coping with problems and adapting to limitations.

   Question: Can occupation construct opportunities for learning that yield mastery and adaptation?

3. As competency is gained and autonomy can be expressed, independence is achieved.

   Question: What is the relationship between competency, autonomy, and independence?

4. Autonomy implies choice and control over environmental circumstances. Thus, opportunities for exerting self-determination should be reflected in intervention strategies.

   Question: Is there a difference in the outcome of persons who exhibit self-determination by exercising choice and control in the design and implementation of occupational therapy services? Does changing the environment influence a person's ability to participate effectively in occupations?

5. Choice and control extend to decisions about intervention, thus identifying occupational therapy as a collaborative process between the therapist and recipient of care. In this collaboration, the patient's values are respected.

   Question: Does a collaborative, client-centered approach promote health and well-being and fewer secondary conditions?

6. Because of its focus on life performance, occupational therapy is neither somatic nor psychological, but concerned with the unity of body and mind in doing.

   Question: What is the relationship of an integrated body-mind approach to care vs. a psychological approach vs. a physical impairment orientation on the person's perception of his or her capacity for life and satisfaction? How does a person's spirituality affect his or her occupations?

It is incumbent on all practitioners in occupational therapy to be familiar with these core principles (Bing, 1991) and use them in assessing and planning occupational therapy services.

IMPACT OF SOCIOCULTURAL FACTORS ON OUR FOCUS ON OCCUPATION

For the past several decades, occupational therapy has been inextricably linked to the medical model of health care. This linkage has fostered the tendency for occupational therapists to measure performance components (e.g. strength, mood, range of movement, pain) as the primary outcome(s) of therapy. Medicine has influenced the history of occupational therapy practice. Beginning in the 1930s, occupational therapy practice became progressively less influenced by a view of function that was holistic and occupation-centered, in favor of practice techniques that emphasized components of function such as muscle strength, range of motion, or disturbed processes of thought. In fact, from the mid-1960s to the mid-1980s in the United States, occupational therapy's reimbursement was directly related to documentation of these performance components. In this orientation, little consideration was given to how these components affected performance in day-to-day living. Findings from research indicate that there is little direct relationship between impairments (or components) and abilities (Badley, 1995). Even today there is little transfer of skills from doing a specific action to being able to apply the action in a sequenced complex task. Fortunately, in the late 1970s, several prominent writers in the field expressed concern for this state of affairs and encouraged a return to the occupation-centered philosophy upon which the profession was first established.

Prominent among these was an article entitled "The Derailment of Occupational Therapy," by Philip Shannon (1977). Shannon wrote that:

   . . . a new hypothesis has emerged that views man not as a creative being, capable of making choices and directing his own future, but as a mechanistic creature susceptible to manipulation and control via the application of techniques. The technique hypothesis, inspired by the principles of reduction-

ism, subverts the occupational therapy hypothesis of man using his hands to influence the state of his own health. (p. 233)

In the same year, Kielhofner and Burke (1977) provided a detailed account of various bases for practice during the first 60 years of occupational therapy. They traced the evolution of guiding principles in the field from its humanistic roots to the competing ideas of the 1980s, noting that the paradigm of reductionism was reflected in three dominant intervention models that continued to influence practice. These were the kinesiological, the psychoanalytic or interpersonal, and the sensory integrative or neurological model. The authors concluded that advancement of the field would require a theoretical approach that went "beyond reductionism" and allowed an understanding of human adaptation, or "social man within a holistic theoretical framework." Today we see the importance of this sift as all of medicine is being challenged to focus on function to foster well-being and participation.

CENTRAL CONCEPTS FOR CONTEMPORARY OCCUPATIONAL THERAPY PRACTICE

What Is Occupation?

Just as good health is often taken for granted, so too are everyday life experiences. The satisfaction of dining with friends and family, enjoying a walk in the park, or gaining a sense of accomplishment from seeing a garden blossom can be diminished by impairments resulting from injury or disease, inability to do an activity, or lack of environmental supports. But they need not be. The remarkable adaptability of the human body, our spirituality, and the power of meaning and self-will provide many ways for people to derive satisfaction from participation in life's occupations despite temporary or permanent functional limitations. When these resources are coupled with the skillful intervention of the occupational therapist, health-related occupational performance limitations can often be overcome.

Occupation is everything that we do in life, including actions, tasks, activities, thinking, and being. Engagement in occupation describes the interaction of the individual with their self-directed life activities. Adolph Meyer (1922) professed that individuals should attain and retain a healthful "rhythm in sleep and waking hours, of hunger and its gratification, and finally the big four—work and play and rest and sleep" (p. 3). Wilcock (1993) challenges us to view "occupation [as] a central aspect of the human experience and unique to each individual" (p. 17). The definition of occupation should be basic to every occupational therapist's vocabulary. Occupation meets the [individual's] intrinsic needs for self-maintenance, expression, and fulfillment within the context of personal roles and environment (Law et al., 1996). Thus, it is through the process of engagement in occupation that people develop and maintain health and well-being (Wilcock, 1998; Law, Steinwender, & LeClair, 1998; Christiansen & Baum, 1991, 1997, 2004).

Occupational Performance

Occupational performance is the doing of occupation in order to satisfy life needs. Recent literature has given more definition to the term occupational performance. Occupational therapy uses the word "function" interchangeably with "performance" and "occupational performance" because occupational therapy's domain is the function of the person in his or her occupational roles. The unique contribution of occupational therapy is that the practitioner creates the opportunity for individuals to gain the skill and confidence to accomplish activities and tasks that are meaningful and productive and in doing so increases their occupational performance (Baum & Edwards, 1995).

- The term occupational therapists use for function is *occupational performance*, or the point when the person, the environment, and the person's occupation intersect to support the tasks, activities, and roles that define that person as an individual (Baum & Law, 1997; Law et al., 1996).

- The concept of occupational performance has become mainstay in the development of models of occupational therapy. It operates as a means of connecting the individual to roles and to the sociocultural environment (Reed & Sanderson, 1999, p.93).

- Performance results from complex interactions between the person and the environments in which he or she carries out activities, tasks and roles (Christiansen & Baum, 1991, 1997, 2004).

- Occupational performance refers to the ability to choose, organize, and satisfactorily perform meaningful occupations that are culturally defined and age appropriate for looking after one's self, enjoying life, and contributing to the social and economic fabric of a community (Canadian Association of Occupational Therapists [CAOT], 1997, p.30).

- Occupational performance results from the dynamic interaction between people, their occupations and roles, and the environments in which they live, work and play (Law et al., 1996).

- Occupational performance consists of meaningful sequences of action in which a person completes an occupational form (Kielhofner, 1995, p.113).

- Occupational performance is the ability to perceive, desire, recall, plan and carry out roles, routines, tasks and sub-tasks for the purpose of self maintenance,

productivity, leisure and rest in response to demands of the internal and/or external environment (Chapparo & Ranka, 1997, p. 58).

- Performance includes both the process and the result of the person interacting with context to engage in tasks (Dunn, Brown, & McGuigan, 1994).

The ideas underlying occupational therapy models of practice that address the inter-relationships between the person, environment, and occupation are not new. In many ways, these ideas are similar to a model (called the ecological systems model) proposed by occupational therapists Howe and Briggs (1982) and share characteristics in common with self-determination theory, formulated by Deci and Ryan (1991). Performance is viewed as the result of complex relationships between the individual as an open system and the specific environments in which activities, tasks, and roles occur. It is important to consider that a complete view of occupational performance must consider the actions, tasks, occupations, and roles of an individual as he or she goes about his or her daily life (Christiansen & Baum, 1997).

David Nelson (1988, 1996) has contributed to our thinking about occupation. Recognizing that people use the term occupation to mean active-doing, as well as that which is done, Nelson proposed including both interpretations in our understanding of occupation. In his schema, occupation is defined as the relationship between an occupational form and occupational performance. Occupational performance consists of the "doing" of occupation, whereas occupational form concerns the context of the doing, or the other elements of a "doing situation," which provide it with purpose and meaning.

There is consensus for the term occupational performance. The next step in our development is for measurement models to evolve that support the occupational therapist in determining the effectiveness of occupational therapy services through the evaluation of occupational performance. The measurement of occupational performance requires the practitioner to employ three strategies: 1) What people do in their daily lives, 2) What motivates them, and 3) How their personal characteristics combine with the environment in which occupations are undertaken to influence successful occupational performance. Such an approach provides a framework for viewing human behavior that combines knowledge about the impairments (components) that impede performance, the environments that support or hinder performance, and the individual needs, preferences, styles, and goals (Christiansen & Baum, 1997; Law et al., 1996).

Occupational therapy practice must place its focus on occupational performance—assisting our clients to become actively engaged in their life activities. Basic to an occupational performance approach are the skills of the therapist to analyze tasks, activities, and occupations and propose and use learning or adaptive strategies to support the individual to perform meaningful occupations.

The environment in which persons live, work, and play make doing and being possible. People conduct their daily lives within many different environments. Some are using the term environment and context interchangeably. Every task and activity has a context—that what is present at the time the activity occurs. The environment exists whether or not an activity occurs. For example a community may offer curb cuts, large font (signage) for its street signs, or verbal cues at crosswalks. That city has created a universal environment which may or may not give context to the performance of a task for an individual.with a particular set of skills or limitations. Occupational performance is always influenced by the characteristics of the environment in which it occurs. In noting this, Rogers (1983) described the qualities of the environment as important "enablers of human performance." In Chapter 2, we discuss the issues of contextual measurement for contemporary occupational therapy practice.

A Client-Centered Approach to Measurement

Over the past two decades, occupational therapists have described the need for a practice based on a client-centered approach to occupational therapy. The national association and occupational therapists in Canada developed client-centered guidelines for occupational therapy (CAOT, 1983, 1997), and now therapists around the world contribute to this perspective.

Client-centered occupational therapy has been defined as "an approach to service which embraces a philosophy of respect for, and partnership with, people receiving services" (Law, Baptiste, & Mills, 1995, p. 253). Such an approach to therapy acknowledges our responsibilities to work in partnership with clients to enable them to find meaning in life through daily occupations. We celebrate everyone's ability to find sources of meaning and bring their resources to the occupational therapy intervention process when using a client-centered approach.

"The goal of the [client-] centered philosophy is to create a caring, dignified, and empowering environment in which [clients] truly direct the course of their care and call upon their inner resources to speed the healing process" (Matheis-Kraft, George, Olinger, & York, 1990, p. 128). Such an approach fosters a partnership with clients to enable them to identify their needs and individualize the services they perceive they will need in order to accomplish their goals. Clients are encouraged to recognize and build on their strengths, using natural community supports as much as possible.

Adolph Meyer (1922) spoke of client-centered concepts in the *Philosophy of Occupation*, yet Carl Rogers was the first person to use the actual term *client-centered* to describe a health care practice that was non-directive and centered on the person's articulated needs (Rogers, 1939). Roger's recognized that a client-centered approach would often be at odds with a medical model approach. Indeed, the client-centered approach has often been criticized for its lack of specific techniques and inherent optimism (Cain, 1990; May, 1983).

Law (1998) has summarized the concepts of client-centered practice inherent in all theoretical discussion of this approach. These concepts include:

- Respect for clients and their families, and the choices they make.
- Clients and families have the ultimate responsibility for decisions about daily occupations and occupational therapy services.
- Provision of information, physical comfort, and emotional support. Emphasis on person-centered communication.
- Facilitation of client participation in all aspects of occupational therapy service.
- Flexible, individualized occupational therapy service delivery.
- Enabling clients to solve occupational performance issues.
- Focus on the person-environment-occupation relationship.

Using these assumptions, clients and therapists can jointly focus on their unique contribution and responsibilities and jointly select measures that will contribute to the decision-making process (Law et al., 1995).

What does a client-centered, occupational therapy practice mean for the way in which we measure occupational performance? The concepts of client-centered practice have the following implications for measurement of occupational performance.

1. Occupational performance issues/problems will be identified by the client and his or her family, not by the therapist or team; if there are issues that do not surface (safety, prevention, or health maintenance), the therapist will communicate these concerns directly to the client and family.

2. Evaluation of the success of therapy intervention will focus on change in occupational performance.

3. Our measurement techniques will enable clients to have a say in evaluating the outcomes of their therapy intervention.

4. Measurement will reflect the individualized nature of people's participation in occupations.

5. Measurement will focus on both the subjective experience and the observable qualities of occupational performance.

6. Measurement of the environment is critical in helping therapists and clients understand the influence of the environment on occupational performance, as well as measuring the effects of changing environmental conditions during the therapy process as well as in the home, the work site, or community that would foster participation.

Client-centered measurement is based on the principle that effective therapy begins with a careful understanding of the individual. An occupational therapy practice based on the concepts of client-centeredness is more likely to engage clients in the occupational therapy process and lead to increased cooperation and satisfaction with therapy (Law, 1998). Any of the occupational therapy models discussed in this chapter provides a framework for clinicians to organize information gained from interviews and formal assessments. These frameworks can form a basis for intervention that is collaborative and client-directed. Such an approach is better able to enlist the personal and spiritual resources necessary to facilitate the healing process (Matheis-Kraft et al., 1990) and is more likely to engage clients in the occupational therapy process, leading to increased adherence and satisfaction with therapy (Law, 1998).

In a client-centered approach, clients and therapists work together to define the nature of the occupational performance problems, the focus and need for intervention, and the preferred outcomes of therapy. Clients will participate at different levels, depending on their capabilities, but all are capable of making choices about how they approach their rehabilitation to improve their capacity for daily life. The occupational therapist must have a fundamental respect for clients' values and visions and for their style of coping without being judgmental, as well as knowledge of the factors that influence occupational performance. It is important for the occupational therapist to plan the first phase of the intervention to seek information from the client about his or her perception of the problem, needs, and goals. Information that is shared builds the occupational performance history, which includes information about the person, the environment, and the occupational factors that require occupational therapy intervention.

In order to be considered client-centered, occupational therapy models must consider the activities, tasks, and roles of the person (Christiansen & Baum, 2004); the organization of services to support the individual as an active participant in his or her care (Blank, Horowitz, & Matza, 1995); and create a partnership that enables individuals to assume responsibility for their own care (Law et al., 1995). Each of these considerations challenges the practitioner to employ measurement strategies that go far beyond, but must include, measurement at the performance component level to fully understand the individual's

capacities for occupational pursuits. The measurement process must be clinically useful and integrated into the intervention process.

A measurement model must allow the client and practitioner to jointly plan intervention. The client's knowledge of his or her condition and experience with the problem must become clear for the relationship to progress (Baum & Law, 1997). Occasionally, intervention planning must occur with a person who has a cognitive deficit or, because of age or intelligence, does not have the capacity for independent decision-making. In this case, a family-centered approach is critical. A family-centered approach is based on the same principles as a client-centered approach, with members of the family providing important information about the client's occupation and their roles and occupations as caregivers.

Why is it important for occupational therapists to use a client-centered approach to therapy measurement and intervention? As well as recognizing the fundamental respect for others inherent in this approach, there is also increasing evidence from research that client-centered practice improves not only the process but also the outcomes of care (Law, 1998). Researchers have shown that a client- or family-centered approach to health services improves adherence to therapy recommendations (King, King, & Rosenbaum, 1996), client satisfaction (Calnan, Katsouyiannopoulos, Ovcharov, Prokhorskas, Ramic, & Williams, 1994; Caro & Derevensky, 1991; Doyle & Ware, 1977; Dunst, Trivette, Boyd, & Brookfield, 1994), and leads to enhanced functional outcomes (Dunst, Trivette, & Deal, 1988; Greenfield, Kaplan, & Ware, 1985; Moxley-Haegert & Serbin, 1983; Rosenbaum, King, Law, King, & Evans, 1998).

Defining Best Practice

Best practice is a professional's decisions and actions based on knowledge and evidence that reflect the most current and innovative ideas available (Dunn, 2000). Many therapists, teams, and agencies engage in "standard practice," which is employing more traditional, routine, and established ways of providing services. This is a perfectly acceptable paradigm for conducting professional business (i.e., the routines or protocols are known and work). It is not the location of practice that determines whether one engages in best practice; therapists can work in traditional or nontraditional settings and use standard or best practices. Best practice is a way of thinking about problems in imaginative ways, applying knowledge creatively to solve performance problems while also taking responsibility for evaluating the effectiveness of the innovations to inform future practices.

Remember: What is best practice today evolves into standard practice in the future. This is how knowledge advances in our discipline. The standard practices of today were best practices of the past that have influenced practice. When someone continues his or her standard practices across too long a time, we would say that his or her practice is out of date and would not stand up to standard practice scrutiny. As your career unfolds, watch for these transitions and recognize their contributions to our evolution as a discipline.

INTERDISCIPLINARY SYSTEMS MODELS FOR PARTICIPATION AND QUALITY OF LIFE

It is important for occupational therapists to understand several key concepts to appreciate fully how occupational therapy fits into the larger context of health care and rehabilitation. Concepts from the WHO, as well as the National Center for Medical Rehabilitation Research (NCMRR) in the United States, are useful here. We acknowledge the pioneering work of Nagi (1976), who was among the first to examine the various causes and consequences of disability.

The traditional approach to medical care has focused on impairments or the loss and/or abnormality of mental, emotional, physiological, or anatomical structure or function. When there is an interruption or interference of normal physiological and developmental processes or structures, a term that is used is pathophysiology (NCMRR, 1993). Impairment includes all losses or abnormalities, not just those attributable to the initial pathophysiology, and also includes pain as a limiting experience (NCMRR, 1993). Institutional-based rehabilitation has traditionally focused on functional limitations or impairments, which have been defined as restrictions or lack of ability to perform an action or activity in the manner or within the range considered normal that results from impairment or failure of an individual to return to the pre-existing level or function (NCMRR, 1993; WHO, 1980). The term *functional limitation* or *impairment* is synonymous with the term performance components used by many occupational therapists. In contrast, disability has been defined as the inability to perform or a limitation in performing socially defined activities and roles expected of individuals within a social and physical environment as a result of internal or external factors and their interplay (NCMRR, 1993).

A social disadvantage or handicap for a given individual results when he or she is not able to fulfill a role that he or she expects or is required to fill. If the environment presents a barrier to the performance of an activity (a non-accessible building, an attitude of discrimination, or a policy that denies access), the barrier is defined as a handicapping situation (Fougeyrollas, Bergon, Cloutier, & St. Michel, 1991). When societal policy, attitudes, and actions or lack of actions create a physical, social, or finan-

cial barrier to access health care, housing, or vocational/avocational opportunities, a term that is used is *societal limitation* (NCMRR, 1993).

The more recent rehabilitation literature has questioned the wisdom of declaring independence as an absolute goal in rehabilitation (Christiansen, 1994; Grady, 1995; Meier & Purtilo, 1994). The term *interdependence* communicates that those in societies depend on collaboration and cooperation and that no community-dwelling individual is truly independent. It also suggests that we can achieve something greater working with others than we can achieve working on our own. The concept of interdependence is embodied within the idea of occupational therapy as a profession. By working in partnership with our clients and their families, we can achieve goals that we could not achieve working independently (Clark, Corcoran, & Gitlin, 1995).

When an occupational therapist approaches problem solving with clients, three sets of information are basic to the plan. Intrinsic factors (i.e., performance components) that must be considered are the neurobehavioral, cognitive, physical, and psychosocial strengths and deficits presented by the person. Extrinsic or environmental factors to be considered include the physical environment, culture, economic, institutional, political, and social context from the perspective of the person. Occupation factors include the self-maintenance, work, school, home, leisure, and family tasks and roles of the person. The unique term used by occupational therapy to express function is *occupational performance*. It reflects the individual's dynamic experience of engaging in daily occupations within the environment (Law & Baum, 1994).

INTERNATIONAL CLASSIFICATION OF FUNCTIONING, DISABILITY, AND HEALTH

A comprehensive rehabilitation model from the WHO has been developed that offers definitions and structures for facilitating communication among health professionals and policy makers. Most health care services have focused on the impairment and disability aspects of the human condition; however, the new International Classification of Functioning, Disability, and Health (ICF) (WHO, 2001) has improved definitions and systems of classification. The ICF puts forward a conceptual framework of body function and structure, activity, participation, and personal and environmental factors (WHO, 2001). Through the worldwide effort to develop this classification, it was recognized that an individual's participation in society is dependent upon the interactive relationships between these elements. This new model will influence data collection that will be used by policy makers to build systems of care that facilitate the independence in persons with disabilities.

Table 1-1

WORLD HEALTH ORGANIZATION'S INTERNATIONAL CLASSIFICATION OF FUNCTIONING, DISABILITY, AND HEALTH

	ICIDH (1980 Version)	*ICF (2002)*
Body	Impairment	Body Function and Structure—"physiological functions of body systems or anatomical parts of the body and their components."
Person	Disability	Activity—"the execution of a task or action by an individual."
Community/society	Handicap	Participation—"involvement in a life situation."
Environment	Not addressed in 1980 version	Environmental Factors—"the physical, social, and attitudinal environment in which people live and conduct their lives."
Personal factors	Not addressed in 1980 version	Personal Factors—"particular background of an individual's life and living (e.g., gender, race, age, fitness)."

Adapted from WHO. (2001). International classification of functioning, disability, and health (ICF). Geneva, Switzerland. Author.

We introduce the ICF here to familiarize the reader with key terms, concepts, and the factors that must be considered at each level. Table 1-1 highlights the key terminology and concepts of the new classification and contrasts the revision to the original 1980 version.

In using a framework such as the ICF to organize measurement, interventions, and services, one issue is critical: occupational therapists must place their primary focus at the level of the person-environment interaction so that occupational performance issues can be assessed and addressed in the occupational therapy plan. Person-environment issues are addressed in the ICF model at the activity, environmental factors, and participation levels. Tables 1-2, 1-3, and 1-4 illustrate how this framework can be used to organize the focus of measurement in occupational therapy. When we do not focus on occupational performance, the contributions of occupational therapy are not made explicit; since no one else has this expertise and emphasis, the result may be that the client must fend for him- or herself with occupational dysfunction that will compromise his or her function, participation, and health.

It is important for all practitioners in occupational therapy to be familiar with these principles and use them in planning services. It is also essential for educators to teach students how to measure the constructs inherent in these principles and for therapists to use occupational performance measurements in daily practice.

OCCUPATIONAL THERAPY MODELS FOR CONSIDERING OCCUPATIONAL PERFORMANCE WITHIN COMMUNITY ENVIRONMENTS

The health system focuses on outcomes because of the need to be accountable, not only to the clients in need of services, but also to the government and/or the third party who provides funding for these services. With a shift in focus toward primary and secondary prevention, it is also important to know if interventions are successful in reducing the impact of secondary problems. Health outcomes are being defined as well-being and quality of life; improved occupational performance is a critical construct in measuring quality of life regardless of the measure that is used. A review of the research examining the relationship between occupation, health, and well-being indicates that occupation is a significant factor in positively influencing a person's subjective and objective health and well-being (Law, Steinwender, & LeClair, 1998).

It is within the context of performance transactions that individuals encounter the objects, people, conditions, and events that stimulate development or maturation. As Kielhofner (1985, p. 41) has suggested, although change is not always grossly apparent, experiences accumulate that reinforce or modify individual characteristics. Over time,

---

Table 1-2

USING THE ICF FRAMEWORK FOR OCCUPATIONAL THERAPY MEASUREMENT

ICF Dimension	*Body Function or Structure*	*Activities*	*Participation*	*Environmental Factors*
Occupational therapy classification	**Performance components**	**Occupational performance**	**Occupational performance; role competence**	**Environmental factors**
Examples of attributes	Attention	Dressing	Community mobility	Architecture
	Cognition	Eating	Education	Attitudes
	Endurance	Learning	Housing	Cultural norms
	Memory	Making meal	Personal care	Economic
	Movement patterns	Manipulation tasks	Play	Geography
	Mood	Money management	Recreation	Light
	Pain	Socialization	Social relationships	Resources
	Range of motion	Shopping	Volunteer work	Health services
	Reflexes	Walking	Work	Institutions
	Strengths	Washing		Social rules
	Tone	Writing		Sound
				Weather

Table 1-3

NEEDS OF POTENTIAL CLIENTS (FOR THE INDIVIDUAL)

Population	*Occupational Need*	*Required Measurement Approach*
Persons with chronic disease	Productive living and quality of life	Person, environment, and occupational influences including family and community participation
Children with chronic or neurological conditions	Opportunity to develop to productive adult	Person, environment, and occupational influences including family and community participation
Individuals with acute injuries	Return to productive living	Person, environment, and occupational influences including family and community participation

---

changes become more evident, although the overall trend may be characterized by periods of varying organization or advancement. As the life cycle progresses, the desired course is one of greater satisfaction within one's environmental circumstances and an increasing sense of fulfillment through life's activities.

People spend most of their waking hours engaged in occupations, which, in addition to dressing and related self-maintenance activities, include other productive and leisure pursuits. Thus, to speak of performance in occupational therapy is to refer to occupational performance. Viewing occupational performance as a transaction between the individual, the occupations he or she does, and the environment provides a useful framework for viewing occupational therapy practice and measuring the occupational performance of our clients. This approach toward organizing information useful to measurement emphasizes the relationships between the person, environment, and occupation.

The following occupational therapy models can be used in a client-centered approach if the therapist places the focus on the client's goals and the client's occupational needs. Each of these models has the potential to evolve into a partnership between the occupational therapist and the client to address the client's goals. These models go far beyond the issues of performance components, but do not

Table 1-4

NEED OF POTENTIAL CLIENTS (FOR SOCIETY)

Population	Occupational Need	Required Measurement Approach
Industry	Productive workers	Capacity for work, person/environment fit
Social security administration	Eligible recipients	Functional capacities evaluation
Hospital/community health system	Healthy communities	Community participation, absence of secondary conditions
Schools	Children with the capacity to learn	School participation
City and county government	Housing and resources for older adults	Capacity for community living
Architecture or engineering firm	Consumers, universal design	Person/environment fit
Retirement communities	Satisfied residents, least support	Person, environment, and occupational influences including family and community participation
Day care facilities (child and adult)	Enhance performance	Person, environment, and occupational influences including family and community participation
University/colleges	Support learning	ADA—disability—access officers

prohibit the therapist working with the client on strategies to address component issues and environmental conditions that can influence the person's occupational performance. As they evolve, it is important that they extend their interventions beyond the clients' immediate needs to help clients develop behaviors that avoid unnecessary secondary conditions and promote health that will support them in doing the things they want to do. Each model can benefit from continued testing, and some require the development of more assessment tools; however, all are currently being studied and offer occupational therapy practitioners guidance in developing innovative and effective client-centered, occupation-based models of practice. We provide an overview of the key measurement issues for these models in comparison to each other; you will see both consistency and uniqueness among the models.

The Ecology of Human Performance Model

The Ecology of Human Performance Model (Dunn, Brown, & McGuigan, 1994) focuses on context and how contextual factors such as physical, temporal, social, cultural, and/or phenomenology can impact the performance of the client. The framework includes person, context, and performance variables and the interaction among them.

They describe a three-dimensional model in which you can only see the person by observing him or her in the context. A client-centered approach is central to the identification of the tasks and activities that the person does. Measurement tools are being developed to support this model; these will ensure a strong orientation to the person-environment interaction and should make client-centeredness very visible in the practice of the clinicians that subscribe to the model. This model helps the practitioner explore specific strategies to overcome the barriers that would limit the client's performance.

Key Measurement Issues

- Tasks and activities that the person does within his or her living context
- Understanding of the social, cultural, and physical environment and its impact on the performance of the client

The Model of Human Occupation

The Model of Human Occupation (MOHO) (Kielhofner, 1992, 1995; Kielhofner & Burke, 1980) evolved from Reilly's Model of Occupational Behavior (Reilly, 1966). The MOHO focuses on occupational functioning and serves to guide practice in the organization or reorganization of occupational behavior. Because it focuses on the client's routines and habits, the client's perspective and motivation for activities must be determined. The person is viewed as a dynamic system influenced by the physical and social environment. MOHO has made significant contributions to occupational therapists' knowledge of clients' roles and how occupation is central to an individual's health. A number of interview measures have been developed to support the model.

Key Measurement Issues

- The routine and habits of the person
- The person's motivation for activities and tasks
- The meaning of the activity and choice of occupations

The Person-Environment-Occupation Model

This transactive Person-Environment-Occupation Model (Law et al., 1996; Strong et al., 1999) considers the person, the occupation, and the environment in an interwoven relationship that views people in their everyday lives. The originators acknowledge that occupational performance cannot be separated from contextual influences, temporal factors, and the physical and psychological characteristics of the person. They place their model in a developmental context recognizing that environments, task demands, activities, and roles are constantly shifting. A Person-Environment-Occupation intervention seeks to enable optimal occupational performance in occupations that are defined as important by the client. The authors of this model have explicitly stated the importance of focusing on the client's goals and sharing the process of the interaction to form a partnership that will assist the client in taking responsibility for his or her own rehabilitation. This model considers the Canadian Occupational Performance Measure (Law, Steinwender, & LeClair, 1998) essential to its implementation; thus, the client's goals become the focus of the intervention.

Key Measurement Issues

- Determine the occupations that a person chooses and the goals for the therapeutic experience
- The physical and psychological characteristics of the person
- Factors in the social, cultural, physical, and institutional environment that support or hinder performance
- Temporal orientation and phase of life

The Person-Environment-Occupation-Performance Model

The Person-Environment-Occupational Performance Model (Christiansen & Baum, 1991, 1997; 2004) recognizes that the person's occupational performance cannot be separated from person-centered and contextual influences. It has operationalized the intrinsic factors (psychological, cognitive, physiological, and neurobehavioral) and extrinsic or environmental factors (physical, cultural, social, and societal policies and attitudes) to understand the capacities of the individual to perform the activities, tasks, and roles that are important to the person. Additionally, the person's self-image, determined from competency, self-concept, and motivation, are considered in the overall plan for care that is driven by the client in a dynamic partnership with the clinician (and perhaps the family and others who are instrumental in the client's life). This approach requires that the practitioner determine the activities, tasks, and roles of the client to use as the central element in planning interventions and requires that the intervention engage the person in meaningful occupations as the process to support recovery or health maintenance. This model also support an occupational performance based approach for organization and population-based approach.

Key Measurement Issues

- The activities, tasks, and roles that are important to the person, organization, or population. The person's view of him- or herself as an occupational being
- Intrinsic factors that support performance. These include the psychological, cognitive, physiological, and neurobehavioral capacities
- Extrinsic or environmental factors that serve as supports or create barriers to occupational performance, including the physical, cultural, and social environment and societal policies and attitudes

The Contemporary Task-Oriented Approach Model

The Contemporary Task-Oriented Approach Model (Mathiowetz & Bass Haugen, 1994) integrates concepts from contemporary motor control, motor development, and motor learning theories. It proposes that occupational and role performance emerges from the interaction of personal characteristics (cognitive, psychosocial, and sensorimotor) and environmental contexts (physical, socioeconomic, and cultural). In this "top-down" approach, evaluation and intervention focus primarily on occupations and roles important to the client and secondarily on any performance components and/or contexts that enable or limit performance. In contrast to earlier neuromotor approaches, this approach emphasizes the importance of the client's goals and natural contexts as major influences on occupational performance.

Key Measurement Issues

- Personal characteristics (cognitive, psychosocial, and sensorimotor)
- The environmental context of the individual (physical, socioeconomic, and cultural)
- The person's goals

The Canadian Model of Occupational Performance

The Canadian Model of Occupational Performance (CAOT, 1997) is a revised and updated version of the model in the Canadian Guidelines for Client-Centered Practice, which was originally published in 1981 (CAOT & Department of National Health & Welfare [DNHW], 1983). The model describes the relationship between persons, their environments and occupations, and the process by which occupational therapists can enable clients to achieve optimal occupational performance. Spirituality, the innate essence of self, is a central construct in the model. This model is designed around processes to guide therapists in helping clients (individuals, groups, and organizations) achieve satisfying levels of occupational performance.

Key Measurement Issues

- Occupations that are meaningful to the client
- The internal resources of the client (physical, affective, cognitive)
- The environment of the client
- Spirituality

A review of these six emerging models indicates their commonality in the measurement of occupational performance. All, either explicitly or implicitly, require a client-centered approach to the identification of the activities, tasks, and roles of the person (occupation). In addition, they consider the personal factors (psychological, cognitive, neurobehavioral, and physiological) and the environment (culture, social, and physical) in which the occupation is performed and the meaning that is attributed to the occupation. All of these constructs are essential to understanding the process to maximize the occupational performance of the individual. If the occupational therapy profession can consistently address the occupational performance needs of the people they serve, the public understanding of occupational therapy's contribution to health

care and society will improve. As we become explicit in our use of occupational performance language, we will also facilitate the advancement of our knowledge to better serve the people who need occupational therapy services.

THE OCCUPATIONAL THERAPY MEASUREMENT PROCESS

Measurement in occupational therapy serves multiple purposes. From an overall practice perspective, measurement is used to improve our decisions regarding specific clients or programs. As professionals, occupational therapists have an obligation to measure the need for service, design interventions based on knowledge gained from measurement, and evaluate the results of interventions. Information gathered through measurement helps occupational therapists to design interventions for individuals or groups and evaluate the outcomes of these programs. Management and policy makers use measurement information to make decisions about the continuance of funding for programs or the need to establish and/or evaluate new policy directions.

What Are Testing and Measurement

Testing has been defined by Educational Research Information Clearinghouse (ERIC) as "gathering and processing information about individuals' ability, skill, understanding, or knowledge under controlled conditions" (ERIC, 2004). Testing involves the collection, appraisal, and classification of information gathered in an organized manner. Such methods or tools for collecting information include naturalistic observation, interview, rating of task performance, and self-report (Christiansen & Baum, 1997). Testing methods and specific tools, whether qualitative or quantitative in nature, are developed and tested to ensure that they can be applied consistently and gather valid information. It is helpful to think of testing or evaluation as an overall approach to gathering knowledge about an attribute. An evaluation process organizes the way in which we learn about a person, his or her family, and the occupational performance issues that bring him or her to receive our services and the way that we evaluate the outcomes of those services. During testing, we need to consider the purpose of gathering information, the context of measurement, and the specific methods to be used.

Measurement is a process that involves an assessment, calculation, or judgment of the magnitude, quantity, or quality of a characteristic or attribute. Measurement is defined as the "process of obtaining a numerical description of the extent to which persons, organizations, or things possess specified characteristics" (ERIC, 2004). In everyday living, we deal with measurements ranging from calculation of time, length, or weight to judgments of quality of life and satisfaction.

Table 1-5

NEEDS AND MEASUREMENT APPROACHES OF POTENTIAL CLIENTS
(FOR THE INDIVIDUAL)

Population	Occupational Need	Required Measurement Approach
Persons with chronic disease	Productive living and quality of life	Person, environment, and occupational influences including family and community participation
Children with chronic occupational or neuro-logical conditions	Opportunity to develop into productive adult	Person, environment, and occupational influences including family and community participation
Individuals with acute injuries	Return to productive living	Person, environment, and occupational influences including family and community participation

---

Occupational Therapy's Testing and Measurement Focus

In this book, we will consider evaluation in occupational therapy from the broad perspective of testing and measurement of person, occupation, and environment. Measurement of occupational performance involves evaluation of self-care, work, other productive pursuits, play, and leisure. Because of the importance of the environment for performance, we also discuss the evaluation of the environmental factors that influence performance. Since the focus of this book is on measurement of occupational performance, we do not discuss in detail or review evaluation tools that assess performance components such as range of motion, mood, endurance, or memory. Performance component testing is important as a means to gather information about why an occupational performance problem is occurring, but, in an occupation-based practice, used to establish capacity and not as the outcome of care. Evaluations of performance components are best used to support occupational performance interventions.

Measurement of occupational performance includes the use of both quantitative and qualitative approaches from the perspective of the client, his or her family or caregiver, and the occupational therapist. As occupational therapists develop an evidence-based practice, a valid measurement process is essential in providing evidence of the effectiveness and efficiency of our services. Our measurement practices need to fit within a client-centered practice where persons, their families, and therapists work in partnership to enhance occupational performance. Our clients expect, and have a right to know and receive, evidence of the outcomes of occupational therapy service provision.

What aspects of occupational performance do occupa-tional therapists evaluate? It depends on the needs of those whom we serve. Tables 1-5 and 1-6 describe some of the needs of potential clients and suggest the issues that occupational therapists need to address from a measurement standpoint.

Implementing a measurement process within an occupational therapy practice is challenging. Currently, the field has few examples of systematic methods of measurement. There are a number of issues therapists must consider when instituting measurement within their practice—lack of time, deciding what to measure, finding an appropriate assessment tool for the measurement process, aggregating measurement information, and using the results of measurement to make decisions about services (Law, King, Russell, MacKinnon, Hurley & Murphy, 1999). These are the issues that we will address in this book.

PLANNING MEASUREMENT STRATEGIES

Occupational therapists must draw upon their knowledge of the individual, organizations, occupation, and the environment as they identify assets and limitations that affect the quality of occupational performance of the people and organizations they serve. A careful consideration of this information and the possible intervention alternatives permit the selection of various strategies for meeting client-centered goals. In each case, the particular application of an intervention process will be unique, since individuals and their circumstances are unique.

Rogers (1982) cautions that a therapeutic program that is right for one person is not necessarily right for another. She suggests that clinical inquiry be individualized and focus on three questions: 1) What is the client's current status in occupational performance? 2) What could be

---

Table 1-6

NEEDS AND MEASUREMENT APPROACHES OF POTENTIAL CLIENTS (FOR SOCIETY)

Population	*Occupational Need*	*Required Measurement Approach*
Industry	Productive workers	Capacity for work, person/environment fit
Social Security Administration	Eligible recipients	Functional capacities evaluation
Hospital/community health system	Healthy communities	Community participation, absence of secondary conditions
Schools	Children with the capacity to learn	School participation
City and county government	Housing and resources for older adults	Capacity for community living
Architecture or engineering firm	Consumers, universal design	Person/environment fit
Retirement communities	Satisfied residents, least support	Person, environment, and occupational influences including family and community participation
Day care facilities (child and adult)	Enhance performance	Person, environment, and occupational influences including family and community participation

---

done to enhance the client's performance? and 3) What ought to be done to enhance the individual's occupational performance?

It is, in fact, the critical analysis of the intrinsic, extrinsic, and occupational factors and planning of intervention for the unique constellation of circumstances represented in each client's story that makes occupational therapy an immensely complex undertaking. Because of this complexity, intervention planning is one of the most challenging and critical skills for therapists to master. As Mattingly and Fleming (1994) point out, what occupational therapists do appears so very simple, but the process of determining what to do is so very complex. Despite its complexities, effective intervention planning can be accomplished if careful attention is devoted to understanding the individual, what it is that he or she wants or needs to do, and the environmental context of the performance.

Occupational therapists face a challenge in trying to integrate person, occupation, and environmental issues in a plan of care. Being able to live a satisfying life is the only thing that matters for the person and the family. For some, living a satisfying life would include developing skills to perform the task; for others it might mean finding or designing an approach that would enable them to perform the task, or they may choose to have someone do it for them. This information must be determined and evaluated in the occupational therapy measurement process.

Goal Identification

The measurement process in occupational therapy begins and ends with occupational performance. In this process, the first step is for the client, his or her family or caregiver, or the organization to identify his or her occupational performance issues and needs. The identification of areas of occupational performance in which the client is experiencing difficulty helps therapists to organize the rest of the measurement process. A detailed decision-making process for this purpose is discussed in Chapter 3.

Another critical aspect of quality evaluation is the person's interests and needs. In client-centered care, professionals demonstrate respect for what the individual and family wish to accomplish. Professionals then consider strengths and barriers to the performance of those tasks that the individual and family have identified. Professionals must depart from traditional expert models that support the professional to direct the course of evaluation and planning in order to provide client-centered care.

Most formal testing that occupational therapists use measures the person's skills and abilities or specific task performance. However, a person's performance can vary considerably in different contexts. For example, a worker may not be able to concentrate with other workers talking but may be able to manage the phone ringing and computer printer sounds quite well. A seamstress will need to use more primitive mending strategies for a clothing repair in a hotel room than in her sewing station. A young child may remember to wipe himself after toileting within the hygiene rituals at home but may be distracted with peers in the early childhood center. Performance is context dependent; we must consider the impact of particular contexts as part of the data gathering process.

Summarizing Measurement Data

Following the identification of occupational performance issues, further evaluation of specific performance areas is often completed in order to review the person's strengths and weaknesses from the perspective of the person, the environment, and occupational factors. Based upon the identified occupational performance issues and a summary of strengths and weaknesses, a list of goals is developed with the client. These should directly relate to each identified problem or need. Short-term goals will often relate to problems identified in performance components or environmental issues. Longer term goals relate to the performance of functional daily occupations related to role performance.

Developing Priorities

Once each problem has an accompanying goal and plan, the vital task of determining priorities must take place. Evaluation initially takes precedence over intervention, since effective treatment is contingent on complete information. Principles of therapeutic management involve the use of activities that are meaningful to the client and incorporate therapeutic principles to support recovery.

Intervention planning includes a logical flow from identified problems to goals to intervention strategies. In essence, the intervention planning process, when performed by the client and therapist together, can be likened to weaving. There is a clear design and guiding principles. The challenge is to combine the warp and weft in a way that captures opportunities for creativity yet yields a satisfactory outcome. The experienced weaver, like the occupational therapist in providing intervention, executes the design with a shuttle that glides smoothly, wasting neither time nor energy in pursuit of the selvage that ends this effort and marks the beginning of yet another challenge. The outcome, or the fabric of the plan, is optimal occupational performance outcomes for the client.

Selecting Intervention Plans and Methods

Here, specific methods and techniques for achieving goals are determined. In achieving short-term goals, the emphasis may be on restoring ability and skills; however, means of reengaging in meaningful occupations must be considered to foster the motivation of the individual and to use the engagement in the recovery process. Longer term goals may be more adaptive in nature, since tasks may need to be performed with restricted underlying ability and skill. As a consequence, compensatory techniques, special equipment, and environmental modification may be necessary to accommodate residual disability. Pelland (1987) has observed that effective intervention plans are balanced in that they address remedial and adaptive goals within and across treatment sessions. For example, in treatment of a grandmother who is recovering from a stroke, one might devote time to compensating for a visual field deficit while enabling her to relearn to bake cookies for her grandchildren—an activity that balances her goals and strategies.

Planning for Further Data Collection

Pelland (1987) also notes the importance of planning for further data collection and documenting these intentions. By including assessment intentions within the overall intervention plan, the therapist ensures that this important aspect of intervention will be addressed. Collecting data during the intervention process is called progress monitoring. When therapists monitor progress systematically, they generate evidence for practice decisions.

Implementing Intervention

Strategies for addressing occupational performance problems tend to fall into five major categories. Two major categories relate to the environment and include making changes in a person's physical, social, and institutional environment and using technology in the form of various devices and aids. A third category focuses on the person and includes various approaches to facilitating the recovery or adaptation of neurological, sensory, and motor deficits. The remaining two categories have principles that warrant specific focus in the text. These include the means of delivering services and strategies that challenge the occupational therapist to take an active role in changing attitudes, policies, and laws that shape the political and social environment. Through strategies of adaptation or compensation, occupational therapy makes it possible for the tasks and roles necessary for optimal participation in the occupations of everyday life.

We have written this book to give practitioners the tools to employ an occupational performance model in evaluating their clients and to form the basis of planning care. We recognize that this approach is a paradigm shift from a traditional medical or social model but we also recognize that such an approach supports the practice guidelines and best practices and will make occupational therapists' unique contributions to care visible and contemporary with the changes in health care.

References

Badley, E. M. (1995). The genesis of handicap: Definition, models of disablement, and role of external factors. *Disability and Rehabilitation, 17,* 53-62.

Baum, C. M. (1995). The contribution of occupation to function in persons with Alzheimer's disease. *Journal of Occupation Science: Australia, 2(2),* 59-67.

Baum, C. M., & Edwards, D. (1995). Occupational performance: Occupational therapy's definition of function. *American Journal of Occupational Therapy, 49,* 1019-1020.

Baum, C. M., & Law, M. (1997). Occupational therapy practice: Focusing on occupational performance. *American Journal of Occupational Therapy, 51(4),* 277-288.

Bing, R. K. (1991). Occupational therapy revisited: A paraphrasic journey. *American Journal of Occupational Therapy, 35(8),* 499-518.

Blank, A. E., Horowitz, S., & Matza, D. (1995). Quality with a human face? The Samuel Planetree model hospital unit. *Journal of Quality Improvement, 21,* 289-299.

Brandt, E. N., Jr., & Pope, A. M. (Eds.). (1997). *Enabling America: Assessing the role of rehabilitation science and engineering.* Washington, DC: National Academy Press.

Burke, J. P. (1977). A clinical perspective on motivation: Pawn versus origin. *American Journal of Occupational Therapy, 31,* 254-258.

Cain, D. J. (1990). Further thoughts on non-directiveness and client-centered therapy. *Person-Centered Review, 5,* 89-99.

Calnan, M., Katsouyiannopoulos, V., Ovcharov, V. K., Prokhorskas, R., Ramic, H., & Williams, S. (1994). Major determinants of consumer satisfaction with primary care in different health systems. *Family Practice, 11(4),* 468-478.

Canadian Association of Occupational Therapists (1997). *Enabling occupation: An occupational therapy perspective.* Ottawa, Ontario: CAOT Publications ACE.

Canadian Association of Occupational Therapists & Department of National Health & Welfare (1983). *Guidelines for the client-centered practice of occupational therapy.* Ottawa, Ontario: Minister of Supply and Services.

Caro, P., & Derevensky, J. L. (1991). Family-focused intervention model: Implementation and research findings. *Topics in Early Childhood Special Education, 11(3),* 66-80.

Chapparo, C & Ranka, J. (1997).

Christiansen, C. (1991). Occupational therapy: Intervention for life performance. In C. Christiansen & C. Baum (Eds.), *Occupational therapy: Overcoming human performance deficits* (pp. 4-43). Thorofare, NJ: SLACK Incorporated.

Christiansen, C. (1994). A social framework for viewing self-care intervention. In C. Christiansen (Ed.), *Ways of Living: Self Care Strategies for Special Needs* (pp. 1-27). Bethesda, MD: American Occupational Therapy Association.

Christiansen, C., & Baum, C. (1991). *Occupational therapy: Overcoming human performance deficits.* Thorofare, NJ: SLACK Incorporated.

Christiansen, C., & Baum, C. (1997). *Occupational therapy: Enhancing function and well-being* (2nd ed.). Thorofare, NJ: SLACK Incorporated.

Christiansen, C., Baum, C., Bass-Haugen, J. (2004). *Occupational therapy: Performance, participation, and well-being* (3rd ed.). Thorofare, NJ: SLACK Incorporated.

Clark, C. A., Corcoran, M., & Gitlin, L. N. (1995). An exploratory study of how occupational therapists develop therapeutic relationships with family caregivers. *American Journal of Occupational Therapy, 49(7),* 587-594.

Deci, R., & Ryan, E. M. (1991). A motivational approach to self-integration in personality. *Nebraska Symposium on Motivation, 38,* 237-288.

Doyle, B. J., & Ware, J. E. (1977). Physician conduct and other factors that affect consumer satisfaction with medical care. *Journal of Medical Education, 52(10),* 793-801.

Dunn, W. (2000). *Best practice occupational therapy.* Thorofare, NJ: SLACK Incorporated.

Dunn, W., Brown, C., & McGuigan, A. (1994). Ecology of human performance: A framework. In M. Perlmutter, C. M. Baum, & D. Edwards for considering the effect of context. *American Journal of Occupational Therapy, 48(7),* 595-607.

Dunst, D. J., Trivette, C. M., Boyd, K., & Brookfield, J. (1994). Help-giving practices and the self-efficacy appraisals of parents. In C. J. Dunst, C. M. Trivette, & A. G. Deal (Eds.), *Supporting and strengthening families (Vol. 1): Methods, Strategies and Practices.* Cambridge, MA: Brookline Books.

Dunst, C. J., Trivette, C. M., & Deal, A. (1988). *Enabling and empowering families: Principles and guidelines for practice.* Cambridge, MA: Brookline Books.

ERIC. (2004). Testing. Retrieved May 3, 2004 from http://www.ericfacility.net/ extra/pub/thessearch.cfm.

Fidler, G., & Fidler, J. (1963). *Occupational therapy: A communication process in psychiatry.* New York: Macmillan.

Fidler, G. S., & Fidler, J. W. (1978). Doing and becoming: Purposeful action and self-actualization. *American Journal of Occupational Therapy, 32,* 305-310.

Fougeyrollas, P., Bergeron, H., Cloutier, R., & St. Michel, G. (1991). The handicaps creation process: Analysis of the consultation and new full proposals. *International ICIDH Network, 4.*

Grady, A. P. (1995). Building inclusive community: A challenge for occupational therapy. *American Journal of Occupational Therapy, 49(4),* 300-310

Greenfield, S., Kaplan, S., & Ware, J. E. (1985). Expanding patient involvement in care: Effects on patient outcomes. *Annals of Internal Medicine, 102,* 520-528.

Howe, M. C., & Briggs, A. K. (1982). Ecological systems model for occupational therapy. *American Journal of Occupational Therapy, 36,* 322-327.

Kielhofner, G. (1985). *A model of human occupation: Theory and application.* Baltimore: Williams & Wilkins.

Kielhofner, G. (1992). *Conceptual foundations of occupational therapy.* Philadelphia: F. A. Davis.

Kielhofner, G. (1995). *A model of human occupation: Theory and application* (2nd ed.). Baltimore: Williams & Wilkins.

Kielhofner, G., & Burke, J. P. (1977). Occupational therapy after 60 years: An account of changing identity and knowledge. *American Journal of Occupational Therapy, 31,* 675-689.

Kielhofner, G., & Burke, J. (1980). A model of human occupation, part one: Conceptual framework and content. *American Journal of Occupational Therapy, 34,* 572-581.

King, G., King, S., & Rosenbaum, P. (1996). Interpersonal aspects of care-giving and client outcomes: A review of the literature. *Ambulatory Child Health, 2,* 151-160.

Law, M. (1998). *Client-centered occupational therapy.* Thorofare, NJ: SLACK Incorporated.

Law, M., Baptiste, S., Carswell, A., McColl, M., Polatajko, H., & Pollock, N. (1998). *Canadian Occupational Performance Measure* (3rd ed.). Toronto, Canada: CAOT Publication.

Law, M., Baptiste, S., & Mills, J. (1995). Client-centered practice: What does it mean and does it make a difference? *Canadian Journal of Occupational Therapy, 62,* 250-257.

Law, M., & Baum, M. C. (1994). A brief occupational therapy history: The importance of occupation of promoting and maintaining health, creating the future: A joint effort. Can-Am Conference, Boston, July.

Law, M., Cooper, B. A., Strong, S., Stewart, D., Rigby, P., & Letts, L. (1996). The person-environment-occupation model: A transactive approach to occupational performance. *Canadian Journal of Occupational Therapy, 63,* 9-23.

Law, M., King, G., Russell, D., MacKinnon, E., Hurley, P., & Murphy, C. (1999). Measuring outcomes in children's rehabilitation: A decision protocol. *Archives of Physical Medicine and Rehabilitation, 80,* 629-636.

Law, M., Steinwender, S., & LeClair, L. (1998). Occupation, health and well-being. *Canadian Journal of Occupational Therapy, 65(2),* 81-91.

Matheis-Kraft, C., George, S., Olinger, M. J., & York, L. (1990). Patient-driven health care works! *Nursing Management, 21,* 124-128.

Mathiowetz, V., & Bass Haugen, J. B. (1994). Motor behavior research: Implications for therapeutic approaches to central nervous system dysfunction. *American Journal of Occupational Therapy, 48(8),* 733-745.

Mattingly, C., & Fleming, M. (1994). *Clinical reasoning: Forms of inquiry in a therapeutic practice.* Philadelphia: F. A. Davis.

May, R. (1983). The problem of evil: An open letter to Carl Rogers. *Journal of Humanistic Psychology, 122,* 10-21.

Meier, R. H., & Purtilo, R. B. (1994). Ethical issues and the patient-provider relationship. *American Journal of Physical Medicine and Rehabilitation, 73(5),* 365-366.

Meyer, A. (1922). The philosophy of occupation therapy. *Archives of Occupational Therapy, 1(1),* 1-10.

Moxley-Haegert, L., & Serbin, L. A. (1983). Developmental education for parents of delayed infants: Effects on parental motivation and children's development. *Child Development, 54,* 1324-1331.

Nagi, S. Z. (1976). An epidemiology of disability in the United States. *Milbank Memorial Fund Quarterly—Health and Society, 54(4),* 439-467.

National Center for Medical Rehabilitation Research (1993). *Research Plan for the National Center for Medical Rehabilitation Research.* National Institutes of Health Publication No. 93-3509.

Nelson, D. (1988). Occupation: Form and performance. *American Journal of Occupational Therapy, 42,* 633-641.

Nelson, D. (1996). Therapeutic occupation: A definition. *American Journal of Occupational Therapy, 50(10),* 775-782.

Pelland, M. J. (1987). A conceptual model for the instruction and supervision of treatment planning. *American Journal of Occupational Therapy, 41(6),* 351-359.

Pope, A. M., & Tarloff, A. R. (1991). *Disability in America: Toward a national agenda for prevention.* Washington, DC: National Academy Press.

Reed, K. & Sanderson, S. (1999). *Concepts of occupational therapy.* Philadelphia: Lippincott Williams & Wilkins.

Reilly, M. (1962). Occupational therapy can be one of the great ideas of 20th century medicine. *American Journal of Occupational Therapy, 16,* 87-105.

Reilly, M. (1966). A psychiatric occupational therapy program as a teaching model. *American Journal of Occupational Therapy, 20,* 61-67.

Rogers, C. R. (1939). *The clinical treatment of the problem child.* Boston: Houghton-Mifflin.

Rogers, J. C. (1982). Order and disorder in medicine and occupational therapy. *American Journal of Occupational Therapy, 36,* 29-35.

Rogers, J. C. (1983). Clinical reasoning: The ethics, science and art. *American Journal of Occupational Therapy, 37,* 601-616.

Rosenbaum, P., King, S., Law, M., King, G., & Evans, J. (1998). Family-centered service: A conceptual framework and research review. *Physical & Occupational Therapy in Pediatrics, 18(1),* 1-20.

Shannon, P. D. (1977). The derailment of occupational therapy. *American Journal of Occupational Therapy, 31(4),* 229-234.

Sharrott, G. W., & Cooper-Fraps, C. (1986). Theories of motivation in occupational therapy. *American Journal of Occupational Therapy, 40(4),* 249-257.

Statistics Canada (2002). *Participation and activity limitation survey: A profile of disability in Canada.* Ottawa, Ontario: Author.

Strong, S., Rigby, P., Stewart, D., Law, M., Letts, L., & Cooper, B. (1999). Application of the person-environment-occupation model: A practical tool. *Canadian Journal of Occupational Therapy, 66(3),* 122-133.

Wilcock, A. (1993). A theory of the human need for occupation. *Occupational Science: Australia, 1(1),* 17-24.

Wilcock, A. (1998). *An occupational perspective of health.* Thorofare, NJ: SLACK Incorporated.

WHO. (1980). *International classification of impairment, disability and handicap.* Geneva, Switzerland: Author.

WHO. (2001). *International classification of functioning, disability, and health (ICF).* Geneva, Switzerland: Author.

Yerxa, E. (1967). Authentic occupational therapy. *American Journal of Occupational Therapy, 21,* 1-9.

2

MEASUREMENT ISSUES AND PRACTICES

Winnie Dunn, PhD, OTR, FAOTA

Chapter 2 provides detailed information about measurement issues necessary for occupational therapists to understand before doing assessments. The importance of maintaining contextual validity in the testing process will be discussed, along with suggestions to ensure that contextual validity is accomplished. Characteristics of specific measurement strategies, issues of clinical utility, and types of assessment tools will be addressed.

SETTING THE FRAMEWORK FOR MEASUREMENT

In order to understand the importance of measurement as a core professional skill, we must recognize why professionals need measurement knowledge for their practice and what the central considerations are when using measurement as a tool in practice.

Why Professionals Need Measurement Knowledge in Practice

There are two primary reasons why professionals need measurement knowledge in practice. First, measurement processes provide convincing evidence about a person's status, competencies, and difficulties for both planning and documenting the effectiveness of interventions. Second, using sound measurement strategies enables professionals to include individuals and their families in the process of selecting the most compatible and effective interventions for them.

Measurement Provides Convincing Evidence

When persons need services from professionals, they have a right to expect the service providers to employ current practices and to report their activities in a systematic manner. Professionals in any discipline have a base of knowledge that enables them to view performance problems from a particular perspective; this base of knowledge is necessary, but not sufficient when providing best practice services. In addition to having mastered knowledge, professionals must find ways to document their decision-making processes for the service recipient and others as appropriate.

Measurement strategies provide the tools to ensure that the process of decision-making can be recorded in a systematic manner. When professionals document their own decision-making processes and the recipient's outcomes, they take responsibility for their work because systematic measurement provides a means for others to scrutinize the professional's work. Solid measurement practices create a mechanism for analysis of the effectiveness and efficiency of the services and, when taken collectively, can inform a profession about ways to advance knowledge and practices in the profession.

Professionals Need to Engage in Evidence-Based Practice

Professionals have another responsibility related to measurement. In addition to recording our decision-making in a systematic manner, we must engage in a practice that is currently being called *evidence-based practice*. Evidence-based practice means that the professional informs the potential service recipient of what the profession knows (or does not know) about the effectiveness of the evaluations and interventions being proposed so that the recipient can make informed decisions about what services are acceptable and what he or she is willing to accept.

Employing evidence-based practices during planning offers professionals an additional way to establish rapport. Occupational therapy professionals have traditionally emphasized rapport-building as an important part of the therapeutic process. When therapists take the additional step to involve service recipients in the process of thinking through the meaning of measurement findings and the options for intervention, a partnership is initiated with the service recipient. This partnership establishes new roles in the therapist-client relationship and invites the service recipient to have an active voice in the therapeutic process. As a partner, the person has a bigger investment in a positive outcome, but also feels permission to speak up about plans that would be incompatible with lifestyle or be too encumbering to carry out each day. "Partners" also offer different perspectives on the meaning of data; the perspective of the person who has had the lived experience is unfortunately frequently discounted in more traditional therapeutic processes.

Central Considerations in the Measurement Process

There are three useful questions to assist therapists in planning their measurement strategies: 1) Will the measurement process generate consistent (reliable) information?, 2) What are the most appropriate measurement parameters?, and 3) Would everyone agree about what you are measuring (validity)? Let's consider each one.

Will the Measurement Process Generate Consistent Information? (Reliability)

When measuring performance, we must be concerned about whether the performance we observe and record is likely to be the same under various circumstances. Would the person perform the same in the morning or afternoon? Would various environments affect performance? Would persistence or endurance make a difference in what you measure and record? When there is a risk of inconsistency, professionals can make the wrong decisions about the best course of action. For example, we could decide that a person is unable to participate in rehabilitation based on the observation that the person participates in therapy sessions in the mornings but cannot maintain arousal during the 1:30 p.m. therapy session. Perhaps different activities would maintain arousal or the lunch meal could be made lighter to keep arousal through the day. We must be cautious in deriving meaning from both consistent and inconsistent information.

The consistency of a measurement process is called reliability, defined by the Educational Resources Information Center as the "extent to which something is consistent, dependable, and stable over repeated trials" (ERIC, 2004a). There are many times that professionals can control some of these factors and not others. It is less important to control all of the factors that may affect consistency; what is more important is to recognize what may affect the consistency of your findings. A simple way to handle consistency in daily practice is to be vigilant about recording factors that may affect consistency as part of measurement documentation. This way, if the team finds inconsistent performance, the related factors are available for comparison. When the team can discuss possible reasons for differences in performance, the team is more likely to increase its accuracy in understanding the person's difficulties and therefore design more effective interventions.

For example, several team members may observe Tom's orientation to present time, place, and person while they are chatting with him throughout the day. The nurse on the rehab unit and Tom's partner both report that he knows he is in the hospital and knows what is happening, while the physical therapist observes that Tom keeps asking what day it is throughout the intervention period. The team discusses this, and hypothesizes that moving him off of the rehab unit floor and being taken to the therapy gym is causing confusion; they decide to be more active in discussing this transition while it is occurring.

Ways that measures document their reliability are reported in this text. This documentation makes it possible for the user to decide whether the measure will be useful. For example, Meenan et al. (1992) report both internal consistency and test-retest reliability on the Arthritis Impact Measurement Scales (AIMS2). Internal consistency is a measure of how much the items are homogeneous within the groups on the test (Portney & Watkins, 2000). If we have a subset of items, we want that subset to measure that single characteristic. For the AIMS2, the authors were able to show that the subsections contained items that reflected that one characteristic (e.g., mobility, walking and bending), and not other characteristic (see Table 11-3 in this text for further details). They also report on test-retest reliability, or the ability to get the same findings with repeated testing (Portney & Watkins, 2000). The AIMS2 reports good ability to get the same results from their participants across two testing opportunities (Meenan et al., 1992).

Would Everyone Agree About What You Are Measuring? (Validity)

Another important consideration in the measurement process is the validity of the measurement (i.e., would everyone agree about what you are measuring?). Validity is defined by the ERIC as the "extent to which something does what it is used or intended to do" (ERIC, 2004b).

There are formal methods for testing validity, and, if professionals select standardized measures, it is important to review the validity features of the measure to be sure that the test is designed to offer the kind of information the professional desires.

The three most common types of validity are *content, criterion,* and *construct validity.* A measure meets content validity when the items look as if they measure what the author says that they measure. Frequently people check content validity by asking experts to judge whether items measure the stated topic. For example, if the test is named 'The Test of Sewing', a judge might expect to see items about thread, needles, stitches and perhaps machines, but not items about gardening. To establish criterion validity, authors compare their items to some external standard. For example, if putting together a test of children's development, the authors might compare their items to well established standards for when children can perform motor, language and cognitive tasks. Developers might also compare their new test to an established test to document criterion validity. Finally, researchers establish construct validity by evaluating their measure in comparison to ideas in a body of knowledge they are trying to characterize. For example, if someone is trying to measure cognitive skills, then the researchers would want to show that people whose cognitive skills are known (i.e., both higher and lower ability) perform consistently with their known skills on the new measure. We call it convergent validity (a type of construct validity) when the new measure is consistent with known constructs. The authors would also want to show that constructs NOT included in the measure would not relate to the new measure. For example, on the cognitive skills test, they would want to show that there is a low relationship to another, different category such as repetitive movement skills. This is called discriminant validity (also a type of construct validity). By showing sameness to consistent knowledge categories, and difference from 'other' categories, researchers establish that the construct of interest is being tested without other things contaminating that construct.

Professionals also face many situations in which standardized measurements are either unavailable or inappropriate. In these cases, qualitative measurement strategies such as interviews, skilled observations, and records reviews must be constructed with validity issues in mind. For occupational therapists, a skilled observation of a person in the kitchen would certainly appear to be a valid way to evaluate food preparation skills. But an occupational therapist could assess sensorimotor, cognitive, and psychosocial skills within this activity as well. When interpreting findings, the therapist would have to consider whether other team members would find it plausible that memory, sequencing, and dexterity could be measured in that activity via skilled observation. It is likely that team members would believe these connections, but would this therapist be free to go one step further and suggest that the person will have trouble with his or her personal hygiene? Some team members would believe this step is a "valid" extension of knowledge, while others might think this step was too big a leap and be unwilling to consider personal hygiene rituals in the intervention plan.

Therapists face a similar "validity" dilemma when they conduct assessments of component skills in isolation from the tasks of daily life. If a therapist measures range of motion and strength, is it "valid" to conclude that the person cannot eat a meal? Perhaps we know that lifting utensils requires certain component skills (under typical circumstances); we might then conclude that anyone who has less than these skills will not be able to eat with utensils. Although there is a sensible relationship here, this logic does not account for less common but successful ways of using utensils and eating. It may be "invalid" to conclude that a person cannot eat with utensils by only testing component skills; persons who have weakness may have constructed a different way to eat that doesn't require the same level of strength. Relationships among task performance, the person's interest in the task, and the skills to perform the tasks must be carefully considered to ensure that professionals construct valid hypotheses and conclusions.

In this text, you will also see many examples of authors reporting validity of the measures. When authors document validity, users can have more confidence that the tools will evaluate what they state as their topic of measurement. For example, the authors of the Leisure Boredom Scale (LBS) report on content, criterion and construct validity (see Table 12-5 in this text). Content validity concerns how successfully the measure covers the topic it is supposed to be testing. The authors of the LBS used typical strategies to determine content validity (i.e., expert judgment) (Iso-Ahola & Weissinger, 1990). Criterion validity is the ability of one measure to reflect the results on another measure of the same ideas. Construct validity is the ability to measure an abstract idea successfully (Portney & Watkins, 2000). For the LBS, the authors used established scales of leisure motivation and satisfaction, reasoning that factors that lead to successful leisure would be poorly related to boredom in leisure. The LBS was negatively related to these scales, and to some of the subscales as well. Positive correlations with frequency and depth of boredom from these comparison scales add additional construct validity evidence to the overall picture.

What Are the Most Appropriate Measurement Parameters?

A critical and often overlooked consideration when setting out to measure performance is identifying the testing strategy that will yield proper information. Sometimes it is most important to know how often a behavior occurs (i.e., frequency); other times how long a behavior lasts is critical to measurement and planning (i.e., duration); still other times, the flexibility of the behavior across time or settings is important (i.e., generalizability). Another set of considerations involves identifying process (i.e., the way the practice is being conducted) and outcome (i.e., what happens as a result of the practice) measurement parameters. Finally, professionals must determine whether they need to measure current status as part of the diagnostic process or for determining the course of intervention planning.

Measurement parameters help professionals characterize behaviors properly. When conducting skilled observations, if a student is yelling out answers during class discussions, the teacher is probably more interested in the number of times (*frequency*) the student interrupts others, rather than how long each interruption takes (*duration*). However, that same teacher needs to know the length of a student's attention for seatwork (*duration*), rather than the number of times the student looks at the paper or workbook (*frequency*). When selecting a formal measurement tool, we have to consider floor and ceiling effects as well. Floor and ceiling effects refer to the bottom and top of the measurement scales respectively. If the person's performance is likely to be at the bottom or top of the measurement scale, there will not be enough items in their range of performance to completely evaluate the person's skills. When the person's actual performance is below the floor of the test, the only possible score is the lowest score on the test; this may be an overestimate of performance. When the person's actual performance is above the ceiling of the test, the only possible score is the highest score on the test; this may be an underestimate of performance. Selecting measurement tools that record an accurate range of successful and challenging behaviors increases the possibility of correct assessment of current performance.

Another key measurement parameter is applicability across situations. In order to measure applicability properly, one must measure across opportunities; one type of opportunity to perform cannot inform professionals about the person's ability to use skills in various ways. For example, if a person can find things in the bedroom at home, we might hypothesize that the person can find things everywhere. However, the bedroom may be so familiar that this situation does not challenge perceptual skills, and when faced with "finding" tasks in other settings, performance deteriorates. Flexibility in using one's skills and the contextual resources to complete tasks is an important performance issue when managing life, and therefore must be a central consideration in measurement.

In the practice of a profession, it is important to measure both the process and the outcomes of the practices. *Process* measurement is directed at evaluating the way that the practices are being carried out; outcome measurement evaluates the product or impact of the practices (Scheirer, 1994). Therapists use process measurement when they wish to know how things are going. Process measures can be very focused, as in feeling tone changes as a person shifts posture, or can be programmatic, as in identifying the effectiveness and efficiency of one's scheduling system. Process measurement enables professionals to "evaluate in action" so they can adjust what they are doing to improve the experience.

Therapists use *outcome* measurement when they wish to know the end result or how things went. Measuring a person's successful transition to community living is a measure of the outcomes of the service system and interdisciplinary providers. Capturing accurate information as outcome data is sometimes a difficult process; it is not uncommon for professionals to "know" that a person made progress, but to have measures they selected indicate "no progress." If professionals select weak or inappropriate outcome measures, they can make the inaccurate conclusion that the services were not effective. They can also incorrectly conclude that services were effective by using very narrow measures of outcome that are not actually representative of the person's skills or satisfaction with daily life. Good outcome measures hold up to tests of validity (i.e., others who look at the performance/results would agree that the measurement strategy is yielding accurate information about that person's therapeutic outcomes and satisfaction with living). We will discuss selection of outcome measures in Chapter 3.

When we begin to apply knowledge about measurement tools within practice, we have to consider whether the measurement device is responsive to changes in the behaviors of interest. Not all measures are appropriate for measuring changes; for instance, some measures are designed for documenting traits that remain relatively the same across time (e.g., global intelligence). It is not appropriate to use trait or status measures for charting progress or planning specific features of an intervention program. For example, the Bruininks-Oseretsky Test of Motor Proficiency (BOTMP) (Bruininks, 1978) is a norm referenced and standardized test, Norm referenced means that the BOTMP has data from a comparison sample of typical children, so we know what is inside and outside of normal expectations. Standardized means that there are specific methods for completing the test procedures. After administering and scoring the BOTMP, the examiner looks up the child's raw score to derive a standard score. The standard score provides a comparison of this child's performance to other children the same age. Although the professional would then know generally about balance, dexterity, etc., the BOTMP does not enable the professional to know how these skills (or lack of skills) are affecting performance or how the child functions with this pattern of skills (i.e., the designation "status") without additional information from parents, the child or the teacher.

We consider a measure responsive to change when that measure will be able to detect changes that are proportional to the person's actual behavioral changes. Responsiveness can be evaluated by looking at the change in scores across time in treated and untreated groups, by calculating effect size or by plotting change compared to chance (Portney & Watkins, 2000). Portney & Watkins (2000) caution that practitioners must understand the behaviors they are measuring so they can determine when changes in behavior are large enough to matter for the person's life. Sometimes, a statistically significant difference in a research study can be due to large samples, and the actual amount of change in the behavior would not matter in daily life performance. Other times a study can report no differences statistically, and yet the behavior difference would be important in the person's life. Statistical tests of significance merely tell us whether the numbers we report are different from a mathematical perspective. In practice, this may not be adequate information for determining whether the difference matters in the lives of the persons we are serving.

The *Activities Scale for Kids* (ASK) (see Table 11-1) is an example of a measure that reports on the measure's sensitivity to change. They measured across a 6-month period, and found that the performance section of the ASK was more sensitive to change than the capability section (Young, Yoshida, Williams, Bombardier, & Wright, 1995). We will discuss selection of outcome measures in Chapter 3, and provide additional examples of measurements that are sensitive to change throughout the book. Other measures are considered performance or criterion measures. These measures provide information about the person's actual performance and skill development and therefore enable the professional to plan appropriate interventions and evaluate their impact on performance. Standardized tests require the professional and person to engage in a predesigned task so that everyone has the same chance to perform. Criterion measures are designed to elicit that person's pattern of performance. Comparisons in a criterion measurement might be with that person's performance previously or with another person in the immediate setting who is more successful (i.e., the gold standard for that task). The *School Function Assessment* (SFA) (see Table 8-2) is a standardized and criterion referenced measure of children's participation in school.

Criterion measurement is especially critical for occupational therapists for two reasons. First, many persons who have disabilities cannot complete the rigors of standardized test protocols and therefore cannot be compared to a national norm. Second, the course of development and performance for persons who have disabilities is different than for persons who do not have disabilities; criterion measures enable professionals to characterize these unique features of performance. For example, a person who has

spasticity subsequent to nervous system trauma will move using very different postural support patterns. This person will never move the way a person who has normal tone can move, so comparing to typical patterns of movement is not useful. In fact, there are some situations in which the spasticity provides extra support for postural control that is not available to persons who have normal tone. Criterion measures provide the means to characterize the functional utility of whatever skills a person has and how these skills are used in day-to-day occupations.

IMPORTANCE OF ENVIRONMENTAL CONTEXT AND ECOLOGICAL VALIDITY IN MEASUREMENT

Persons conduct their daily lives within the larger environment and in particular environmental contexts. Even when conducting an evaluation in a medical center clinic, the environmental context in that situation will have an influence on the person's performance. Sometimes the unfamiliar furniture and equipment will distract the person; the fact that the therapist is setting expectations for performance might cause the person anxiety. Without knowing the person's life, the therapist might construct a confusing context for the person. On the other hand, the therapist's engaging behavior could facilitate performance in areas that the person more typically performs poorly due to lack of interest (Dunn, 1997). We cannot derive meaning about the person's performance without considering the environmental context in which we asked the person to perform. In Chapter 1, we reviewed the frameworks in occupational therapy that include environment in their conceptualization of occupational performance.

A Framework to Measure Performance within a Person's Environment

There are four key assumptions essential to this understanding: 1) persons and the environments in which they live are unique and dynamic, 2) contrived environmental contexts are different than natural environmental contexts, 3) occupational therapy practice involves promoting self-determination and inclusion of persons with disabilities in all aspects of society, and 4) independence means meeting your wants and needs (Dunn, McClain, Brown, & Youngstrom, 1997).

Essential Assumptions of Performance

Persons and the environmental contexts in which they perform occupations are unique and dynamic. When conducting an evaluation, we cannot understand a person without understanding the person's environment. For each occupation, the environmental context includes physical, social, cultural, and temporal features (Christiansen & Baum, 1991, 1997; Dunn, Brown, & McGuigan, 1994; Law Cooper, Strong, Stewart, Rigby, & Letts, 1996). Even within the same family (a social and cultural environment), siblings experience life differently and develop unique interests and skills. We must consider each person's unique skills and abilities and how environmental factors influence that person's experiences. The interaction between the person and the environment forms the basis of the meaning that persons derive from their life experiences.

The person-environment interaction is dynamic. The environmental context changes when persons do occupations and changes in the environment affect how persons react as well. For example, we set up our closets to facilitate our own dressing rituals. Our performance changes when our clothing and accessories are arranged differently (i.e., when staying at a friend's house). We must also remember that persons have a range of performance abilities depending on the cues and supports or barriers they experience under different environmental circumstances.

During the evaluation process, we determine the person's performance range, not just the person's skills and difficulties. As described in Section I, the performance range is evaluated based on what the person wants or needs to do. Although we must know what the person's skills and difficulties are, this knowledge is inadequate without knowing what the person is interested in and where the person is likely to be conducting various aspects of daily life.

Contrived and natural environmental contexts are different. Occupational therapists work in a variety of service systems designed for specialized services (e.g., clinical settings, acute-care settings). When we conduct evaluations in these specialized settings, we must factor in the potential differences in performance that would occur in more natural settings (i.e., the workplace or home). Sometimes the person will perform better in contrived settings because contrived settings control some features of the environment that might be disruptive to the person. This control might enable us to see optimal performance, but therapeutic interventions must be based on typical performance needs, not optimal ones. Conversely, we might incorrectly decide that the person cannot perform when we evaluate in contrived environments, because that person needed such familiarity to provide cues and supports for better performance. Ultimately, what matters to the person is the ability to perform during daily life; therefore, we must be vigilant at discovering as much as we can about the person's desired and actual performance in natural settings.

Best practice occupational therapy promotes self-determination and inclusion of persons with disabilities in all aspects of society. In occupational therapy services we want to enable persons to live satisfying lives. Therefore,

we must find out what persons and their families want and need to do as the first step in the comprehensive evaluation processes. In its position paper on inclusion, the American Occupational Therapy Association (AOTA) (1996) states that occupational therapy personnel must advocate for all persons to have access to all the community environments that will enable them to live satisfying lives. Therefore, a comprehensive evaluation might include visiting the workplace to identify possible adaptations or speaking to peers and supervisors about routines of the day that support or create barriers to performance (Dunn, 1997).

Independence means meeting your wants and needs. Independence occurs when persons are able to manage their lives to get what they want and need. Traditionally, independence meant that persons had to actually perform the tasks of interest, yet some have taken a stand that all persons make decisions about how they want to use their resources, and this might include employing someone else to complete a necessary task (e.g., getting clothing pressed), adapting the environment to make the task easier (e.g., using a jar opener), or asking for help from others. The salient feature is the person's ability to know what needs to be done and finding a way to get it done; the person doesn't need to actually do the task to be considered independent (AOTA, 1996).

When conducting a comprehensive evaluation with persons who have performance needs, occupational therapists must explore adaptations in the task or environment that might support performance. We all use adaptations to support daily life (e.g., pencil grips, step stools). When persons have disabilities, there is a temptation to consider typical adaptations such as these as indications that the person has the problem. A more progressive view is that the environment might need to be adjusted to make task performance easier for those who perform in that context. When we make activity or environmental adaptations, we acknowledge that the person's skills and abilities can remain the same, and the person can still improve performance.

Supporting Interaction Between Persons and Their Environmental Context

Some persons have limited skills, abilities, or experience (e.g., arthritis, developmental disability, mental illness). When a person has limited personal skills, this will also limit the possibilities when the person interacts within different environments (Dunn et al., 1997). The person may not be able to take advantage of cues and supports of each environment. A child who has developmental delays has the same environmental context as other children in the preschool but may not be able to take advantage of these cues to guide appropriate behavior. For example, the other children might quickly notice the cues that it is snack time, but the child with developmental delays may not understand these cues and be slower to join the other children. Often the person who has more limited skills displays a more limited performance range.

The environmental context can also be limited. Each time a person tries to do something without adequate equipment or supplies, that person has a limited environmental context (Dunn et al., 1997). When support within an environment is limited, the performance range is also smaller. Even with good skills and abilities, when the environmental support is limited, the interaction between the person and environment will produce a limited performance range. A conductor will not be able to demonstrate those skills without an environment that contains an orchestra.

Sometimes both person skills and experience and environmental supports are diminished (i.e., a person who has a disability and who lives in an impoverished setting). The performance range can be very restricted in this situation. Occupational therapists must attend to both person and environmental variables in comprehensive evaluation to ensure that all factors related to the performance range are considered (Christiansen & Baum, 1991, 1997; Dunn, 1997; Law et al., 1996).

Comprehensive Measurement Using a Performance in Environmental Context Perspective

Occupational therapists are concerned with performance in daily life; therefore the most important aspect of any occupational therapy evaluation is performance (Dunn, 1997). When using a performance within environmental context perspective in comprehensive evaluation, performance has two features: 1) what the person wants and needs to do, and 2) assessment of actual performance. To determine what the person wants and needs to do, we talk to the person and significant others (e.g., the family, friends, other care providers, a coworker, boss, minister, neighbors). Our goal is to find out what matters in the person's life. When evaluating actual performance, occupational therapists have several strategies available, including conducting interviews about how performance looks in the natural settings and how satisfying that performance is for the person. We can also observe the person's task performance, either informally or with formal assessments.

Evaluation of Person Variables

Comprehensive evaluation also requires consideration of the person's skills, abilities, and experiences. Occupational therapists examine sensorimotor, cognitive, and psychosocial features of the person's performance. We evaluate these features to determine which person variables seem to contribute to or create barriers to desired performance. There are many formal and informal methods of evaluating performance components; other references address the details of performance component assessments (e.g., Asher & Norman, 1989; Cook, 1991).

The performance within context perspective enables us to determine possible barriers and supports to participation. The interaction between these environmental variables and the person's performance is what determines the meaning the person derives from his or her own experiences.

Evaluation of the Environmental Context

Occupational therapists employ skilled observations and interviews to identify the physical, social, cultural, and temporal features of relevant environments (Dunn, Brown, & McGuigan, 1994; Letts et al., 2003). The physical features of the environmental context include the objects, terrain, layout, and structures of the environment. Social features include the persons, interaction styles, and relationships, while culture includes the expectations of stakeholders (e.g., family, community, ethnic groups, office). Temporal features of an environmental context include expectations related to age, calendar time, and stage of disability.

Although the occupational therapy literature has consistently included environments as a key feature of performance, we have evaluated specific environmental contexts far less than person and performance variables. When evaluating environments, we must consider physical, social, cultural, and temporal features of the environments of interest. Then, we must identify the possible supports and barriers to participation. Finally, we must collaborate with the service recipient to identify the meaning of performance within each particular environmental context. Other sections of this text contain an analysis of environmental assessments available to professionals (see Chapter 17).

Many professionals use ecological assessments to evaluate the features of the environment. In an ecological assessment, professionals record the typical way that activities occur in a particular environmental context; then, the professional records what the person of interest does to complete the tasks. Finally, the evaluation team designs possible ways to bridge the gap between typical performance and the person's current performance strategies.

Supports and Barriers to Participation

Evaluation of environmental context also includes consideration of how environmental features support or create barriers to participation. Each person reacts to environmental variables differently; what might provide supports to one person can be a barrier to performance for another person. For example, the noise in the street may only provide background noise for one person but may be so distracting for another person that it would be hard to concentrate on homework. Peers may successfully compel one adolescent to work harder on a group project and may have no impact on another young person. Gathering objective data about the environmental context is necessary but not sufficient to make decisions about performance; we must identify the impact of those features on the person's performance.

Identifying Meaningfulness

Experienced professionals can collect information and hypothesize about the meaning of occupations, tasks and activities for persons. However, we cannot know meaning for others without interacting with them about their lived experiences. When inquiring about what a person wants and needs to do, we can also ask why those occupations are important or satisfying, or why doing them in a certain way or in a certain place is significant (Dunn, 1997). We can listen for the presence or absence of daily routines, ask about how unexpected events affect the person's performance, and identify how the person establishes priorities. This information informs us about what is meaningful to the persons we are serving and their families. Performance has different meaning when it occurs in relevant environments. When a person has poor performance in a nonrelevant environmental context, this may only indicate lack of meaningfulness of the task in that context, not lack of skill for performance (Dunn, 1997).

THE CHALLENGE OF INTEGRATING PERSON, PERFORMANCE, AND ENVIRONMENTAL CONTEXTUAL DATA

Living a satisfying life is the only thing that matters for the person and family in person-centered service provision. For some persons, living a satisfying life would include developing one's own skills, but for other persons it might mean finding or designing environmental contexts that can support desired task performance or selecting alternative life goals. During the evaluation process, professionals must organize information and insights around the actual life the person wants to live even if services will be provided in a center or agency (e.g., hospital, clinic, senior citizen center, or shelter).

For example, it doesn't matter what the child's visual perceptual scores are on a standardized test if visual perception is not interfering with daily life activities of interest to the child and family. We only pursue visual perception testing when the teacher, child, and/or family express concern about life situations that require strong visual perceptual skills. For example, if a child wishes to participate with the family's winter leisure activity of puzzle construction and has been displaying frustration (e.g., outbursts, shoving pieces off the table), it is appropriate to suspect visual perception may be a barrier to this desired social-

ization experience. In this example, we also recognize that participating with family members has some inherent qualities that must be considered as well. The child may feel that this is a desirable way to get parental attention; the child might also feel pressure to compete with siblings. The type of picture on the puzzle and the family's puzzle strategies (e.g., sorting pieces by colors, by edges) will change the situation and supports for the child. Best practice occupational therapy would require that the therapist know as much of this information as possible to design the most successful intervention. Evaluation of visual perception is irrelevant without first considering the person's desired performance and then considering contextual features that may impact performance.

SELECTING MEASUREMENT CRITERIA

When selecting the criterion for particular measurements, there are five factors to consider: 1) Relevance to the person's life, 2) Comparisons to external standards, 3) Application of formal evidence criteria, 4) Which measures will capture the important changes, and 5) What levels of change are important.

Relevance to the Person's Life

The most important criterion when designing a measurement strategy is relevance. There are many measurement strategies available to us that are technically correct but would yield results that are irrelevant to the person's performance needs or desires in his or her daily life. For example, although it might be interesting to know a person's level and type of perceptual and memory skills, this information might initially be peripheral to the person's desire to cook. When someone tells us he or she wants to cook, and we then measure his or her performance by asking him or her to match pictures, draw shapes, or repeat numbers, the service recipient is likely to be confused about the relationship between the two sets of tasks. This does not mean that perceptual and memory skills are unimportant for cooking, but the connection between them is elusive to the consumer when component skills are tested in isolation from the desired performance. Meeting the criterion of relevance would occur if the therapist listened to the person describe cooking methods and frustrations, or if the therapist watched a cooking task. Then, as perceptual and memory issues arose out of the interaction, their relationship to the desired outcome would be clear for everyone.

Comparisons of Performance to External Standards

Sometimes it is important to be able to describe a person's performance in relation to other performance.

Professionals can make comparisons between the person's earlier and current performance, between the service recipient and successful performers in the environmental context of interest, and between the service recipient and a standard performance of a like group.

Comparing to Self

It is most common and appropriate to compare a person's performance currently to that same person's performance at an earlier time or in another place. If a person can handle money and change for a purchase within the community center, we might want to know if that person can handle money as effectively at convenience or grocery stores. If we have been working together with a man so he can dress himself, we will want to compare his current abilities with his performance at an earlier time. The "compare to self" paradigm is most often used to measure a person's progress in achieving performance goals and to determine the effectiveness of intervention strategies.

Comparing to Typical Models

Another measurement standard that can be used in some settings is the comparison to typical models. This means that the professional collects information about a typical performer and compares that to the performance of the service recipient in that same environmental context. School programs lend themselves readily to this type of measurement criteria. When conducting a skilled observation of the student who has been referred for assessment, the therapist can also record data on another student in the classroom who is successful at the tasks of interest. It is important to avoid the best performer; it is better to select a student who is successful in the midrange of the classroom.

The advantage of this measurement criterion is that it enables professionals to frame the person's performance in the very environment that will be used. There is also an opportunity to be reminded of the range of behaviors that peers use while getting things done.

For example, a worker may be having difficulty getting work completed, and the supervisor thinks it's because he is up roaming around the office "all the time." However, by collecting data on another worker, the therapist can determine whether roaming around is typical behavior of many workers in this work environment. If many workers roam around and still get their work finished, then the therapist has the opportunity to provide insight about other behaviors that might be interfering with productivity. Perhaps for other workers, roaming around occurs when they have work to delegate to others, and for the target worker, roaming does not advance the work product. Knowing this can help the supervisor frame the work expectations to ensure higher work product.

Comparing to Typical Models in a Standard Sample

A more traditional external standard is a normative sample of individuals whose performance is considered collectively. Professionals are using a standard sample when they look up a person's raw score on a table to determine a standard score for that level of performance. The standard scores are derived from calculations of the scores of all the persons in a particular category (e.g., all 20- to 25-year-old males); the standard score that the person receives represents that person's performance in relation to all other persons in the category.

Professionals need to understand which scale is being used for the standard score. If a standard scale has a mean of 100 and a standard deviation of 10, then we can interpret the person's standard score by comparing to this scale. A score of 80 would be two standard deviations below the average and is likely a cause for some concern, while a 95 would be considered within average limits. However, if a standard score scale is based on a mean of 50 and a standard deviation of 10, a score of 80 would be three standard deviations above the mean, while a 95 would be even higher, representing less than 1% of the population.

There are advantages and disadvantages of standard sample comparisons. Standard score comparisons are most appropriate as measures of status or to establish eligibility for particular services. They are typically not appropriate for charting performance progress or for planning particular intervention strategies. Because the comparison is to an established behavioral pattern, it is sometimes easier to hypothesize about the person's performance in relation to a cohort group. However, standard measures also require a more prescribed performance from the person being assessed, and this is not always possible. If a person cannot complete tasks on a standard measure in the prescribed way, it is inappropriate to compare the performance to the standard scores.

As with each measurement issue, the professional has the responsibility to select strategies and tasks based on the purpose of the measurement activities. Each of these parameters are important for certain aspects of measurement and will enhance the data available when used correctly.

Using Measurement Information for Evidence-Based Practice

The ultimate application of measurement skills and principles to practice is in using information gathered from measurement to partner with the service recipients in selecting the best course of action. When service recipients and professionals can collaborate about the meaning of information and the ways to work toward a desired outcome, everyone is successful. Measurement data provide the tools for this collaboration.

Professionals engage in evidence-based practice when they actively inform the persons they are serving about the known (and unknown) benefits and risks of the intervention options. Engaging in evidence-based practice creates a vulnerability for the professional, but the process of exposing costs, benefits, and unknown factors opens the communication process as well. Service recipients are more likely to question a decision to proceed in a certain way when they understand the parameters of that plan of action. Evidence-based practice also offers the opportunity for persons to be more committed to the process of their own therapy, because they will feel like a part of the process, rather than a passive beneficiary. In addition, it provides a mechanism for professionals to think systematically and take responsibility for the relationships between plans and the person's desired outcomes.

For example, a therapist interviewed Alan, a man who wanted to improve his personal hygiene. She observed the personal hygiene ritual; and noticed that Alan did not use toothpaste and hairbrush. Although it was possible that Alan did not know about these aspects of personal hygiene, these two items were put away in the drawer, so the therapist suspected that Alan might need some way to remember to use these items. In a follow-up, Alan demonstrated the ability to use the toothpaste and hairbrush, so the therapist focused her planning on the issue of remembering the parts of the personal hygiene ritual for Alan.

When she met with Alan, she presented several options. She discussed a skills training approach, which would incorporate Alan learning a pattern of performance during hygiene. She told him that skills training had been shown to be successful with young adults with mental illness, but that professionals had not been able to show that skills training generalized to other patterns of task performance. Since Alan wanted to have paid work, he wanted to learn strategies for remembering the parts of the activity. The therapist also discussed cognitive retraining with Alan. She explained this approach had also been successful for improving the cognitive skill (in this case, memory), but application within daily life environments had not been tested.

The therapist also discussed adaptive strategies for supporting his task performance, such as making a list of the parts of the hygiene ritual that Alan could post or making a mat of the necessary tools on the counter to remind Alan what he needs to do in the morning. The therapist explained that adaptive strategies have been shown to support performance of desired tasks because they are designed with that task in mind. In order for this adaptive strategy to be helpful with new tasks, Alan and others would have to consider adaptations to those tasks; Alan might discover adaptive strategies that are always (or

never) helpful, and he might narrow down the field of adaptations over time.

Alan decided he wanted to work on his memory skills separate from the hygiene tasks. He wanted to use adaptations for getting "regular stuff" done and work on memory to "make himself better." The therapist, caseworker, Alan, and his brother all met to hear about the plans, and the interventions proceeded.

Employing best practices in measurement is the first step to employing evidence-based practices in the course of providing services. The data from forward thinking measurement strategies (as presented throughout this book) provides the information for current planning with individuals and the evidence for emerging best practices in the future.

The Challenges of Providing Evidence-Based Practice

There are three challenges in providing evidence-based practice. The professional must: 1) keep apprised of current literature, 2) develop effective communication strategies, and 3) understand how to evaluate the evidence available in the literature.

Keeping Current

Professionals must be apprised of current and innovative practices and the supports and challenges to those practices in the literature if they wish to engage in evidence-based practice. With the huge amount of professional literature published each month, this can seem overwhelming. It is sometimes very helpful to participate in a journal club, in which the participants take turns bringing articles to read and discuss. With technology more streamlined, professionals can also periodically conduct a search within a library system or on the Internet for current references of interest. Another strategy is to share abstracts of articles as a method of scanning for those that might inform you about your practice considerations. The team of professionals has the collective responsibility to stay current on knowledge that impacts your practice.

An example of keeping current is to review the Cochrane Collaboration databases. These reviews of studies inform professionals about the current knowledge and practices related to particular diagnoses and conditions. A limitation of the Cochrane Collaboration data is that the types of studies they accept into their databases are restricted to clinical trials. There are currently not many clinical trial studies in occupational therapy, so inferences must be made from the more general information provided.

There are several ways to obtain information. Universities have databases that enable you to search professional literature. You can search medical and health literature (e.g., PubMed, Cinahl) resources, or educational resources (e.g., ERIC). There are also other Web sites that provide information (e.g., Bottomlines, Cochrane collaboration) in a summarized way. For occupational therapists, OTSeeker (www.otseeker.com) provides a comprehensive searchable database of systematic reviews and randomized controlled trials applicable to occupational therapy.

Communicating as Partners

When engaging in evidence-based practice, professionals must find ways to clearly articulate their decision-making processes and options. This includes describing the pros and cons of certain choices and presenting a range of alternatives for a positive outcome, since the decision to proceed rests collectively in the hands of the professional and other interested parties (e.g., the person, family, other team members). Evidence-based practice changes the role of the "expert" in the assessment and intervention process; professionals are expert in their fields, and the service recipients are experts in living their lives. Communication must therefore be jargon free, and the professionals must distinguish factual information (i.e., data) from interpretive information that the professionals derive from their experience and knowledge. In this form of conducting practice, professionals acknowledge and welcome the possibility that the intervention decisions will evolve from the communication and typically are not designed prior to the collaboration (although possibilities are presented from various perspectives as part of the interpretive process in measurement).

Evaluating Evidence

The process of evaluating the evidence available about a particular topic to decide the best course of action is complex and beyond the scope of this chapter and this book. There are some general strategies that professionals can use to guide their thinking processes. First, professionals must decide how similar their service recipients are to the participants in a particular study (e.g., similar ages, performance difficulties, diagnosis). This does not mean that the study participants have to be exactly like your service group, but that they are similar on issues that matter to the problem. For example, there are many diagnoses that involve hand weakness; regardless of diagnosis, if the study addresses the interference of hand weakness, it may be applicable to your service group.

Second, you must decide how much is convincing. If everyone in the study made huge gains, this is easy to incorporate into your thinking, but this rarely happens in research. One way to evaluate "how much is convincing" is to see whether the statistical tests were significant; researchers will tell you this in the results. However, sometimes measurement data can be "clinically significant" (i.e., important for practice decisions) separate from statistical significance. For example, Kientz and Dunn (1997)

reported on the Sensory Profile results with children who had autism. Although many items reached statistical significance, the researchers determined that, for practice, therapists needed to only consider items that were different by more than one raw score point on the Sensory Profile scale (i.e., 1 to 5) because parents could only report whole points on the scale. Ottenbacher (1986) discusses the opposite issue (i.e., when the statistical test reveals no significance, but the change in the study is of utmost importance to practice). For example, small changes in postural control can make a very big difference in performance, but the number that is used to characterize the change is so small that the calculations do not reveal this importance. Sometimes, researchers select the wrong parameters for measurement and therefore mask a result that may be important to practice. For these situations, therapists must ask, "Would the changes reported make a difference to the persons I serve?" Professional practice requires ongoing reflection about the meaning of information for the process and outcomes of serving persons who have performance needs.

SUMMARY

The process of measurement is a complex one. Therapists must consider the process through which they design an assessment strategy and select measurement tools. With the guidance of this chapter, therapists can create a best practice method for making solid practice decisions.

REFERENCES

American Occupational Therapy Association (1996). *Position paper on inclusion.* Rockville, MD: Author.

Asher, K., & Norman, J. (1989). Why is word recognition impaired by disorientation while the identification of single letters is not? *Journal of Experimental Psychology, 15(1),* 153-163.

Bruininks, R. H (1978). *Bruininks-Oseretsky Test of Motor Proficiency.* Circle Pines, MN: American Guidance Service.

Christiansen, C., & Baum, C. (1991). *Occupational therapy: Overcoming human performance deficits.* Thorofare, NJ: SLACK Incorporated.

Christiansen, C., & Baum, C. (1997). *Occupational therapy: Enabling function and well-being* (2nd ed.). Thorofare, NJ: SLACK Incorporated.

Cook, D. G. (1991). The assessment process. In W. Dunn (Ed.), *Pediatric occupational therapy: Facilitating effective service provision* (pp. 35-74). Thorofare, NJ: SLACK Incorporated.

Dunn, W. (1997, April). A conceptual model for considering the impact of sensory processing abilities on the daily lives of young children and their families. *Infants and Young Children.*

Dunn, W., Brown, C., & McGuigan, A. (1994). The ecology of human performance: A framework for thought and action. *American Journal of Occupational Therapy, 48(7)*, 595-607.

Dunn, W., McClain, L., Brown, C., & Youngstrom, M. J. (1997). The ecology of human performance; Contextual influences on occupational performance. In M. Neidstadt & E. Crepeau (Eds.), *Willard & Spackman's occupational therapy.* Philadelphia: Lippincott.

ERIC. (2004a). Reliability. Retrieved May 3, 2004 from http://www.ericfacility.net/extra/pub/thessearch.cfm.

ERIC. (2004b). Validity. Retrieved May 3, 2004 from http://www.ericfacility.net/extra/pub/thessearch.cfm.

Iso-Ahola, S. E., & Weissinger, E. (1990). Perceptions of boredom in leisure: Conceptualization, reliability, and validity of the Leisure Boredom Scale. *Journal of Leisure Research, 22*, 1-17.

Kientz, M., & Dunn, W. (1997). A comparison of children with autism and typical children on the sensory profile. *American Journal of Occupational Therapy, 51*, 530-537.

Law, M., Cooper, B., Strong, S., Stewart, D., Rigby, P., & Letts, L. (1996). The person-environment-occupational model: A transactive approach to occupational performance. *Canadian Journal of Occupational Therapy, 63(1)*, 9-23.

Letts, L., Rigby, P., & Stewart, D., et al. (2003). *Using environments to enable occupational performance.* Thorofare, NJ: SLACK Incorporated.

Meenan, R. F., Mason, J. H., Anderson, J. J., Guccione, A. A., & Kazis, L. E. (1992). The content and properties of a revised and expanded Arthritis Impact Measurement Scales health status questionnaire. *Arthritis and Rheumatism, 35*, 1-10.

Ottenbacher, K. (1986). Use of applied behavioral techniques and an adaptive device to teach lip closure to severely handicapped children. *American Journal of Occupational Therapy, 90(5)*, 535-539.

Portney, L. G., & Watkins, M. P. (2000). *Foundations of clinical research: Applications to practice.* Upper Saddle River, New Jersey, Prentice Hall.

Scheirer, M. (1994). Designing and using process evaluation. In J. Wholey, H. Hatry, & K. Newcomer (Eds.), *Handbook of practical program evaluation* (pp. 40-68). San Francisco: Jossey-Bass.

Young, N. L., Yoshida, K. K., Williams, J. I., Bombardier, C., & Wright, J. G. (1995). The role of children in reporting their physical disability. *Archives of Physical Medicine and Rehabilitation, 76*, 913-918.

3

GUIDING THERAPIST DECISIONS ABOUT MEASURING OUTCOMES IN OCCUPATIONAL THERAPY

Mary Law, PhD, OT Reg. (Ont.), FCAOT; Gillian King, PhD; and Dianne Russell, MSc

The process of deciding how to measure occupational performance is challenging to occupational therapists for several reasons. First, while it is common for therapists in their educational programs to learn to administer many different assessments, it is less common for such evaluations to be learned as part of an overall measurement approach. Placing the use of assessments within a person, occupation, and environment measurement framework helps to organize our thinking about how we use measurement in practice. Second, therapists often have difficulty deciding what specific attribute(s) to measure. For example, a client has identified that he or she wants to be able to go shopping. What are the occupational performance attributes that are important in the occupation of shopping but are causing him or her difficulty—is it moving around a store, managing money, or selecting the groceries? Is the problem in performance related to where he or she will shop? The area of performance difficulty leads to a decision about the attribute for measurement. Finally, once a decision has been made about the attribute(s) to measure, what specific assessment tool is the best to use? Considerations of ease of use, time, psychometric characteristics, and cost are central to this decision.

This chapter presents a decision-making process that occupational therapists can use to guide the process of the measurement of occupational performance. In this section, we outline the decision-making process, list key questions to ask at each stage of the measurement process, and discuss important issues to consider as part of this process (Tables 3-1 to 3-7). For example, Law, King, Russell, Murphy, and Hurley (1999) discuss two foci for measure-

ment: 1) for an individual and/or his or her family, and 2) for a therapy program or service. Reflective questions for therapists to consider are listed for each stage of the measurement process. Although this decision-making process may seem long initially, we have purposefully described it in detail to enable student occupational therapists to learn the measurement process in a step-by-step fashion. As therapists become more skilled in measurement, they will find that the process flows smoothly from the identification of occupational performance issues to further assessment to intervention and outcome measurement.

MEASURING OCCUPATIONAL PERFORMANCE OUTCOMES FOR A PERSON AND/OR HIS OR HER FAMILY

I. Identification of Occupational Performance Issues by the Person

The first stage in the measurement process requires an occupational therapist to identify the client's perspectives about the reasons for referral to occupational therapy and the issues to be addressed during occupational therapy intervention. The goal is for the therapist to learn about the client, his or her occupations, and any difficulties he or she is having in performing the occupations that he or she needs to, wants to, or is expected to do (Law, Baptiste, Carswell, McColl, Polatajko, & Pollock, 1998; Law, Baum & Dunn, 2004).

Table 3-1

MEASURING OCCUPATIONAL PERFORMANCE OUTCOMES—STAGE I

<u>Stage in the Measurement Process</u>	<u>Key Questions</u>
Identification of occupational performance issues by the person	• How will I enable the person to identify the occupational performance issues that are the reasons for seeking occupational therapy services? • Is the client able to complete this assessment? If not, who has the best information about these issues? (see Table 3-2) • What assessment method will I use? • Where will I do the assessment? • Why am I evaluating occupational performance—to screen; to identify that there are occupational performance issues; to describe the person's status in performing occupations that they need to, want to or are expected to do? • Is the assessment method reliable and valid? • Is the assessment method clinically useful? • Is the assessment method valid for client(s) with this type of problem? • How will the results of this assessment of occupational performance issues guide decisions about further assessment and occupational therapy intervention?

How is this identification of occupational performance issues accomplished? Since it is the person's perspective and experiences that are most important, this information is best gained through an interview, narrative, or other self-report method with the person receiving occupational therapy services. Several methods used to enable a person to identify occupational performance issues are discussed in detail in Chapter 7. If the person is unable to participate in the identification of occupational performance issues, it is necessary to find an alternative source of information. This could be a family member, friend, or caregiver (see Stage II of this measurement process).

Therapists need to ensure that there is time and a suitable place for such assessment. For example, it is very difficult for a person to identify occupational performance issues quickly in a rushed outpatient clinic. In such a situation, finding a quieter room and more time will facilitate a more positive experience and lead to a more valid identification of issues.

The primary purpose of this stage of the measurement process is to identify occupational performance issues that will be the focus of intervention. This stage serves as a screening process. If the person is competent to respond and does not identify any occupations that they need to do and are having difficulty in performing, then occupa-

tional therapy services are not required. It may be that occupational therapy services will be required at a later time, or they are not necessary at all. If there are occupational performance issues identified, then this stage of the process serves to describe the status of the person's performance from their perspective. Using this information, the therapist can begin to make hypotheses about the reasons for performance difficulties. Decisions about further assessment of specific performance areas, components, and environmental conditions flow directly from these hypotheses.

Some of the reflective questions at this stage of the process center on the clinical usefulness, reliability and validity, and the applicability of the assessment to specific populations. These topics have already been discussed in some detail in Chapter 2, and specific methods to critically review measurement tools regarding these properties are described later in this chapter. However, it is important for therapists to consider the clinical utility and psychometric properties of a quantitative measure at every stage of the measurement process. If a measure has not been shown to provide consistent (reliable) and accurate (valid) information, its use in identification of occupational performance issues is not warranted. It is often tempting for a therapist to use a home-grown checklist or make a few changes to a

> **Table 3-2**
>
> ## MEASURING OCCUPATIONAL PERFORMANCE OUTCOMES—STAGE II
>
> | *Stage in the Measurement Process* | *Key Questions* |
> |---|---|
> | Identification of occupational performance issues for this person by another individual or group | • Why has another person or group identified potential occupation performance issues?
• Have I discussed this issue with the person and their family?
• What assessment method will I use?
• Why am I evaluating occupational performance—to screen for issues, or to describe occupational performance status?
• Is the assessment method reliable and valid?
• Is the assessment method clinically useful?
• Is the assessment method valid for use with client(s) with this type of problem?
• How will the results of this assessment of occupational performance issues guide decisions about occupational therapy assessment and intervention? |

published measure before using it. Checklists and adapted measures are not reliable or valid unless extensively tested, so a therapist using them will never be certain if the information that they are obtaining is accurate. Likewise, there are specific methods to ensure that qualitative assessments are consistent and dependable (see Chapter 5).

II. Identification of Occupational Performance Issues for This Person by Another Individual or Group

Because family and friends are so often central to the occupational therapy service plan, they are included in this stage of the process. In fact, in instances such as young children or persons with significant cognitive impairments, family or friends are the primary source of information about a person's occupational performance. In other situations, another service provider may be the source of issue identification. For example, a service provider in a skilled nursing facility may indicate a need for assistance with feeding a resident or transferring him or her from a wheelchair to a toilet. In Chapter 7, methods to assess occupational performance from the perspective of others are described in detail.

III. Further Assessment of Specific Occupational Performance Areas

Once the person, family, or others have identified the occupational performance issues that will be the focus of occupational therapy intervention, further assessment of

these specific performance attributes is often required. For example, a 26-year-old woman recovering from a brain injury resulting from a motor vehicle accident wants to be able to look after her apartment, cook meals, do laundry, shop for groceries and household items, and get around her community. Using an assessment of instrumental activities of daily living, the therapist assesses actual performance in these activities. This assessment provides specific information about the woman's initial level of performance so that intervention can focus on appropriate tasks and provide a comparison for future assessments of progress during therapy. The information from such an assessment also contributes to the clinical reasoning process about why performance difficulties are occurring.

IV. Assessment of Environmental Conditions and Performance Components

Using information from the referral for occupational therapy services, the person's (or other's) identification of occupational performance issues and further assessment of occupational performance attributes, the therapist forms a hypothesis about the reasons for the difficulties in occupational performance. To confirm this hypothesis, assessment of specific performance components and/or environmental conditions that are barriers to performance are often required. For example, information about strength and range of motion of a worker with a hand injury is important in planning intervention. If the parents of a 3-

Table 3-3

MEASURING OCCUPATIONAL PERFORMANCE OUTCOMES—STAGE III

Stage in the Measurement Process	*Key Questions*
Further assessment of specific occupational performance areas	• What specific occupational performance attribute(s) will I assess? • What assessment method will I use—individualized or standardized; quantitative or qualitative? • Who will complete the assessment? • Where will the assessment occur? • What is the age of the person? • Is the assessment method reliable and valid? • Is the assessment method clinically useful? • How will I use the results of this assessment?

Table 3-4

MEASURING OCCUPATIONAL PERFORMANCE OUTCOMES—STAGE IV

Stage in the Measurement Process	*Key Questions*
Assessment of environmental conditions and performance components	• What specific aspects of the environment and performance components are potential barriers to performance and need further assessment? • Who will complete the assessment? • Where will the assessment occur? • Is the assessment method reliable and valid? • Is the assessment method clinically useful? • How will I use the results of this assessment to focus occupational therapy intervention?

year-old girl with spina bifida want their daughter to be able to play on an outdoor playground in her neighborhood, information about the physical accessibility of the playground is necessary before planning intervention.

The purpose for the assessment of performance components and environmental conditions is to provide information about the reasons for performance difficulty and help to identify the focus of intervention. The most important consideration is how further information will contribute to knowledge about the person and help determine the focus of therapy intervention. Is the time taken for these assessments worth the benefit gained from increased knowledge? Let's consider the young girl and the outdoor playground. If a physical accessibility assessment indicates that the playground is fully accessible, then the focus of intervention would be on ensuring that the girl had sufficient outdoor mobility to use the playground. If, however, the playground is not accessible, then the most beneficial focus of intervention will be on changing the playground

environment to increase accessibility for all children with disabilities.

V. Selection of Outcome Measures

One of the most challenging decisions in measurement is deciding what specific assessment tool(s) to use for the evaluation of occupational performance. Issues of theoretical compatibility, specific purpose for measurement, clinical utility, reliability, and validity are important to consider.

First, let's consider where you might look to find an appropriate outcome measure for use in a specific clinical situation. Potential sources of information include textbooks (including this text), published test critiques, journals, and published reviews of measures in the occupational therapy field. (See the references at the end of this and other chapters, as well as the book indices, for more information about these sources.)

Table 3-5

MEASURING OCCUPATIONAL PERFORMANCE OUTCOMES—STAGE V

Stage in the Measurement Process	*Key Questions*
Selection of assessments to use	• Where do I look to find measures to use?
	• Does this assessment fit with my theoretical approach to occupational therapy?
	• What is the purpose of this assessment—to describe a person's status, to predict future performance, to evaluate change in performance over time?
	• What is the cost of the assessment?
	• How long does it take to administer?
	• How much training do I require before I can administer the assessment in a reliable manner?
	• Is there a manual available to guide the assessment?
	• How easy is it to administer the assessment, score it and interpret the results?
	• Does the assessment have evidence of reliability—over time, between raters?
	• Does the assessment have evidence of validity—content, criterion and construct?
	• If I am using the assessment to evaluate change over time, does it have evidence of responsiveness?

Occupational therapists use theory and models of practice to guide their clinical practice. In Chapter 1, we described several theoretical approaches to occupational therapy practice that use a person-environment-occupation perspective as the way of understanding occupational performance and planning occupational therapy services. Using one of these approaches leads to the use of assessments that measure a person's occupational performance in the context of his or her everyday life. In selecting assessment tools to use, a therapist will want to ensure that the assessment measures occupational performance from this broad perspective so that the assessment fits with his or her approach to practice.

In current health care practice, therapists have a limited amount of time for measurement. It is important to use assessments that provide useful information in as short a time as possible. One must also consider whether doing an assessment initially will save or increase time later on in the occupational therapy intervention process. For example, the identification of specific occupational performance issues by the client may take longer initially but can lead to more focused further assessment and intervention, thus saving time in the long run. Other issues of clinical utility to consider include the availability and cost of an assessment manual, training required to learn the assess-

ment, and ease of administration, scoring, and interpretation. Clinical utility is often overlooked by developers of measures, but it is one of the most significant influences on actual use of an outcome measure in a clinical situation.

Finally, it is important to review the reliability and validity of a measure. It is here that the purpose for using a particular outcome measure will guide decisions about which measure is best. Do you want the assessment to describe the current status of a person, to predict his or her performance in the future, or to assess change in performance over time? If you wish to describe a person's current status, you will want evidence that the measure is reliable between observers and can discriminate between persons who do or do not have performance difficulties. For prediction of performance in the future, a measure should have reliability between observers and over time and evidence that it can accurately predict future performance. In the increasingly important area of evaluation of change over time, a measure needs to have reliability between observers and over time as well as evidence that it is sensitive to and will pick up actual changes in performance over time (Law, 1987). Use of the measurement review form in Appendix D will aid therapists in evaluating the clinical utility, reliability, and validity of an outcome measure.

Table 3-6

MEASURING OCCUPATIONAL PERFORMANCE OUTCOMES—STAGE VI

Stage in the Measurement Process	*Key Questions*
Carry out the assessment	• How do I ensure a contextually accurate assessment? • How do I ensure a reliable assessment?

Table 3-7

MEASURING OCCUPATIONAL PERFORMANCE OUTCOMES—STAGE VII

Stage in the Measurement Process	*Key Questions*
Interpret measurement results	• How do I involve my client in assessment interpretation? • Am I trained to interpret the assessment results? • Do I need assistance in analyzing trends in assessment data? • Who will receive the assessment results? • What will occur based on the assessment results?

VI. Carry Out the Assessment

The next stage in the measurement process is the actual use of the assessment. Whether that assessment is used for initial identification of occupational performance issues or further assessment of components or environmental conditions, there are several important factors to consider.

Research on assessment practices indicates that the environmental location or context of the assessment has a significant influence on the validity of the findings (Park, Fisher, & Velozo, 1993; Sbordone, 2003). Performance of specific activities is dependent on the environment where performance takes place, so an assessment is best if carried out where the activity will be done most often by that person. With an increased emphasis on community-based interventions and concerns about the lack of generalization of acquired skills, it is most appropriate to measure outcomes in home and community environments. When this is not possible, the therapist must remember that the observed performance accurately reflects function only in the testing environment.

As we have learned earlier, it is important for outcome measures to have evidence of consistency or reliability. However, information that a measure has excellent reliability does not mean that you, as the therapist using the measure, will be able to administer it in a reliable manner. To ensure consistency in your measurement practices, take the time to learn and practice each new assessment tool that you begin using. Work with your colleagues to train each other. Test consistency (reliability) between therapists by both administering an assessment with the same client(s) and compare the agreement between your scores. To test consistency with yourself for assessments involving scoring of performance, one suggested method is to videotape clients performing the assessment, score these tapes a few weeks apart, and compare the agreement between scores. The limitation of this method is that scoring an assessment on a videotape is not the same context as scoring with a person right there with you. However, if you score the assessment at the same pace as you would in real life, the use of videotapes can tell you about your consistency while minimizing the measurement burden for the client.

VII. Interpret Measurement Results

Interpreting and communicating the results of measurement to your client and others is the last step in the measurement process. Each time an assessment is completed, a therapist spends time making sense of the information and how it informs the therapy process. Do the results of the assessment indicate that the person is having difficulty performing certain tasks? Are there specific performance components (e.g., organizing, planning) that are barriers to performance? This information is discussed with the client, the family, and others such as the rehabilitation team. Decisions are made about what therapy should be provided, or if it has already been provided, was it successful?

USING THE DECISION-MAKING PROCESS FOR A PERSON

Let's use an example to consider how this decision-making process is implemented in occupational therapy practice. Mrs. Talbot recently had a stroke, affecting the left side of her body. She was in the hospital for 10 days and is now returning home. While she is able to move around her house using a cane and can dress and feed herself, she and her family are concerned about her ability to look after herself on a day-to-day basis.

I. Identification of Occupational Performance Issues by the Person

The occupational therapist uses the Canadian Occupational Performance Measure (COPM) (Law et al., 1998) to enable Mrs. Talbot to identify the occupational performance issues most important to her as she returned home. Through this assessment, she identifies making meals, housework, taking the bus to the grocery store, grocery shopping, and working in her garden as the five most important issues to her. Doing the COPM with Mrs. Talbot took about 40 minutes. By the end of that time, both the therapist and Mrs. Talbot knew what the focus of occupational therapy intervention will be.

II. Identification of Occupational Performance Issues for This Person by Another Individual or Group

The occupational therapist, with Mrs. Talbot's permission, contacts her son and daughter-in-law after the first visit in order to ask them about their concerns for their mother. In this instance, the concerns of the son are very similar to those of Mrs. Talbot.

III. Further Assessment of Specific Occupational Performance Areas

Mrs. Talbot wants to focus on household activities initially. The therapist uses the Performance Assessment of Self-Care Skills (PASS) (Rogers, Holm, Goldstein, McCue & Nussbaum., 1994) to assess her performance in the activities of meal preparation, finances, use of the telephone, shopping, and housekeeping. The results of this assessment indicate that performance is decreased in the area of meal preparation and shopping.

IV. Assessment of Environmental Conditions and Performance Components

Mrs. Talbot indicates that making meals is the first task she wants to focus on in occupational therapy interven-

tion. Using the Kitchen Task Assessment (KTA) (Baum & Edwards, 1993), the occupational therapist assesses Mrs. Talbot's cognitive abilities to plan and carry out a cooking task. Through observation during this assessment, the therapist is also able to identify any limitations in performance caused by movement difficulties. The results of this assessment indicate that Mrs. Talbot can plan and organize a cooking task without difficulty. She does, however, have problems in carrying out tasks requiring the use of both hands together. It is also difficult for her to move around the kitchen to obtain cooking utensils. Using this information, the therapist and Mrs. Talbot develop an intervention plan that includes making changes to the organization of her kitchen and the use of some adaptive strategies for two-handed activities.

V. Selection of Outcome Measures

As we have seen in Stages II, III, and IV of this example, the occupational therapist chooses specific assessment tools to use with Mrs. Talbot. The decision to use the specific assessments is based on the therapist's theoretical model of practice and her knowledge of the psychometric properties of different assessments. This occupational therapist uses a client-centered approach to occupational therapy assessment and intervention. The use of the COPM fits with this perspective as it enables a client to identify the occupational performance issues that are most important to him or her at a particular time. The therapist, through reading the COPM manual, knows that the COPM has good to excellent test-retest reliability and excellent validity in detecting change over time.

This therapist uses a person-environment-occupation approach to practice that focuses on the assessment of client-identified tasks within his or her own environment. Both PASS and KTA assessments enabled the therapist and Mrs. Talbot to determine the reasons for difficulties in performance. For example, in meal preparation, the primary difficulties relate to the environmental layout of her kitchen and performance of two-handed activities.

VI. Carry Out the Assessment

In this example, performing the assessments in a contextually appropriate location is easy since Mrs. Talbot is seen in her home. Prior to using the assessments cited in this example, the occupational therapist has ensured that she received appropriate training in assessment administration. In the case of the COPM, she worked with a colleague and used the COPM training video to learn how to do the measure. For the other assessments, she and her colleagues had practiced together before using them with a client.

Table 3-8

EVALUATION OF OUTCOMES FOR A PROGRAM—STAGE I

Stage in the Measurement Process	_Key Questions_
Identification of occupational performance goals for the program	• What are the overall goals/mission of your organization? • What are the long-term goals for the program (in occupational performance terms)? • Who is involved in delivering the program? • Who are the clients who receive the program? • What specific occupational performance attribute(s) do want to assess? • Who will be the respondent(s) for the assessment? • Who has the best information about these issues? • How will the results of this assessment of occupational performance issues guide decisions about occupational therapy intervention?

VII. Interpret Measurement Results

After each assessment is completed, the therapist shows Mrs. Talbot the results, carefully pointing out areas of performance that are accomplished without difficulty and areas in which performance is decreased. A short, easily understandable report on the results of each assessment is given to Mrs. Talbot, along with a copy for her son and the home-therapy program. When the therapist and Mrs. Talbot feel that intervention directed toward improving meal preparation is completed, the COPM is used for Mrs. Talbot to rate change in performance. Again, these results are shared with her, her son, and other members of the home-therapy team.

MEASUREMENT OF THE DECISION-MAKING PROCESS—EVALUATION OF OUTCOMES FOR A PROGRAM

When developing a measurement approach to evaluate the outcomes of an occupational therapy intervention program, there are additional issues to consider (Tables 3-8 to 3-11). Programs usually include groups of clinical activities that are delivered in a package to a specific group of clients. For example, a day program for seniors with dementia often includes a variety of activities designed to engage group members in occupation and thus maintain everyday functioning. In evaluating outcomes for the program, the primary interest is in information about the average amount of change in clients who participate in the program. The outcomes that are measured relate to the specific goals of the program, rather than to the specific goals of each client.

I. Identification of Occupational Performance Goals for the Program

The first stage in the measurement process for evaluation of a program requires those who are running the program to identify the long-term occupational performance goals of the program. Designing an evaluation strategy for a program takes time and is best started by a review of the mission of the organization and the goals of the program (Letts et al., 1999). Reviewing the mission of the organization providing the program provides a direction for the types of outcomes that will be measured. For example, if the mission of the program is to facilitate community integration, the outcomes that will be measured for program evaluation will focus on attributes that reflect integration into the community. It is important at this stage to specifically describe who delivers the program and which clients receive the program. It is also important to ensure that people in the program are delivering services in a consistent manner. All of this information will help you to decide the feasibility of evaluating the program. The resources, both time and people, that are required to evaluate a program are often overlooked in the enthusiasm to get started. It is important to include all stakeholders, both service providers and clients, in the process of developing an evaluation of a program. Without this inclusion, implementation of changes based on the evaluation results will be more difficult.

Table 3-9	
EVALUATION OF OUTCOMES FOR A PROGRAM—STAGE II	
Stage in the Measurement Process	*Key Questions*
Selection of assessment tool(s) to use	• Where do I look to find assessment tool(s) to use?
	• Does this assessment fit with the program's theoretical approach to occupational therapy?
	• Will this assessment fit with my purpose—to describe a person's status prior to entry into a program, or to evaluate change in performance over time?
	• What is the cost of the assessment?
	• How long does it take to administer?
	• How much training do I require before I can administer the assessment in a reliable manner?
	• Is there a manual available to guide the assessment?
	• How easy is it to administer the assessment, score it and interpret the results?
	• Does the assessment have evidence of reliability—over time, between raters?
	• Does the assessment have evidence of validity—content, criterion, and construct?
	• If I am using the assessment to evaluate change over time, does it have evidence of responsiveness?

Following a review of the mission and the structure of the program, the long-term occupational performance goals and attributes to be measured are specified. For example, a program to provide therapy services to children with disabilities in schools has a long-term goal of improving the children's function within the school environment. The specific attributes to be measured in this situation include functional mobility, handwriting, and socialization. Once the specific attributes have been selected, the most appropriate respondents for the assessment are identified. For example, in a school therapy program, do you want to measure outcomes from the perspective of teachers, therapists, parents, or the children themselves (if old enough)? Outcome assessment from a perspective of teachers or therapists is often completed, while the perspective of parents or children receiving those services is not gathered as often.

II. Selection of Assessment Tool(s) to Use

In selecting appropriate assessment tools for the evaluation of programs, many of the issues to consider are the same as a measurement process for individuals. Issues of theoretical compatibility, the specific purpose of the assessment, clinical utility, reliability, and validity all influence the selection of the assessment to use. (You can refer back to Stage V of the individual decision-making process for a discussion of these issues.) The use of standardized assessment tools that have previously been used in the evaluation of programs is recommended. Using individualized tools such as goal attainment scaling is more difficult in evaluating programs as aggregation of individualized data is difficult to interpret.

III. Carry Out the Assessment

The goal for measurement in the evaluation of a program is to do outcome assessment in the context (place) that will most accurately reflect a person's performance. In evaluating the outcomes of a school therapy program, the most appropriate context in which to do the evaluation is in the school itself. On the other hand, for a program focused on community reintegration, evaluation is best done out in the community rather than in the location of the program.

If more than one person is administering assessments in evaluating a program, it is important to ensure a satisfactory level of agreement between evaluators. At a minimum, agreement between evaluators on at least five assessments

---

Table 3-10

EVALUATION OF OUTCOMES FOR A PROGRAM—STAGE III

Stage in the Measurement Process	*Key Questions*
Carry out the assessment	• How do I ensure a contextually accurate assessment? • Have I shown that the evaluators can administer the assessment tool(s) in a consistent (reliable) manner? • Have I developed a process/forms for data collection?

Table 3-11

EVALUATION OF OUTCOMES FOR A PROGRAM—STAGE IV

Stage in the Measurement Process	*Key Questions*
Interpret assessment results	• How will you be aggregating assessment results across clients? • Am I trained to interpret the assessment results? • Do you need assistance in analysing trends in assessment data? • How do I involve my clients in assessment interpretation? • Who will receive the assessment results? • What will occur based on the assessment results?

---

should be calculated and be over 75%. For large evaluations, reliability statistics for evaluators should be calculated.

Before beginning the evaluation, a data collection process is developed. A data collection form can be developed to capture the relevant information for the evaluation of the program. This process works best if it is simple, accessible, and short.

IV. Interpret Measurement Results

Once the assessment information for a program evaluation is collected, the next step is analysis and interpretation of the data. Decisions to be made at this stage include how the data will be aggregated and analyzed. Often, program evaluations simply calculate average change for each client and for the group. These results can be displayed in charts or graphs so that they are easily interpreted. If further statistical analysis is desired, you may need to seek out other resources, such as a statistician to help with that analysis.

It is essential to communicate the results of your outcome measurement to the program clients and other stakeholders (e.g., managers, funders). They will want to know if, overall, there are positive changes in the attributes that are measured. Are the results of the evaluation consistent with the goals of the program? Finally, you and others involved in the evaluation can address how the program should be changed based on the evaluation results. It is at this point that one needs to be creative and look at options for change supported by the data that are gathered. Any decisions about change are communicated to the clients, families, service providers, and others involved with the program. For the results of a program evaluation to have impact, it is important to use the information that is collected to improve the effectiveness of the program.

USING THE DECISION-MAKING PROCESS FOR A PROGRAM

How would the decision-making process for outcome measurement with programs be implemented in an example occupational therapy program? Consider the school-based therapy program discussed earlier. You work in a program providing occupational therapy services to children ages 5 to 12 in the school system. The overall mission of this program is to maintain and enhance functioning of the children within the school. The program is delivered by three therapists within a school district.

I. Identification of Occupational Performance Goals for the Program

The goals for the program are improved functioning in the school setting, as indicated by changes in ability to move around the school, do classroom activities, and socialize with other children and school staff.

II. Selection of Assessment Tool(s) to Use

Based on a review of the measurement literature, you determine that the School Function Assessment (SFA) (Coster, Deeney, Haltwanger & Haley, 1998) is the most appropriate measure to use to evaluate your program. The SFA is a relatively new measure that focuses on children's abilities in a school setting and has been well supported in terms of reliability and validity.

III. Carry Out the Assessment

All of the therapists in the program attend a course focused on using the SFA. You then train with each other and together administer the assessment to a few children. This enables you to compare results and ensure that all of you are administering and scoring the assessment in a consistent manner. During the course of 1 year of the program, the SFA is administered to each child in the program before he or she begins occupational therapy and after therapy is finished. By the end of 1 year, you have results from 85 children.

IV. Interpret Measurement Results

The data from the SFA, as well as demographic information such as age, referral problem, and diagnosis, is recorded on a data collection form. Using a computer spreadsheet, you calculate the average scores of the group of children before and after therapy, enabling you to determine the average change in scores on the SFA. These change scores are graphed according to age and referral problem to determine if there are differences in outcomes according to these factors. If you wish to do further analysis, you will contact someone who is more knowledgeable about statistics. The written results from this evaluation are shared with the families, the schools, and the school administrators.

THE CRITICAL REVIEW OF MEASURES

Occupational therapists, in selecting measures to use in their practice, want to use the best available measures in their practice. To ensure this, it is important to determine the clinical utility, standardization, reliability, and validity of potential measures. How can therapists find out information about measures? The most obvious choice is to find a critical review of a measure. Sources of these types of reviews include textbooks (Law, Baum, & Dunn, 2000; Van Deusen & Brunt, 1998) or measurement review books (Murphy, Plake, Impara & Spies, 2002; Plake & Impara, 2001). The Internet is also a source of information about measures. An example is the Educational Resource Information Clearinghouse (ERIC), which has published reviews on the Internet. Finally, there is educational software (available on CD-ROM) that provides critical reviews of outcome measures used in rehabilitation (Law, King, MacKinnon, et al., 1999).

There is always a chance that a critical review of a measure is not available. It is important, therefore, that students and therapists develop an understanding of the process of reviewing a measurement tool. To aid in this process, we have provided rating forms for this purpose that have been developed and tested over the past 19 years. The rating forms and accompanying guidelines were used in the review of all measures described in this book and can be used by students and therapists to review measures for their practice. See Appendix D for Outcome Measures Rating Forms and Guidelines. These forms can be downloaded from the CanChild Centre for Childhood Disability Research at McMaster University Web site: www.fhs.mcmaster.ca/canchild.ca (look under subject index for measures and multimedia).

REFERENCES

Baum C. M., & Edwards, D. (1993). Cognitive performance in senile dementia of the Alzheimer's type: The Kitchen Task Assessment. *American Journal of Occupational Therapy, 47(5)*,431-436.

Coster, W., Deeney, T., Haltwanger, I., & Haley, S. (1998). *The school function assessment.* San Antonio, TX: The Psychological Corporation.

Law, M. (1987). Criteria for the evaluation of measurement instruments. *Canadian Journal of Occupational Therapy, 54*, 121-127.

Law, M., Baptiste, S., Carswell, A., McColl, M., Polatajko, H., & Pollock, N. (1998). *Canadian occupational performance measure* (3rd ed.). Ottawa, Ontario: CAOT Publications.

Law, M., Baum, C., & Dunn, W. (2000). *Measuring occupational performance: Supporting best practice in occupational therapy.* Thorofare, NJ: SLACK Incorporated.

Law, M., Baum, C., & Dunn, W. (2004). Occupational performance assessment. In C. Christensen and C. Baum (Eds.), *Occupational therapy: Enabling function and well-being* (3rd ed). Thorofare, NJ: SLACK Incorporated.

Law, M., King, G., MacKinnon, E., Russell, D., Murphy, C., & Hurley, P. (1999). *All about outcomes. Version 1.0.* (CD-ROM). Thorofare, NJ: SLACK Incorporated.

Law, M., King, G., MacKinnon, E., Russell, D., Murphy, C., & Hurley, P. (1999). *All about outcomes-Adult.* (CD-ROM). Thorofare, NJ: SLACK Incorporated.

Law, M., King, G., Russell, D., MacKinnon, E., Hurley, P., & Murphy, C. (1999). Measuring outcomes in children's rehabilitation: A decision protocol. *Archives of Physical Medicine and Rehabilitation, 80(6),* 629-636.

Letts, L., Law, M., Pollock, N., Stewart, D., Westmorland, M., Philpot, A., & Bosch, J. (1999). *A programme evaluation workbook for occupational therapists: An evidence-based practice tool.* Ottawa, Ontario: CAOT Publications.

Murphy, L. L.,Plake, B. S., Impara, J.C. & Spies, R.A. (Eds.). (2002). *Tests in print VI.* Buros Institute of Mental Measurements. Lincoln, NE: University of Nebraska Press.

Park, S., Fisher, A. G., & Velozo, C. A. (1993). Using the Assessment of Motor and Process Skills to compare performance between home and clinical settings. *American Journal of Occupational Therapy, 48,* 519-525.

Plake, B. S., & Impara, J. C. (2001). *The fourteenth mental measurements yearbook.* Lincoln, NE: University of Nebraska Press.

Rogers, I. C., Holm, M. B., Goldstein, G., McCue, M., & Nussbaum, P. D. (1994). Stability and change in functional assessment of patients with geropsychiatric disorders. *American Journal of Occupational Therapy, 48,* 914-918.

Sbordone, R.J. (2003). Limitations of neuropsychological testing to predict the cognitive and behavioral functioning of persons with brain injury in real-world settings. *NeuroRehabilitation. 16(4),* 199-201.

Van Deusen, I., & Brunt, D. (Eds.). (1998). *Assessment in occupational therapy and physical therapy.* Orlando, FL: W. B. Saunders.

SECTION II

MEASUREMENT IN OCCUPATIONAL THERAPY

In Section 2, we review occupational performance measures. We have organized this section to assist the reader in locating appropriate measures and to provide a conceptual framework for making the transition to occupational performance measurement in practice. We have not included all measures available in the universe, but rather have selected the best measures available in each topic area (i.e., chapters). We have also provided cross-reference lists in the Appendices, which organize the measures alphabetically, by area of occupational performance, by author, and by World Health Organization's International Classification of Functioning, Disability and Health (ICF) mapping.

THE PERSON-ENVIRONMENT-OCCUPATION FRAMEWORK

In Section 1, we discussed several frameworks from the occupational therapy literature that characterize occupational performance in context. One of these is the person-environment-occupation (PEO) framework (Law et al., 1996); this framework illustrates the relationship among the person, the task, and the environment using a Venn diagram. In this diagram, each of these three variables is represented by a circle; the three circles intersect so that there are seven unique "spaces," which are numbered on the following diagrams.

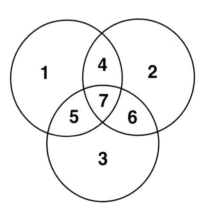

To assist the reader, we have included a diagram next to each measure title. We have highlighted the "space" that each measure primarily evaluates so that you can scan through sections if you need a particular type of measure.

Space 1 illustrates the person variables alone. Measures of performance components would fit here. We are not addressing this form of measurement in this text.

Space 2 illustrates the environmental variables alone. This would include measures of the features of the environment, such as are included in Chapter 16.

Space 3 illustrates the occupation variables alone. There are only a few measures of this type in this book.

Space 4 represents the intersection of person and environment. Measures in this category will inform you about how the person fits into or responds to environmental conditions. Various chapters include measures of this type.

Space 5 represents the intersection of person and occupation. Measures in this category will inform you about the person's interests and needs for occupational performance. Various chapters will introduce these measures to you.

Space 6 represents the intersection of occupation and the environment. Measures in this category address the capacity of environments to support particular tasks and the match between tasks and environments. This classification is not used in this book.

Space 7 represents the intersection of all three variables, occupational performance. Many of the measures in this section capture this relationship, and therefore are very useful tools for intervention planning in natural environments.

THE FIVE KEY ACTIONS FOR BEST PRACTICE MEASUREMENT

Let's return to the five key actions that we believe occupational therapists must implement when conducting assessments, reporting findings, and interpreting measurement information for intervention planning. As you recall from the introduction to Section I, these five actions enable occupational therapists to take advantage of wisdom from other disciplines, create an organized approach, and provide a framework for best practice by taking an occupation-centered, evidence-based approach to measurement.

Because we believe that these are so critical to effective measurement, we discuss the actions here in relationship to the selection of outcomes measures in occupational therapy. We will revisit them in each of the chapters in this section to demonstrate how these actions can be applied.

Mine the Gold

Many disciplines are concerned with how persons interact with environments to perform tasks. Occupational therapists must take a broad view of the problems of performance, and in doing so, can gain more insight about how to address these problems effectively. "Mining the gold" is finding out what other disciplines have to say, what they have found in research, and what they have produced that will advance occupational therapy thinking and practices.

Become Systematic

It has been difficult for occupational therapists to provide evidence for their teams and service recipi-

ents with an occupational performance focus. Therapists have felt worried to report all observational or interview data when others are reporting their findings in a different manner. The measures in this section will provide ways to keep an occupational performance focus and provide systematic data about status and progress. Many of these measures formalize observation and interview data, and therefore provide a mechanism for embellishing findings with qualitative information. Being systematic means creating an explicit plan that enables others to see how and why you are doing what you do. When others cannot see the relationships between what you say you do and what you actually do, our professional practices take on a "folklore" perspective.

Use Evidence in Practice

With changes in service systems and mechanisms for funding services comes increased pressure to demonstrate the efficacy of professionals' practices. Consumers of services are also becoming more informed about their needs and options through media, technology, and an increased awareness of one's responsibility to participate in decision-making about one's life and health. The trend in the literature to provide "evidence-based" services encourages professionals to 1) keep current on what is known about a particular problem, 2) apply knowledge to the practices a professional engages in, and 3) clearly inform the recipient and family what we know and don't know about interventions. These steps ensure that the service recipient understands the benefits and risks of each choice; it is also helpful to discuss ways to evaluate effectiveness during intervention so that changes can be made if needed.

Make Occupational Therapy Contribution Explicit

Many of the measures we have included in this section come from other disciplines. Although we acknowledge the wisdom from others (in mining the gold), occupational therapists must also clearly articulate the unique occupational therapy perspective when using these measures. We look at problems and solutions differently than any other discipline; when we don't clearly communicate that occupation-focused perspective, we miss opportunities to inform others about our contribution. For example, social workers are concerned about the environment for performance but may be more focused on the sociocultural features and may need the perspectives of occupational therapy to consider the physical and temporal features that are facilitating or creating barriers to performance.

Engage in Occupation-Based, Client-Centered Practice

As we discussed in Section I, we are proposing that it is necessary and possible to have occupational therapy practice evolve so that it is centrally focused on occupational performance and demonstrates value for client-centered practice. This means that we address problems that the person and family identify, things that will enable and enhance daily living. We do not spend resources addressing issues that are not important to either the occupational performance or the person's and family's priorities about how they wish to live their lives. The measures in this section will enable occupational therapists to create their practice to incorporate these principles easily.

The Measure Analysis Worksheets

The authors have analyzed each measure using the critical review format that is outlined in Chapter Three and reproduced in Appendix E. This method was used to assist in comparisons and selection of the best tool for a situation. Components include:

- Title
- Source
- Important References
- Purpose
- Type of Client
- Focus
- Sensitivity to Change
- Clinical Utility
- Standardization
- Reliability
- Validity
- Scale Construction
- Strengths
- Weaknesses
- Overall Utility

4

Establishing the Integrity of Measurement Data

Identifying Impairments That Can Limit Occupational Performance and Threaten the Validity of Assessments

Carolyn Baum, PhD, OTR/C, FAOTA; Monica Perlmutter, MA, OTR/L; and Winnie Dunn, PhD, OTR, FAOTA

Context for Measuring Performance

Throughout this text, we emphasize the importance of the person's self-selected performance in daily life as the central feature of occupational therapy measurement. Occupational therapists are trained to identify factors that may limit the person's capacity to engage in his or her occupations. Occupational therapists don't just watch someone do something and deem it successful or unsuccessful; occupational therapists observe the person, the environment, and the task to determine what contributes to successful performance and what limits the person's capacity for performance.

Occupational therapists must develop their measurement skills to recognize the impact impairments may or not have on an individual's ability to engage in activities and tasks. The use of assessments goes beyond simple identification of impairments. Therapists must identify impairments that may affect an individual's performance during assessments, while participating in intervention and also those that will require ongoing management or accommodation in order to maximize performance. For example, if a person has difficulty participating in an assessment or performing a task, possible underlying causes may be decreased visual acuity, hearing loss, depression, memory loss, or low literacy. The validity of our occupational therapy assessment may be threatened by such impairments that would interfere with the individual's ability to demonstrate his or her capacity. Fortunately our body of knowledge enables us to make adjustments to accommodate for particular impairments; we just need to recognize what the factors might be.

Fisher (1998) encourages occupational therapists to employ a top-down approach to the identification of occupational performance problems. Although a top-down approach is a good one, it does not always take into consideration the need to understand how impairments can influence performance-based tests. Information about the sensory, cognitive, and motor capacities of our clients can give the practitioner more confidence in our occupational performance assessment findings and adds an important dimension to the development of a client- and family-centered plan. Occupational therapists' knowledge of anatomy, neuroscience, and physiology prepares practitioners to assess and identify impairments that could create an excess disability (i.e., an unnecessary disability) for our clients and their families.

Impairment level measurements can be useful in several ways. First, it would be important to determine impairments that may affect the client's performance prior to the diagnostic assessment. For example, a child's performance on the Bruininks-Oseretsky Test of Motor Proficiency (BOTMP) (Bruininks, 1978) may be affected by unidentified low vision; an adult who is experiencing depression may not perform optimally on a test involving cognition.

Second, in some instances, it may be beneficial to assess impairments at the performance component level prior to an occupational performance assessment. For example, if you were initiating occupational therapy at an assisted living center and there were minimal records about the residents, you may want to do a screening to determine the person's vision, hearing, cognition, presence of depression, and if the person is literate. This information could assist the occupational therapist with interpreting functional assessments and could form the basis of resident profiles. This information could also assist with program development and identify issues that needed to be referred to medical and or community resources.

In most occupational therapy encounters, it is best to measure impairments at the performance component level as a follow-up to performance-based assessment. For example, after watching a client prepare a meal, the therapist might have several hypotheses about why the individual had trouble locating utensils and seemed confused and cautious with the tasks. The therapist could follow up with assessments that screen for vision, audition, literacy, cognitive skills, praxis, and/or sequencing in an effort to identify specific abilities and limitations that might be impacting the client's performance.

In this chapter, we will focus on methods of identifying impairments that can limit occupational performance. This will require an understanding by the family or careprovider to learn how to accommodate problems that can not be remediated and also may threaten the validity of the occupational therapy assessments. Our intention is to share examples of this type of measurement to encourage greater attention to identifying problems that might limit a client's performance on the occupational therapy assessment and those that must be taken into account in context of treatment planning. A note of caution: measuring a person's performance in terms of impairments alone is not acceptable. The ultimate focus of occupational therapy measurement is on how the impairment impacts a person's everyday life.

Key Issues in Considering Impairments That May Impact Performance When Administering Assessments

Engagement in occupation requires skills and abilities. Occupational therapists may refer to these skills and abilities as performance components of intrinsic or person factors. Clients think of them as problems that limit what it is that they want or need to do. Many people that occupational therapists serve have long-standing developmental, chronic, or neurological conditions that impact their occupational performance. Occupational therapists must use knowledge of the client's abilities to assist him or her in developing strategies to accomplish his or her goals. Many of the interventions occupational therapists use are dependent on memory, attention, vision, audition, senso-

ry receptors, and the ability to read. Occasionally such impairments may have gone unrecognized, either because they are thought to be a condition associated with the person's status, such as, aging (Branch, Horowitz, & Carr, 1989) or the person has not called the impairment to the attention of his or her health or educational professionals. An occupational performance assessment approach requires the practitioner to identify impairments that can interfere with the individual's occupational performance. as they may limit an the person's ability to perform the activities, tasks, and roles that are central to his or her life. Additionally many impairments (vision, cognition, audition for example) can benefit from medical management. The occupational therapist can call these impairments to the attention of the client's primary physician or recommend that the client seek additional medical help or community resources.

As we strive to implement evidence-based practice, standardized tests play an important role in our clinical and research protocols. We must ask the questions: Can the client see the task, hear the directions, read, and retain the instructions? Is it possible that the client's performance could be influenced by depression? Could it be that the person's depression is confounding the planning process? The occupational therapist must have access to this information prior to implementing client-centered intervention strategies. If a person has an unrecognized visual, auditory, motor, psychological cognitive or language problem, or cannot read, the validity of the assessment will be threatened and the absence of such information will produce data that implies excess disabilities. It is the occupational therapist's role to raise issues regarding the conditions that would limit the function of the client to the health care or educational team and work with them to enable the person to accomplish the goals that will help the person do what is important and has meaning. Let's consider each of these issues separately.

Issues Related to Acuity

When a person has less than optimal function in the sensory receptors, it is harder to capture the information needed to determine a persons capacity for activities and tasks. Hearing and vision can be corrected in most situations, but in other situations, there remains some residual losses that make it harder to hear or see optimally. In measuring occupational performance, it is critical for therapists to consider whether the person can hear directions, see objects that need to be manipulated, and feel the shape and texture (i.e., tactile sensation) of things as performance is occurring. If therapists do not consider acuity, decisions about performance can be skewed. A therapist might observed that a man cannot make his lunch; one reason for this could be that the man does not see the meat and cheese slices with sufficient detail to separate them and make the sandwich. The therapist might also document concerns that safety could become a factor if the man needs to use a knife to cut a tomato for his sandwich.

When therapists hypothesize, do they hypothesize or determine via assessment that acuity or hearing loss could be affecting performance, as these can introduce adjustments to reduce the impact of the sensory loss on the performance required in the assessment. For example, amplification devices, magnifiers and better lighting can help. If tactile sensation is suspected to be less than optimal, therapists can pair tactile input with auditory or visual cues, or can touch more firmly to get the person's attention.

Issues Related to Language

Although the technical details about language are typically addressed by colleagues from other disciplines, the functions that language affords to performance is central to occupational therapists. Language includes reading, writing, talking and listening. Each of these skills can affect occupational performance and performance on standardized testing. Occupational therapists need to consider how all these aspects of language might have an impact on the measurement selected for assessment. Language is part of most assessment procedures, even when it is not the focus of the assessment. Giving simple instructions requires listening skills; asking the person to respond requires listening and talking to form an answer, even if the topic is about activities of daily living.

When therapists are concerned that language could be interfering with performance on other tasks, they can make sure instructions are available in multiple forms (e.g., verbally and written). They can also compare demonstrated performance to verbally instructed performance. Therapists can also create a practice session to check the persons' ability to complete the required tasks separate from the actual assessment.

Modest changes in language, particularly with naming objects, have been identified in the normal aging population (Kirshner & Bakar, 1995). Even slight changes may interfere with the individual's ability to effectively communicate with family, friends, and physicians. Literature on more severe language disorders in healthy older adults does not exist. The deficits may not occur in this population. However, if a deficit exists, function would certainly be affected. Aphasia is a group of language deficits in which the individual has difficulty with language comprehension and/or expression (Duchek, 1991). Such a deficit would severely hamper an individual's ability to communicate effectively and maintain independence.

Issues Related to Cognition

Cognition is the way information is processed and structured in the brain as it supports the performance of everyday life. Cognition involves the mechanisms of com-

prehension and production of language, pattern recognition, task organization, reasoning, attention, and memory (Duchek, 1991; Duchek & Abreu, 1997). Cognition encompasses many interrelated processes: the act of thinking, perceiving objects, recognizing objects, solving problems, and ability to judge one's own actions and the events around him or her (Duchek, 1991). Cognition is critical for independence—planning a meal, including shopping, cooking, and serving, planning and maintaining a garden, paying bills, performing car maintenance, and taking medicine all require high levels of cognitive function.

Sometimes, therapists are testing these aspects of cognition; however, at other times, the focus of assessment is on movement, task completion or participation, and in these cases, we don't want cognition to interfere with our ability to know about these other functions. For example, when testing a child's ability to complete personal hygiene tasks, therapists would have to consider whether the child's perceptual or executive function might be interfering with the child's ability to get the tools and supplies needed from the drawers. In school, this same child might have trouble completing a math test not because of math skills per se, but because he cannot keep his place on the page to finish the test efficiently. If we want to know whether the child has the technical skills in both personal hygiene and math, we have to first identify that perception or difficulties in organization or sequencing might be interfering, and then set into place some strategies to reduce the impact of perception difficulties so we can know the child's skills.

Cognitive problems are often first recognized by alterations in memory. An older person misplaces keys and has difficulty remembering names and recalling everyday events. These events can be very upsetting for an individual (Dublin, 1992) and may or may not be indicative of permanent cognitive impairment. Memory and attention impairments produce deficits that have a great impact on occupational performance. Activities such as following medication routines, keeping appointments, performing self-care and instrumental tasks, driving, and social interaction are predicated on the ability to remember and attend to the task.

Agnosia is a cognitive and perceptual deficit in which the person is unable to recognize familiar objects perceived by visual, tactile, proprioceptive, and/or auditory senses. Zoltan (1996) tells us that there is a disruption between the input and the stored description of the object. This deficit can take several different forms and interfere with recognizing faces or objects, identifying colors, perceiving spatial relationships, and recognizing sounds. Language naming deficits are often one of the first signs of early stages of dementia and have been found to be a good predictor of progression of senile dementia of the Alzheimer's type (Knesevich, LaBarge, & Edwards, 1986).

In addition, there is evidence that naming abilities decline slightly with advancing age (Van Gorp, Satz, Kiersch, & Henry, 1986).

Unilateral visual neglect is usually associated with a neurological deficit. It limits the person's ability to perceive, respond, or attend to stimuli (Lin, 1996). Usually, neglect is associated with a neurological episode; however, its presence in a community sample is currently not known. Neglect can affect any channel of input such as visual, auditory, tactile, or olfactory, and is expressed in several modes of output such as manual, ocular, navigational, and verbal (Halligan & Marshall, 1994). The presence of neglect would not only confound performance on tests, it would severely limit a person's independence and present difficult problems for the family.

Issues Related to Motor Impairments

Many assessments require motor responses regardless of the fact that the assessment is not about motor performance. Some tests have obvious motor requirements, but even pointing is a motor act that is challenging for some people with motoric challenges. Additionally, eye movements, head turning, and mouth movements can also be challenging for some people, and might be imbedded into an assessment and be hard to discern from the overall plan of the assessment. Since movement is so routine for so many people, it is easy to overlook what the motor aspects of an assessment might be. We discussed oral responses as part of language above, but talking also requires motor movements, and this aspect of movement needs to be considered as well. It is possible to consider the impact of motor skills within an assessment by asking the person to perform the tasks in two ways, one in the standardized manner, and again with another mode of responding that either eliminates motor performance, or in most cases, changes or reduces the motor requirements. We can ask for a verbal response instead of pointing.

Issues Related to Psychosocial Status

Probably the most elusive factor to consider is the person's psychosocial status. We all have the experience of being 'off the game', knowing that we have not performed to our capacity on a particular day, sometimes due to fatigue or hunger, and other times due to competing thoughts of anxiety or depression. In this area more than others, establishing rapport with the person being evaluated can provide an anchor point for considering the person's psychosocial condition. Asking the person how they felt about their performance is also a strategy that can become part of the interpretation process. When therapists feel that a person's psychosocial status is interfering, changing the time for assessment can also reduce the impact on the performance standard. Mood can have an effect on memory function and may impact many areas of daily function as well. Depression is a disorder that is commonly seen in older adults (Yesavage et al., 1983) yet it is more and more being reported in children. Depression is thought to be associated with increased risk of disability and loss of independence (Alexopoulos Vrontou, Kakuma, Meyers, Young, Klausner, et al.. 1996). Individuals with depression often experience low motivation, have difficulty in planning ahead, exhibit self-neglect, and have poor attention and memory problems (Austin, Mitchell, Wilhelm, et al., 1999) all of which compromise occupational performance.

All of these key factors can affect performance, and therapists have the responsibility to ensure that they have done everything to ensure valid assessment data by minimizing the impact of these components. To illustrate how to consider these factors, we will discuss assessment of older adults and children.

RECOGNIZING PERFORMANCE IMPAIRMENTS IN OLDER ADULTS

The assessment of older adults should include a consideration of the aging process and the impact this may have on the older adult's optimal performance. Central to such an assessment is an assessment of factors that, though they may be associated with aging, are also manageable with medical and/or environmental attention.

Presbycusis, or hearing loss, effects one-third of individuals over the age of 65 (Bess, Lichtenstein, Logan, Burger, & Nelson, 1989; Mulrow et al., 1990) and many younger persons who have jobs and leisure interests that expose them to loud noises. Hearing loss could be due to degeneration of the acoustic nerve and sclerosing of the ossicles in the ear (Dublin, 1992). Hearing loss makes it difficult for individuals to accomplish their daily activities (Dargent-Molina, Hays, & Breart, 1996).

Diminished visual acuity, or the ability of the eye to determine fine detail at high contrast, is another common problem (Bonder & Goodman, 1995). As a person ages, the cornea flattens, increasing the amount of astigmatism, and decreased pupil diameter slows the pupillary response to light (Rubin, Bandeen-Roche, Prasada-Rao, Fried, & SEE Project team., 1994). The iris increases in rigidity, causing the pupil to become smaller. As a result, older adults need additional lighting to read. Thickening of the lens, or presbyopia, can occur in individuals in their 50s (Hayflick, 1998). This makes it difficult to focus on objects, and many individuals require bifocals. In some persons, the lens yellows and color vision is impaired (Ainlay, 1988). Glare, or decrease in visibility of an object due to other light sources in the field (Rubin et al., 1994), is a common complaint of older adults. These changes can be associated with a decrease of self-sufficiency in daily activities because the individuals have difficulty judging the distance of a curb, finding a sign, reading in dim light, and performing activities that require accurate vision (Rubin et al., 1994).

Cognition, which has been previously discussed, is central to retaining independence in the older adult. According to an American Association of Retired Persons (AARP) survey, 89% of retired Americans prefer to remain in their current residences as long as possible. Current statistics report that only 5% of the older population resides in nursing homes. That proportion, however, increases with age such that 20% of individuals over 80 live in nursing homes (Mynatt, Essa, & Rogers, 2000); much of this can be attributed to a poor cognitive status. Occupational therapists are being called on to assess the capacity of an individual to remain in community settings. Such an assessment is heavily dependent on cognitive capacity.

Literacy interferes with the capacity of individuals to live independently and would also contribute to poor performance on tests where reading is required. Low literacy can affect the person's ability to perform self-care activities, may interfere with self-esteem, increase frustration levels, and increase the risk for developing health problems (Meade & Thornhill, 1989). Nearly 40 to 44 million people in the United States have low literacy (Parker, Baker, Williams, & Nurss, 1995). Literacy supports reading and writing to engage in social interaction, to follow medical routines, and to participate in leisure activities (Rigg & Kazemek, 1983). People with low reading ability have difficulty with instructions and may ask fewer questions to avoid humiliation (Hussey & Gilliard, 1989). While the number of adults experiencing illiteracy is unknown, many have not completed the 8th grade (Rigg & Kazemek, 1983), and it is impossible to know the reading competencies of individuals educated over 60 years ago. This being the case, we have to wonder why education materials are often developed at or above the 10th grade reading level (Meade & Thornhill, 1989). Given the prevalence of low literacy in our society, occupational therapists should routinely consider literacy and plan interventions accordingly.

Limiting the Impact of Impairments

People need to be able to carry out the activities of their daily lives based upon their needs and preferences. Wilcock (1993) suggested that the adult has three major occupations: 1.) to provide for the immediate bodily needs of sustenance, self-care, and shelter; 2.) to develop skills, social structures, and superiority over predictors and the environment; and 3.) to increase personal capacities to enable maintenance and development of the organism. While it is difficult to categorize individuals and their unique patterns of activity, it is clear that impairments that

affect vision, audition, language, memory, and mood will make the activities more difficult and may threaten occupational performance.

How Can Impairments Be Identified?

The Functional Impairment Battery (FIB), a battery of eight standardized tests, provides the therapist with useful information for interpreting assessment findings, for intervention planning, and helping the client seek help to resolve impairments like vision, hearing, and depression (Perlmutter, 1998; Perlmutter, Baum, & Edwards, 1998). The FIB includes the following constructs: visual acuity, audition, visual neglect, anomia, aphasia, memory, depression, and literacy.

When considering the use of the FIB, practitioners should investigate the information that may already be available in their setting. For example, speech pathologists and neuropsychologists may evaluate some of these constructs. There is no need to duplicate testing. It is our experience that vision, audition, memory, depression, and literacy are not often assessed in a formalized way and will require the occupational therapist to collect data for use in treatment planning.

The FIB includes eight assessments that can identify impairments that may limit the individual's potential for success in assessments and interventions. Existing measures were included based on the following criteria: 1.) appropriateness for the neurological population, 2.) established reliability and validity, 3.) clinical utility, 4.) brevity and ease of administration, and 5.) portability for use in hospital and community settings. Each of the measures included in the FIB met all five criteria, with the exception of the audition test, which is undergoing standardization. It should be noted that the FIB is a screening battery and not a diagnostic procedure. The references for the FIB measures are at the end of the chapter.

While the initial version of the FIB is designed for older adults in a U.S. population, colleagues in other cultures may want to choose comparable measures that are standardized in their environments and for the age range of their populations.

The tests included in the FIB can all be administered by occupational therapists, as they are in the public domain. However, the FIB offers an opportunity for certified occupational therapy assistants and other health professionals to participate in the testing. It is not of consequence who administers the FIB; it matters that occupational therapists and other health professionals know how the identified impairments affect the client's performance.

The first section of the FIB examines specific visual impairments, including visual acuity and visual-spatial neglect. The following tests were used to measure these constructs.

Corrected near vision and visual acuity is measured with a near vision card (Ferris, Kassoff, Bresnick, & Bailey, 1982). The vision card is held 14 inches away from the person's eyes; persons are allowed to use both eyes and wear glasses. The distance equivalent of the last line read is recorded as the person's visual acuity level. A score of over 20 to 70 is considered indicative of a visual impairment.

Unilateral visual neglect is measured by the Rivermead Behavioral Inattention Test (BIT) line-crossing task. This is a valid and reliable test that was developed for use with individuals with stroke (Wilson, Cockburn, & Halligan, 1987). Standard verbal and scoring instructions are used to administer the test. A score of 36 or greater indicates functional impairment.

The second section of the FIB addresses audition and self-perception of functional communication and employs measures that can be administered by non-specialists.

Audition is measured by a new test that is being standardized (Popelka, 1997). This test assesses the individual's capacity for hearing a combination of high- and low-pitched sounds without the benefit of lip reading. Persons are asked to repeat the sounds sa, se, si, so, and su, while the person vocalizing the sounds blocks the view of his or her lips. An audiologist recommended this test after a comprehensive literature search did not produce a measure that met the criteria for the battery. It is portable and low-tech. A score of 4 or less indicates a functional impairment.

Language is assessed by two measures that incorporate aspects of comprehension, expression, naming, identifying, and recognizing objects. Aphasia is measured with the shortened form of the Frenchay Aphasia Screening Test (FAST) (Enderby, Wood, Wade, & Hewer, 1987). The shortened form of the FAST assesses comprehension and expression by having the subject follow increasingly difficult instructions and point to a series of objects. Subjects are also asked to describe what is seen in a second picture and name as many animals in 60 seconds as possible. The correlation of the FAST and the Functional Communication Profile was=40.90. It also has strong inter-rater (w=0.97) and test-retest (w=0.97) reliability. The maximum score is 20; less than 13 indicates potential impairment. Anomia is measured with the Consortium to Establish a Registry for Alzheimer's Disease (CERAD) version of the Boston Naming Test (Morris et al., 1989). Subjects are asked to name 15 objects, which are presented in line drawings. Internal consistency has been established between the CERAD and four alternative versions and the original 60-item test (r=0.97 to 0.98) (Mack, Freed, Williams, & Henderson, 1992). Construct validity was established and was found to discriminate between Alzheimer's disease and non-demented older adults (Williams, Mack, & Henderson, 1989).

Memory, concentration, and orientation are measured with the Short Blessed Test, or Short Orientation-Memory-Concentration Test (Katzman, Brown, Fuld, Peck, & Schimmel, 1983). This six-item test includes questions regarding orientation, a memory phrase, counting backward, and reciting the months of the year backward. It has been validated as a measure of cognitive impairment in older adults and reliably discriminates between mild, moderate, and severe cognitive deficits. The maximum score is 33, and a score of 9 or more indicates a cognitive impairment.

Functional literacy is measured with the Rapid Estimate of Adult Literacy in Medicine (REALM) (Davis, Long, Jackson, et al., 1993). It is designed for use in public health and primary care settings to estimate reading grade levels for people who read below the ninth grade reading level. It can be administered in less than 5 minutes. The REALM correlates with the Peabody Individual Achievement Test-Revised (r=0.97) and the Slosson Oral Reading Test-Revised (r=0.96) (Davis et al.). Inter-observer (r=0.99) and test-retest (r=0.98) reliability is high. The possible score is 0 to 66. A score indicating less than ninth grade reading level (60) was identified as the cut off for a functional reading impairment.

Depression is measured with the Geriatric Depression Scale Short Form (GDS-SF) (Alden, Austin, & Sturgeon, 1989), specifically designed and validated with the older population (Yesavage et al., 1983). Subjects answer 15 yes/no questions about feelings, interests, activities, and hopes. The short 15-item version correlates highly with the original 30-item test (r=0.84). Construct validity was determined by examining the performance of the GDS with the Hamilton Rating Scale for Depression and the Zung Self Rating Scale (Austin et al., 1999; Yesavage et al., 1983). Test-retest reliability was 0.85. The range of possible scores is 0 to 15. A score of greater than 5 indicates probable depression.

Table 4-1 presents a case study showing how the FIB informs an occupation-based approach to assessment and client-centered plan.

RECOGNIZING PERFORMANCE IMPAIRMENTS IN CHILDREN USING INTERDISCIPLINARY ASSESSMENT DATA

It is equally important to identify the performance component impairments that limit a child's function and engagement in occupation. Since teams are required to conduct comprehensive assessments, data collected by other professionals can be informative about the child's skills and limitations. Records are constructed differently in various settings, so you will need to find out what is available in your setting. Here are some examples to get you started.

Table 4-1

ASSESSING THE IMPAIRMENT ISSUES OF AN OLDER ADULT

Mrs. Wheeler is a 68-year-old woman who suffered a stroke 6 months ago. After 2 weeks of inpatient rehabilitation she went home. She recently visited her physician and indicated that she was having difficulties doing what she needed to do at home and that she was no longer leaving her home. She was referred for an in-home visit by an occupational therapist.

Mrs. Wheeler lives in a home that is accessed by five steps to the front door and four to the back. Her daughter visits 2 to 3 times a month and she has little social support other than those visits. The occupational therapist wants to understand Mrs. Wheeler's goals and her occupational history prior to helping her make a plan, so she decides to administer the FIB to get a sense of the issues that will be central to understanding her limitations when performance based assessments like the Activity Card Sort and the COPM are administered. The FIB takes 15 to 20 minutes.

Assessments (FIB)	*Result*	*Implications*
Lighthouse Near Acuity Card	20/80 with glasses on	Low vision and the physician needs to know she needs a referral for visual services
Rivermead Behavior Inattention Test	43/54	Probable left neglect
Simple Audition Test	3/5	Probable hearing loss
Short Blessed	10/28	Mild cognitive loss and may not retain new information, poor concentration and a possible safety risk
FAST (comprehension and expression)	19/20	Language is within normal limits
Boston Naming Test	10/14	Some limit in naming—may indicate mild cognitive loss
REALM	155 (7.7 grade reading level)	Needs simply written instruction
GDS (Geriatric Depression Scale)	8	Probable depression and the physician needs to know

Equipped with this information, the OT proceeds to administer the ACS, COPM, and other relevant measures. The following adjustments we made in administering the assessments.

- Speaking in a loud tone of voice and positioning across from the Mrs. Wheeler so she can benefit from lip reading and gestures.
- Use of clear, simple terminology in view of literacy level.
- Repeating and clarifying directions as needed to facilitate cognitive processing.
- Positioning ACS cards in the right visual field to enable Mrs. Wheeler to attend to the testing materials.
- Use of the enlarged version of the COPM rating cards that were also placed in the right visual field.

Information from the FIB allowed the occupational therapist to gain more accurate evaluation results and get a clear understanding of Mrs. Wheelers capacity and limitations and how they will be considered in her client-centered plan. It will also give the OT information to share with Mrs. Wheeler's daughter, particularly how the impairments impact on her mothers occupational performance and how they must be managed in strategies to foster her mother's participation and help her in assuming or managing the caregiving process. Some impairments were found that must be reported to the referring physician for further management.

For the school-aged child, information regarding performance component impairments is most likely to come from psychologists, educators, and speech-language pathologists who are members of the educational team in schools. When occupational therapists familiarize themselves with assessments used by other team members, they can derive substantial information about performance strengths and concerns before conducting any assessments of their own. The following measures should provide valuable information for the occupational therapist to understand the child's capacity and limitations that might affect occupational performance.

The Kaufman Assessment Battery for Children (KABC) (Kaufman & Kaufman, 1983) is a nationally standardized intelligence test. It was designed to yield useful information about children's factual knowledge and their ability to solve unfamiliar problems. There are three scales on the KABC: the sequential processing scale and the simultaneous processing scale, which make up the mental processing component of the test, and the achievement scale, which assesses factual knowledge and skills (i.e., reading, vocabulary, arithmetic). The sequential processing scale evaluates serial and temporal order problem-solving, while the simultaneous processing scale evaluates gestalt and spatial problem-solving.

The KABC items can provide occupational therapists with information about visual and auditory processing, kinesthesia, visual-motor integration, attention span, memory, sequencing, categorization, concept formation, problem-solving, generalization of learning and self-control. In general, poor performance on the sequential subtests indicates difficulty with cognitive and organizational components, while poor performance on the simultaneous subtests indicates difficulty with perceptual skills (Dunn, 1994). If your team uses the KABC, take time to meet with your colleague who administers this test to identify how these performance components manifest themselves in the KABC subtests.

The Wechsler Intelligence Scales (Wechsler, 1991) are the most widely used intelligence scales with children. There is a version for young children and one for school-aged children; they both yield a verbal scale, a performance scale, and a full scale intelligence score. The verbal scale subtests and items focus on language and auditory processing, while the performance scale subtests and items focus on visual perceptual and motor processing (Dunn, 1994).

As with the KABC, the pattern of scores on the Wechsler scales can indicate performance component strengths and concerns for therapists who are familiar with the performance requirements on each subtest. Sattler (1992) provides an excellent reference if this is a routine test employed by your agency.

The Woodcock Johnson Psycho-Educational Battery (Woodcock & Johnson, 1977) is a nationally standardized comprehensive battery of tests that evaluates three constructs: cognitive ability, achievement, and interest. The cognitive section is similar to other tests of intelligence described previously, and the achievement section tests the content areas found in a typical school curriculum. Evaluators don't always give the interest section, which probes the person's academic and non-academic preferences. The Woodcock Johnson Psycho-Educational Battery has achievement and cognition sections, which are useful for diagnostic processes that require differential performance between the person's capacity and his or her performance in specific areas (e.g., the diagnosis of a learning disability). It also provides similar information regarding performance components as found in the KABC and the Wechsler Intelligence Scales.

There are a number of language assessments used with children; consult your colleagues in speech-language pathology to identify the specific measures and their characteristics. Because language is a cognitive and psychosocial function, we can derive information about many of the cognitive and psychosocial performance components within the domain of concern of occupational therapy from these test data. Most of them will provide information about auditory processing, oral motor control and praxis, attention span, memory, sequencing, categorization, concept formation, problem-solving, generalization of learning, social conduct, self-expression, and self-control.

There are a number of formal assessments available to occupational therapists to measure performance component function in children. Many of the tests that occupational therapists use measure sensorimotor performance components (e.g., BOTMP [Bruininks, 1978], Developmental Test of Visual Motor Integration [Hammill, 1996], Motor Free Test of Visual Perception [Colarusso & Hammill, 1996], and Sensory Integration and Praxis Tests [Ayres, 1989]). The Buros Mental Measurement Yearbook (Impara & Plake, 1998) is a good resource for reviewing the features of these and other assessments. We should not forget that children also have visual acuity problems, auditory limitations, depression, and, depending on their age, problems with literacy. Any of these impairments will interfere with occupational performance and should be addressed in the planning phase of services.

THE IMPACT OF SENSORY PROCESSING ON PERFORMANCE

The way in which a person responds to sensory information in daily life can have a substantial effect on occupational performance. Assessment of sensory processing enables the occupational therapist to include consideration of these effects in intervention planning. Dunn and colleagues have developed a comprehensive research program investigating sensory processing Dunn, 1994, 1997, 1999, 2000). We have included information on the three sensory profiles in this chapter so that occupational therapists can use these assessments in their practice (Tables 4-2 through 4-4). Although the importance of sensory processing is introduced in the pediatric section of this chapter the Adult Sensory Profile is a very valuable tool to use with adults to understand the role that sensory processing plays in the occupational performance and occupational choices of people across the life span.

SUMMARY

Although we have focused on school-aged children and older adults, all individuals served by occupational therapy may have impairments that could limit their occupational performance. To focus on occupational performance, the practitioner needs to help individuals eliminate barriers that limit the achievement of their goals. It seems so simple to provide a new prescription for their glasses, brighter lights for reading, a volume speaker on the phone, or a medical intervention for depression. The only problem is that health professionals may not have recognized the impairment. If the practitioner can recognize the impairments that are limiting the person's occupational performance, strategies can be used to remove barriers that create excess disabilities.

Occupational therapists need to join with colleagues to assist in building healthier communities. This includes helping the family to foster an environment to support independence and decrease the costs of secondary conditions. If we can remove or minimize barriers that limit a persons' capacity to do that which he or she feels is important, we will help him or her achieve their goals, and his or her occupational performance will be maximized.

REFERENCES

Ainlay, S. C. (1988). Aging and new vision loss—Disruptions of the here and now. *Journal of Social Issues, 44(1)*, 70-94.

Alden, D., Austin, C., & Sturgeon, R. (1989). A correlation between the geriatric depression scale long and short forms. *Journal of Gerontology, 44*,124-125.

Alexopoulos, G. S., Vrontou, C., Kakuma, T., Meyers, B. S., Young, R. C., Klausner, E., et al. (1996). Disability in geriatric depression. *American Journal of Psychiatry, 153*, 877-885.

Austin, M. P., Mitchell, P., Wilhelm, K., et al. (1999). Cognitive function in depression: A distinct pattern of frontal impairment in melancholia? *Psychological Medicine, 29(1)*,73-85.

Ayres, A. J. (1980). *Sensory integration and praxis tests.* Los Angeles: Western Psychological Services.

Ayres, A.J. (1989). *Sensory integration and praxis tests.* Los Angeles: Western Psychological Services.

Beery, K. E. (1997). *Developmental test of visual motor integration.* NJ: Modern Curriculum Press.

Bess, F. H., Lichtenstein, M. J., Logan, S. A., Burger, M. C., & Nelson, E. (1989). Hearing impairment as a determinant of function in the elderly. *Journal of American Geriatric Society, 37*, 123-128.

Bonder, B. R., & Goodman, G. (1995). Preventing occupational dysfunction secondary to aging. In C. L. Trombly (Ed.), *Occupational Therapy for Physical Dysfunction* (4th ed., pp. 391-404). Baltimore: Williams & Wilkins.

Branch, L. G., Horowitz, A., & Carr, C. (1989). The implications for every day life of resident self-reported visual decline among people over age 65 living in the community. *The Gerontologist, 29(3)*, 359-365.

Brown, C., Cromwell, R., Filion, D., Dunn, W., & Tollefson, N. (In revision). Sensory processing in schizophrenia: Missing and avoiding information.

Brown, C. & Dunn, W. (1999). *The adult sensory profile.* Kansas City, Ka: Department of Occupational Therapy Education, University of Kansas Medical Center.

Brown, C., Tollefson, N., Dunn, W., Cromwell, R., & Filion, D. (In press). The Adult Sensory Profile: Measuring patterns of sensory processing. *American Journal of Occupational Therapy.*

Bruininks, R. H. (1978). *Bruininks-Oseretsky test of motor proficiency.* MN: American Guidance Service.

Colarusso, R. P., & Hammill, D. D. (1996). *The motor-free test of visual perception.* Novato, CA: Academic Therapy Publications.

Dargent-Molina, P., Hays, M., & Breart, G. (1996). Sensory impairments and physical disability in aged women living at home. *International Journal of Epidemiology, 25*, 621-629.

Davis, T. C., Long, S. W., Jackson, R. H., et al. do you need the rest of the authors? (1993). Rapid estimate of adult literacy in medicine: A shortened screening instrument. *Family Medicine, 25*, 391-395.

Dublin, S. (1992). The physiologic changes of aging. *Orthopedic Nursing, 11*, 45-50.

Duchek, J. (1991). Cognitive dimensions of performance. In C. Christiansen & C. M. Baum (Eds.), *Occupational therapy: Overcoming human performance deficits* (pp. 283-303).Thorofare, NJ: SLACK Incorporated.

Duchek, J. M., & Abreu, B. C. (1997). Meeting the challenges of cognitive disabilities. In C. Christiansen & C. Baum (Eds.), *Occupational therapy: Enabling function and well-being.* (2nd ed.). Thorofare, NJ: SLACK Incorporated.

Dunn, W. (1994). Tests used by other professionals. In W. Dunn (Ed.), *Pediatric occupational therapy.* Thorofare, NJ: SLACK Incorporated.

Dunn, W. (1997). The impact of sensory processing abilities on the daily lives of young children and their families: A conceptual model. *Infants and Young Children, 9(4)*, 23-35.

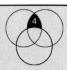

Table 4-2

SENSORY PROFILE

Source	The Psychological Corporation, Therapy Skill Builders, 555 Academic Court, San Antonio, TX, 78204-2498; (phone) 1-800-211-8378
Important References	Dunn, W. (1997). The impact of sensory processing abilities on the daily lives of young children and their families: A conceptual model. *Infants and Young Children, 9(4)*, 23-35.
	Dunn, W. (1999). *Sensory Profile user's manual*. San Antonio, TX: The Psychological Corp.
	Dunn, W., & Brown, C. (1997). Factor analysis on the Sensory Profile from a national sample of children without disabilities. *American Journal of Occupational Therapy, 51(7)*, 490-495.
	Dunn, W., & Westman, K. (1997). The Sensory Profile: The performance of a national sample of children without disabilities. *American Journal of Occupational Therapy, 51(1)*, 25-34.
	Ermer, J., & Dunn, W. (1998). The Sensory Profile: A discriminant analysis of children with and without disabilities. *American Journal of Occupational Therapy, 52(4)*, 283-290.
Purpose	• The Sensory Profile was developed to measure children's responses to sensory events in daily life.
Type of Client	• The Sensory Profile is appropriate for all children ages 3 to 10 years (an infant toddler version) and an adult version are in development). There have been studies on children without disabilities and children with autism, ADHD, Fragile X, tic disorders, and sensory modulation disorders.
Clinical Utility	
Format	• The Sensory Profile consists of 125 items organized into three sections: sensory processing, modulation, and behavior and emotional responses. The subsections are as follows:
	Sensory Processing: Auditory processing, visual processing, vestibular processing, touch processing, multisensory processing, and oral sensory processing.
	Modulation: Sensory processing related to endurance/tone, modulation related to body position/movement, modulation of movement affecting activity level, and modulation of sensory input affecting emotional responses.
	Behavior and Emotional Responses: Emotional/social responses, behavior outcomes of sensory processing, and items indicating thresholds for responses.
Procedures	• Caregivers report the frequency their child engages in each behavior (n=125) using a 5-point Likert scale. Examiners calculate a score for each of the 14 sections (see above) and for nine factors (see Dunn & Brown, 1997) indicating the child's level of responsivity to sensory input. Examiners then plot total raw scores to determine the child's performance as "typical," "probable difference," and "definite difference"; these score categorizations are based on a national sample of children without disabilities (see below).
Completion Time	• It takes 15 to 20 minutes for the caregiver to complete the Sensory Profile, and 30 minutes for the examiner to score the Sensory Profile.
Standardization	• The test manual (Dunn, 1999) provides information on all the samples used in the studies to date. Dunn & Westman (1997) reported on a national sample of 1115 children without disabilities who were 3 to 10 years old. This sample was used to identify patterns of typical performance and as a comparison group for children with various disabilities.

continued

Table 4-2 (continued)

SENSORY PROFILE

Reliability

Internal Consistency
- The researchers calculated the coefficient α (i.e., Cronbach's) for each section to analyze relationships (i.e., item-to-item, item-to-category, and item-to-factor correlation). The item-to-category (i.e., each item to its own group) correlation ranged from 0.47 to 0.91. The coefficients for other relationships (e.g., items to other categories) are lower than these ranges, suggesting that the items in the current categories are related to each other. These relationships need to be investigated further.

Inter-Rater
- Caregivers complete the Sensory Profile. The only instructions they are given come at the beginning of the caregiver questionnaire and outline how to mark each item. It is interesting to note that caregivers of children with a particular disability report characteristic patterns of performance for that group that are different from other groups of caregivers who have children with other disabilities.

Intra-Rater
- Not reported.

Test-Retest
- Not reported.

Validity

Content
- The authors report three methods for establishing content validity. First, the author and others conducted a literature review to compile items about sensory processing (Ayres, 1980). Second, they conducted an expert review by having 8 therapists experienced in applying sensory integration theory to practice review the items and make recommendations. These therapists also conducted the first pilot study of the Sensory Profile (Dunn, 1994) to determine whether children without disabilities displayed these behaviors. Third, the author conducted a category analysis to determine the way that experienced therapists (n=155) would categorize Sensory Profile items. These data provided the organizational structure for the current Sensory Profile.

Criterion
- The author demonstrated convergent and discriminant validity in a correlation study between the School Function Assessment (SFA) and the Sensory Profile. Researchers calculated correlations between the sections of the SFA (i.e., accommodation items, n=21; assistance items, n=21; and performance groupings, n=21) and the Sensory Profile sections (n=14) and factor scores (n=9). In this sample of 16 children, some clear patterns emerged. As expected, there were many significant correlations between the Sensory Profile's Factor 9 (fine motor/perceptual) and the three sections of the SFA (n=18 with assistance items, n=12 with accommodation items, n=5 with performance groupings). Factor 9 contains items that describe product-oriented behaviors (e.g., writing is illegible, has trouble staying between the lines when writing, has difficulty putting puzzles together). Although this is certainly validation that the SFA items are tapping work product, this is not particularly informative about the relationship between sensory processing and performance at school. However, other patterns are informative about the sensory features of performance at school. Although some might have hypothesized that school tasks with a more "sensorimotor performance" emphasis would be correlated with the Sensory Profile, this did not occur. The most notable relationships that emerged were those between the behavior regulation and positive interaction sections of the SFA and the sections and factors on the Sensory Profile.

Construct
- The author tested construct validity on the Sensory Profile by administering it and the Children's Autism Rating Scale (CARS) (Kientz & Dunn, 1997) to children with autism. The CARS is a checklist that aids in the diagnosis of autism; it has sections that address the key features of this disorder (e.g., social interaction, communication), including sensory processing (e.g., auditory processing). The Sensory Profile correlated with sections of the CARS that tap sensory responsiveness and processing, lending support to the idea that the Sensory Profile taps the construct of sensory processing

continued

Table 4-2 (continued)

SENSORY PROFILE

Clinical	• The author also reports on clinical validity (i.e., the utility of the measure in assessment/practice). The author and others tested groups of children with and without disabilities to determine whether the Sensory Profile could delineate among the groups based on the children's responses to sensory events in daily life. The author and others tested children with autism, ADHD, Fragile X, Asperger's syndrome, tic disorders, and sensory modulation disorders and found unique patterns in scores for each group.
	• The author and others (Ermer & Dunn, 1997) conducted a discriminant analysis to determine the Sensory Profile's ability to categorize children by their diagnosis. In the study, the authors used the ADHD group, the autism group, and the group of children without disabilities. The Sensory Profile was able to discriminate these groups with 89% accuracy.
Strengths	• Includes caregivers in the measurement/assessment process.
	• Links sensory processing with daily life.
	• Based on a theoretical model.
	• Research used in development and refinement.
	• Scores provide guidance for intervention planning.
	• Research findings are promising for discriminating groups and performance patterns.
Weaknesses	• Examiner must understand theoretical model to interpret results effectively.
	• Scoring may seem complicated until examiner is familiar with it.
	• Requires other data to derive meaning for performance needs.
	• Needs more construct validity research.

Dunn, W. (1999). *Sensory profile user's manual.* San Antonio, TX: The Psychological Corp.

Dunn, W. (2000). *Clinical edition of the infant toddler sensory profile.* San Antonio, TX: The Psychological Corp.

Dunn, W. (2002). *The infant toddler sensory profile.* San Antonio, TX: Psychological Corporation.

Dunn, W., & Brown, C. (1997). Factor analysis on the Sensory Profile from a national sample of children without disabilities. *American Journal of Occupational Therapy, 51(7),* 490-495.

Dunn, W. and D. Daniels (2001). Initial development of the Infant Toddler Sensory Profile. *Journal of Early Intervention, 25(1),* 27-41.

Dunn, W., & Westman, K. (1997). The Sensory Profile: The performance of a national sample of children without disabilities. *American Journal of Occupational Therapy, 51(1),* 25-34.

Enderby, P. M., Wood, V. A., Wade, D. T., & Hewer, R. L. (1987). The Frenchay aphasia screening test: A short, simple test for aphasia appropriate for non-specialists. *International Rehabilitation Medicine,* 166-170.

Ermer, J., & Dunn, W. (1997). The Sensory Profile: A discriminant analysis of children with and without disabilities. *American Journal of Occupational Therapy, 52(4),* 283-290.

Fisher, A. G. (1998). Uniting practice and theory in occupational framework. 1998 Eleanor Clarke Slagle Lecture. *American Journal of Occupational Therapy, 52,* 509-521.

Ferris, FL, Kassoff, A, Bresnick, GH & Bailey, I (1982). New visual acuity charts for clinical research. *American Journal of Ophthalmology, 94,* 91-96.

Halligan, P., & Marshall, J. (1994). Current issues in spatial neglect: An editorial introduction. *Neuropsychological Rehabilitation, 4(2),* 103-110.

Hammill, D. (1996). *Test of Visual-Motor Integration.* Austin, TX: Pro-Ed.

Hayflick, L. (1998). How and why we age. *Experimental Gerontology. 33(7-8),* 639-653.

Hussey, L., & Gilliard, K. (1989). Compliance, low literacy, and locus of control. *Nursing Clinics of North America,* 24(3), 605-611.

Impara, J. C., & Plake, B. S. (1998). *The thirteenth mental measurements yearbook.* Lincoln, NE: Buros Institute of Mental Measurements.

Katzman, R., Brown, T., Fuld, P., Peck, A., Schechter, R., & Schimmel, H. (1983). Validation of a short orientation-memory-concentration test of cognitive impairment. *American Journal of Psychiatry, 140,* 734-739.

Kaufman, A., & Kaufman, N. (1983). K-ABC: *Kaufman assessment battery for children.* Circle Pines, MN: American Guidance Service.

Kirshner, H. S., & Bakar, M. (1995). Syndromes of language dissolution in aging and dementia. *Comprehensive Therapy, 21,* 519-523.

Table 4-3

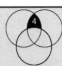

ADULT SENSORY PROFILE

Source	Brown, C., & Dunn, W. (1999). Department of Occupational Therapy Education, 3033 Robinson, University of Kansas Medical Center, 3901 Rainbow Boulevard, Kansas City, KS, 66160-7602.
Important References	Brown, C., Tollefson, N., et al. (2001). The Adult Sensory Profile: Measuring patterns of sensory processing. *American Journal of Occupational Therapy, 55*, 75-82.
	Brown, T., Cromwell, R., et al. (2002). Sensory processing in schizophrenia: Missing and avoiding information. *Schizophrenia Research, 55(1-2)*, 187-195.
Purpose	• The Adult Sensory Profile was developed to measure adult's responses to sensory events in daily life.
Type of Client	• Appropriate for all adults.
Clinical Utility	
Format	• The Adult Sensory Profile consists of 60 items organized into six sections: taste/smell, movement, visual, touch, activity level, and auditory. The examiner can calculate scores based on responsivity as well (i.e., sensory seeking, sensory avoiding, low registration, and high responding [sensitivity]).
Procedures	• The individual completes the form by reporting the frequency he or she engages in each behavior (n=60) using a 5-point Likert scale. Examiners calculate a score for four quadrants, based on the theoretical model developed by Dunn (1997), which indicates the individual's level of responsivity to sensory input. There are four sub-scales for scoring: sensation seeking, sensation avoiding, poor registration, and sensitivity to stimuli.
Completion Time	• It takes 10 to 15 minutes for the individual to complete the Adult Sensory Profile, and 5 to 10 minutes for the examiner to score.
Standardization	• Brown and Dunn (1999) report on a factor analysis with 615 adults ranging from 17 to 79 years: 38.8% of the sample were males, and 61.2% of the sample were females. This sample was used to identify patterns of typical performance.
Reliability	
Internal Consistency	• The researchers calculated the coefficient alpha (i.e., Cronbach's) for each of the four sub-scales to analyze relationships (i.e., item-to-item, item-to-category, and item-to-factor correlation). The item-to-category (i.e., each item to its own group) correlations were as follows: sensory sensitivity, 0.81; sensation avoiding, 0.66; poor registration, 0.82; and sensation seeking, 0.79. The other relationships (e.g., items to other categories) are lower than these ranges, suggesting that the items in the current categories are related to each other.
Intra-Rater	• Not reported.
Inter-Rater	• Individuals complete the Adult Sensory Profile on themselves. The only instructions they are given come at the beginning of the questionnaire, which outline how to mark each item.
Test-Retest	• Not reported.
Validity	
Content	• The authors report the following methods for establishing content validity. First, the authors used the work on the child version of the Sensory Profile to develop items for adults. Second, they conducted an expert review by having eight peers sort the items by the quadrants; these reviewers sorted all but one of the items correctly.

continued

Table 4-3 (continued)

ADULT SENSORY PROFILE

Construct

- Brown and Dunn (1999) tested construct validity on the Adult Sensory Profile by administration and skin conductance measures. In one study, they compared four groups of young adults who had the highest scores on the four quadrants. Results indicated a clear pattern of skin conductance performance for each group, supporting Dunn's model of sensory processing (Dunn, 1997). In another study, Brown and Dunn (1999) compared mentally healthy adults with adults who had schizophrenia and adults who had bipolar disorder. She reported differences among the groups and the presence of skin conductance patterns that can be associated with the four quadrants in Dunn's model.

Strengths

- Includes individual in the measurement/assessment process.
- Links sensory processing with daily life.
- Based on a theoretical model.
- Research used in development and refinement.
- Scores provide guidance for intervention planning.
- Research findings are promising for discriminating groups and performance patterns.

Weaknesses

- Examiner must understand theoretical model to interpret results effectively.
- Scoring is not yet developed for easy interpretation.
- Requires other data to derive meaning for performance needs.
- Needs more research.

Knesevich, J., LaBarge, E., & Edwards, D. (1986). Predictive value of the Boston Naming Test in mild senile dementia of the Alzheimer type. *Psychiatry Research, 14*, 255-263.

Lin, K. (1996). Right-hemispheric activation approaches to neglect rehabilitation poststroke. *American Journal of Occupational Therapy, 50(7)*, 504-515.

Mack, W. J., Freed, D. M., Williams, B. W., & Henderson, V. W. (1992). Boston Naming Test: Shortened versions for use in Alzheimer's disease. *Journal of Gerontology: Psychological Sciences, 47*, 154-158.

Meade, C., & Thornhill, D. (1989). Illiteracy in healthcare. *Nursing Management, 20(10)*, 14-15.

Morris, J. C., Heyman, A., Mohs, R. C., et al. (1989). The consortium to establish a registry for Alzheimer's disease (CERAD). Part I. Clinical and neuropsychological assessment of Alzheimer's disease. *Neurology, 39*, 1159-1165.

Mulrow, C. C., Aguilar, C., Endicott, J., et al. (1990). Association between hearing impairment and the quality of life of elderly individuals. *Journal of American Geriatric Society, 38(1)*, 45-50.

Mynatt, E. D, Essa, I., & Rogers, W. (2000). Increasing the opportunities for aging in place. In *Proceedings of the ACM Conference on Universal Usability (CUU 2000; Washington D.C.)*. New York: ACM Press, 65-71.

Parker, R., Baker, D., Williams, M., & Nurss, J. (1995). The test of functional health literacy in adults: A new instrument for measuring patients' literacy skills. *Journal of General Internal Medicine, 10*, 537-541.

Perlmutter, M. (1998). The development of the Functional Impairment Battery. Paper presented at the meeting of the World Federation of Occupational Therapy, Montreal, Canada.

Baum, MC, Perlmutter, M & Edwards, D (Summer, 2000). Measuring function in Alzheimer's Disease. *Alzheimer's Quarterly*, 44-61.

Popelka, G. R. (1997). High and low pitched sounds: A screening tool. Unpublished manuscript.

Rigg, P., & Kazemek, F. (1983). Literacy and elders: What we know and what we need to know. *Educational Gerontology, 9*, 417-424.

Rubin, G. S., Bandeen-Roche, K., Prasada-Rao, P., Fried, L., & SEE Project Team. (1994). Visual impairment and disability in older adults. *Optometry and Visual Science, 71*, 750-760.

Sattler, J. M. (1992). *Assessment of children*. San Diego: Jerome M. Sattler Inc.

Van Gorp, W., Satz, P., Kiersch, & Henry, R. (1986). Normative data on the Boston Naming Test for a group of normal older adults. *Journal of Clinical and Experimental Neuropsychology, 8*, 702-705.

Wechsler, D. (1991). *The Wechsler intelligence scale* (3rd ed.) (WISC-III). San Antonio, TX: The Psychological Corp.

Wilcock, A. (1993). A theory of the human need for occupation. *Occupational Science: Australia, 1(1)*, 17-24.

Williams, B. W., Mack, W., & Henderson, V. W. (1989). Boston Naming Test in Alzheimer's disease. *Neuropsychologia, 27(8)*, 1073-1079.

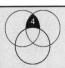

Table 4-4

INFANT TODDLER SENSORY PROFILE

Source
The Psychological Corporation, Therapy Skill Builders, 555 Academic Court, San Antonio, TX, 78204-2498; (phone) 800-211-8378

Important References
Dunn, W. (1997). The impact of sensory processing abilities on the daily lives of young children and their families: A conceptual model. *Infants and Young Children, 9(4)*, 23-35.

Dunn, W., & Daniels, D. (2001). Initial development of the Infant Toddler Sensory Profile. *Journal of Early Intervention, 25(1)*, 27-41.

Dunn, W. (2002). *The Infant Toddler Sensory Profile*. San Antonio, TX: Psychological Corporation.

Purpose
- The Infant Toddler Sensory Profile was developed to measure infant and toddler responses to sensory events in daily life.

Type of Client
- Children from birth to 3 years.

Clinical Utility

Format
- The Infant Toddler Sensory Profile consists of 36 items for infants birth to 6 months of age and 48 items for children 7 months to 3 years of age. The questionnaire is divided into six sections: general processing, auditory processing, visual processing, vestibular processing and oral sensory processing. In addition to these scores, examiners can calculate quadrant scores, which are 4 types of sensory processing based on Dunn's model of sensory processing. Cut scores are based on data from 589 infants and toddlers without disabilities.
- There is a Spanish version as well.

Procedures
- Caregivers report the frequency their child engages in each behavior using a 5-point Likert scale.

Completion Time
- It takes 15 to 20 minutes for the caregiver to complete.

Standardization
- Researchers studied 589 children without disabilities who ranged in age from birth to 36 months. The standardization sample represents children from across the country, includes ethnic groups, families of various incomes and from various sized communities. In a study of children in Spanish speaking homes, the score patterns were comparable to the national sample, suggesting that this test can be used with this sample as well. Cut scores represent 1.0 SD (probable difference scores) and 2.0 SD (definitely difference scores), and identify whether the child's sensory processing is the same as or different from peers.
- Researchers have also studied children with various disabilities, and shown that children in disability groups have different sensory processing patterns than peers without disabilities.

Reliability
- Researchers established test-retest reliability and calculated internal consistency for the Infant Toddler Sensory Profile.

Internal Consistency
- The Alpha coefficient values for the quadrant scores on the Infant Toddler Sensory Profile range from 0.42 to 0.86 for the children 7 to 36 months. For the infants birth to 6 months of age, the alpha coefficients ranged from 0.17 to 0.83.

Test-Retest Reliability
- Researchers tested 32 children 2 to 3 weeks apart, and obtained 0.86 reliability for the sensory processing section scores, and 0.74 for the quadrant scores.

Validity
- Researchers established content, convergent and discriminant validity on the Infant Toddler Sensory Profile.

continued

Table 4-4 (continued)

INFANT TODDLER SENSORY PROFILE

Content	• The authors used the work in the Sensory Profile to design the the Infant Toddler Sensory Profile. They have adapted items to more accurately reflect the activities of younger children and have used experts to provide feedback and evidence about the integrity of the items to reflect Dunn's model of sensory processing (Dunn, 1997).
Convergent and Discriminant	• Researchers conducted an evaluation of the Infant Toddler Sensory Profile and the Infant Toddler Symptom Checklist. They found that some items on the two measures were highly correlated with each other (i.e., convergent validity) and other items were not correlated with each other (i.e., discriminant validity).
Strengths	• Includes caregivers in the measurement/assessment process.
• Links sensory processing with daily life.
• Based on a theoretical model.
• Research is being used in development and refinement.
• Scores provide guidance for intervention planning.
Weaknesses	• Examiner must understand theoretical model to interpret results effectively.
• Requires other data to derive meaning for performance needs.
• Research needs to be completed.

Wilson, B., Cockburn, J., & Halligan, P. (1987). *Behavioural Inattention Test* (pp. 11, 14). London, England: Thames Valley Test Co.

Woodcock, R. W., & Johnson, M. B. (1977). *The Woodcock-Johnson Psychoeducational Battery*. Austin, TX: Pro-Ed.

Yesavage, J. A., Brink, T. L., Rose, T. L., et al. (1982-83). Development and validation of a geriatric depression screening scale: A preliminary report. *Journal of Psychiatric Research, 17(1),* 37-49.

Zoltan, B. (1996). *Vision, perception, and cognition* (3rd ed.). Thorofare, NJ: SLACK Incorporated.

Editors' Notes for Chapter 5

Mine the Gold

Qualitative assessment methods have been developed by social science disciplines to facilitate the exploration of persons' lived experience. Occupational therapists use these approaches to explore the meaningfulness of occupation in everyday life.

Become Systematic

The use of qualitative methods enables therapists to dependably identify important themes in their clinical observations and in the occupational stories told to them by clients and the clients' families.

Use Evidence in Practice

Gathering and using knowledge about how each person finds meaning through occupation enables the client to identify therapy goals and facilitates active participation in the therapy process.

Make Occupational Therapy Contribution Explicit

By systematically exploring the experiential aspects of occupation, occupational therapists contribute to knowledge about persons' day-to-day lives and how engagement in occupation leads to health and well-being.

Engage in Occupation-Based, Client-Centered Practice

The use of narrative and observational methods assist therapists in ensuring a focus on occupations that are meaningful to clients.

USING QUALITATIVE MEASUREMENT METHODS TO UNDERSTAND OCCUPATIONAL PERFORMANCE

Mary Corcoran, PhD, OTR(L), FAOTA

INTRODUCTION

Occupational therapists continue to feel the effects of increasingly greater demands from organizations, payers and decision makers for clinical outcomes to justify occupational therapy intervention. The costs of health care in the United States and many other countries are spiraling upward at an unprecedented pace. At the same time, access to information and demographic changes has resulted in better informed clients who expect individualized outcomes that return them to meaningful roles. This has proven to be a source of tension for the occupational therapy profession. On one hand, reimbursable parameters for clinical outcomes often remain narrowly focused on self-care and mobility components of performance; but on the other hand, the profession and many consumers are beginning to understand the power of occupation-based practice.

As a profession, occupational therapy has no option but to focus on convincing payers and the public at large about the value of occupation. Until that time, the strategies used by therapists to imbue the therapeutic process with meaning and relevance, such as collaborating with clients, will be regarded as untested and less important. Unfortunately, the temptation exists to minimize the focus of occupational therapy to those variables that *can* be measured, instead of what *should* be measured. Further, many occupational therapists have learned to simply not document the strategies used to create a client-centered experience. The result is missed opportunities to illustrate the complexity and depth of human occupation and its impact on health, document the importance of therapeutic goals that fall outside the areas of self-care and mobility, and enrich our understanding of occupation-based therapy.

Occupation-based therapy absolutely depends on an accurate understanding of the client's occupational profile and performance. Although many therapists strive to obtain this information for every client, two nagging questions persist. How do we know that the right questions are being asked, and how do we ensure that we have conducted and interpreted our observations and interviews accurately? This measurement dilemma is compounded by the fact that often there are few rating scales or tests that quickly and accurately assess many of our concepts of interest. When measurement tools do exist they may be lengthy to administer, making them impractical in a busy practice setting. In addition, many concepts that are central to occupation, such as habits, role balance, and meaning, are difficult to measure without a precise definition that clearly distinguishes each concept from similar concepts. To make matters worse, even defining the specific aspects of the occupational therapy process (or what we do as therapists) can be challenging, as evidenced by the many permutations of a practice framework in the United States over the past two decades. How can we measure occupational performance, therapeutic processes, and intervention outcomes that reflect our rich traditions in the absence of operational definitions?

Qualitative research designs and data analysis methods are a natural choice when clinical questions include concepts that are not well-defined and, are therefore difficult to measure. These methods also fit well into a busy practice setting. In fact, occupational therapists are already widely using two data collection methods that are central to qualitative research: observation and interviews. The problem with use of qualitative methods to assess occupation is that techniques to assure rigorous use are not well understood by many health care providers. Without understanding how to conduct interviews and observations to assure trustworthiness, the therapist runs the risk of missing important information or being criticized for using an unscientific approach to assessment. Therefore, the purpose of this chapter is to help therapists refine and expand their use of qualitative methods to systematically assess occupational performance, validate practice, and build new knowledge. To this end, material will be presented to:

- Define qualitative methods.
- Discuss the application of qualitative methods to practice.
- Describe the process for analyzing narrative data.
- Introduce the use of mixed methods (integrating qualitative and quantitative data) in occupational therapy.

This chapter is not meant to be a substitute for texts on therapist-client interaction, in-depth interviewing, or qualitative research methods. In fact, those seeking an exhaustive presentation of qualitative research or any of its attributes should look elsewhere. Rather, the chapter provides selected introductory material about the nature of qualitative research and adding rigor to the use of observation and interview techniques during the occupational therapy process. This information is offered as a way of reliably gaining insight about a client's occupational profile and supporting occupation-based practice.

WHY USE A QUALITATIVE APPROACH TO UNDERSTAND OCCUPATION?

We have been fortunate in our profession to count among our members a number of highly skilled qualitative researchers. These researchers, such as Elizabeth Yerxa and Betty Hasselkus, not only add to the body of literature but also issue a call to action for the use of qualitative methods as *a relevant, ethical, and realistic way of knowing...*" (Yerxa, 1991, pg. 199). Many in the occupational therapy and occupational science literature have turned to qualitative methods as the natural choice for understanding occupation.

What are the characteristics of occupation that lend themselves to study from a qualitative perspective (Cook, 2001)?

1. Occupation is complex and nuanced.
2. Occupations are processes in that they are the means to an end (activity) and involve active doing.

3. Occupations are meaningful and therefore can only be understood from the participant's perspective. Similarly, occupations are an individual experience at a particular time. Although the individual may be engaging in an occupation within a group of individuals who are all doing exactly the same thing, the experiences of each are unique.

4. Occupations are dynamic, changing, and developing over time even, in subtle ways, from day to day.

5. Occupations are formed by cultural backgrounds; they are shaped by personal interests, desires, and values.

6. Occupations are highly influenced by environment, including physical, social, spiritual, cultural, personal, temporal, and virtual environmental contexts.

Thus we have an ethical and scientific responsibility to study occupation using methods that preserve the specific environmental context, clarify meaning and complexity, and reflect a basis in cultural beliefs and values. Occupational therapy researchers have responded to that responsibility with a variety of designs to study, including use of life history by Frank (1984), grounded theory by Hasselkus (1987), single-case research by Price-Lackey & Cashman (1996), and ethnography by Clark (1993), Jonsson, Keilhofner, and Brell (1997), and Frank, Bernardo, Tropper, Noguchi, Lipman, Maulhardt, et al., (1997). In fact, occupational therapy is a profession with a rich heritage of qualitative study. A prominent example is Florence Clark's Eleanor Clarke Slagle lecture (1993) in which she offered a narrative analysis of Penny Richardson, an active, intelligent woman who struggles to regain occupational health after a stroke. Clark's purpose in her lecture was to offer a unique design for scientific inquiry in occupational science, a design based in the ethnographic tradition. In doing so, she drew on a substantial history of research within and outside the field of occupational therapy that seeks the meaning of occupation in the "...deep richness of mundane affairs" (Kielhofner, 1982, p. 162).

In order to gain this insight into the meanings associated with occupation, the tradition of qualitative (or naturalistic) research must be understood. In particular, what is a naturalistic tradition, how is it different from an experimental tradition, and what strategies are used to increase our ability to trust the results (trustworthiness)?

NATURALISTIC RESEARCH TRADITION

A naturalistic research tradition seeks to gain an in-depth and complex understanding of some poorly understood phenomena within a particular group. This understanding cannot be generalized beyond the individuals who participated in the study but does offer rich insight that *may* have compelling implications for a larger group.

Table 5-1		
COMPARISON OF NATURALISTIC AND EXPERIMENTAL TRADITIONS		
Characteristics	*Naturalistic*	*Experimental*
Type of reasoning	Inductive	Deductive
Epistemology	Holistic perspectives	Logical positivism
Purpose	Reveal complexity and meanings; Generate theory	Predict, explain, test theory
Research process	Spiral	Linear
Setting	Naturalistic	Controlled
Role of the investigator	Involved; subjective	Uninvolved; objective
Type of data	Pictures; text; observation	Numbers
Sources of accuracy	Strategies to assure trustworthiness	Validity and reliability
Use of writing	Analysis	Dissemination

Table 5-1 lists several ways that a naturalistic tradition is different from an experimental tradition.

While it is beyond the scope of this chapter to discuss all these differences, several of particular relevance are examined here.

Purpose: Complexity and Meaning vs Predicting and Explaining

The client's choices about activities, competence, environment, and every other aspect of occupation set the parameters for occupational therapy - therefore it is reasonable that an approach must be adopted that will clarify those expectations and desires. In her book entitled *Qualitative Research in Occupational Therapy* (2001), Dr. Joanne Cook provides a compelling connection between the values, beliefs, and language of occupational therapy and qualitative research. Cook asserts that understanding the complexities and nuances of occupation requires the in-depth and context-based approach of naturalistic inquiry. Occupational therapy and qualitative research are also congruent in terms of their very purpose, which is to *understand* feelings, attitudes, experiences, and behaviors, as opposed to *predicting* behaviors. Cook (2001, pg 7) quotes Maxwell (1996 regarding the purposes of research for which a qualitative approach is appropriate. The purposes of a qualitative approach are to:

- Understand the meaning for participants in the study of the events, situations, and actions they are involved with and of the accounts that they give of their lives and expectations.
- Understand the particular environmental context within which the participants act and the influence that this environment has on their actions.

- Identify unanticipated phenomena and influences and generate new grounded theories about the latter.
- Understand the process by which events and actions take place.

Thus, qualitative research methods are an appropriate choice for learning about the meanings of life events, from the participant's perspective, in such a way as to preserve the complexities and environmental context.

The Setting: Natural vs Controlled

Investigators using naturalistic designs study things in their natural settings, as opposed to an experimental tradition where a natural setting is not necessarily desirable. For example, if you were administering a highly standardized test to a group of children, you would want a controlled classroom setting with minimal distractions. If you test the child in his home, any unusual occurrence, such as a pet entering the room or a sibling playing with an attractive toy, can introduce confounding variables and change the outcome of the test.

In a naturalistic study, the natural setting is necessary because investigators want to describe social occurrences in order to make sense of them and the meanings people associate with them (Denzin & Lincoln, 1994). For example, to describe the experience of caring for a spouse with dementia at home, Corcoran interviewed caregiving husbands and wives to understand caregiving style (ways of thinking about and conducting care tasks) (Corcoran, 2003). These middle-class, Caucasian spouses were interviewed in their homes in order to understand care as it occurred everyday in that particular setting. The environment (both physical and social) was a vital part of understanding what and why caregivers made the decisions they did. For example, one woman who was caring for her husband talked about his inability to help her in the kitchen as he used to do. She was very upset about this change in her husband and talked about how fixing a meal together was meaningful to their relationship. Now that meaningful activity was gone and the woman was sure that this was a sign that her husband was one step closer to death. As she showed the interviewer around the kitchen, she pointed out her new mini-blinds which replaced the "ugly roll-up type of blind." The interviewer noticed the glare from this new window covering and made a notation about it. When the last research visit was completed just 2 weeks later, the interviewer suggested to the woman that she close the mini-blinds whenever she worked in the kitchen with her husband. This suggestion was based on the possibility that her husband was susceptible to the glare created by the mini blinds and unable to see well in the kitchen. Although the outcome of this suggestion is not known, one can be sure that without visiting the woman in her home, the suggestion may not have occurred to the interviewer. Interviewing in the home provided an opportunity to observe what was happening and rely less on being told what was happening.

Type of Data: Words vs Numbers

The potential sources of data are quite extensive, but how the data are managed once collected is different in a qualitative versus a quantitative study. The purpose of data management is to convert "raw" data into a form that lends itself to analysis. If the purpose of analysis is to predict or explain behavior (or other phenomena) the type of study is probably quantitative and data are reduced to numbers. However, if the purpose of the study is to understand more about the meanings associated with events (or other phenomena), the type of study is probably qualitative and data are reduced to words. The two examples that follow help to illustrate that difference.

An occupational therapist wants to know what differences exist in types of leisure activities of individuals with stroke in comparison to individuals with brain injury. He interviews a large number of clients and asks each to "Tell me about your leisure activities during the past month".

Example #1

In order to predict type of leisure activities based on diagnosis, the occupational therapist would use a quantitative design and analyze his data with statistical tests. Statistical tests require numbers, so the occupational therapist would need to assign numerical codes to the different types of leisure activities that emerged from the interviews. Let's say the occupational therapist assigns the following codes to the information he collected through interviews.

0 = No leisure activities are reported

1 = More than 50% of reported activities primarily involve playing sports

2 = More than 50% of reported activities primarily involve games or puzzles

3 = More than 50% of reported activities are primarily passive

4 = More than 50% of reported activities are primarily social

If the occupational therapist sorts the data in terms of diagnosis, the result of analysis would be a comparison of types of activities reported by individuals with stroke to leisure activities reported by individuals with brain injury.

Example #2

In order to understand the meanings associated with these leisure activities, the occupational therapist would sort the phrases (retained as words) into several categories. Let's say the occupational therapist hears the following types of information.

Activities that stretch my abilities:
- Sports
- Puzzles

Activities that help me relax:
- Visiting with friends and family
- Listening to music
- Reading the paper/book

Activities that are done for fun:
- Building model cars
- Playing games

Activities that pass the time:
- Watching television
- Surfing the internet

Again, keeping track and sorting by diagnosis, the result of analysis would indicate the meaning associated with leisure activities of individuals with stroke and individuals with brain injury. They are the same activities, but different questions yielded different outcomes.

See the difference? In example one, the data were reduced to numbers and the results answered the question of *what* was done for leisure. In example two, data were reduced to phrases and the results answered the question of *why* participants engaged in leisure activities. One approach is not better than the other; they are simply different questions.

Sources of Accuracy: Trustworthiness vs Validity and Reliability

The mix of observation and interview discussed in the caregiving style study (previously) actually increases the validity of the results because it provides a way to check on conclusions from two sources, what was seen and what was heard. This technique for increasing the validity of qualitative inferences is one type of *triangulation*. Triangulation is a method used by qualitative researcher to "...get a better fix on the subject matter at hand" (Denzin & Lincoln, 1994, p. 2). An interesting example of triangulation is found in historical analysis in which data are collected from archival materials, including letters, photographs, diaries, books, films, and manuscripts. Triangulation consists of a range of interconnected approaches, including many forms of observation and interview, which enable the researcher to view the phenomena from several angles. Interviews can involve anything from one-on-one conversations to group discussions, and formats range from completely open-ended to highly structured. Likewise, observations take many forms, ranging from photographs or field notes of naturally occurring social scenes to simulated interactions in role plays. If a therapist cannot travel to a client's home, there are any number of creative methods for understanding the physical attributes of the home, including floor plans, photographs, and videos.

What other principles of qualitative research, such as triangulation, exist and can potentially be applied to practice? Traditionally these include credibility, transferability, dependability, and confirmability. Each is defined below.

Credibility involves establishing that the results of the qualitative inquiry are credible or believable from the perspective of the participant in the research. Because the purpose of qualitative research is to describe or understand the phenomena of interest from the participant's eyes, the participants are the only ones who can legitimately judge the "correctness" of the results. One popular way to assure credibility is called *member checking*. With member checking, the results of the analysis are communicated to the participants so they can clarify, refute, revise, or verify.

Transferability refers to the degree to which the results of qualitative research can be transferred to other contexts or settings. From a qualitative perspective, transferability is primarily the responsibility of the one doing the transferring. The qualitative researcher can and should enhance transferability by doing a thorough job of describing the participants, research context, and the assumptions that guided the research. The person who wishes to "transfer" the results to a different context is then responsible for making the judgment of how sensible the transfer is.

Dependability emphasizes the need for the researcher to account for the ever-changing context within which research occurs. The researcher is responsible for describing the changes that occur in the setting and how these changes affected the way the researcher approached the study.

Confirmability refers to the degree to which the results could be confirmed or corroborated by others. There are a number of strategies for enhancing confirmability. The researcher can document the procedures for checking and rechecking the data throughout the study. Another researcher can take a "devil's advocate" role with respect to the results, and this process can be documented. The researcher can actively search for and describe negative instances that contradict study conclusions, also known as looking for "disconfirming cases." And, after the study, one can conduct a data audit that examines the data collection and analysis procedures and makes judgments about the potential for bias or distortion.

From the above strategies, one would correctly take away the impression that qualitative questions require the researcher to make many notes and reflect on similarities and differences in the context. These notes are not always used by others to "check" on the veracity of the findings, so one additional strategy for assuring trustworthiness includes use of multiple interviewers who are also involved in analysis. Teams of interview-researchers spend many hours talking about what they are hearing and seeing, then coming to a consensus as to what it all means. Many readers would consider these team approaches to be among the most reliable of qualitative designs.

Role of the Investigator: Involved and Subjective vs Uninvolved and Objective

Many new researchers and others using qualitative methods worry about injecting too much of their own viewpoint and assumptions into the data analysis. This concern is rooted in the fact that quantitative studies require the investigator to remain totally objective in order to avoid introducing bias to the study. In fact, the most highly controlled and valid design is considered the randomized two-group double blind study, in which everyone, including the investigator has no idea of group assignment until the end of the study. Although controlling for bias is important and addressed through mechanisms such as those in the preceding paragraph, the qualitative investigator must take a very involved and subjective role in the research process. The qualitative investigator chooses those topics with which he has familiarity, if not substantial expertise. This expertise allows the investigator to draw on a bank of knowledge to direct questions and interpret data. Further, and perhaps more importantly, the investigator becomes a research tool in that his expertise and experiences lead to insightful, creative, and informed hunches. In qualitative research, the investigator maintains a careful balance between inserting himself into the data and forcing the data to his will.

Robert Stake, the author of a classic text on case study research (Stake, 1995), discusses six common researcher roles seen in qualitative work. Notice how well these researcher roles overlap with the roles occupational therapists often assume in a therapeutic relationship. Perhaps this overlap further reflects one of the points in this chapter; there is a natural and consistent purpose between qualitative research and occupational therapy. The investigator's primary purpose, according to Stake (1995, pg. 105), is reflected in the following roles:

1. *Teacher*: Learn what the target audience needs to know, then inform, sophisticate, increase competence, socialize, or liberate the group.

2. *Evaluator*: Give careful attention to data's merits and shortcomings based on a specific set of criteria.

3. *Theorist*: Use the uniqueness of the data to illustrate a solution, or new understanding for the data.

4. *Advocate*: Discover the best arguments against assertions and provide data to counter them.

5. *Biographer*: Chronicle a life history explored against a thematic network (i.e., a set of issues).

6. *Interpreter*: Recognize and substantiate new meaning: Find new connections and make them comprehensible to others.

Up to this point, the content of this chapter has reasoned that much of occupational therapy and occupational science involves minimally defined and understood concepts, and that measuring these concepts calls for applying qualitative approaches to occupational therapy practice. An overview of selected principles of qualitative research has been presented (purpose, setting, data type, sources of accuracy, and researcher roles) as the basis for applying these principles in practice.

PRACTICE-BASED USES FOR QUALITATIVE APPROACHES

Despite the long tradition of "special harmony" between occupational therapy and qualitative study (Kielhofner, 1982, p. 162), the range of possible ways that qualitative designs can be applied to everyday practice has not been fully explored. However, qualitative methods are already an important clinical tool in occupational therapy. In this section, use of qualitative methods to support four practice-related efforts will be described. They are 1) evaluation and treatment planning; 2) case studies; 3) clinical reasoning; and, 4) program evaluation.

Evaluation and Treatment Planning

Therapists are probably most familiar with the use of qualitative methods to gather information for purposes of evaluation and treatment planning, such as interviewing to understand a client's goals. For example, how often have you asked a new client "What is a typical day like for you?" Occupational therapists gather vital insight into routines, activity choices, performance, social systems, and resources with just this one simple interview question. This is one example of many informal ways that occupational therapists use the basics of qualitative methods in everyday practice. Another example is careful observation. Occupational therapists watch clients engaged in daily activities in order to understand issues such as safety, fatigue, problem solving, and performance. Thus, much of the information used to evaluate performance and plan treatment are qualitative methods. Later, we'll talk about principles for improving the trustworthiness of these methods.

Case Studies

In another familiar clinical application, qualitative methods are used in case studies to gather relevant occupational performance and profile data, which is derived at least partially from interviews and observations. Case reports are a regular feature in the major occupational therapy journals around the world and are valued for their ability to illustrate complex and dynamic relationships. Think about how occupational therapists choose the best illustration of occupation or a change in occupation. Oftentimes, the case is chosen because it is classic—the person in the case demonstrates characteristics or are residing in contexts that are typical of the situation encountered. Other cases are chosen because they are so unusual, either in terms of the presenting circumstances or the outcomes. Both these decisions are similar to the goals of a qualitative study, which might involve quoting a typical informant or looking for a disconfirming case.

Clinical Reasoning

Qualitative methods have also been used on an informal basis to guide clinical reasoning. For example, ethnographic principles can be used as a framework by which an occupational therapist can identify and describe occupation from the client's perspective, including its meaning (Gitlin, Corcoran, & Eckhardt, 1995). "Ethnography is the work of describing a culture. The central aim of ethnography is to understand another way of life ..." (Spradley, 1980, pg. 3). Culture as the basis of occupation was a relationship recognized by the founders of the profession (Dunton, 1918, in Bonder, Martin, & Miracle., 2004) although the ability to understand and apply cultural concepts to therapeutic interventions remains a contemporary topic of discussion (Bonder et al., 2004). Occupational therapy is one of only a few health professions to actively shape clinical decisions based on the client's beliefs and meanings. For this reason, many occupational therapists function as informal ethnographers without really being aware of the connection. Occupational therapists conduct these ethnographies in several settings. Therapists engage in narrative analysis with each other over lunch and between treatment sessions, sharing clinical successes and puzzles in an effort to better understand their clients' occupational performance. Clark (1993) named these lunchroom discussions "occupational storytelling," which she describes as important to understanding the "spirit of the survivors with whom they [occupational therapists] work" (p. 1074). Mattingly and Fleming (1994) also speak of storymaking between occupational therapist and client during which a future story is created for the client. This type of storytelling is crucial for building a therapeutic partnership between client and therapist, and for guiding the clinical reasoning of the occupational therapist. In the beginning, the therapist's contribution to the story may be sketchy and largely based on past experiences and technical knowledge. Over time, details that individualize the story are added so that, in the best cases, the client's unique experiences and meaning shape the intervention.

Evaluating Programs

While most therapists are familiar with qualitative data for describing single cases and puzzling through practice issues, fewer are aware of the clinical application of qualitative methods to evaluate clinical programs. Most of the time, the goal of program evaluation is to determine whether the program is effective. While effectiveness is often measured by calculating a numerical change score, qualitative methods are a useful approach when tests and surveys are not appropriate. Sometimes, the effectiveness of a program can only appropriately be understood from the viewpoint of the individuals who experienced it. In these cases, data would be gathered through focus groups, open-ended questions, or individual interviews. The evaluator would sort the responses in terms of "themes" or types of experience or opinions expressed. In doing so, the evaluator performs a thematic analysis, a grandiose term for organizing, reducing, and describing the data (Schwandt, 2001). In program evaluation, qualitative methods can be used alone or in combination with quantitative (numerical) data, and may even help to elucidate findings on a survey or questionnaire. Besides testing a program's effect, it is also important to understanding how a program was implemented, the participants' opinions, unexpected effects, and the program's strengths and weaknesses from a number of perspectives (Gitlin, Corcoran, & Martindale-Adams, 2000; Patton, 1987). This information,

which is critical to replication, is sometimes only available in narrative form through interviews or observations.

Patton (1987) identified five types of program evaluations that have particular relevance to the clinic and can be at least partially conducted through qualitative methods. *Process evaluations* measure the internal operations of the program, including how the clients accessed and moved through the program, client-therapist interactions, and program strengths and weaknesses. Because the evaluator is interested in how the program operated, detailed information is required from clients, therapists, and program administrators. The evaluator is looking for information about formal and informal activities that give the program its character. A second type of program evaluation involves outcomes that are highly individualized. *Evaluating individualized outcomes* is necessary when a range of effects and experiences can be appropriately expected. Usually, this type of evaluation involves interview and observation of the client before, during, and after the program. The evaluator is seeking evidence of the effect of the program for that particular client. A third type of program evaluation includes detailed case studies of *unusual circumstances*. While there are many reasons for presenting cases as an example of usual treatment, new knowledge about the program can be gained from an in-depth study of situations that were not typical (outstanding successes, unusual failures, or dropouts). A qualitative approach helps the evaluator to understand the unique set of circumstances at play in unusual cases as the basis for making programmatic changes. *Program implementation information* is the fourth type of potential evaluation data. If a program is not implemented as it was designed, predicted outcomes may not be achieved. Therefore, it is important to gather data about what the therapist actually did in treatment and compare this information to the intended treatment. Qualitative data are especially appropriate to program implementation evaluation because few program designers can accurately anticipate the effect of client characteristics and contextual attributes on treatment implementation. *Quality improvement* is the fifth type of program evaluation that can be partially conducted through qualitative methods. While it is important to know how much adaptive equipment was issued and how long clients were treated, the evaluator will also want to know more about how clients experienced or were affected by treatment. For instance, it would be a useful indicator of quality to know if and how clients used strategies introduced as part of their occupational therapy experience.

Use of qualitative methods to evaluate occupational performance and clinical programs can result in rich information that falls between and beyond the points on a standardized scale. The next section overviews broad decisions and methods for applying a qualitative approach to measurement in occupational therapy practice.

Principles for Applying Qualitative Methods to Occupational Therapy Practice

For discussion purposes, this section is organized according to six broad principles related to the use of qualitative methods to evaluate occupational performance and clinical programs. They are:

- Choose the most knowledgeable informants
- Ask the right questions, watch the right behaviors
- Keep the setting natural
- Document your observations or interview information
- Analyze your data for themes
- Confirm your findings

Each of these topics is represented by a wealth of conceptual and technical information in the literature. In fact, books are available that address each one of these questions in detail. The purpose of the following discussion is to provide a broad overview of how to approach these questions and to pique interest in learning more. Therapists who are committed to applying qualitative methods to practice are encouraged to read any of a number of excellent publications on the topic, especially Miles and Huberman (1994) or Denzin and Lincoln (1994). The occupational therapy literature also contains many excellent examples of a qualitative approach to exploring occupation. In fact, in a 5-year period from 1999 to 2004, there have been 34 articles reporting qualitative research published in the *American Journal of Occupational Therapy* alone. Other occupational therapy journals from around the world, especially Canada, United Kingdom, and Australia, also have a strong record of publishing qualitative studies. Contemporary studies include descriptions of parental perspectives (Cohn, Miller, & Tickle-Degnen, 2000; Farber, 2000; Pierce, 2000; Cohn, 2001; Segal, Mandich, Polatajko, & Cook, 2002; Cronin, 2004), the experiences of individuals with mental health issues (Rebeiro, Day, Semeniuk, O'Brien-Bed, & Wilson, 2001; Duncombe, 2004), adaptations of adults with physical disabilities (Thoren Jonsson, Moller, & Grimby, 1999; Spencer, Hersch, Shelton, Ripple, Spencer, Dyer, & Murphy, 2002; Neville-Jan, 2003; Chan & Spencer, 2004; Barker, Reid, & Cott, 2004), and perspectives on occupational therapy by practitioners and students (Hammel et al., 1999; Dubouloz, Egan, Vallerand, & von Zweck, 1999; Cusick, 2001; Walker, 2001; Lyons & Crepeau, 2001; Lawlor, 2003; Scheerer, 2003)..

Finally, it is highly recommended that therapists seek out and partner with a researcher who is familiar with qualitative methods. It is not necessary that this person is an occupational therapist, but his or her knowledge of technique will be beneficial to develop the therapist's approach and answer questions.

Choose the Most Knowledgeable Informants

In clinical application of qualitative methods, this is often the easiest question to answer. Informants are knowledgeable sources of information that can provide an insider's perspective (Crabtree & Miller, 1992). In the clinic, this would obviously include the client as the recipient of occupational therapy services. However, the richness and detail of qualitative methods is partially due to the fact that information is gathered from many sources; plus this serves as a triangulation strategy. So it is important to think about others, such as family, who may be good informants by virtue of having a unique perspective on the questions at hand.

To develop a list of potential informants, keep clearly in mind what you want to know. For instance, if you are questioning the benefits of occupational therapy for a particular individual, you may wish to interview only one other person in addition to the individual receiving treatment. However, if you want to know the strengths and weaknesses of an occupational therapy program, then the list grows longer. First, think about the types of individuals who are in a position to comment knowledgeably. Your list may include clients, family members, interventionists, clerical staff, and administrators. Second, since you cannot interview everyone on the list, think about which individuals within each type will provide information that is unique. You may want to speak with the most satisfied and least satisfied clients. In qualitative designs, the investigator looks for informants that will represent a wide range of experiences. Don't forget to ask each of your informants to recommend someone for an interview who feels differently about the topic than he or she does. This strategy, called *snowballing*, provides entry into those valuable disconfirming cases.

Ask the Right Questions; Watch the Right Behaviors

As with all aspects of research, deciding how to gather information must be driven by the clinical question and the amount of time the therapist has available. To decide among the range of possible data collection techniques, the occupational therapist must keep his or her questions clearly in mind. To do otherwise usually adds time and effort to the project without adding substantial gain. After a short list of appropriate data collection techniques has been developed, the occupational therapist must carefully examine each for its costs in terms of time and materials. For instance, data collection and analysis from interviews with five clients for 30 minutes each over a 2-month time frame may be more cost-effective than videotaping 10 hours of treatment. While videotaping sounds easier, it represents a high initial cost in materials, and analysis is time-consuming. It is important to remember when choosing a method that in-depth information can be effectively collected with just a few well-chosen interview questions or observations, as opposed to a large number (as would be needed in a quantitative-type study).

As has been indicated, qualitative methods yield non-numerical data. These data may be in the form of observations, interviews, or other visual information. Each is discussed in more detail below.

Observation is a vital part of the therapeutic process. Occupational therapists constantly observe their clients for many reasons, including assessment of progress, motivation, response to therapy, adverse effects, and level of challenge. Deciding what, when, and how to observe must be driven by the clinical questions asked. In addition, the therapist may either participate in the activity being observed while making notes about observations, or stand back and observe without participating. The determinant for participation or non-participation depends on the extent to which the observed phenomena can occur or will be changed by the occupational therapist's presence. For example, think about observations of self-feeding with or without the occupational therapist's presence. If the therapist wants to observe for the effect of a particular piece of adaptive equipment on performance, he or she will want to participate. However, if the therapist wants to see how well the client uses the equipment independently at lunch, the occupational therapist should not be involved.

Interviews can proceed in a number of ways depending on many factors, including setting, allotted time, complexity of information being sought, and characteristics of the informant and interviewer. Interviews raise a host of critical decisions to consider thoughtfully, especially decisions about the setting, interview questions, and interviewer's actions. As always, it is important to remind yourself of the question since it establishes the purpose, goals, and direction of the interview. Next, it may help to consider the informant's characteristics. Children require short, simple questions or the opportunity to look at objects (pictures, toys) that are relevant to the discussion. Based on your knowledge of the informant, plan other aspects of the interview, including order of the questions, their level of complexity, and needed attributes of the setting.

An important but often overlooked consideration is the interviewer's approach, including how friendly, talkative, and casual the interviewer appears. Interviewers must avoid asking questions in such a way as to promote or suggest a particular response, labeled a leading question. An example of a leading question is "Did that make you upset?" instead of "How did that make you feel?" The therapist as an interviewer also has a special challenge to avoid: offering treatment advice during the interview. If information comes up that could potentially lead to a therapeutic suggestion, make a note and return to it during a treatment session. A final consideration involves the interviewer's actions during the interview. Although we will discuss documenting information in more detail below, it is important to consider what the interviewer will be doing during the interview, such as taking extensive field notes or audiotaping the interview.

Decisions about interviews also include interview format and content. Format refers to the plan for organizing data collection, ranging from group interviews to individual interviews. With a limited amount of time, interviews may be done in groups. A focus group format is especially popular but requires special knowledge since this format combines expertise in interviewing with expertise in group dynamics. Anyone wishing to use a focus group approach should refer to a number of excellent texts, especially Krueger (1994) and Morgan and Krueger (1998). Interviews may also be conducted in other formats, such as one-on-one, small group, telephone, or internet interviews. However, each of these formats introduces other decisions. For example, use of telephone or internet interviewing may lack depth since the atmosphere does not involve direct human contact.

Interview content refers to the composition of the questions or what is being asked and their order. In an open-ended interview, a few carefully chosen *stem* questions or statements are posed to the participants to establish the topic, such as "Describe your morning routine." The interviewer then uses probes to get more in-depth and detailed information about the participant's response to the stem question. Probes are questions that ask for clarification ("Tell me more about how that goes"), similarities ("What other situations make that happen?"), dissimilarities ("How is that different from other mornings?"), and description ("Can you give me some examples of when that happens?"). Some qualitative researchers regard the probes as more important than the initial stem question, so practitioners should be very familiar and comfortable with their use. An alternative to the use of stem questions is an invitation to the informant to tell a story that illustrates a significant experience. The practitioner can then use probes to delve more deeply for meaning. For example, interviewing parents of a child with a disability may include a request to relate a story about an event when the child's disability did not influence how things went.

Visual data can be gathered from sources other than interview and observation. Potential sources of narrative data may be found in archival material (photographs, recordings, film, diaries) or more contemporary materials, such as informant logs. A good source of visual data for therapists to consider is medical records, in particular evaluations or discharge summaries from key team members.

Keep the Setting Natural

While it is not always possible to interview someone in the environment where an activity primarily occurs, this is the ideal. In the caregiving style study mentioned previously, some spouses were concerned about the reactions of other family members, so the interview was conducted in local coffee shops or a library. The interviewer attempted to get as close to the natural setting as possible, both because information could be provided by seeing the immediate area of an informant's home, and also out of courtesy to the caregiver. On these occasions, caregivers were asked to bring photo albums of recent events so that the interview could involve clarifying and understanding aspects of the environmental context.

For those occupational therapists who do not work in the community, a few strategies may be helpful:

- Make generous use of visuals such as photographs, videotapes, or floor plans. Ask the client to look at the visuals with you and tell you what you're seeing. Remember that environments are dynamic, so ask about times when the picture might look different, such as on a busy day.

- When interviewing, try to talk in an area that is private, but comfortable as opposed to institutional. The point is to make the client comfortable enough to trust you with his innermost feelings and concerns. Sometimes the best place is the client's room when no staff or other patients are around.

- Remove any symbols that will remind the client of the institution or your position as a health care provider, such as a white lab coat or a medical records file.

In an institutional setting, sometimes just one member of the team conducting a home visit can have a large effect on treatment planning and problem solving. Consider a proposal to the administration of the institution for a home visit for each client that meets certain criteria, such as lacking a full-time caregiver.

Document Your Observations or Interview Information

There are a number of choices about how to record qualitative data. As with all choices in qualitative research, data collection methods should be guided by what the occupational therapist wants to know (the clinical question). It is usually not important for the purposes of clinical evaluation to have information recorded verbatim, so the expense of audio- or videotaped data collection may not be justified. The occupational therapist may choose to use *field notes* if the information sought is very focused, such as a review of a typical daily routine to understand use of pacing. Field notes are familiar to most therapists as a method for documenting the contents of an interview or observations and the therapist's impressions. A safe method is to take field notes and audiotape so that information can be verified from a number of sources. Be aware however, that your plans for audiotaping need to be approved by the compliance officer at your institution or the institutional review board. No matter what the recording method chosen, be sure to accurately record the date and client initials in notes and on tape labels. Preserve the informant's confidentiality by using his or her initials only and by locking materials in a secure place. Destroy these tapes as soon as their information has been used.

Analyze Your Data for Themes

By far, the best way to become familiar with drawing conclusions from qualitative data is by working with someone who has experience in the area of qualitative data analysis. There are many computer software programs that make qualitative analysis manageable (for an overview of several strategies, see Miles & Huberman, 1994). These programs are useful, flexible, and powerful tools that save time and expand the interviewer's ability to explore the data. However, for everyday clinical practice, these programs may not be necessary or even feasible. For decades, qualitative analysis was conducted by sorting index cards containing text into piles based on similarities. Later, highlighters made it possible to color-code information to reflect themes. Practitioners may find that it is sufficient to keep a running log or journal that summarizes the emerging themes.

If you take nothing else away from this chapter regarding analysis, the most important point to understand is that collecting and analyzing data are simultaneous tasks. Never make the mistake of collecting information without attempting to understand what you are seeing and hearing. Qualitative designs are spiral, so that analysis of data leads to refinement of understanding, and that refinement leads to more focused and relevant data collection.

According to Wolcott (1994), the purpose of qualitative analysis to transform data from their original form (transcripts of interviews, videotapes) to new knowledge. This transformation occurs as a result of three overlapping processes: description, analysis, and interpretation (Wolcott, 1994). These processes do not particularly proceed in a linear fashion because the process of analysis may reveal the need for further description, and so on. In description, data are described generally through a summarizing narrative; a short memo that attempts to capture the gist of what is being said. To get started, think about answering the basic questions of who, what, when, and where. Morse and Richards (2002) also talk about describing data in terms of gathering material that relate to selected topics of interest to the researcher (or occupational therapist), such as daily routines or social outings.

Description provides the groundwork for analysis, during which data are examined for concepts or themes among key elements and relationships. Analytic coding is used to identify and define "common threads that run through the data" (Morse and Richards, 2002, pg. 113). By identifying themes, a researcher begins to understand what is important or meaningful about the topic. The third process involved in transforming data is interpreting themes for meanings and implications. In this process, the themes are compared and contrasted so to develop an overarching theory about what is happening it this study. For example, in the caregiving study, the themes appeared to be related to the concept of control. Thus, when the caregiving style study was completed, the three styles that emerged were different in terms of the amount, focus, and strategies of control (Corcoran, 2004).

An important contribution to transforming data comes from the insights and hunches of anyone who reviews or collects the data. These insights and hunches are captured in memos to oneself that are documented immediately as they occur. Often, memos from another person who is in contact with the client provides a vital idea that can jump start an analysis in interesting and new directions.

Confirm Your Findings

Earlier in this chapter, information was presented regarding strategies that can help a researcher delve below the surface to reveal interesting and important information, as well as to assure trustworthiness. Many of those strategies can and should be used by occupational therapists who are interviewing or observing for clinical reasons. Triangulate the data by finding several perspectives on the same phenomena. For example, you could ask a family member about the same events or behaviors on which the client commented, not as a way of confirming or refuting but just simply to get a more nuanced picture of that event. Alternately, you could interview and observe the same actions, thereby getting an idea of how the client talks about performance and then carries out the activity. If necessary, use simulation or role play. A third way of triangulating data is by asking another staff member to interview the client. This may not be as feasible in a busy setting, but if you keep the questions brief and focused, it may be possible in a short amount of time. Finally, triangulate by testing the same skills or performance areas that the client has told you about. For example, using Baum, Edwards, and Morrow-Howell's (1993) Functional Behavioral Profile will help to better understand the behaviors you are observing when an individual with dementia engages in a daily activity.

Not only is it important and entirely possible to triangulate data, it is equally necessary to confirm the data. Talk with the client about your findings so that she can comment, correct, or modify. Finally, occupational thera-

pists can address transferability by changing the context for performance and making note of the effect. For instance, it is much simpler to practice relaxation in a quiet room than it is in a bustling cafeteria.

AN EXAMPLE OF QUALITATIVE MEASUREMENT

The following example is an actual study conducted in 1999 that involved a partnership between a group of home care occupational therapists and the author of this chapter. A discussion of this pilot effectiveness study is offered to illustrate several points. First, occupational therapists in the study use a semi-structured interview process to collect information about their client's occupational performance. This means that stem questions are asked of all informants but the interviewer chose probe question to follow-up and search for deeper meaning. Second, the study attempted to further define concepts identified in Mattingly and Fleming's (1994) previous qualitative study of clinical reasoning. This illustrates the dynamic fit between experimental-type and qualitative research traditions; by defining concepts that could be counted. Third, the study uses a set of open-ended questions as part of the program evaluation strategy. As a result, the investigators gained critical information about the occupational therapy program itself that could be used to further refine the program. Fourth, in analysis, qualitative and quantitative data were integrated for a deep understanding of who benefited from the occupational therapy program and how.

A Pilot Study of Home Care

The purpose of the 18-month Home Care pilot study (Corcoran & Johnson, 1999), funded by the American Occupational Therapy Foundation, was to identify and validate occupational therapy's unique contribution to functional health of 96 home care clients and, therefore, to the viability of home care agencies under prospective payment. Initially, the group of occupational therapists and researchers met for 4 days to design the study. In the course of those discussions, it became apparent that each therapist in the group used a therapeutic process that was unique in significant ways, such as how and when treatment goals were developed. Wishing to maintain the ability to individualize treatment, the group decided to define and implement broad concepts about best practice to conduct occupational therapy in the home. The next task was difficult—defining best practice.

The group spent an entire day talking about the behaviors that occupational therapists exhibit when engaged in best practice. As the day progressed, it became apparent that the group was naming thinking and action behaviors that sounded very much like three occupational therapy clinical reasoning domains identified by Mattingly and Fleming (1994). The group found that, to date, little had been done to operationalize each clinical reasoning domain. In other words, the literature did not help clarify what the occupational therapist is actually doing and thinking when engaged in the three domains of procedural, interactive, and conditional reasoning. While promising work has been conducted to examine use of these concepts in pediatric occupational therapy (Burke, 1997), no study has attempted to date to systematically examine the use of these concepts in home care. Using Burke's study and our own experiences, the group spent several hours defining the indicators of each domain. For example, procedural reasoning was demonstrated when the occupational therapist considered the relative merits of specific techniques (e.g., neurodevelopmental treatment, sensory integration, group dynamics) that might be used to address a particular occupational performance problem. Likewise, interactive reasoning was reflected in thinking about how to best approach the client with suggestions, given that person's emotional, social, motivational and psychological needs. These indicators of clinical reasoning were developed into a checklist which was used to record use of principles within these three clinical reasoning domains. The checklist left room for comments and the occupational therapists were encouraged to write about their feelings.

In analyzing the data regarding the three different types of reasoning, the occupational therapists reported use of reasoning within each domain on every visit. However, even though they used the three types of reasoning at the same level, the qualitative data showed differences in their perceptions of each domain. The occupational therapists pointedly talked about their struggles and successes interacting with clients and the reasoning that accompanied that effort. They talked about the relative ease of knowing what to do (procedural reasoning) as opposed to *how* to motivate and involve clients (interactive reasoning). They tried to identify use of conditional reasoning (e.g., developing working hypotheses) but were unfamiliar with the principles comprising this domain and grew frustrated. Those who were newer to the profession appeared to assign equal importance to procedural and interactive reasoning.

In the pilot study, functional measurement and program evaluation involved a battery of structured, semi-structured, and open-ended interviews directed at the clients. An example of structured interviews includes the Outcomes Assessment Information Set (OASIS), developed by Shaughnessy, Schlenker, and Hittle. (1994). The semi-structured portion of the interview includes the Client and Clinician Assessment of Performance (CCAP), developed and pilot-tested by Gitlin and Corcoran (2005). The interview also included open-ended questions to elicit the client's perspective on his or her functional health and satisfaction with progress in therapy. These open-ended questions are asked post-treatment only.

Looking at the experience of home care from the clients' perspectives, we were again able to integrate the qualitative and quantitative data. Using the only statistical analysis in the study, the pre- and post-intervention scores on the CCAP for 439 problems addressed in occupational therapy (i.e., self-care, leisure, and work related issues) were found to have improved significantly in rating of assistance needed (p<0.001) and satisfaction (p<0.001). However, without a control group, the improvement cannot be credited to occupational therapy. In addition, no significant change was found when statistically analyzing the numerical scores on the OASIS. At the post-occupational therapy interview, clients talked about the personal meaning they felt related to achieving individual goals. One prominent theme was getting out of the house to socialize, run errands, or shop. Another theme included being able to do things right, such as getting into the shower after weeks of sponge bathing or resuming responsibility for cooking instead of receiving home delivered meals.

A great deal was accomplished with this mixed methods effort. The therapists were able to define an elusive concept (best practice) and put it into action for their home care clients. To evaluate this best practice program, qualitative data were collected about the clients' perspectives on this experience. Clients identified the types of activities that were meaningful for them, which in turn can direct new efforts at best practice. Despite the fact that the program could not be validated on a standardized scale (OASIS) the therapists still had quality indicators of their effectiveness because they were systematic about how they conducted this study.

WHERE DO WE GO FROM HERE?

Clinical questions come in many forms and may be asked about an individual client or a whole group. Hopefully, the reader understands from this chapter that the clinical question determines the type of measurement approach taken and details about data collection and analysis. When clinical research questions involve underdeveloped concepts, therapists should consider the merits and feasibility of applying a qualitative approach. A qualitative approach is useful for examining questions ranging from an individual's occupational preferences to program evaluation. With their skilled use of observation and interview, occupational therapists are in a unique position to use qualitative inquiry in everyday practice. A substantial literature on naturalistic research methods is available to further inform practitioners, and contact with an experienced researcher is highly recommended. With practice, therapists may find themselves publishing case studies that illustrate clinical phenomena and, hopefully, designing more opportunities to examine occupation through the use of qualitative approaches.

REFERENCES

Barker, D. J., Reid, D., & Cott, C. (2004). Acceptance and meanings of wheelchair use in senior stroke survivors. *American Journal of Occupational Therapy, 58(2)*, 221-230.

Baum, C. M., Edwards, D. F., & Morrow-Howell, N. (1993). Identification and measurement of productive behaviors in senile dementia of the Alzheimer type. *The Gerontologist, 33(3)*, 403-408.

Bonder, B. R., Martin, L., & Miracle, A. W. (2004). Culture emergent in occupation. *American Journal of Occupational Therapy, 58*, 159-168.

Burke, J. P. (1997). *Frames of meaning: An analysis of occupational therapy evaluations of children.* Ann Arbor, MI: UMI Dissertation Information Service.

Chan, J., & Spencer, J. (2004). Adaptation to hand injury: An evolving experience. *American Journal of Occupational Therapy, 58(2)*, 128-139.

Clark, F. (1993). Occupation embedded in a real life: Interweaving occupational science and occupational therapy. Eleanor Clarke Slagle Lecture, *American Journal of Occupational Therapy, 47(12)*, 1067-1078.

Cohn, E. S. (2001). Parent perspectives of occupational therapy using a sensory integration approach. *American Journal of Occupational Therapy, 55(3)*.

Cohn, E., Miller, L. J., & Tickle-Degnen, L. (2000). Parental hopes for therapy outcomes: Children with sensory modulation disorders. *American Journal of Occupational Therapy, 54(1)*.

Corcoran, M. A. (2003). Strategies and styles of spouse caregivers. In Doka, K (Ed) *Living with grief: Alzheimer's disease.* Washington DC: Hospice Foundation of America.

Corcoran, M. A. (2004). *Caregiving styles of spouses who provide dementia care.* Minneapolis, MN: AOTA annual conference.

Corcoran, M.A., & Johnson, K. V. (1999). *Creating academic-clinical partnerships: A pilot study of home care.* Seattle, WA: AOTF Research Symposium, AOTA annual conference.

Cook J. V. (2001). *Qualitative research in occupational therapy: Strategies and experiences.* Albany NY: Delmar.

Cronin, A. F. (2004). Mothering a child with hidden impairments. *American Journal of Occupational Therapy, 58(1)*, 83-92.

Crabtree, B. F., & Miller, W. L. (1992). *Doing qualitative research.* Newbury Park, CA: Sage Publications.

Cusick, A. (2001). The experience of clinician-researchers in occupational therapy. *American Journal of Occupational Therapy, 55(1)*.

Denzin, N. K., & Lincoln, Y. S. (1994). *Handbook of qualitative research.* Newbury Park, CA: Sage Publications.

Dubouloz, C.J., Egan, M., Vallerand, J., & von Zweck, C. (1999). Occupational therapists' perceptions of evidence-based practice. *American Journal of Occupational Therapy, 53(5)*.

Duncombe, L. W. (2004). Comparing learning of cooking in home and clinic for people with schizophrenia. *American Journal of Occupational Therapy, 58(3)*, 272-278.

Farber, R. S. (2000). Mothers with disabilities: In their own voice. *American Journal of Occupational Therapy, 54(3)*.

Frank, G. (1984). Life history model of adaptation to disability: The case of a "congenital amputee." *Social Science of Medicine, 19(6)*, 639-645.

Frank, G., Bernardo, C., Tropper, S., Noguchi, F., Lipman, C., Maulhardt, B., et al. do you need al the authors? (1997). Jewish spirituality through actions in time: Daily occupations of young orthodox Jewish couples in Los Angeles. *American Journal of Occupational Therapy, 51(3)*, 199-206.

Gitlin, L.N., Corcoran, M. A., & Eckhardt, S. (1995). Understanding the family perspective: An ethnographic framework for providing occupational therapy in the home. *American Journal of Occupational Therapy, 49(6)*.

Gitlin, L. N., Corcoran, M. A., Martindale-Adams, J., Malone, C., Stevens, A., & Winter, L. (2000). Identifying mechanisms of action: Why and how does intervention work? In R. Schultz (Ed.), *Intervention approaches to dementia caregiving.* CITY, STATE: Oxford Press.

Gitlin, L. N., & Corcoran, M. A. (in press). *An occupational therapy guide to helping caregivers of persons with dementia: The Home Environmental Skill-building Program (ESP).* Bethesda MD: AOTA Press.

Hammel, J., Royeen, C. B., Bagatell, N., Chandler, B., Jensen, G., Loveland, J., & Stone G. (1999). Student perspectives on problem-based learning in an occupational therapy curriculum: A multiyear qualitative evaluation. *American Journal of Occupational Therapy, 53(2)*.

Hasselkus, B. R. (1987). *Family caregivers for the elderly at home: ethnography of meaning and informal learning.* Ann Arbor, MI: UMI Dissertation Information Service.

Jonsson, H., Kielhofner, G., & Borell, L. (1997). Anticipating retirement: The formation of narratives concerning occupational transition. *American Journal of Occupational Therapy, 51(1)*, 49-56.

Kielhofner, G. (1982). Qualitative research: Part two — Methodological approaches and relevance to occupational therapy. *Occupational Therapy Journal of Research, 2*, 150-164.

Krueger, R. A. (1994). *Focus groups: A practical guide for applied research* (2nd ed.). Newbury Park, CA: Sage Publications.

Lawlor, M. C. (2003). Gazing anew: The shift from a clinical gaze to an ethnographic lens. *American Journal of Occupational Therapy, 57(1)*.

Lyons, K. D., & Crepeau, E. B. (2001). The clinical reasoning of an occupational therapy assistant. *American Journal of Occupational Therapy, 55(5)*.

Mattingly, C., & Fleming, M. (1994). *Clinical reasoning: Forms of inquiry in a therapeutic practice.* Philadelphia: F. A. Davis.

Miles, M. B., & Huberman, A. M. (1994). *Qualitative data analysis* (2nd ed.). Newbury Park, CA: Sage Publications.

Morgan, D. L., & Krueger, R. A. (1998). *The focus group kit* (Vol. 1-6). Newbury Park, CA: Sage Publications.

Morse, J. M., & Richards, L. (2002). *Readme first for a user's guide to qualitative methods.* Thousand Oaks, CA: Sage Publications.

Neville-Jan, A. (2003). Encounters in a world of pain. An autoethnography. *American Journal of Occupational Therapy, 57(1).*

Patton, M. Q. (1987). *How to use qualitative methods in evaluation.* Newbury Park, CA: Sage Publications.

Pierce, D. (2000). Maternal management of the home as a developmental play space for infants and toddlers. *American Journal of Occupational Therapy, 54(3).*

Price-Lackey, P., & Cashman, J. (1996). Jenny's story: Reinventing oneself through occupation and narrative configuration. *American Journal of Occupational Therapy, 50(4),* 306-314.

Rebeiro, K. L., Day, D. G., Semeniuk, B., O'Brien-Bed, M.C., & Wilson, B. (2001). Northern initiative for social action: An occupation-based mental health program. *American Journal of Occupational Therapy, 55(5).*

Scheerer, C. R. (2003). Perceptions of effective professional behavior feedback: Occupational therapy student voices. *American Journal of Occupational Therapy, 57(2).*

Schwandt, T.A. (2001). *Dictionary of qualitative inquiry.* (2nd ed). Thousand Oaks, CA: Sage Publications.

Segal, R., Mandich, A., Polatajko, H., and Cook, J.V. (2002). Stigma and its management: A pilot study of parental perceptions of the experiences of children with developmental coordination disorder. *American Journal of Occupational Therapy, 56(4).*

Shaughnessy, P., Schlenker, R. E., & Hittle, D. F. (1994). *A study of home health care quality and cost under capitated and fee-for-service payment systems.* Denver, CO: Center for Health Policy Research.

Spencer, J., Hersch, G., Shelton, M., Ripple, J., Spencer, C., Dyer, C.B., & Murphy, K. (2002). Functional outcomes and daily life activities of African-American elders after hospitalization. *American Journal of Occupational Therapy, 56(2).*

Spradley, J.P. (1980). *Participant observation.* New York, NY: Holt, Rinehart, and Winston.

Stake, R.E. (1995). *The art of case study research.* Thousand Oaks, CA: Sage Publications.

Thoren Jonsson, A.L., Moller, A., & Grimby, G. (1999). Managing occupations in everyday life to achieve adaptation. *American Journal of Occupational Therapy, 53(4).*

Walker, K.F. (2001). Adjustments to managed health care: Pushing against it, going with it, and making the best of it. *American Journal of Occupational Therapy, 55(2).*

Wolcott, H. F. (1994). *Transforming qualitative data.* Newbury Park, CA: Sage Publications.

Yerxa, E. (1991). Seeking a relevant, ethical, and realistic way of knowing for occupational therapy. *American Journal of Occupational Therapy, 45(3),* 199-204.

Editors' Notes for Chapter 6

Mine the Gold

The notion of client-centered practice has a rich history in the psychology literature, dating back to the 1950's, which informs occupational therapists' approach to assessment.

Become Systematic

This chapter provides information to permit therapists to make an informed decision about the selection of measures that assess occupational performance from a client-centered perspective.

Use Evidence in Practice

Evidence is accumulating supporting the use of these measures in a variety of population and client groups and settings. Examples of applications in practice, research, and program evaluation may be found.

Make Occupational Therapy Contribution Explicit

This chapter deals with one of the core concepts and key approaches in occupational therapy practice.

Engage in Occupation-Based, Client-Centered Practice

Occupation-focus and client-centered approach are the hallmarks of the four measures reviewed in this chapter.

6

MEASURING OCCUPATIONAL PERFORMANCE USING A CLIENT-CENTERED PERSPECTIVE

Mary Ann McColl, PhD, OT Reg. (Ont.) and Nancy Pollock, MSc, OT Reg. (Ont.)

INTRODUCTION

This chapter reviews four measures designed to assess occupational performance using a client-centered approach. Assessment often represents a therapist's first interaction with a client and, therefore, it takes on considerable importance in establishing the focus on occupational performance and the parameters of the therapeutic relationship (Baum & Law, 1997; Pollock, 1993; Pollock & McColl, 1998a).

The four measures covered in this chapter are all based on the following definition of occupational performance. Occupational performance is defined differently in Canada and the US. Although these two definitions are entirely compatible, they have differences in components and terminology that have implications for measurement. In Canada, we define occupational performance as the individual's experience of being engaged in self-care, productivity, and leisure (Canadian Association of Occupational Therapists [CAOT], 1997). Alternatively, in the US, occupational performance is defined as consisting of activities of daily living, instrumental activities of daily living, education, work, play, leisure and social participation (American Association of Occupational Therapists [AOTA], 2002). Optimal occupational performance implies a balance among performance areas.

These definitions recognize that occupational performance is made up of two components: one objective, observable component (the behaviors associated with occupation) and one subjective, experiential component (the cognitive and affective experiences associated with these behaviors). In order to measure occupational performance, we must also capture these two aspects—the actual doing of an occupation and the personal experience, meanings, and feelings associated with it. For example, in measuring productivity, we can watch someone do his or her job, address the boss, interact with work colleagues, and perform specific job functions. Through observation, we can obtain information about the objective aspects of this individual's productivity. However, to obtain the full picture, we also need to hear from the individual about the experience of his or her productivity: what is the workplace like for the individual, how challenging are the demands of the job, how does it fit with his or her goals for future productivity, how satisfying is the job, how do co-workers affect his or her ability to do the job?

Classroom Activity

To illustrate these ideas, choose an occupation you performed yesterday. Can you classify it as self-care, productivity, or leisure? Were you involved with others or did you do this alone? Was it something you did by choice or out of obligation? Did you enjoy yourself? How would your day have been different if you hadn't done this occupation? Would anyone else have cared? What role(s) were you fulfilling?

This chapter focuses on measuring the subjective aspect of occupation, using a client-centered approach. For every occupation, there is the observable component, what you actually did, and then many layers of meaning and context associated with the occupation. Occupation is a particularly personal construct that can only be fully assessed using client-centered measures. A client-centered approach to assessing occupational performance is one where the therapist not only places the client's perspective first, but in fact recognizes it as the only perspective that is important. While it is not always possible to have the client as the primary respondent (e.g., a young child, it is preferable). Caregiver perspectives are important, but are not proxies for the client's perspective.

There are a number of assumptions of the client-centered approach that may assist us in understanding its implications for assessment of occupational performance. The first assumption of client-centered assessment is that clients know what they want in terms of their occupational performance. This assumption allows therapists to trust clients to identify the problems that interfere with optimum occupational performance (Dickerson, 1996). For therapists who function from a client-centered perspective, there is no question of conflict between the problems that the therapist identifies and those that the client identifies, because the therapist understands his or her job in assessment as uncovering the problems for which the client is seeking help.

A second assumption of the client-centered approach is that the only relevant frame of reference for therapy is that of the client. While the therapist may have knowledge and expertise about certain aspects of disability and therapy, he or she can never fully understand the values, beliefs, and experiences of the client, and must therefore accept the client's reports as the most relevant source of information. This assumption is consistent with our understanding of occupational performance not simply as an objective phenomenon that can be observed and measured, but also as a subjective phenomenon that must be understood from the perspective of the person experiencing it. This assumption requires that assessment within a client-centered approach focus on the use of self-report methods.

Furthermore, this assumption suggests that the more open-ended the assessment is, the greater the opportunity to hear the client's unedited, uncensored experience of occupation. Much meaning and information is conveyed in the way a question is answered—the words chosen, the tone in which a response is delivered, the time taken to produce a response. All of these factors tell us something about our client and his or her occupational performance. Consider the difference between the following two answers to the question "How are things going for you at work these days?"

- "I hate that place!"
- "Not so well, actually. I've been having trouble getting up for it each day."

Both are admittedly negative responses, but they are significantly different in the emotional tone conveyed and the amount of information exchanged. Now compare both of these with a less open-ended format, where the same clients are asked to rate their productivity as positive, neutral, or negative. Both would say negative, but we would fail to capture the qualitative differences in their two experiences of occupational performance.

The third assumption of the client-centered approach is that the therapist cannot actually promote change; he or she can only create an environment that facilitates change. The most valuable role for the therapist is to support the client through the changes he or she wishes to make, with information, ideas, suggestions, resources, and trust in his or her ability to succeed in making the desired change. The implication of this assumption for assessment is slightly more oblique, but it has to do with the nature of the therapeutic relationship and the extent to which this is largely established during the assessment. To the extent that a therapist develops and maintains a client-centered approach throughout assessment, a relationship is established where a client understands that the therapist is not going to take over the process, assume sole responsibility for the success of therapy, nor impose his or her will on the client. The dominance of professionals in the process of assessment and therapy has been shown to be, in fact, counter-therapeutic (Goodall, 1992). Professional dominance creates dependency, disempowerment, and perhaps even institutionalization. Instead, a therapeutic relationship is established in which the therapist shows belief in the potential of the client, enthusiasm about his or her ability to achieve goals and overcome problems, and offers knowledge and experience that may be marshalled to help.

ADVANTAGES AND DISADVANTAGES OF THE CLIENT-CENTERED APPROACH TO ASSESSING OCCUPATIONAL PERFORMANCE

The client-centered approach for assessing occupational performance has a number of advantages over other approaches. The main advantage is its tendency to enhance the sense of mastery and control among clients (Emener, 1991; Goodall, 1992). This is accomplished in a number of ways: through communication of interest in the client's perceptions of his or her problems, through the therapist's commitment to assist the client with those problems, and through the therapist's communication of confidence in the client's ability to identify and solve problems.

A second advantage of the client-centered approach to assessing occupational performance is the extent to which it supports an individualized approach to therapy (Brown, 1992). Because clients identify occupational performance problems that are pertinent to their unique circumstances and context, occupational therapy interventions become explicitly framed in the context of that individual's life.

The third advantage of the client-centered approach is the opportunity that it presents for the therapist's own personal and professional growth and development. Unlike the traditional model, where the therapist is the expert and people are learning from him or her, the client is the expert in the client-centered model. Thus, client-centered therapy provides an opportunity for the therapist to learn more about occupational performance from each new client.

There are, of course, also disadvantages to assessing occupational performance from a client-centered perspective. Some clients appear to expect therapists to tell them what their problems are. For these clients, a therapist who will not take this role may be perceived as less skilled, less effective, or less cooperative (Jaffe & Kipper, 1982; Schroeder & Bloom, 1979; Wanigaratne & Barker, 1995).

A second disadvantage of client-centered assessment is that it may not be acceptable to all therapists. Rogers (1965) admits that the success or failure of client-centered therapy is often a function of the therapist's personality and his or her respect for others and belief in their resourcefulness and adaptiveness.

A third disadvantage of the client-centered approach is the need for more assessments that support this approach to measuring occupational performance. A number of reviews of the literature show that there are few occupational therapy assessments that are suitable for application in a client-centered practice (Pollock, 1993; Pollock, Baptiste, Law, McColl, Opzoomer, & Polatajko et al., 1990; Trombly, 1993).

ASSESSMENT METHODS

This chapter reviews four measures for occupational performance that fulfill the following four criteria:

1. They measure all areas of occupational performance.

2. They capture the client's perspective on occupational performance.

3. They are widely used by occupational therapists in practice, education, and research, and there is recent information on their current usage.

4. Evidence is available on their psychometric properties.

This is by no means an exhaustive list of available methods for measuring occupational performance, but rather an overview of four measures that are compatible with client-centered practice. Other measures of occupational performance are included elsewhere in the book; for example, the Occupational Questionnaire is covered in Chapter 14, as part of occupational balance, and the Assessment of Occupational Functioning is discussed in Chapter 12, particularly as it pertains to occupational roles.

OCCUPATIONAL PERFORMANCE HISTORY INTERVIEW

The Occupational Performance History Interview (OPHI) (Kielhofner & Henry, 1988) was originally a three-part measure comparing past and present occupational performance. It consisted of: 1) a scaled questionnaire covering these content areas: organization of daily routines, life roles, interests, values and goals, perceptions of ability and responsibility, and environmental influences; 2) a life history narrative form used to summarize qualitative findings from the interview; and 3) a life history patterns rating completed by a therapist. The original OPHI was designed to be used in conjunction with the Model of Human Occupation (MOHO) (Kielhofner, Mallinson, Crawford. Nowak, Rigby, Henry, & Walens, 1998), however, it has also been shown to be amenable to use in practice based on other frameworks (Kielhofner, Henry, Walens, & Rogers, 1991). The OPHI, like any interview, is dependent on the therapist's skill at establishing rapport and eliciting information. The scaled questions are rated by the respondent, the narrative history is composed jointly by the therapist and respondent, and the life patterns are rated by the therapist. Reliability studies showed the original OPHI to be moderately stable, with high utility reported by therapists for assessing occupational performance (Kielhofner & Henry, 1988; Kielhofner et al., 1991).

Based on Rasch analysis of the 42 items of the scaled questionnaire, a second version of the OPHI was developed, called the OPHI-II (Kielhofner et al., 1998) (Table 6-1). The OPHI-II has three subscales representing occupational identity, occupational competence, and occupational behavioral settings (Mallinson, Mahaffey, & Kielhofner, 1998). Together these three scales examine the client's ability to sustain behavior patterns that are satisfying and productive, to maintain a positive occupational identity and to understand the impact of the environment on the individual (Kielhofner et al., 1998). This version of the OPHI is based specifically on concepts from the MOHO and requires at least a basic knowledge of the model. Increased specificity in the rating scales with the OPHI II has contributed to the reliability of the measure. International studies using the OPHI-II have shown that the three subscales are valid measures across cultures and languages (Kielhofner, Mallinson, Forsyth, & Lai, 2001).

OCCUPATIONAL SELF-ASSESSMENT

Table 6-2, the Occupational Self-Assessment (OSA) (Baron, Kielhofner, Iyenger, Goldhammer, & Wolenski, 2002) is a self-report measure that assists the client in establishing the priorities for change and goals for therapy. It captures the client's perceptions of their occupational competence and the impact of their environments on

Table 6-1

OCCUPATIONAL PERFORMANCE HISTORY INTERVIEW II

Source	Kielhofner, G. Mallinson, T., Crawford, C., Nowak, M., Rigby, M., Henry, A., & Walens, D. (1998). *The Occupational Performance History Interview* (Version 2.0) OPHI-II. Chicago, Il: Model of Human Occupation Clearinghouse.
Purpose	• The OPHI-II is designed to assess three constructs of occupational adaptation: occupational identity, occupational competence, and the impact of occupation behavior settings.
Type of Client	• Occupational therapy clients who are capable of responding to an in-depth interview.
Clinical Utility	
Format	• Semi-structured interview; administered by occupational therapist.
	• Rating scales: 3 scales—occupational identity, occupational competence, occupational behavior settings.
Procedures	• Life History Narrative: qualitative data from interview.
	• Therapist interviews client and completes rating scales and Life History Narrative.
Completion Time	• Approximately 1 hour.
Reliability	
Internal Consistency	• Not reported.
Observer	• Rater separation statistics indicated that raters have the same degree of severity and leniency.
Test-Retest	• Not reported.
Validity	
Content	• Using RASCH analysis methods, strong evidence that test items captured underlying traits. Low percentage of misfit statistics (8% to 9%) indicate validity across different subjects.
Criterion	• Not reported.
Construct	• Separation statistics indicate OPHI-II detects meaningful differences between persons and levels of competence.
Strengths	• OPHI-II can be readily learned through the manual, and used with a wide variety of clients. Validity evidence is stronger than the original OPHI.
Weaknesses	• Therapist rather than client assigns the scores.

their occupational adaptation. The OSA is another measure based on the MOHO (Kielhofner, 1995). Unlike the OPHI-II, the clients rate themselves through a questionnaire rather than the therapist deciding on the rating. In this regard, the OSA is a more client-centered measure. The OSA is a two-part measure that includes 21 items about occupational performance and eight items about the environment. All items are self-report, and, like the COPM, the OSA scores both performance and importance. A large international study using Rasch analysis confirms the unidimensionality and construct validity of the four subscales (Kielhofner & Forsyth, 2001).

CANADIAN OCCUPATIONAL PERFORMANCE MEASURE

Table 6-3, the Canadian Occupational Performance Measure (COPM) (Law et al., 1998), is a semi-structured interview aimed at identifying problems in occupational performance. The COPM was designed to correspond to the Canadian Model of Occupational Performance (CAOT, 1981, 1991, 1997). The COPM has three sections: self-care (activities of daily living and instrumental activities of daily living), productivity (education and work), and leisure (play, leisure, and social participation). The COPM offers two scores: performance and satisfac-

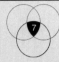

	Table 6-2
	OCCUPATIONAL SELF-ASSESSMENT
Source	Baron, K., Kielhofner, G., Ienger, A., Goldhammer, V., & Wolenski, J. (2002). *Occupational Self-Assessment Version 2.1.* Chicago: Model of Human Occupation Clearinghouse.
Purpose	• The OSA was designed to measure self-rated occupational performance and environmental adaptation, according to the Model of Human Occupation.
Type of Client	• All occupational therapy clients who can self-report.
Clinical Utility	
Format	• Two-part questionnaire, with 3 response options for each question.
Procedures	• Self-administered.
Completion Time	• 10 to 20 minutes.
Reliability	
Internal Consistency	• Not reported.
Observer	• Self-administered.
Test-Retest	• Not reported.
Validity	
Content	• Using Rasch analysis, no item misfits indicating that all four scales have internal
Criterion	validity. Scales valid for most subjects and order of item calibrations performed as
Construct	expected .
Strengths	• OSA performed well across different languages and cultures in an international study.
Weaknesses	• None noted.

tion with performance, both of which are self-rated by the client. In addition, identified occupational performance problems are weighted in terms of the importance of those activities. This serves to establish the client's priorities and leads very naturally into goal setting and treatment planning. The COPM has been used with a broad spectrum of clients in a wide variety of setting. It has been officially translated into 22 languages and is used in over 35 countries. The COPM has been shown to have good reliability, with values in the range of 0.80 for both the performance and satisfaction scales (Law et al, 1998). It has also been shown to be highly responsive to change, and approximately 10 published studies support its validity relative to various well-known measures. A review article has recently been published summarizing the results of approximately 85 research articles published in the last 10 years involving the COPM (Carswell et al., 2004).

Recently, there have been two new measures published, based on the structure of the COPM. The Self-Identified Goals Assessment (SIGA; Link-Melville, Baltic, Bettcher & Nelson, 2002) incorporates fixed alternative questions in an effort to increase ease of administration and to decrease administration time. The Client-Oriented Role Evaluation (Toal-Sullivan & Henderson, 2004) focuses on roles, and assesses each in terms of importance, performance and satisfaction with performance. Both of these measures have

had initial pilot work conducted, and the test authors recommend further psychometric evaluation.

OCCUPATIONAL CIRCUMSTANCE ASSESSMENT INTERVIEW AND RATING SCALE

Table 6-4, the Occupational Circumstances Assessment-Interview and Rating Scale (OCAIRS) (Deshpande, Kielhofner, Henriksson, Haglund, Olson, Forsyth, & Kulkarni, 2002) represents another instrument based on the MOHO frame of reference. It is derived from the Occupational Case Analysis Interview and Rating Scale (Kaplan & Kielhofner, 1989), and is aimed at assessing occupational adaptation and participation. Assessment with the OCAIRS involves a 40-minute interview to collect information on participation, personal causation, values and goals, interests, roles, habits, skills, and social and physical environments. Subsequent to the interview, the therapist completes a rating scale that defines areas of strength and weakness in terms of occupational adaptation, requiring an additional 15 minutes. This provides a profile of strengths and weaknesses relative to occupational performance. However, to obtain a score, it is necessary to submit the profile to a computer scoring procedure.

Table 6-3

THE CANADIAN OCCUPATIONAL PERFORMANCE MEASURE

Source	Law, M., Baptiste, S., Carswell, A., McColl, M. A., Polatajko, H. & Pollock, N. (1998). *The Canadian Occupational Performance Measure*. (3rd ed.). Toronto: CAOT.
Purpose	• The COPM was developed to be compatible with the Canadian Guidelines for client-centered practice (CAOT, 1981, 1991). It offers a measure of occupational performance that is based on a client-centered approach to practice.
Type of Client	• All occupational therapy clients.
Clinical Utility	
Format	• Administered in three sections corresponding to self-care, productivity and leisure.
	• Scores for performance and satisfaction with occupational performance.
Procedures	• Semi-structured interview, focusing on problem identification.
Completion Time	• Average of 30 to 40 minutes.
Reliability	
Internal Consistency	• 0.56 (performance); 0.71 (satisfaction) (Law et al., 1998).
Observer	• Not reported.
Test-Retest	• In the range of 0.80 for both subscales (Carswell et al., 2004).
Validity	
Content	• Based on the process of development (Law et al., 1998).
Criterion	• Based on relationships with a number of widely used measures and constructs—
Construct	for a review, see Carswell et al., 2004.
Strengths	• Clients find COPM helpful in identifying their problems; Therapists and other professionals find information helpful and unique; Intensifies focus on occupational performance in therapy.
Weaknesses	• Requires good interviewing skills to administer. Can be time consuming if focus on problem parameters, instead of just on problem identification.

The original OCAIRS was designed for use as a discharge planning tool for short-term psychiatric patients, but the current version is recommended for use with a wider range of clients. It has also been used successfully as a screening tool for occupational therapy services in acute mental health services. Results from the OCAIRS have been shown to compare very favorably with those on the Assessment of Occupational Functioning, and this is offered as proof for both of concurrent validity (Brollier, 1988). Studies by the authors and colleagues have shown moderate levels of inter-rater reliability and discriminant validity (Brollier, Watts, Bauer, & Schmidt, 1989; Haglund & Henriksson, 1994; Haglund, Thorell, & Walinder, 1998).

COMPARISONS OF THE FOUR MEASURES

The four measures reviewed have a number of notable similarities and some differences that make them more or less applicable in certain situations. An examination of the domains covered, the methods of administration, scoring, and psychometric properties highlight the commonalities and the differences.

Domain

At the most basic level, all four instruments clearly measure occupational performance: the COPM has three sections entitled self-care, productivity, and leisure; the OPHI-II and the OSA deal with occupational functioning and environmental impact; and the OCAIRS deals with occupational adaptation and participation.

Administration

All four measures are self-report to some extent, thus making them compatible with the client-centered approach. The measures differ in whether the client does the rating or the therapist completes the rating scales. On the COPM, clients identify problems and rate importance, performance, and satisfaction; on the OSA, clients rate performance and importance of occupational functioning

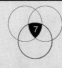

Table 6-4

OCCUPATIONAL CIRCUMSTANCES ASSESSMENT-INTERVIEW AND RATING SCALE (OCAIRS)

Source	Deshpande, S., Kielhofner, G., Henriksson, C., Haglund, L., Olson, L., Forsyth, K., & Kulkarni, S. (2002) *Model of Human Occupation*. Chicago: Clearinghouse.
Purpose	• The OCAIRS was designed to gather information on client's occupational adaptation.
Type of Client	• All occupational therapy clients who can participate in an interview.
Clinical Utility	
Format	• Semi-structured interview and therapist-scored rating scales.
Procedures	• Client is interviewed and therapist assigns ratings regarding strengths and weaknesses.
Completion Time	• Interview 40 minutes, rating scales 15 minutes.
Reliability	
Internal Consistency	• Not reported.
Observer	• Good inter-rater reliability; ICC=0.88 to 0.96.
Test-Retest	• Not reported.
Validity	
Content	• Content validity based on previous research with former version of OCAIRS.
Criterion	• Related positively to Assessment of Occupational Functioning (AOF).
Construct	• Discriminant validity—Differentiates different types of psychosocial dysfunction using Global Assessment Scale.
Strengths	• Overcomes weaknesses of previous version of OCAIRS. Effective screening for OT services.
Weaknesses	• Requires good interviewing skills to administer. Can be time consuming if focus on problem parameters, instead of just on problem identification.

and importance and availability of certain environments. On the OPHI-II, therapists rate the client's occupational identity, competence and behavior settings, and on the OCAIRS, therapists rate occupational adaptation according to four categories. Differences in the administration process may dictate which measure to use depending on the client population and the degree of structure required.

All four measures have in common that they are fairly demanding, with administration times typically between 30 minutes and an hour. The one exception is the OSA, which appears to take less time, at 10 to 20 minutes. However, in all cases, therapists and clients are quick to point out that the information dividends make the time investment worthwhile.

Scoring

Each of the measures has at least the potential to provide numerical total scores. The COPM yields scores for performance and satisfaction that can be used to compare outcomes before and after intervention. The OPHI-II

yields scores reflecting the client's occupational identity, competence and behavior settings. The OSA offers four ordinal scores representing performance and importance of occupational competence and environment. The OCAIRS yields a profile of occupational functioning, and scores can be computer-generated if needed.

Psychometric Properties

There is evidence of psychometric acceptability for all four measures, making them all worthy of consideration for applications in practice, management, and research.

CLIENT-CENTERED ASSESSMENT WITH CHILDREN

The ability to understand the subjective experience of children is often more difficult given their level of cognitive and language development. A recently developed measure has been shown to be useful with young children. The Perceived Efficacy and Goal Setting System (PEGS)

Table 6-5

PERCEIVED EFFICACY AND GOAL SETTING SYSTEM (PEGS)

Source	Missiuna, C., Pollock, N., & Law, M. (2004). *The perceived efficacy and goal setting system.* San Antonio, TX: PsychCorp.
Purpose	• The PEGS was developed as a goal-setting instrument for use with young children.
Type of Client	• Children ages 5 to 10 years.
Clinical Utility	
Format	• Children self-assess their perceived efficacy using pictures of daily activities and then set goals. Parallel parent and teacher questionnaires can be used.
Procedures	• Interview and questionnaire.
Completion Time	• Average of 15 minutes.
Reliability	
Internal Consistency	• Excellent Alpha coefficient 0.91 (Missiuna, 1998).
Observer	• Not reported.
Test-Retest	• Adequate Pearson coefficient 0.77 (Klein & Magill-Evans, 1998).
Validity	
Content	• Excellent based on the process of development (Missiuna et al., 2004).
Criterion	• Adequate—expected correlations with other related measures of performance and self efficacy (Missiuna et al., 2004).
Construct	• Excellent, hypotheses supported in validation study (Missiuna et al., 2004).
Strengths	• Children require a cognitive level of at least five years of age.
Weaknesses	• Children enjoy doing the PEGS. Therapists reported value as a negotiating tool and for increasing parent and teacher understanding of the scope of OT practice.

(Missiuna, Pollock, & Law, 2004) is designed for use with young children ages 5 to 10 years. Using pictures of children performing typical daily activities, the child rates their perceived efficacy in performing those activities and then using these responses, sets goals for therapy. Within the test items are activities representing the areas of self-care, productivity and leisure. Parallel teacher and parent questionnaires allow for caregiver perspectives to be included. The PEGS has just been published, so is not yet in wide use, but a more detailed review of the PEGS is included in Table 6-5.

ISSUES ARISING IN CLIENT-CENTERED ASSESSMENT OF OCCUPATIONAL PERFORMANCE

This chapter has reviewed four measures of occupational performance that are compatible with the client-centered approach to occupational therapy. As Frank (1996) states, "what really matters is that the work of understanding patients' lives is done well" (p. 252). Four issues that frequently arise in the use of client-centered

measurement of occupational performance are time, client insight, who the client is, and contextual fit.

With regard to time, occupational therapists frequently state that they do not have time for occupational performance assessments, since they are already heavily burdened with assessments of performance components. Therapists may feel that measures of occupational performance are an add-on to their already busy assessment schedule. The use of client-centered methods to identify the occupational performance problems should in fact save time, as they serve to focus on areas meaningful to the client and actively engage them in the therapeutic process from the outset. These methods free the therapist from more "comprehensive" or time-consuming assessment batteries that gather a great deal of data but may hold little relevance for the client.

A second issue frequently raised is client insight. All of the methods of client-centered assessment of occupational performance rely on the clients to articulate their occupational performance issues. It is important that we not make assumptions about a client's level of insight or ability to understand his or her own problems. Clinicians have been surprised on more than a few occasions by the ability of a client, previously thought to be incompetent, to articulate his or her needs. If we are to work with clients from a client-centered perspective, it is essential that we hear their perspective, regardless of our initial assessment of their cognitive functioning. As discussed earlier, the subjective experience of occupational performance is a key part of the assessment and can only be understood from the client's view. Furthermore, if we are to help people make changes in their occupational performance through therapy, we must respect their assessment of where their problems lie.

This raises a third issue, which is the importance of being clear about who the client is in client-centered practice. Our automatic assumption is that it is the person whose name is on the referral—the individual with a disability who has been recommended for occupational therapy. In many cases, this is true; however, there are a number of instances where it is not. By definition, a client is someone who is seeking the advice of a professional. In the therapeutic context, we would add a further idea to the definition—that a client is someone who wishes to make a change through a process of therapy. In most instances, our clients will be people with disabilities who wish to solve problems relating to their occupational performance, with the assistance of an occupational therapist. However, in some instances, individuals with disabilities will not be the ones in whom we expect to see change. This is an important idea to be clear about when discussing client-centered assessment, because if we are to assess our client (i.e., the person or environment in whom we seek to facilitate change), we must accurately identify the client and choose assessments that are appropriate to him, her, or it (the environment).

Here are three examples in which the client, or the person seeking to make a change, may not be the person whose name is on the referral.

Example #1

Imagine that you are working with a couple, one of whom has an irreversible cognitive disability, such as Alzheimer's disease. It is unlikely that you would seek to make changes in the way the ill spouse functions, but rather in the way the well spouse functions.

1. Who, then, is "the client?"
2. What might be the focus of therapy?
3. How does the decision about the identity of the client determine how your therapy will proceed?

The most appropriate focus for assessment would be the well spouse. Since he or she is the one who seeks to make changes through therapy, by definition, then, he or she becomes the client, and occupational therapy focuses

on issues around how to manage the ill spouse, how to best adapt the environment to promote healthy occupational performance, how to enlist support to sustain his or her own daily occupations. The identification of the client is the first step in pursuing a therapeutic agenda.

Example #2

Imagine you have a client with a disability who is having difficulty obtaining appropriate accommodations in the workplace. Which of the following would be an appropriate locus for change?
- The physical environment?
- The co-workers?
- The management?
- The job requirements?

Any or all of the above possibilities are appropriate targets for therapy, following an environmental approach to therapy. Your client remains the worker who has a disability, while all of these possible elements of his or her environment become potential areas where changes in the environment could help to enhance occupational performance.

Example #3

Imagine you are asked to see a child who is having difficulties at school. Recognizing the importance of the relationship with the parents and the teacher in achieving a successful outcome, you acknowledge the need to involve them all in the assessment process. At this point, which of the following two routes is preferable?

1. Treat the parents and teacher as informants about the child. If this were the case, who would be the focus of our questions? Who would we actually interview? In whom would we hope to see occupational changes?
2. Treat the child, parents, and teacher all as clients. In this case, whose occupational performance would we assess? Who would set therapy goals and timelines? How would you decide on priorities?

Either scenario is a perfectly reasonable approach for occupational therapy. In the first instance, you would interview all possible informants about the child's occupational performance, seeking their unique perspectives on the child's problems and capabilities. In the second instance, you would interview each informant about his or her own occupational performance.

A fourth issue to consider is the environmental context in which the therapist works. Client-centered therapy is difficult to practice in a system dominated by profession-als. The therapist needs to examine the values that guide his or her practice and look at the system within which he or she is working. Pragmatic issues such as team philoso-phies, reporting requirements, and limitations on length of stay can make it very challenging for the therapist striving to practice in a client-centered manner. It is important to analyze these factors and be aware of obstacles that may exist in the current system. Therapists also need to exam-ine whether they are truly interested in assessing occupa-tional performance or whether they have a fairly circum-scribed role that focuses on particular areas of function (e.g., practice in a hand clinic, where the emphasis is on impairments or performance components). Awareness of the "fit" of the practice model can go a long way toward overcoming barriers.

SUMMARY

The measurement of occupational performance requires attention to both the observable components of occupational performance (i.e., what the person actually does) and the subjective, experiential component (i.e., the meaning, importance, satisfaction, and temporal qualities of the occupational performance within the individual's life context). Four measures of occupational performance from a client-centered perspective have been reviewed. These measures share many commonalities, but are dis-tinct as well and may be more or less applicable in differ-ent situations.

Client-centered practice is based on a number of assumptions that differ from other models of practice. It is important to reflect on the implications of these assump-tions on the assessment process and the relationship with the client. Differences in philosophy, values, and context will impact on the use of these measures of occupational performance with clients and should be considered in the therapist's decision-making process.

ACKNOWLEDGMENTS

The authors acknowledge the assistance of Gary Kielhofner and of the other COPM authors (Sue Baptiste, Anne Carswell, Mary Law, and Helene Polatajko) in the preparation of this chapter.

REFERENCES

AOTA. (2002). Occupational therapy practice framework: Domain and process. *American Journal of Occupational Therapy, 56,* 609-639.

Baron, K., Kielhofner, G., Ienger, A., Goldhammer, V. & Wolenski, J. (2002). *Occupational self-assessment. Version 2.1.* Chicago: Model of Human Occupation Clearinghouse

Baum, C. M., & Law, M. (1997). Occupational therapy practice: Focusing on occupational performance. *American Journal of Occupational Therapy, 51(4),* 277-288..

Brollier, C. (1988). A concurrent validity study of two occupa-tional therapy evaluation instruments: AOF and OCAIRS. *Occupational Therapy in Mental Health, 8(4),* 49-60.

Brollier, C., Watts, J., Bauer, D., Schmidt, W. (1989). A concur-rent validity study of two occupational therapy evaluation instruments: The AOF and OCAIRS. *Occupational Therapy in Mental Health, 8(4),* 49-59.

Brown, S. J. (1992). Tailoring nursing care to the individual client: Empirical challenge of a theoretical concept. *Research in Nursing and Health, 15,* 39-46.

Canadian Association of Occupational Therapists (1981). *Occupational therapy guidelines for client-centered prac-tice* (1st ed.). Toronto, Ontario: Author.

Canadian Association of Occupational Therapists (1991). *Occupational therapy guidelines for client-centered prac-tice* (2nd ed.). Toronto, Ontario: Author.

Canadian Association of Occupational Therapists (1997). *Enabling occupation.* Ottawa: CAOT Publishing.

Carswell, A., McColl, M.A., Baptiste, S., Law, M., Polatajko, H., Pollock, N. (2004). The COPM: A research and clinical review. *Canadian Journal of Occupational Therapy, 71(4),* 210-222.

Dickerson, A. E. (1996). Should choice be a component in occu-pational therapy assessments? *Occupational Therapy in Health Care, 10(3),* 23-32.

Emener, W. G. (1991). Empowerment in rehabilitation: An empowerment philosophy for rehabilitation in the 20th century. *Journal of Rehabilitation, 57(4),* 7-12.

Frank, G. (1996). Life histories in occupational therapy clinical practice. *American Journal of Occupational Therapy,* 251-264.

Goodall, C. (1992). Preserving dignity for disabled people. *Nursing Standard, 6(35),* 25-27.

Haglund, L. & Henriksson, C. (1994). Testing a Swedish version of OCAIRS on two different patient groups. *Scandinavian Journal of Caring Sciences, 8,* 223-230.

Haglund, L., Thorell, L-H. & Walinder, J. (1998). Assessment of occupational functioning for screening of patients in occu-pational therapy in general psychiatric care. *Occupational Therapy in Mental Health, 18(4),* 193-206.

Henry, A., Baron, K., Mouradian, L., Curtin, C. (1998). Brief or new: Reliability and validity of the self-assessment of occu-pational functioning. *Canadian Journal of Occupational Therapy,* not a full reference; not in the text.

Jaffe, Y., & Kipper, D. A. (1982). Appeal of rational-emotive and client-centered therapies to first-year psychology and non-psychology students. *Psychological Reports, 50,* 781-782.

Kaplan, K., & Kielhofner, G. (1989). *The occupational case analysis interview and rating scale.* Thorofare,NJ: SLACK Incorporated.

Kielhofner, G. (1995). *A model of human occupation: Theory and application* (2nd ed.). Baltimore: Williams & Wilkins.

Kielhofner, G., & Forsyth, K. (2001). Measurement properties of a client self-report for treatment planning and documenting occupational therapy outcomes. *Scandinavian Journal of Occupational Therapy, 8,* 131-139.

Kielhofner, G., & Henry, A. D. (1988). Development and investigation of the Occupational Performance History Interview. *American Journal of Occupational Therapy, 42,* 489-498.

Kielhofner, G., Henry, A. D., Walens, D., & Rogers, E. S. (1991). A generalizability study of the Occupational Performance History Interview. *Occupational Therapy Journal of Research, 11,* 292-306.

Kielhofner, G., Mallinson, T., Crawford, D., Nowak, M., Rigby, M., Henry, A. & Walens. (1998). *User's manual for the OPHI-II.* Chicago, IL: Model of Occupational Performance Clearinghouse.

Kielhofner, G., Mallinson, T., Forsyth, K., & Lai, J. (2001). Psychometric properties of the second version of the Occupational Performance History Interview (OPHI-II). *American Journal of Occupational Therapy, 55,* 260-267.

Law, M., Baptiste, S., Carswell, A., McColl, M .A., Polatajko, H., & Pollock, N. (1994). *The Canadian Occupational Performance Measure* (2nd ed.). Toronto, Ontario: CAOT Publications.

Law, M., Baptiste, S., Carswell, A., McColl, M. A., Polatajko, H., & Pollock, N. (1998). *The Canadian Occupational Performance Measure.* (3rd ed.). Toronto, Ontario: CAOT Publications.

Link-Melville, L., Baltic, T.A., Bettcher, T.W., Nelson, D. (2002). Patients' perspectives on the self-identified goals assessment. *American Journal of Occupational Therapy, 56,* 650-659.

Mallinson, T., Mahaffey, L., & Kielhofner, G. (1998). The Occupational Performance History Interview: Evidence for three underlying constructs of occupational adaptation. *Canadian Journal of Occupational Therapy, 65(4),* 219-228.

Missuna, Pollock, & Law. (2004). *The perceived efficacy and goal setting system.* San Antonio, TX: PsychCorp.

Pollock, N. (1993). Client-centered assessment. *American Journal of Occupational Therapy, 47,* 298-301.

Pollock, N., Baptiste, S., Law, M., McColl, M. A., Opzoomer, A., & Polatajko, H. (1990). Occupational performance measures: A review based on the guidelines for client-centered practice. *Canadian Journal of Occupational Therapy, 57(2),* 82-87.

Pollock, N., & McColl, M. A. (1998). Assessment in client-centered practice. In M. Law (Ed.). *Client-centered occupational therapy.* Thorofare, NJ: SLACK Incorporated.

Rogers, C. (1965). *Client-centered therapy: Its current practice, implications and theory.* Boston: Houghton-Mifflin Co.

Schroeder, D. H., & Bloom, L. J. (1979). Attraction to therapy and therapist credibility as a function of therapy orientation. *Journal of Clinical Psychology, 35,* 683-686.

Toal-Sullivan, D., & Henderson, P. R. (2004). Client-Oriented Role Evaluation (CORE): the development of a clinical rehabilitation instrument to assess role change associated with disability. *American Journal of Occupational Therapy,* 58(2);211-20.

Trombly, C. (1993). Anticipating the future: Assessment of occupational function. *American Journal of Occupational Therapy, 47,* 253-257.

Wanigaratne, S., & Barker, C. (1995). Clients' preferences for styles of therapy. *British Journal of Clinical Psychology, 34,* 215-222.

Editors' Notes for Chapter 7

Mine the Gold

Social scientists and educators have studied the perspectives and contributions of others to the overall picture of performance. Constructs such as stress and caregiver burden inform us about the social environment of performance.

Become Systematic

Because family and other care providers are emotionally involved, we can hear their concerns about not taking advantage of the opportunity to incorporate their perspectives in systematic planning.

Use Evidence in Practice

Each of these measures provides comparison groups so you can determine the level of risk for disruptions to performance and track changes in behaviors with your interventions.

Make Occupational Therapy Contribution Explicit

Occupational therapists frequently have multiple cohorts as their clients within a family/community system. These measures acknowledge your interest in the social context as part of performance outcomes.

Engage in Occupation-Based, Client-Centered Practice

Occupational performance is a dynamic process that requires supports from cohorts in the family/community of interest. These measures enable us to acknowledge the client's support system and to obtain information that is valuable for intervention planning.

OCCUPATIONAL PERFORMANCE: MEASURING THE PERSPECTIVES OF OTHERS

Dorothy Edwards, PhD and Carolyn Baum, PhD, OTR/C, FAOTA

Humans live in a social context: a clan, a tribe, or family; some are connections of chance and others connections of choice (Howard, 1978). When occupational performance deficits occur, not only does the individual have to alter the processes that support the activities, tasks, and roles of daily life, but the family structure, tasks, and routines will change.

The household provides the context for a great deal of caregiving (Pruchno, 1990). In fact, data from the National Long-Term Care Survey shows that 85% of the care received by elders with impairments is provided by the family (Brody, 1990). Most family caregivers balance a number of other work and family responsibilities in addition to providing care and/or support to a dependent family member; these additional demands must be considered by the occupational therapist in planning services.

The providers of care, spouses, partners, siblings, children, or friends are critical to the long-term recovery of persons served by occupational therapy. Often these caregivers become our clients, too. Who are the caregivers? Pruchno (1990) studied individuals caring for elders at home. Fifty-one percent of the caregivers were spouses (12.5% husbands, 38.5% wives). Forty-five percent were children (38.5% daughters, 6.5% sons), and 4.5% were others. Nearly 70% of the sample was married. Cicirelli (1983) demonstrated that adult children provide significant social and community support; however, help with maintenance of daily life was not as frequent because of competing responsibilities such as family and jobs. Birkel and Jones (1989) reported that household insularity is associated with a downward spiral of performance and motivation affecting all household members.

How does the occupational therapist identify the family members' issues? To fully understand occupational performance, the individual's characteristics, the environment, the nature of and meaning of the occupations that the individual wants or needs to perform, and the impact these factors have on others must be understood. When the family is, or perceives that it has been, excluded in the care planning process, it may not acquire the skills to enable loved ones to achieve higher levels of occupational performance.

There continues to be some controversy about proxy report, or accepting a family member's rating of the performance of an individual. The use of proxy respondents is common in epidemiological research (Nelson, Longstreth, Koepsell, & Van Belle, 1990). However, until very recently, little has been published about the reliability of proxy respondents in evaluating functional capacity and even less in evaluating occupational performance. It is very important to differentiate between proxy reports and caregiver reports. We often rely on the caregiver's perceptions of the occupational performance of a family member. The Functional Behavior Profile (FBP) (Baum, Edwards, & Morrow-Howell, 1993), for example, records the caregiver's observations and impressions about the client's ability to perform tasks, solve problems, and engage in social interaction. A proxy report, on the other hand, records the family member's estimate of the client's evaluation of his or her own performance.

Segal, Gilliard, and Schall (1996) examined the reliability of proxy responses to the Functional Independence Measure (FIM) with 25 stroke patients following stroke. They found overall agreement for total scores (ICC, or intra-class correlation 40.91). The ICC for the physical dimension scores was 0.94 and 0.52 for the cognitive dimension scores. Dorman, Waddell, Slattery, Dennis, and Sandercock (1997) evaluated the reliability of friends and relatives of 152 stroke patients on the EuroQol, a measure of health related quality of life. The mobility and self-care scales agreement between proxy and subject was 80% and 76% for social functioning; however, agreement was less accurate in describing pain and emotional status. Sneeuw, Aaronson, deHaan, and Limburg (1997), using the Sickness Impact Profile (SIP) with a sample of 437 persons interviewed 6 months after their first stroke, reported similar findings. Intraclass correlation coefficients were used. Good to excellent agreements (ICCs>0.60) were found for ambulation, body care and movement, mobility, household management, and recreation and pastimes. The eating scale had the lowest agreement (0.43).

Todorov and Kirchener (2000) examined differences between self-reports and proxy reports of disabilities among more than 50,000 respondents to the National Health Interview Survey on Disability. This representative continuing nationwide household survey of adults aged 18 and older. They found systematic differences between self and proxy reports of disabilities. For younger persons (18 to 65 years of age) proxy respondents were likely to under-report difficulties, while for older persons, proxies were likely to over-report disabilities. They also found that the highest levels of agreement were associated with disabilities that were visible as opposed to problems that were not obvious in the course of normal social interaction. This study did not include any information from clinical observations or performance based assessments.

Few studies compare actual performance to self-reports and proxy ratings. In one important study, Joan Rodgers and colleagues (2003) determined the level of agreement between self-report, proxy report, and performance testing in the clinic and the participants' homes with a sample of community dwelling older women with arthritis. Proxy reports were obtained from spouses, daughters, and friends of the participant. The proxy reporters spent on average, almost 40 hours per week with the participant. They found the highest levels of agreement between self-report, proxy report and in-home performance based testing for measures of personal care, cognitive Instrumental Activities of Daily Living (IADL) and functional mobility. In these domains, the authors concluded that when older adults are unable or unwilling to provide disability data, information from proxies who are knowledgeable about daily living habits may be reliably substituted. The authors also stress that when proxy information is used, it is essential to ascertain their level of familiarity with the elders daily routines.

Parents are assumed to be the best source of information about their children, yet few studies have actually examined the accuracy of compared parental reports. Waters, Brown and Fitzpatrick (2003), examined parent and adolescent agreement on physical, emotional, mental and social health and well being in a representative sample of 2096 parent child dyads. Overall, they found high levels of agreement for physical health. Significant parent child differences were observed for social health, school enjoyment and performance ratings.

In a study of 37 children with central nervous system tumors, the greatest agreement on the Lansky Play-Performance Scale and the Karnofsky Performance Scale occurred between parents and children; physiotherapists and physicians agreed less well on cognition, emotion, and pain (Glaser, Davies, Walker, & Brazier, 1997). In a large epidemiological study, Whiteman and Green (1997) examined the agreement between parents and children, concluding that the level of agreement is highly dependent on the type of information sought and the way the questions are asked. A large study of health related quality of life in pediatric bone marrow transplant survivors (Parsons, Barlow, Levy, Supran, & Kaplan, 1999) found that children's self-reported health status was more highly correlated with physician's disease severity ratings than parental reports. However, parent reports of mental health and quality of life were concordant with the child's ratings of the same domains.

The adult and children studies consistently find that proxies are best at reporting on observable phenomena, such as performance of activities of daily living (ADL) and IADL tasks, and less accurate at reporting the internal or emotional states of the client. Actually having a family observation of an individual's performance is quite helpful in planning care. If there is a gap between the family's observation and the objective testing of the practitioner, the discrepancy identifies the factors that need to be discussed in planning for discharge and follow-up care.

There are three basic areas of inquiry central to the occupational therapist's approach to planning follow-up care: 1) the caregiver's readiness to assume the role of caregiver, 2) the caregiver's observation of the occupational performance of the family member, and 3) the caregiver's perception of stress and burden of care. Each of these must be considered in building a client-centered plan of care that will require the participation of the family.

The following assessments (Tables 7-1 through 7-7) were chosen to address these questions. They should be administered after institutional discharge and after the family has some experience managing the loved one at home. An occupational performance approach requires the practitioner to address the needs and expectations of others as they influence the performance of the client. The following measures will help the occupational therapist bring others with their observations, capacities and commitment into the plan of care.

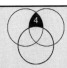

Table 7-1

PARENTING STRESS INDEX (PSI)

Source	Psychological Assessment Resources, Inc., PO Box 998, Odessa, FL, 33556, (phone) 800-331-TEST
Important References	Abidin, R. R. (1995). *Parenting Stress Index: Professional manual* (3rd ed.). Odessa, FL: PAR.
	Abidin, R. R., Jenkins, C. L., & McGaughey, M. C. (1992). The relationship of early family variables on children's subsequent behavioral adjustment. *Journal of Clinical Child Psychology, 21,* 60-69.
	Beckman, P. J. (1991). Comparisons of mothers' and fathers' perceptions of the effect of young children with and without disabilities. *American Journal of Mental Retardation, 95,* 585-595.
	Esdaile, S. A., Greenwood, K. M. (2003). A comparison of mothers' and fathers' experience of parenting stress and attributions for parent child interaction outcomes. *Occupational Therapy International, 10(2),* 115-126.
	Innocenti, M. S., Huh, K., & Boyce, G. C. (1992). Families of children with disabilities: Normative data on parenting stress. *Topics in Early Childhood Special Education, 12,* 403-427.
	Thomas, K. A., Renaud, M. T., & Depaul, D. (2004) Use of parenting stress index in mothers of preterm infants. *Advances in Neonatal Care. 4(1),* 33-41.
Purpose	• Designed to assess stressful parent-child systems and the impact of intervention.
Type of Client	• Parents of children ranging in age from 1 month to 12 years.
Clinical Utility	
Format	• Self-administered 120-item test booklet, with Likert scale response choices.
	• Three additive sources of stress are evaluated: 1) Child characteristics (distractibility/hyperactivity, adaptability, reinforces parent, demandingness, mood, acceptability); 2) Parent characteristics (competence, isolation, attachment, role restriction, depression, spouse, total stress, and life stress); and 3) Situational/demographic life stress.
	• A 36-item short form derived from the long form has also been validated.
	• Test poses no difficulty for persons with a fifth grade or higher education.
Procedures	• Responses are recorded in the test booklet, then either scoring templates or a computer scoring program are used to create scale scores. Items may be read to the respondent.
Completion Time	• The average completion time is about 20 minutes for the long form and 10 minutes for the short form.

continued

The measures included in this chapter were selected to illustrate different approaches to the assessment of occupational performance from the perspective of significant others in the client's life. Each of the scales meets the necessary criteria for reliability and validity. Each will also enable an occupational therapist to obtain important information about the client. Several of the scales, such as the Parenting Stress Index (PSI) (see Table 7-1), are very well established; while other scales, such as the FBP (see Table 7-7) and the School Function Assessment (SFA) (see Table 7-2), which were developed by occupational therapists are emerging as important clinical tools for practice.

Table 7-1 (continued)

PARENTING STRESS INDEX

Standardization	• The original normative sample was comprised of 2633 mothers recruited from well child pediatric clinics. Ethnic and socioeconomic groups were proportionately represented. Data were also collected from a similarly representative sample of 200 fathers. A Spanish version of the test was developed using 233 Hispanic parents in New York.
Reliability	
Internal Consistency	• Not reported.
Observer	• Rater separation statistics indicated that raters have the same degree of severity and leniency.
Test-Retest	• Not reported.
Validity	
Content	• Using RASCH analysis methods, strong evidence that test items captured underlying traits. Low percentage of misfit statistics (8 to 9%) indicate validity across different subjects.
Criterion	• Not reported.
Construct	• Separation statistics indicate OPHI-II detects meaningful differences between persons and levels of competence.
Strengths	• OPHI-II can be readily learned through the manual, and used with a wide variety of clients. Validity evidence is stronger than the original OPHI.
Weaknesses	• Therapist rather than client assigns the scores.

Table 7-2

SCHOOL FUNCTION ASSESSMENT (SFA)

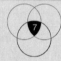

Source	Psychological Corporation, Skill Builders Division, 555 Academic Court, San Antonio, TX, 78204, (phone) 800-228-0752
Important References	American Occupational Therapy Association (1997). *Occupational therapy services for children and youth under the Individuals with Disabilities Education Act.* Bethesda, MD: Author.
	Coster, W. (1998). Occupation centered assessment of children. *American Journal of Occupational Therapy, 52,* 337-344.
	Davies, P. L., Soon, P. L., Young, M., & Clausen-Yamaki, A. (2003). Validity and reliability of the school function assessment in elementary school students with disabilities. *Physical and Occupational Therapy in Pediatrics, 24(3),* 23-43.
Purpose	• This scale is used to measure a student's performance of functional tasks that support his or her participation in the academic and social aspects of an elementary school program. It was designed to facilitate collaborative program planning for students with a variety of disabling conditions.
Type of Client	• Child enrolled in elementary school. Assesses participation, task supports, and activity performance.
Clinical Utility	
Format	• The rating scales are administered to respondents who are familiar with the student's typical performance. Teachers, OTs, PTs, and SLPs as well as classroom and therapy assistants may serve as respondents.

continued

Table 7-2 (continued)

SCHOOL FUNCTION ASSESSMENT (SFA)

Procedures	• The rating form has 26 scales; each scale is scored using a 4- or 6-level rating, depending on the item. For example, functional activities ratings range from 1 (does not perform) to 4 (consistent performance). • The assessment is completed by the team, either under the supervision of a coordinator who contacts individual team members and records their scores, or by the team collaboratively completing the assignment together.
Completion Time	• Completion time is not reported.
Standardization	• Pools of items were developed by reviewing existing standardized and nonstandardized tests, published literature on the requirements for successful school performance, and published and unpublished curricula for students with disabilities. A set of 539 items was submitted to expert reviewers. IRT analysis was then computed. A reduced set of items was then tested with a sample of 363 students with disabilities, drawn from 112 sites in 40 states and Puerto Rico. Criterion and cut-off scores were then developed using a sample of 318 non-disabled students.
Reliability	
Internal Consistency	• Coefficient alpha's ranged from 0.92 to 0.98. Fit statistics using IRT methods were also computed. The fit statistics confirmed the coherence of the items within each scale.
Test-Retest	• Test-retest studies were conducted using intervals ranging from 2 to 4 weeks. Reliability coefficients (both Pearson's r's and intraclass coefficients) ranged from 0.80 to 0.99. The lowest coefficients were on the task support items.
Validity	
Content	• Two content validity studies were completed. The first used a sample of 30 content experts who were asked to rate the comprehensiveness and relevance of the items. A second study involved a field trial of the SFA with 40 students. Related service professionals assessed students and then provided an evaluation of the relevance, comprehensiveness, and usefulness of the items and ratings scales.
Construct	• A series of Rasch, multiple regression, and IRT analyses tested each aspect of construct validity. The scales were found to have excellent predictive and discriminative power.
Overall Utility·	• The SFA was very carefully developed and appears to be a very practical and empirically robust measure. The scale was designed to reflect current models of function and special education legislation. It will help organize the input from a number of different sources into an assessment used to plan and evaluate interventions for school-aged children. The manual is informative and easy to read. • This is a new assessment with content that is well-referenced. However, as it is new, the scale itself is not yet referenced in any scholarly publications.

Table 7-3

COPING INVENTORY FOR CHILDREN

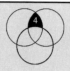

Source	Scholastic Testing Service, Inc.
Important References	Williamson, G., Szczepanski, M., & Zeitlin, S. (1993). Coping frame of reference. In P. Kramer & J. Hinojosa (Eds.), *Frames of reference in pediatric occupational therapy* (pp. 395-436). Baltimore: Williams & Wilkins.
	Williamson, G., & Zeitlin, S. (1990). Assessment of coping and temperament: Contributions to adaptive functioning. In E. D. Gibbs & D. M. Teti (Eds.), *Interdiscipinary assessment of infants: A guide for early intervention professionals* (pp. 215-226). Baltimore: Paul H. Brookes.
	Williamson, G. , Zeitlin, S., & Szczepanski, M. (1989). Coping behavior: Implications for disabled infants and toddlers. *Infant Mental Health Journal, 10*, 3-13.
	Zeitlin, S. (1985). *Coping inventory.* Bensenville, IL: Scholastic Testing Service, Inc.
	Zeitlin, S., & Williamson, G. (1990). Coping characteristics of disabled and nondisabled young children. *American Journal of Orthopsychiatry, 60*, 404-411.

Purpose
- To assess the coping style of children 3 years and older.

Type of Client
- Children 3 years and older.

Clinical Utility

Format
- A questionnaire that may be completed by a professional or a parent.
- Children's styles of coping are rated in two categories: 1) Coping with Self (confidence, task persistence, generalization of learning, creativity and originality, sense of self-worth, and expression of personal needs), and 2) Coping with the Environment (curiosity, awareness of feelings of others, resiliency following disappointment, ability to follow instructions, awareness of/response to social expectations, acceptance of warmth and support from others).

Procedure
- The rater scores the child's behaviors on a 5-point rating scale, in which 1 is "not effective" and 5 is "consistently effective across situations." Effectiveness means that the behavior is 1) appropriate for situations, 2) appropriate for the child's developmental age, and 3) used successfully by the child.
- The manual encourages ratings based on the child's context, so as to include cultural expectations as part of the rating.

Completion Time
- It takes approximately 30 minutes to complete the inventory.

Reliability
- Inter-rater reliability coefficients 0.80 to 0.94 for the two categories.

Validity
- A series of studies (see references) provide construct and content validity.

Overall Utility
- Excellent tool for not only assessing coping skills, but also providing information to family and team members about the child's strategies, and offers a perspective about the child's reactions to environmental demands that is not available from other tools.

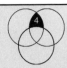

Table 7-4

EARLY COPING INVENTORY

Source	Scholastic Testing Service, Inc.
Important References	Williamson, G., Szczepanski, M., & Zeitlin, S. (1993). Coping frame of reference. In P. Kramer & J. Hinojosa (Eds.), *Frames of reference in pediatric occupational therapy* (pp. 395-436). Baltimore: Williams & Wilkins.
	Williamson, G., & Zeitlin, S. (1990). Assessment of coping and temperament: Contributions to adaptive functioning. In E. D. Gibbs & D. M. Teti (Eds.), *Interdisciplinary assessment of infants: A guide for early intervention professionals* (pp. 215-226). Baltimore: Paul H. Brookes.
	Williamson, G. , Zeitlin, S., & Szczepanski, M. (1989). Coping behavior: Implications for disabled infants and toddlers. *Infant Mental Health Journal, 10,* 3-13.
	Zeitlin, S. (1985). *Coping inventory.* Bensenville, IL: Scholastic Testing Service, Inc.
	Zeitlin, S., & Williamson, G. (1990). Coping characteristics of disabled and nondisabled young children. *American Journal of Orthopsychiatry, 60,* 404-411.
Purpose	• To assess the coping style of children 3 years and younger.
Type of Client	• Infants and toddlers.
Clinical Utility	
Format	• May be completed by a professional or a parent.
	• Examines children's styles of coping in three categories (16 items in each category =48 items): 1) sensorimotor organization (behaviors that regulate psychophysiological functions and integrate sensory and motor information), 2) reactive behaviors (actions that enable the child to respond to demands of the environment), and 3) self-initiated behaviors (self-directed, autonomously generated actions that meet personal needs and provide interaction opportunities).
Procedures	• The rater scores the child's behaviors to yield three different types of scores: an adaptive behavior index, a coping profile (using a 5-point rating scale), and a list of most and least adaptive coping behaviors.
Completion Time	• It takes approximately 30 minutes to complete the inventory.
Reliability	• Inter-rater reliability coefficients 0.80 to 0.94 for the categories.
Validity	• A series of studies (see references) provide construct and content validity.
Overall Utility	• This is an excellent tool for not only assessing coping skills, it provides information to family and team members about the child's strategies, and offers a perspective about the child's reactions to environmental demands that is not available from other tools.

Table 7-5

Vineland Adaptive Behavior Scales (VABS)

Source	American Guidance Service Inc., 4201 Woodland Rd., Circle Pines, MN, 55014, (phone) 800-328-2560
Important References	Beail, N. (2003). Utility of the Vineland Adaptive Behavior Scales in diagnosis and research with adults who have mental retardation. *Mental Retardation, 41(4)*, 286-289.
	Fenton, G., D'Ardiac, Valente D., Del Vecchio, I., Fabrizi, A., Bernabei, P. (2003). Vineland Adaptive Behavior profiles in children with autism and moderate to developmental delay. *Autism, 7(3)*, 269-87.
	Middleton, H. A., Keene, R. G., & Brown, G. W. (1990). Convergent and discriminant validities of the Scales of Independent Behavior and the Revised Vineland Adaptive Behavior Scales. *American Journal on Mental Retardation, 94*, 669-673.
	Rosenbaum, P., Saigal, S., Szatmari, P., & Hoult, L. (1995). Vineland Adaptive Behavior Scales as a summary of functional outcome of extremely low-birthweight children. *Developmental Medicine and Child Neurology, 37*, 577 586.
Purpose	• To assess the adaptive behaviors of children with disabilities.
Type of Client	• Children from birth to 18 years.
Clinical Utility	
Format	• Activities of daily living, cognition, language, play, and social competency from another person's perspective.
Procedures	• The rater may be a parent, health professional, or a teacher. The rater scores the child's behaviors after conducting an interview with the respondent. Scoring is completed using a 3-point rating scale. The manual and instructions are excellent but training is required before a person can administer this measure.
Completion Time	• It takes approximately 20 to 30 minutes to complete this measure, but longer to score it.
Reliability	
Internal Consistency	• 0.78 to 0.94.
Inter-Rater	• 0.96.
Test-Retest	• 0.77 to 0.98.
Validity	
Content	• Has been established through a review of the literature to identify items and through subsequent factor analytic techniques.
Construct	• Many studies have been completed with this measure. Results indicate that scores on the VABS follow a developmental progression and that the VABS successfully differentiates children with and without difficulties in adaptive behavior.
Criterion	• Studies indicate moderate correlations with the Kaufman Assessment Battery and high correlations between the VABS and other measures of adaptive behavior.
Overall Utility	• This is an excellent tool the assessment of adaptive behavior skills in children and youth. The manual provides extensive guidance for administration and interpretation, including guidance for structuring the assessment interview. Users are cautioned that the scoring and interpretation of the scores is time-consuming and requires training.

Table 7-6

MEMORY AND BEHAVIOR PROBLEMS CHECKLIST: REVISED

Source	Teri, L., Truax, P., Logsdon, R., Zarit, S., Uomoto, J., & Vitaliano, P. (1992). Assessment of behavioral problems in dementia. *Psychology and Aging, 7,* 622-631.
Important References	Baum, C. M. (1995). The contribution of occupation to function in persons with Alzheimer's disease. *Journal of Occupation Science: Australia, 2(2)*, 59-67.
	Teri, L., Borson, S., Kiyak, A., & Yamagishi, M. (1989). Behavioral disturbance, cognitive function, and functional skill. *Journal of the American Geriatrics Society, 37,* 109-116.
	Zarit, S., & Zarit, J. (1983). Cognitive impairment. In P. M. Lewinson & L. Teri (Eds.), *Clinical Geropsychology* (pp. 38-81). Elmsford, NY: Pergamon Press.

Purpose
- This scale is a caregiver report measure of behavioral problems in older adults. The scale was developed for use with persons with dementia but can be used with any older adult with suspected cognitive impairment.
- The scale also assesses the caregiver's reaction or emotional response to the specific behavioral problem. In this way it is both a measure of problem behaviors and caregiver burden.
- The scale was designed to be useful for both clinical and research settings. It enables clinicians and researchers to pinpoint areas of disturbance and target intervention goals for patients and caregivers.

Type of Client
- Older adult and his or her caregiver. The scale was developed and standardized on a sample of older adults evaluated by a geriatric and family services clinic at the University of Washington School of Medicine. Persons with and without dementia were included. The caregivers in the study were all family members. The scale has also been used in institutional settings with non-family paid caregivers.

Clinical Utility

Format
- The revised version of the scale consists of 24 items; both the frequency of the problem behavior is recorded and the caregiver's reaction to the behavior is rated using 5-point Likert ratings. The scale provides subscale scores for memory-related problems, disruptive behaviors, and depression.
- The previous version of the scale also included ADL and IADL performance. The earlier version of the scale has 30 items and uses the same format and rating scales.

Procedures
- The scale is designed as a paper and pencil measure to be completed by caregivers. It can also be read to caregivers as part of a face-to-face or telephone interview.

Completion Time
- The scale takes approximately 10 minutes to complete.

Standardization
- The original 30-item scale was supplemented with an additional 34 items developed by authors. The items all represent easily observed specific behaviors representative of memory-related problems, depression, and disruptive behaviors. This 64-item measure was administered to 201 consecutive patients and their accompanying caregivers who participated in a comprehensive physical, psychological, and neuropsychological assessment at the University of Washington. The mean age of the patient was 74; 65% were female; the sample was socioeconomically diverse.

Reliability

Internal Consistency
- Coefficient alphas were computed for the frequency and reaction scores for each dimension (memory-related problems, depression, and disruptive behaviors). They ranged from 0.67 to 0.89.

continued

Table 7-6 (continued)

MEMORY AND BEHAVIOR PROBLEMS CHECKLIST: REVISED

Test-Retest	• Test-retest reliability for the new scale has not been reported. Studies conducted with the original version used intervals ranging from 2 to 4 weeks. Reliability coefficients (both Pearson r's and intraclass coefficients) ranged from 0.80 to 0.99.
Validity	
Content	• The first item reduction was conducted by a group of professional raters who grouped the items into the three theoretical content areas. Then, the items were independently sorted by three experts into the three areas. Agreement was needed between two of the three raters for an item to be retained. Forty-seven items were retained.
Construct	• The 47 items were subjected to principal components analysis with a varimax rotation. The 19 items with loadings of less than 0.36 were deleted. A second set of factor analyses were computed using the reduced item set. Three factors accounting for 53% of the variance were derived.
Overall Utility	• This scale is one of the most widely used measures documenting problem behaviors in older adults. It is an easy to use, easy to score, reliable, and valid method of assessing the overall level of behavioral problems and the degree of specific areas of behavioral dysfunction. It also provides an index of caregiver reactivity.

Table 7-7

FUNCTIONAL BEHAVIOR PROFILE

Source	Dr. Carolyn Baum, Program in Occupational Therapy, Box 8505, Washington University School of Medicine, 4444 Forest Park Blvd., St. Louis, MO, 63108.
Important References	Baum, C. M., Edwards, D. F., & Morrow-Howell, N. (1993). Identification and measurement of productive behaviors in senile dementia of the Alzheimer type. *The Gerontologist, 33*, 403-408.
	Kovach, C. R., & Henschel, H. (1996). Planning activities for patients with dementia: a descriptive study of therapeutic activities on special care units. *Journal of Gerontological Nursing, 22(9)*, 33-38.
	Baum, C. M., & Edwards, D. F. (2000). Documenting productive behaviors: Using the Functional Behavior Profile to plan discharge following stroke. *Journal of Gerontological Nursing, 26(4)*, 34-43.
	Baum, C. M., Perlmutter, M., & Edwards, D. F. (2000). Measuring function in Alzheimer's disease. *Alzheimer's Care Quarterly, 1(3)*, 44-61.
	Baum, C. M., & Edwards, D. F. (2003). What persons with Alzheimer's disease can do: A tool for communication about daily activities. *Alzheimer's Care Quarterly, 4(2)*, 108-118.
Purpose	• This scale is used to provide information to clinicians and caregivers about the remaining capabilities of persons with cognitive loss. Information of residual capacities can be used for the development of treatment plans or to structure caregiver education.
Type of Client	• Adults with cognitive impairments. The test was developed for persons with Alzheimer's disease. The scale has also been used with persons with stroke and head injury in both community and hospital settings.

continued

Table 7-7 (continued)

FUNCTIONAL BEHAVIOR PROFILE

Clinical Utility

Format
- Caregivers are asked to report productive behaviors (ability to perform tasks, solve problems, and socially interact with others) using a 5-point Likert scale.
- The 27 items represent three domains: problem-solving, task performance, and socialization. Each item is scored from 0 (never) to 4 (always)—the lower the score, the poorer the performance. Scores are summed by domain.

Procedures
- This paper and pencil measure can be used as part of a face-to-face interview or completed independently by the caregiver.
- The rating scales are administered to persons familiar with the patient's/client's behavior. Any caregiver who has been able to observe behavior over time should be able to answer the questions

Completion Time
- The questionnaire takes 15 minutes or less to complete.

Standardization
- The test was modeled after the Comprehensive Occupational Therapy Evaluation (COTE) developed for the assessment of psychiatric patients (Brayman et al., 1976).
- The item pool was developed after extensive family interviews with caregivers participating in the family support group sponsored by the Memory and Aging Project at the Washington University Alzheimer's Disease Research Center. A set of 51 items was administered to 106 family caregivers. Principal component analysis with a varimax rotation was used. Three composite scales were created.
- The manual is informative and easy to read.

Reliability

Internal Consistency
- Coefficient alphas ranged from 0.94 to 0.96.

Test-Retest
- Test-retest studies were not conducted.

Validity

Content
- Content validity is reflected in the loadings of the items with the three factors. The loadings ranged from 0.50 to 0.82. Simple structure was achieved for 23 of the 27 items. The four items loading on more than one factor can be explained by the complexity of the behavior being evaluated.

Construct
- Construct validity was determined through comparison with three measures commonly used to assess persons with dementia: the Blessed Dementia Scale, the Memory and Behavior Problems Checklist, and the Katz ADL Scale. Each of these scales relies on a caregiver's report of functional status. Correlations ranged from 0.66 to 0.86.

Overall Utility
- Easy to administer scale that yields information that can be used for treatment planning, caregiver education and training, and research.
- Sensitive to the differences in capacity associated with progression of dementia even at the earliest, most mild stage. It is a practical and empirically robust measure.
- Differs from other functional measures in that it records what the patient/client can do rather than what he or she can't do.
- The scale can be used in community, long-term care, and inpatient treatment settings, by family members, friends, or paid caregivers. The scale is easily scored and interpreted, providing meaningful information for the support of persons with cognitive impairment.

REFERENCES

Abidin, R. R. (1995) *Parenting Stress Index: Professional manual* (3rd ed.). Odessa, FL: Psychological Assessment Resources.

Abidin, R. R., Jenkins, C. L., & McGaughey, M. C. (1992). The relationship of early family variables on children's subsequent behavioral adjustment. *Journal of Clinical Child Psychology, 21*, 60-69.

American Occupational Therapy Association (1997). *Occupational therapy services for children and youth under the Individuals with Disabilities Education Act.* Bethesda, MD: Author.

Baum, C. M. (1995). The contribution of occupation to function in persons with Alzheimer's disease. *Journal of Occupation Science: Australia, 2(2)*, 59-67.

Baum, C. M., Edwards, D. F., & Morrow-Howell, N. (1993). Identification and measurement of productive behaviors in senile dementia of the Alzheimer type. *The Gerontologist, 33(3)*, 403-408.

Baum, C. M., & Edwards, D. F. (2000). Documenting productive behaviors: Using the Functional Behavior Profile to plan discharge following stroke. *Journal of Gerontological Nursing, 26(4)*, 34-43.

Baum, C. M., Perlmutter, M., & Edwards, D. F. (2003). Measuring function in Alzheimer's disease. *Alzheimer's Care Quarterly, 1(3)*, 44-61.

Baum, C. M., & Edwards, D. F. (2003). What persons with Alzheimer's disease can do: A tool for communication about daily activities. *Alzheimer's Care Quarterly, 4(2)*, 108-118.

Beckman, P. J. (1991). Comparisons of mothers' and fathers' perceptions of the effect of young children with and without disabilities. *American Journal of Mental Retardation, 95*, 585-595.

Birkel, R. C., & Jones, C. J. (1989). A comparison of the caregiving networks of dependent elderly individuals who are lucid and those who are demented. *Gerontologist, 29(1)*, 114-119.

Brayman, S. J., Kirby, T. F., Misenheimer, A. M., & Short, M. J. (1976). Comprehensive occupational therapy evaluation scale. *American Journal of Occupational Therapy, 30*, 94-100.

Brody, E. M. (1990). The family at risk. In E. Light & B. D. Lebowitz (Eds.), *Alzheimer's disease treatment and family stress: Directions for research* (pp. 2-49). New York: Hemisphere.

Cicirelli, V. G. (1983). A comparison of helping behavior to elderly parents of adult children with intact and disrupted marriages. *The Gerontologist, 23*, 619-625.

Coster, W. (1998). Occupation centered assessment of children. *American Journal of Occupational Therapy, 52*, 337-344.

Dorman, P. J., Waddell, F., Slattery, J., Dennis, M., & Sandercock, P. (1997). Are proxy assessments of health status after stroke with the EuroQol questionnaire feasible, accurate and unbiased? *Stroke, 28*, 1883-1887.

Glaser, A. W., Davies, K., Walker, D., & Brazier, D. (1997). Influence of proxy respondents and mode of administration on health status assessment following central nervous system tumors in childhood. *Quality of Life Research, 6(1)*, 43-53.

Howard, J. (1978). *Families.* New York: Simon and Schuster.

Innocenti, M. S., Huh, K., & Boyce, G. C. (1992). Families of children with disabilities: Normative data on parenting stress. *Topics in Early Childhood Special Education, 12*, 403-427.

Kovach, C. R., & Henschel, H. (1996). Planning activities for patient's with dementia: A descriptive study of therapeutic activities on special care units. *Journal of Gerontological Nursing, 22(9)*, 33-38.

Middleton, H. A., Keene, R. G., & Brown, G.W. (1990). Convergent and discriminant validities of the Scales of Independent Behavior and the Revised Vineland Adaptive Behavior Scales. *American Journal on Mental Retardation, 94*, 669-673.

Nelson, L. M., Longstreth, W. T., Jr., Koepsell, T. D., & Van Belle, G. (1990). Proxy respondents in epidemiologic research. *Epidemiological Review, 12*, 71-86.

Parsons, S.K., Barlow, S.E., Levy, S.L., Supran, S.E. & Kaplan. (1999). Health related quality of life in pediatric bone marrow transplant survivors: according to whom? *International Journal of Cancer (Supplement), 12*, 46-51.

Pruchno, R. A. (1990). Alzheimer's disease and families: Methodological advances. In E. Light & B. D. Lebowitz (Eds.), *Alzheimer's disease treatment and family stress: Directions for research* (pp. 174-197). New York: Hemisphere.

Rodgers, J.C., Holm, M.B., Beach,S., Schulz, R., Cipriani,J., Fox, A., & Starz, T. (2003). Concordance of four methods of disability assessment using performance in the home as the criterion method. *Arthritis and Rheumatism, 49*, 640-647.

Rosenbaum, P., Saigal, S., Szatmari, P., & Hoult, L. (1995). Vineland Adaptive Behavior Scales as a summary of functional outcome of extremely low-birthweight children. *Developmental Medicine and Child Neurology, 37*, 577-586.

Segal, M. E., Gilliard, M., & Schall, R. (1996). Telephone and in-person proxy agreement between stroke patients and caregivers for the functional independence measure. *American Journal of Physical Medicine & Rehabilitation, 75(3)*, 208-212.

Sneeuw, K. C., Aaronson, N. K., deHaan, R. J., & Limburg, M. (1997). Assessing quality of life after stroke. The value and limitations of proxy ratings. *Stroke, 28(8)*, 1541-1549.

Teri, L., Borson, S., Kiyak, A., & Yamagishi, M. (1989). Behavioral disturbance, cognitive function, and functional skill. *Journal of the American Geriatrics Society, 37*, 109-116.

Teri, L., Truax, P., Logsdon, R., Zarit, S., Uomoto, J., & Vitaliano, P. (1992). Assessment of behavioral problems in dementia. *Psychology and Aging, 7*, 622-631.

Thomas, K. A., Renaud, M. T., & Depaul, D. (2004). Use of the parenting stress index in mothers of preterm infants. *Neonatal Care, 4(1)*, 33-41.

Toderov, A. M., & Kirchener, C. (2000). Bias in proxies reports of disability: Data from the National Health Interview Survey on Disability. *American Journal of Public Health, 90*, 1248-1253.

Waters, E., Stewart-Brown, S., & Fitzpatrick, R. (2003). Agreement between adolescent self-report and parent ratings of health and well being. *Child Care, Health and Development, 29*, 501-509.

Whiteman, D., & Green, A. (1997). Wherein lies the truth? Assessment of agreement between parent proxy and child respondents. *International Journal of Epidemiology, 26(4)*, 855-859.

Williamson, G., Szczepanski, M., & Zeitlin, S. (1993). Coping frame of reference. In P. Kramer & J. Hinojosa (Eds.), *Frames of reference in pediatric occupational therapy* (pp. 395-436). Baltimore: Williams & Wilkins.

Williamson, G., & Zeitlin, S. (1990). Assessment of coping and temperament: Contributions to adaptive functioning. In E. D. Gibbs & D. M. Teti (Eds.), *Interdisciplinary assessment of infants: A guide for early intervention professionals* (pp. 215-226). Baltimore: Paul H. Brookes.

Williamson, G. , Zeitlin, S., & Szczepanski, M. (1989). Coping behavior: Implications for disabled infants and toddlers. *Infant Mental Health Journal, 10*, 3-13.

Zarit, S., & Zarit, J. (1983). Cognitive impairment. In P. M. Lewinson & L. Teri (Eds.), *Clinical geropsychology* (pp. 38-81). Elmsford, NY: Pergamon Press.

Zeitlin, S. (1985). *Coping inventory*. Bensenville, IL: Scholastic Testing Service, Inc.

Zeitlin, S., & Williamson, G. (1990). Coping characteristics of disabled and nondisabled young children. *American Journal of Orthopsychiatry, 60*, 404-411.

Editors' Notes for Chapter 8

Mine the Gold

The World Health Organization acknowledges the importance of participation as an indicator of health and well being. There is an increasing emphasis on participation in criteria for funding healthcare outcomes and educational programs as well.

Become Systematic

By using participation measures consistently in practice, we inform our clients and colleagues that this is a central feature of occupational therapy practice. By linking other measurement data to participation data, we demonstrate our clinical reasoning processes, and demonstrate our unique perspective as occupational therapists.

Use Evidence in Practice

Evidence from occupational therapy literature on participation indicates that we can characterize aspects that support or interfere with a child's or adults' ability to participate in specific situations. Evidence from other disciplines indicates that it is important to measure both the person's methods of participating and their experiences with participation in their life.

Make Occupational Therapy Contribution Explicit

Occupational performance is the central construct of occupational therapy. By measuring participation directly, therapists are clearly indicating the purpose of occupational therapy practice, and other information can serve to inform the participation focus.

Engage in Occupation-Based, Client-Centered Practice

The concept of participation clearly reflects the importance of the person's experience with daily life. With a focus on participation, therapists are less likely to contrive activities that are inconsistent with that person's actual life pattern.

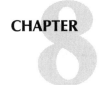

MEASURING PARTICIPATION

Mary Law, PhD, OT Reg. (Ont.), FCAOT; Winnie Dunn, PhD, OTR, FAOTA;
and Carolyn Baum, PhD, OTR/C, FAOTA

INTRODUCTION

Participation has been a central concept to occupational therapy since our profession began in the early 1900s. One of the founders of occupational therapy, Adolph Meyer, spoke eloquently about how persons used their time and organize themselves in order to participate in occupations across the lifespan (Meyer, 1922). In 1977, Tristam Engelhardt stated:

"occupational therapy does not seem to be bound to the concept of disease, instead it focuses upon the success of individuals in finding fulfillment through human activity. [By] viewing humans as engaged in activities, realizing themselves through their occupation, occupational therapy supports a view of the whole person in function and adaptation [and participation]." (p.666)

Participation is derived from the Latin words *participatus* (meaning "part") and *capere* (meaning "to take") (Merriam-Webster Dictionary, 2004). As defined today, participation means taking part in something, sharing, being involved, or experiencing something (Free Dictionary, 2004). From an occupational therapy perspective, participation can be defined as taking part in the occupations of everyday life. Participation is the ultimate goal of occupational therapy intervention.

Over the past two decades, participation has become a central and important concept in the field of health and disability worldwide. The World Health Organization (WHO), in revising their classification of disability, focused on participation as the important goal for persons

with health. The areas of participation described within the International Classification of Functioning (ICF) include Learning & Applying Knowledge, General Tasks and Demands, Communication, Movement, Self Care, Domestic Life Areas, Interpersonal Interactions, Major Life Areas, and Community, Social and Civic Life.

A person's participation does not occur in isolation, thus can only be considered in relationship to that person's skills and abilities and the environment in which he or she lives. In the ICF, the complexity of participation is recognized by stressing the interrelationships between body function and structure, activity, personal factors, and environmental characteristics (WHO, 2001). In occupational therapy, the complexity of participation in occupations is acknowledged in all occupational therapy theoretical models which emphasize the transactional relationships between person, occupations, and environment.

The WHO's conceptual model for disability and health emphasizes participation, and the Person Environment Occupation (PEO) model we are using in this text also focuses on participation as the result of the interaction of person, occupations and environments. Figure 8-1 illustrates the similarities in these conceptual models by superimposing them; the unique contributions of occupational therapy's perspective about occupation is notable.

PARTICIPATION AND OCCUPATIONAL PERFORMANCE

This book focuses on issues and strategies to measure occupational performance. As described in Chapter 1, occupational performance is the result of a person's effort

Figure 8-1. International Classification of Functioning and Disability (ICF).

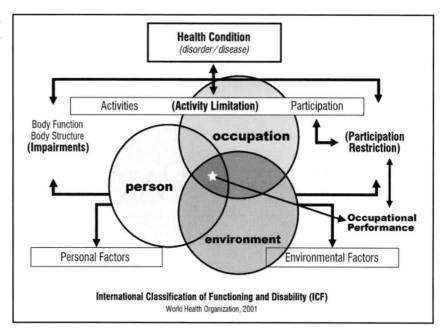

to engage in activities central to daily living which include, but are not limited to, activities of self care (e.g., grooming, bathing, feeding), productivity (e.g., vocational pursuits, maintaining a home, communicating with others) and leisure (e.g., play, hobbies, recreational activities). Occupational performance is a term unique to the profession of occupational therapy to describe how a person functions in his or her environment (American Occupational Therapy Association [AOTA], 1995).

Occupational therapists do not separate the physical act of doing from the meaning or purposeful intent of the act. When examining occupational performance, occupational therapists strive to understand how the dynamic relationship between person, environment & occupation, as well as a person's developmental stage, culture and societal roles impact on his or her ability to perform the tasks and activities that are important to the person. Defined simply, successful occupational performance occurs when a person is able to complete a task or activity in a manner that achieves the goal of the task or activity, while satisfying the person. Occupational therapists understand occupational performance to be the point at which the "person, environment and occupation intersect to support the tasks, activities and roles that define that person as an individual" (Baum & Law, 1997). As detailed in Chapter 5 (McColl & Pollock, 2005), occupational performance has both objective, observable components and subjective, experiential components.

What then is the relationship between occupational performance and participation? Both of these terms are used to describe and classify important concepts. Participation has been defined as involvement in a life situation whereas occupational performance describes the

act of doing an occupation and the experience of those moments in time. One can see that these descriptions share many similarities. In fact, as occupational therapists, our goal is to enable a person's participation in occupations that they want or need to do (Law, Steinwender, & LeClair, 1998).

From the point of view of measurement, an outcome of participation is very similar to the outcome of occupational performance. While the ICF specifies 10 categories of participation, most occupational therapy conceptual models classify occupational performance into three primary categories—self-care, productivity/work, and leisure (Canadian Association of Occupational Therapists [CAOT], 1997; AOTA, 2002). The majority of items within the WHO participation categories would fit into these three categories of occupational performance (see Figure 4-2). We will discuss the similarities further on page 105.

PARTICIPATION, QUALITY OF LIFE, AND HEALTH

Participation in occupations meaningful to a person has a direct and substantial impact on health and quality of life for children, adults, and older adults (Freysinger, Alessio, & Mehdizadeh, 1993; Larson & Verma, 1999; Law, Steinwender & LeClair, 1998). Anne Wilcock (1998) details how participation in occupations been a vital part of humankind throughout history. It it through participation in everyday occupations that people grow and develop, connect with other humans, make a living, learn, contribute to society, and enjoy life (Menec & Chipperfield, 1997; Statistics Canada, 2002; Stewart, Reid, & Mangham, 1997).

MEASURING PARTICIPATION

The assessment of participation is challenging. As Law (2002) states:

"Because participation in occupations is complex, weaving a pattern across time and space, capturing its essence through measurement is challenging. Think about it. Participation in occupations has several dimensions - a person's preferences and interests, what they do, where they do it, with whom they do it, and how much they enjoy and find it satisfying. In considering person, environment and occupation, the measurement of participation occurs at the transactions among these domains" (p. 642).

Many assessments of participation have been accomplished through population-based time use surveys. Information from these surveys contributes to our knowledge about how populations in different countries spend their time (Larson & Verma, 1999; United Nations, 2004). Occupational therapists can use this information to augment their knowledge about typical patterns of occupational performance. These surveys, however, are not as useful in doing assessments for individual clients or groups because they provide general conclusions about what is typical. Occupational therapy intervention is designed to address the specific issues that a particular client or group exhibits, and so measurement must uncover those specific characteristics.

Csikszentmihalyi (1990) has used individual strategies for identifying patterns of participation. He asked participants to record their experiences at randomly selected times triggered by a pager signal. His work led him to conclude that people need a balance of task difficulty and personal skill during participation to experience what he termed 'flow'. During flow, persons are absorbed in their activities and are not aware of time passing. His work provides us with insight about characteristics of successful participation, and also demonstrates a way to measure the experience of participation as it is occurring. However, this strategy for collecting information requires an expanse of time that may not be feasible in many practice settings. Additionally, occupational therapists are also concerned with personal strategies people use to engage in their occupations, and this measurement strategy does not provide a means for uncovering these data.

Because of the personal nature and complexity of participation, most participation measures have used self-report or proxy report formats. Such a measurement strategy fits with a social model of disability and acknowledges the intimate relationships between participation and the environment. The majority of participation measures focus more on the observable characteristics of participation, rather than a person's subjective experiences. Few measures assess the broad nature of participation including what is done, where participation takes place, how often it occurs, and how enjoyable the person finds it.

PARTICIPATION MEASURES REVIEWED IN THIS CHAPTER

The task of choosing participation measures for reviewing this chapter was difficult. There are very few measures which have been developed specifically to focus on participation as defined by the WHO (2001). On the other hand, there are many measures which include some or all of the items and categories found within the participation dimension of the ICF. For example, dozens of quality of life measures exist within the health and social sciences literature. Because of these challenges, we develop criteria to guide the selection of measures to be reviewed within the chapter.

All measures reviewed within the chapter cover a broad range of participation categories within the ICF (Tables 8-1 to 8-9). Thus, an assessment of ADL activities is not included because it covers only one category. Distinguishing between ADL, IADL and participation measures was easier than differentiating participation from leisure and community integration measures. There remains some overlap between measures reviewed in this chapter and in Chapters 6, 11, and 15. Chapter 6 focuses on client-centered measures of occupational performance; the results of these assessments often identify participation issues. For example, a client may identify participation in several occupations on the Canadian Occupational Performance Measure (COPM), For full reviews of these client-centered measures, go to Chapter 6. Chapter 11 focuses on measures that primarily assess leisure activities while Chapter 15 focuses on community integration measures that emphasize social integration. Tables for a few measures have been duplicated across Chapters 8, 11, and 16 to ensure the completeness of each chapter.

The other criteria used to select measures for this chapter include the following:

1. Currently available and in use in occupational therapy practice, education, and/or research.

2. Fit with a client-centered approach to occupational therapy practice.

3. Non-categorical in nature, not focused on one diagnosis.

4. Evidence of recent research about the measure or using it in a study.

5. Evidence of acceptable psychometric properties.

6. Observable or self-report, but focused on the nature and experience of participation.

Table 8-1

CHILDREN'S ASSESSMENT OF PARTICIPATION AND ENJOYMENT (CAPE)

Source	Psychological Corporation, Skill Builders Division, 555 Academic Court, San Antonio, TX, 78204, (phone) 800-228-0752.
Important References	Law, M., Finkelman, S., Hurley, P., Rosenbaum, P., King, S., King, G., & Hanna, S. (2004). The participation of children with physical disabilities: Relationships with diagnosis, physical function, and demographic variables. *Scandinavian Journal of Occupational Therapy, 11(4), 156-162.*
	King, G., Law, M., King, S., Rosenbaum, P., Kertoy, M., & Young, N. L. (2003). A conceptual model of the factors affecting the recreation and leisure participation of children with disabilities. *Physical and Occupational Therapy in Pediatrics, 23,* 63-90.
Purpose	• To capture children/youth's participation in and enjoyment of day-to-day activities outside of mandated school activities.
Type of Client	• Children and youth aged 6 years to 21 years of age. It is not recommended for children or youth who do not understand the task of sorting and categorizing activities.

Clinical Utility

Format
- Contains 55 items that are divided into 5 types of activity, or scales: Recreational (12 items), Active Physical (13 items), Social (10 items), Skill-based (10 items), and Self-improvement/Educational (10 items).
- Items can also be categorized into one of two domains: informal (40 items) or formal activities (15 items).
- The CAPE measures 5 dimensions of participation: diversity (number of activities), intensity (frequency—scale ranges from 0 to 7), with whom (7 possible responses), where (6 possible responses) and enjoyment (scale ranges from 0 to 5).

Procedures
- Self-administered version: Children are asked to look at drawings of children performing 55 different activities and identify on a Likert-type scale if they have performed each activity in the last 4 months, how often, with whom they performed the activity and their level of enjoyment.
- Interviewer-assisted version: Phase 1—child completes (alone or with parent) short questionnaire about whether they have performed each of the 55 activities in the past 4 months, and if so, how often. Phase 2—The interviewer asks the following questions for each activity the child has performed: who he or she performed the activity with, where he or she performed the activity and how much he or she enjoyed the activity.
- Scoring: The CAPE provides overall participation scores, scale scores, and domain scores. From these scores, it can also provide 8 additional scores for each of the dimensions of interest.

Completion time
- Phase 1 generally takes 25 to 30 minutes to complete. Phase 2 takes an additional 20 to 30 minutes.

Standardization
- The CAPE can be self-administered, or interviewer-assisted. The manual provides comprehensive instructions, but training would be beneficial.

Reliability

Test-Retest
- For overall participation and formal and informal domains, ICCs for diversity and intensity scores ranged from 0.67 to 0.86, indicating adequate to good reliability. ICCs for enjoyment ranged from 0.12 (active physical activities) to 0.73 (recreational activities), indicating poor to good reliability.

continued

Table 8-1 (continued)

CHILDREN'S ASSESSMENT OF PARTICIPATION AND ENJOYMENT (CAPE)

	• Intensity scores for five scales (types of activities) ranged from 0.72 to 0.81 (good reliability).
	• Enjoyment scores had low reliability, except for recreational activities.
Internal Consistency	• Cronbach's alpha was calculated for the domains and scales of the CAPE. Values ranged from poor to adequate: a=0.32 (Skill-based activities) to a=0.62 (social activities).
Validity	
Content	• Items were drawn from an extensive literature review, reviewed by a group of experts, and the initial draft of the CAPE was piloted with a small sample.
Construct	• Overall, domain and scale scores were compared with scores on measures of different constructs obtained from a longitudinal study of predictors of children's participation. There were small to moderate, but significant correlations between CAPE participation intensity and enjoyment scores and relevant outcome variables (r<0.01).
	• Comparisons between the CAPE intensity and enjoyment scores and the Preferences for the Activities of Children (PAC) preference scores were conducted. Correlations ranged from 0.22 to 0.61, which supported discriminant validity.
	• The CAPE was shown to discriminate between boys and girls for intensity and enjoyment, as well as between children with and without disabilities and between age groups for intensity.
Criterion	• Not reported
Overall utility	
Research	• Can be used to examine and compare the participation patterns of children and youth with or without disabilities, including changes over time.
	• It can be used as an outcome measure in a recreational program evaluation.
Clinical	• Provides useful information to a clinician about the type, intensity and enjoyment of activities their client has experienced.
	• Can be used to assess the effectiveness of intervention focused on improving the frequency, intensity and/or enjoyment of participation of children in various extra-curricular activities.
Strengths	• Theoretically based on the WHO-ICF. Is a very comprehensive measure of participation.
	• User-friendly for children; captures the child's perspective of their own participation patterns.
	• Culturally sensitive. Pictures are gender-neutral, not culturally specific and include children with physical disabilities.
	• Different methods of administration allow for greater flexibility of use in clinical and research setting.
Weaknesses	• It is a complex tool that requires a solid understanding by the clinician prior to administration.
	• It is lengthy to complete.
	• Additional psychometric testing is required to examine categorization of domain activities and scales.

Table 8-2

SCHOOL FUNCTION ASSESSMENT (SFA)

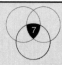

Source	Psychological Corporation, Skill Builders Division, 555 Academic Court, San Antonio, TX, 78204, (phone) 800-228-0752
Important References	AOTA. (1997). *Occupational therapy services for children and youth under the Individuals with Disabilities Education Act.* Bethesda, MD: Author.
	Coster, W. (1998). Occupation centered assessment of children. *American Journal of Occupational Therapy, 52,* 337-344.
	Davies, P. L., Soon, P. L., Young, M., & Clausen-Yamaki, A. (2004). Validity and reliability the school function assessment in elementary school students with disabilities. *Physical and Occupational Therapy in Pediatrics, 24(3),* 23-43.
Purpose	• This scale is used to measure a student's performance of functional tasks that support is or her participation in the academic and social aspects of an elementary school program. It was designed to facilitate collaborative program planning for students with a variety of disabling conditions.
Type of Client	• Child enrolled in elementary school. Assesses participation, task supports, and activity performance.
Clinical Utility	
Format	• The rating scales are administered to respondents who are familiar with the student's typical performance. Teachers, OTs, PTs, and SLPs as well as classroom and therapy assistants may serve as respondents.
	• The rating form has 26 scales; each scale is scored using a 4- or 6-level rating, depending on the item. For example, functional activities ratings range from 1 (does not perform) to 4 (consistent performance).
Procedures	• The assessment is completed by the team, either under the supervision of a coordinator who contacts individual team members and records their scores, or by the team collaboratively completing the assignment together.
Completion Time	• Completion time not reported.
Standardization	• Pools of items were developed by reviewing existing standardized and nonstandardized tests, published literature on the requirements for successful school performance, and published and unpublished curricula for students with disabilities. A set of 539 items was submitted to expert reviewers. IRT analysis was then computed. A reduced set of items was then tested with a sample of 363 students with disabilities, drawn from 112 sites in 40 states and Puerto Rico. Criterion and cut-off scores were then developed using a sample of 318 non-disabled students.
Reliability	
Test-Retest	• Test-retest studies were conducted using intervals ranging from 2 to 4 weeks. Reliability coefficients (both Pearson's r's and intraclass coefficients) ranged from 0.80 to 0.99. The lowest coefficients were on the task support items.
Internal Consistency	• Coefficient alpha's ranged from 0.92 to 0.98. Fit statistics using IRT methods were also computed. The fit statistics confirmed the coherence of the items within each scale.

continued

Table 8-2 (continued)

SCHOOL FUNCTION ASSESSMENT (SFA)

Validity

Content
- Two content validity studies were completed. The first used a sample of 30 content experts who were asked to rate the comprehensiveness and relevance of the items. A second study involved a field trial of the SFA with 40 students. Related service professionals assessed students and then provided an evaluation of the relevance, comprehensiveness, and usefulness of the items and ratings scales.

Construct
- A series of Rasch, multiple regression, and IRT analyses to test each aspect of construct validity. The scales were found to have excellent predictive and discriminative power.

Criterion
- Not established.

Overall Utility
- The SFA was very carefully developed and appears to be a very practical and empirically robust measure. The scale was designed to reflect current models of function and special education legislation. It will help organize the input from a number of different sources into an assessment used to plan and evaluate interventions for school-aged children. The manual is informative and easy to read.
- This is a new assessment with content that is well-referenced. However, as it is new, the scale itself is not yet referenced in any scholarly publications.

REFERENCES

AOTA. (1995). Position Paper: Occupational performance: Occupational therapy's definition of function *American Journal of Occupational Therapy, 49(190)*, 1019-1020.

AOTA. (1997). *Occupational therapy services for children and youth under the Individuals with Disabilities Education Act.* Bethesda, MD: Author.

AOTA. (2002). Occupational therapy practice framework: Domain and process. *American Journal of Occupational Therapy, 56*, 609-639.

Barbara, A., & Whiteford, G. (2005) The Clinical Utility of the Han-dicap Assessment and Resource Tool: An investigation of its use with the aged in hospital. *Australian Occupational Therapy Journal,* in press.

Baum, C. M. (1995). The contribution of occupation to function in persons with Alzheimer's disease. *Journal of Occupation Science: Australia, 2(2)*, 59-67.

Baum, C. M., & Edwards, D. F. (2001) *The Washington University Activity Card Sort.* St. Louis: PenUltima Press.

Baum C. M., Perlmutter, M., & Edwards, D. F. (2000). Measuring function in Alzheimer's disease. *Alzheimer's Care Quarterly,* 1(3):44-61.

Baum, C. M., & Edwards, D. F. (2001) *The Washington University Activity Card Sort.* St. Louis: PenUltima Press.

Baum, C., & Law, M. (1997). Occupational therapy practice: Focusing on occupational performance. *American Journal of Occupational Therapy, 51(4)*, 277-88.

CAOT (1997). *Enabling occupation: An occupational therapy perspective.* Ottawa, Ontario: CAOT Publications ACE.

Christiansen, C., & Baum, C. (1997). Person-environment occupational performance: A conceptual model for practice. In Christiansen, C., & Baum, C. *Occupational therapy: Enabling function and well-being* (2nd ed.). SLACK Incorporated: Thorofare, NJ.

Coster, W. (1998). Occupation centered assessment of children. *American Journal of Occupational Therapy, 52*, 337-344.

Csikszentmihalyi, M. (1990). *Flow: The psychology of optimal experience.* New York: Harper and Row.

Darzins, P., Bremner, F., & Smith, R. (2002). *Outcome Measures in Rehabilitation Phase 2. Report to the Department of Human Services.* Retrieved April 6, 2005 from http://www.health. vic.gov.au/subacute/outcomefinal.pdf·

Darzins, P. (2003). *Section 10.8 The Handicap Assessment and Resource Tool (HART) and the ICF, in ICF Australian User Guide, Version 1.0.* Retrieved April 6, 2005 from http://www.aihw.gov.au/publications/dis/icfaugv1/modules/ugmod_108.pdf.

Davies, P. L., Soon, P. L., Young, M., & Clausen-Yamaki, A. (2004). Validity and reliability of the school function assessment in elementary school students with disabilities. *Physical and Occupational Therapy in Pediatrics, 24(3)*, 23-43.

Dijkers, M. (1991). Scoring CHART: Survey and sensitivity analysis. *Journal of the American Paraplegia Society, 14*, 85-86

Dijkers, M. P. J., Whiteneck, G. & El-Jaroudi, R. (2000). Measures of social outcomes in disability research. *Archives of Physical Medicine and Rehabilitation, 81(12)*, Suppl 2, S63-80.

References continued on page 118

Table 8-3

PEDIATRIC ACTIVITY CARD SORT (PACS)

Source	Canadian Occupational Therapy Association, CAOT publications ACE, Canadian Association of Occupational Therapists, CTTC Building, 3400-1125 Colonel By Drive, Ottawa, Ontario, Canada, K1S 5R1, (Web) www.caot.org
Important References	Mandich, A., Polatojko, M., Miller, L., & Baum, C. (2004). *Pediatric Activity Card Sort*. Ottawa, Ontario: CAOT Publications ACE.
Purpose	Measures child's level of occupational engagement in a range of activities (including play) and participation at a particular point in time. Can be used to initiate goal setting for occupational therapy intervention.
Type of Client	Children between the ages of 6 to 12 years of age with various diagnoses and physical disabilities (e.g., developmental coordination disorder (DCD), Asperger's Syndrome, etc.).
Clinical Utilities	
Format	• Consists of cards (depicting personal care, school/productivity, hobbies/social activities, and sports) and a scoring sheet.
Procedures	• Administered by occupational therapists or certified occupational therapy assistants to either children or their parents. Examiners show cards and ask whether (and how frequently) children engage in activities depicted. Children identify their five most important activities and five activities they want to do.
Completion Time	• Can be administered in 15 to 20 minutes. More time may be required for elaboration of activities.
Standardization	• Criterion referenced.
Reliability	
Test-Retest	• Studies are currently being conducted.
Internal Consistency	• Studies are currently being conducted.
Validity	
Content	• Activities were identified initially through observation and experiences of the authors with children, literature search, and review of existing occupational therapy assessments.
	• Five steps were taken for instrument validation: first, item validation was undertaken with 13 children between the ages of 6 to 12 years; second, parents corroborated their children's (n=11) reports (Bowman, 1999). Next, the instrument was shown to be sensitive to age (Horn & Williams, 2000). Finally, the PACs was shown to detect differences in occupational profile between children with DCD and typically-developing children (n=10; ages 6 to 10).
Clinical utility	
Research	• Can be used to explore occupational engagement.
Clinical	• Can be used in a variety of practice areas such as schools, pediatric facilities or private practice.
Strengths	• Occupation-based assessment supporting a client-centered approach.
	• Photographs are appealing to children.
	• Good tool for research.
Weaknesses	• New instrument; limited evidence for reliability or validity.

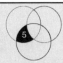

Table 8-4

ACTIVITY CARD SORT (ACS)

Source	Dr. Carolyn Baum, Program in Occupational Therapy, Box 8505, Washington University School of Medicine, 4444 Forest Park Blvd, St. Louis, MO, 63108
Important References	Baum, C. M., & Edwards, D. (2001). *Activity Card Sort*. St. Louis, MO: Washington University at St. Louis.
	Katz, N., Karpin, H., Lak, A., Furman, T., & Hartman-Maeir, A. (2003). Participation in occupational performance: Reliability and validity of the Activity Card Sort. *Occupational Therapy Journal of Rehabilitation, 23(1)*, 10-17.
	Sachs, D., & Josman, N. (2003). The Activity Card Sort: A factor analysis. *Occupational Therapy Journal of Rehabilitation, 23(4)*, 165-74.
Purpose	• Original version (older adult version) was designed to capture activity level of individuals with Alzheimer's Disease in instrumental, leisure, and social activities; has been used with many different adult populations.
	• Institutional version can be used to establish functional treatment goals with a client.
	• Recovering version of ACS allows clinicians to record changes in activity patterns.
Type of Client	• Adults with and without cognitive loss. A youth and children's version has been developed and is currently undergoing research. It is described elsewhere in this chapter.
Clinical Utility	
Format	• Can be performed with client, or with a parent or caregiver.
	• Has a Q-sort methodology (rank order procedure using piles or groups of objects). The client or his or her informant sorts photographs of people performing various activities into groups so that a general history of their participation in each activity can be obtained.
	• Photographs categorized into four domains: 1) instrumental activities, 2) low-demand leisure activities, 3) high-demand leisure activities, and 4) social activities. Clients do not group photographs according to these domains.
Procedures	• The client or his/her caregivers are asked to sort 80 photograph cards, one at a time, into groups. The groups vary, depending on the version of the tool being used.
	• In the healthy older adults version, cards are sorted into the following categories: 1) never done, 2) not done as an older adult, 3) do now, 4) do less, and 5) given up.
	• In the institutional version (hospital, rehab, long term care facility), the cards are sorted into two groups: 1) done prior to illness and 2) not done.
	• In the recovering version, the categories include 1) not done in the last 5 years, 2) gave up due to illness, 3) beginning to do again, and 4) do now.
Scoring	• The sum total of current activities is divided by the sum total of previous activities. This provides a percent of retained activity level.
Completion Time	• Average completion time is 20 minutes. More time is required if the clinician asks probing questions about activities retained, lost, or desired.
Standardization	• The photographs can be tailored to the specific population of interest (i.e., different ages and cultures).
	• An Israeli version has been developed. Some pictures were removed and added from the original version of ACS. The final Israeli version is reported to have 88 pictures.

continued

Table 8-4 (continued)

ACTIVITY CARD SORT (ACS)

Reliability

Test-Retest
- Baum & Edwards (2001) reported a test-retest coefficient of 0.897 in a sample of 20 older adults living within the community.

Internal Consistency
- The Israeli version of the ACS had high internal consistency for IADL and social-cultural activities (a=0.82 and 0.80) and moderate internal consistency for low and high physical leisure activities (a=0.66 and 0.61).

Validity

Content
- Two content validity studies have been completed.
- The photographs were shown to an initial sample of 120 older adults, and then a second sample of 40 older adults (both samples were from the United States). After the sample provided feedback, 7 additional activities were added to the original ACS to bring the total of the second edition of the ACS to 80.

Construct
- Israeli study examined the ability of the ACS to differentiate between healthy adults, healthy older adults, spouses or caregivers of individuals with Alzheimer's, individuals with multiple sclerosis and stroke survivors (1 year post-stroke). The ACS differentiated well between groups with regard to total retained activity level and individual activity areas (p<0.001).
- Factor analysis of Israeli version of the ACS found young and older adults (n=184) classify activities into domains that are different than those suggested by the author. However, the authors in this study modified the scoring scale from the original version. This does not compromise the use of the ACS as a clinical tool, but should be considered when using the tool in research for the purpose of examining the categorization and underlying dimensions of occupational performance.

Criterion
- A significant but moderate Pearson correlation coefficient was found between the Israeli version of the ACS category "doing now" and the number of hours a person reported being active on the Occupational Questionnaire (r=0.54).

Overall Utility

Research
- Useful for research directed at examining the occupational performance patterns of different age and diagnostic groups, as well as between genders.

Clinical
- Can be used as a guide for setting functional treatment goals with the client.
- The institutional version allows the therapist to create a pre-admission status for treatment planning and triggers ideas for intervention that include the person's prior experiences and interests.
- The recovering version allows clinicians to record changes in activity patterns, although the ability of the tool to detect change in performance has not been formally tested.

Strengths
- Allows client to describe how he/she engages in a variety of activities, but is also useful for individuals who have difficulties with speech or speaking English.
- The format is non-threatening, easy to understand and supports client-centered practice.
- Photographs can be modified based on the need of the population being assessed.

Weaknesses
- Has been adapted with minimal difficulty for a variety of populations, some cards from the original version suggest the focus is for a Christian population (i.e., reading the bible, going to church)
- Should not be the sole outcome measure used to establish treatment goals. The percentage score is somewhat arbitrary, as there is no standard for comparison.
- More research is necessary to determine whether the scores capture a change in behavior.

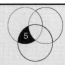

Table 8-5

LONDON HANDICAP SCALE

Source	Medical Outcomes Trust, 235 Wyman St. Suite 130, Waltham, MA, 02451, (phone) 784-890-4884, (web) www.outcomes-trust.org.
Important References	Dubuc, N., Haley, S., Ni, P., Kooyoomjian J., & Jette A. (2004). Function and disability in late life: comparison of the Late-Life Function and Disability Instrument to the Short-Form-36 and the London Handicap Scale. *Disability & Rehabilitation, 26(6),* 362-70.
	Lo, R., Harwood, R., Woo, J., Yeung F., & Ebrahim, S. (2001).Cross-cultural validation of the London Handicap Scale in Hong Kong Chinese. *Clinical Rehabilitation, 15(2),* 177-185.
	Harwood, R. H., & Ebrahim, S. (2000a). Measuring the outcomes of day hospital attendance: a comparison of the Barthel Index and London Handicap Scale. *Clinical Rehabilitation, 14(5),* 527-31.
	Harwood, R. H., & Ebrahim, S. (2000b). The London handicap scale. *Journal of Neurology, Neurosurgery & Psychiatry, 69(3),* 406.
	Jenkinson, C., Mant, J., Carter, J., Wade, D., & Winner, S. (2000). The London handicap scale: A re-evaluation of its validity using standard scoring and simple summation [see comment]. *Journal of Neurology, Neurosurgery & Psychiatry. 68(3),* 365-367.
Purpose	• Measures the effects of disease or disability on participation. Serves as a general measure of disability.
Type of Client	• Adolescents and adults with and without disabilities.
Clinical Utility	
Format	• Based on 6 dimensions of handicap identified in ICIDH. Respondents identify their perceived level of disadvantage in 6 dimensions: mobility, orientation, occupation, physical independence, social integration and economic self-sufficiency.
	• Scoring: Each dimension has a 6 point rating scale, ranging from "none" (no disadvantage) to "extreme" (extreme disadvantage). A final score of 100 indicates no disadvantage, a score of 0 indicates maximum disadvantage. The authors of the instrument advise using a weighted system to calculate final scores, however, Jenkinson et al. (2000) found that scores could be accurately calculated without the weighted system, just by adding the respondent's raw scores.
Procedures	• Can be self-administered or via interview (with client or proxy). Completion Time 10 to 15 minutes.
Standardization	• Has been translated into Chinese.
Reliability	
Test-Retest	• Good to excellent. Studies found test-retest coefficient of 0.70 for 2 months and 0.91 for 2 weeks.
Internal Consistency	• Excellent. Cronbach's alpha has consistently scored at 0.80 or higher.
Validity	
Content	• Based on ICIDH (1980).
Construct	• Good. Studies have found correlations between the LHS and age, impairment, motor disability, depression and anxiety, cognitive impairment and life satisfaction (Dubuc, Haley, Ni, Kooyoomjian, & Jette, 2004; Jenkinson, Mant, Carter, Wade, & Winner, 2000).

continued

Table 8-5 (continued)

LONDON HANDICAP SCALE

	• Good convergent validity. Studies have found strong correlations between LHS and other measures that examine similar constructs such as the Rankin and the Functional Abilities Index. Responsiveness Was found to be more responsive to change than the Barthel Index in a day hospital program for individuals attending 10 or more sessions (Harwood & Ebrahim, 2000).
Overall Utility	
Research	• Designed as an epidemiological tool—particularly for randomized clinical trials.
	• Can also be used in cost analysis of different programs for health policy development.
Clinical	• Measure clinical outcomes and treatment effectiveness.
Strengths	• Although based on initial ICIDH framework, still conceptually linked to ICIDH-2.
	• Demonstrates strong psychometric properties thus far.
Weaknesses	• No inter-rater reliability studies completed. Therefore, it is difficult to comment on accuracy of proxy response.
	• Floor effects may exist in populations with mild to moderate level of disability (i.e., they may have a score indicating no disadvantage, when in fact one exists.)

Dubuc, N., Haley, S., Ni, P., Kooyoomjian J., & Jette A. (2004). Function and disability in late life: comparison of the Late-Life Function and Disability Instrument to the Short-Form-36 and the London Handicap Scale. *Disability & Rehabilitation, 26(6)*, 362-70.

Engelhardt, H. T. (1977). Defining occupational therapy: The meaning of therapy and the virtues of occupation. *American Journal of Occupational Therapy, 31(10)*, 666-672.

Everard, K. M., Lach, H. W., Fisher, E. B., Baum, C. M. (2000). Relationship of activity and social support to the functional health of older adults. *Journal of Gerontology: Social Sciences, 55B(4)*, S208-S212.

Free Dictionary. *Participation*. Retrieved from www.thefreedictionary.com, August 5, 2004.

Freysinger, V. J., Alessio, H., & Mehdizadeh, S. (1993). Re-examining the morale-physical health-activity relationship: A longitudinal study of time changes and gender differences. *Activities, Adaptation and Aging, 17(4)*, 25-41.

Hall, K. M., Dijkers, M., Whiteneck, G., Brooks, C. A., & Stuart Krause, J. (1998). The Craig Handicap Assessment and Reporting Technique (CHART): Metric properties and scoring. *Topics in Spinal Cord Injury Rehabilitation, 4(1)*, 16-30.

Harwood, R., H., & Ebrahim, S. (2000a).Measuring the outcomes of day hospital attendance: a comparison of the Barthel Index and London Handicap Scale. *Clinical Rehabilitation, 14(5)*, 527-31.

Harwood, R. H., & Ebrahim, S. (2000b).The London Handicap Scale. *Journal of Neurology, Neurosurgery & Psychiatry, 69(3)*, 406.

Jenkinson, C., Mant, J., Carter, J., Wade, D., & Winner, S. (2000). The London handicap scale: A re-evaluation of its validity using standard scoring and simple summation. *Journal of Neurology, Neurosurgery & Psychiatry. 68(3)*, 365-367.

Katz, N., Karpin, H., Lak, A., Furman, T., & Hartman-Maeir, A. (2004). Participation in Occupational Performance of Instrumental, Social-Cultural and Leisure Activities: Reliability and Validity of the Activity Card Sort (ACS). *Occupational Therapy Journal of Research, 23(1)*, 10-17.

King, G., Law, M., King, S., Rosenbaum, P., Kertoy, M., & Young, N. L. (2003). A conceptual model of the factors affecting the recreation and leisure participation of children with disabilities. *Physical and Occupational Therapy in Pediatrics, 23*, 63-90.

Larson, R. W., & Verma, S. (1999). How children and adolescents spend time across the world: Work, play, and developmental opportunities. *Psychological Bulletin, 125(6)*, 701-736.

Law, M. (2002). Participation in the occupations of everyday life. *American Journal of Occupational Therapy, 56*, 640-649.

Law, M., Baptiste, S., Carswell, A., McColl, M., Polatajko, H., & Pollock, N. (1998). *Canadian occupational performance measure.* (3rd ed.). Ottawa, Ontario: CAOT Publications.

Law, M., Finkelman, S., Hurley, P., Rosenbaum, P., King, S., King, G., & Hanna, S. (in press). The participation of children with physical disabilities: Relationships with diagnosis, physical function, and demographic variables. *Swedish Journal of Occupational Therapy*.

Law, M., Steinwender, S., & LeClair, L. (1998). Occupation, health and well-being. *Canadian Journal of Occupational Therapy, 65(2)*, 81-91.

References concluded on page 120

Table 8-6

LIFE HABITS ASSESSMENT (LIFE-H)

Source	Centre interdisciplinaire de recherche en réadaptation et intégration sociale, 525 boul. Wilfrid Hamel Québec Canada G1M 2S8
Important references	Dijkers, M. P. J., Whiteneck, G., & El-Jaroudi, R. (2000). Measures of social outcomes in disability research. *Archives of Physical Medicine and Rehabilitation, 81(12),* Suppl 2, S63-80.
	Lepage, C., Noreau, L., Bernard, P., & Fougeyrollas, P. (1998). Profile of handicap situations in children with cerebral palsy. *Scandinavian Journal of Rehabilitation Medicine, 30(4),* 263-72.
Purpose	• To identify factors impeding the accomplishment of life habits for people with disabilities.
Type of Client	• Adults or children with disabilities.
Clinical Utility	
Format	• Long version 3.0: 240 life habits are categorized into 32 categories, which are organized into twelve domains (nutrition, fitness, personal care, communication, housing, mobility, responsibility, interpersonal relations, community, education, employment, recreation).
	200+ items are relevant for children. If an item is not part of the daily life of a child, then it is not incorporated into his/her raw score.
	Respondent rates the level of his/her accomplishment of each item ("no difficulty,""some difficulty," "accomplished by substitution," and "not accomplished"), the amount of assistance they require to complete each item ("no assistance," "technical aid," "adaptation," and "human assistance"), and their overall satisfaction with their performance of each item (5-point scale from "very dissatisfied" to "very satisfied").
	• Short version: 69 life habits
	• Scoring: responses from the accomplishment and assistance subscales are combined to form a 9-point scale.
Procedures	• Questionnaire format.
Completion Time	• Not indicated.
Standardization	• Available in French and English.
Reliability	
Test-Retest	• Good for adults and children: ICC=0.74 for small sample of adults with SCI. ICC= 0.73 for small sample of children (Lepage, Noreau, Bernard, & Fougeyrollas, 1998).
Internal Consistency	• Not reported.
Validity	
Content	• 12 rehabilitation experts judged the items to be appropriate.
Construct	• Comparison of LIFE-H and CHART: Physical domains correlated highly (r=0.76), mobility, occupation, and social domains had fair to low correlations (r=0.33, 0.36, and 0.14 respectively).
Criterion	• Not reported.

continued

Table 8-6 (continued)

LIFE HABITS ASSESSMENT (LIFE-H)

Overall utility

Research
- Measure clinical outcomes and treatment effectiveness.
- Identify level of disability in a sample.

Clinical
- To assess level of handicap in adults and children.
- Identify needs.
- Development of treatment plans.
- Track functioning over time.
- Measure clinical outcomes and treatment effectiveness.

Strengths
- Conceptually linked to the ICIDH-2.
- Cross-cultural measurement of disability.

Weaknesses
- Some items are worded so that people with physical or sensory disabilities typically score low (e.g., "eating with utensils or hands" or "listening to the radio").

Lepage, C., Noreau, L., Bernard, P., & Fougeyrollas, P. (1998). Profile of handicap situations in children with cerebral palsy. *Scandinavian Journal of Rehabilitation Medicine, 30(4)*, 263-72.

Lo, R., Harwood, R., Woo, J., Yeung F., & Ebrahim, S. (2001). Cross-cultural validation of the London Handicap Scale in Hong Kong Chinese. *Clinical Rehabilitation, 15(2)*, 177-185.

McColl, M., & Pollock, N. (2005). Measuring occupational performance using a client-centered perspective. In M. Law, C. Baum & W. Dunn, eds., *Measuring occupational performance.* (2nd ed.). Thorofare, NJ: SLACK Incorporated.

Menec, V. H., & Chipperfield, J. G. (1997). Remaining active in later life. The role of locus of control in seniors' leisure activity participation, health, and life satisfaction. *Journal of Aging and Health, 9(1)*, 105-125.

Merriam-Webster. (2004). *Merriam-Webster online dictionary.* Retrieved from http://www.m-w.com/ August 5, 2004.

Meyer, A. (1922). The philosophy of occupation therapy. *Archives of Occupational Therapy, 1(1)*, 1-10.

Rintala, D., Hart, K., & Fuhrer, M. (1993). *Handicap and spinal cord injury: Levels and correlates of mobility, occupational and social integration.* Proceedings of American Spinal Injury Association Meeting.

Sachs, D., & Josman, N. (2003). The Activity Card Sort: A factor analysis. *OTJR: Occupation, Participation and Health, 23(4)*, 165-176.

Smith, R., Darzins, P., Steel, C., Murray, K., Osborne, D., & Gilsenan, B. (2001). *Outcome Measures in Rehabilitation. Report to the Department of Human Services.* Retrieved April 6, 2005 from http://www.health.vic.gov.au/subacute/outcome_phase1.pdf.

Statistics Canada. (2002). *Participation and activity limitation survey: A profile of disability in Canada.* Ottawa, Ontario: Author.

Stewart, M., Reid, G., & Mangham, C. (1997). Fostering children's resilience. *Journal of Pediatric Nursing, 12(1)*, 21-29.

United Nations. (2004). Allocation of time and time use. Retrieved from http://unstats.un.org/unsd/demographic/sconcerns/tuse/ December 30, 2004.

Vertesi, A., Darzins, P., Edwards, M., Lowe, S., & McEvoy, E. (2000). Development of the Handicap Assessment and Resource Tool (HART). *Canadian Journal of Occupational Therapy, 67*, 120-127.·

Whiteneck, G. (1987). Outcome analysis in spinal cord injury rehabilitation. In M. Fuhrer (Ed.), *Rehabilitation outcomes: Analysis and measurement.* Baltimore: Paul H. Brookes.

Whiteneck, G., Charlifue, S., Gerhart, K., Overholser, D., & Richardson, G. (1992). Quantifying handicap: A new measure of long-term rehabilitation outcomes. *Archives of Physical Medicine and Rehabilitation, 73*, 519-526.

Wilcock, A. A. (1998). Reflections on doing, being and becoming. *Canadian Journal of Occupational Therapy, 65*, 248-257.

WHO. (1980). *International Classification of Impairment, Disability and Handicap.* Geneva, Switzerland: World Health Organization.

WHO. (1998). *International Classification of Impairment, Disability and Handicap—ICIDH2.* Geneva, Switzerland: World Health Organization.

WHO. (2001). *International Classification of Functioning, Disability and Health.* Geneva, Switzerland: World Health Organization.

Table 8-7

CRAIG HANDICAP ASSESSMENT AND REPORTING TECHNIQUE (CHART)

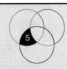

Source	Dave Mellnick, Craig Hospital Research Department, 3425 S. Clarkson Street, Englewood, CO, 80110, (phone) 303-789-8202, (Web) www.craighospital.org.
Important references	Dijkers, M. (1991). Scoring CHART: Survey and sensitivity analysis. *Journal of the American Paraplegia Society, 14*, 85-86.
	Hall, K. M., Dijkers, M., Whiteneck, G. Brooks, C. A., & Stuart Krause, J. (1998). The Craig Handicap Assessment and Reporting Technique (CHART): Metric properties and scoring. *Topics in Spinal Cord Injury Rehabilitation, 4(1)*, 16-30.
	Rintala, D., Hart, K., & Fuhrer, M. (1993). *Handicap and spinal cord injury: Levels and correlates of mobility, occupational, and social integration.* Proceedings of American Spinal Injury Association Meeting.
	Whiteneck, G. (1987). Outcome analysis in spinal cord injury rehabilitation. In M. Fuhrer (Ed.), *Rehabilitation outcomes: Analysis and measurement*. Baltimore: Paul H. Brooks.
	Whiteneck, G., Charlifue, S. Gerhart, K., Overholser, D., & Richardson, G. (1992). Quantifying handicap: A new measure of long-term rehabilitation outcomes. *Archives of Physical Medicine and Rehabilitation, 73*, 519-526.
	WHO. (1998). *International Classification of Impairment, Disability and Handicap—ICIDH2*. Geneva, Switzerland: World Health Organization.
	WHO. (1980). *International Classification of Impairments, Disability and Handicap.* Geneva, Switzerland: World Health Organization.
Purpose	• To measure the level of handicap experienced by an individual in a community setting.
Type of Client	• Designed for clients with spinal cord injuries. The Revised CHART has also been used in research for people with traumatic brain injury, stroke, multiple sclerosis, amputations, and burns.
Clinical Utility	
Format	• Twenty-seven questions belonging to 5 subscales: 1) physical independence, 2) mobility, 3) occupation, 4) social integration, and 5) economic self-sufficiency. There are 2 to 7 items per subscale. Subscales correspond to 5 of 6 areas of handicap identified by ICIDH (WHO, 1998).
	• Scoring: Each subscale has a maximum score of 100 points, which corresponds to typical performance of average person without disability. High subscale and total scores indicate less handicap. The maximum economic self-sufficiency score corresponds to U.S. median income.
Procedures	• Self-report questionnaire that asks client to indicate time spent performing items. Can also be completed by caregiver as a proxy.
Completion Time	• Estimated to be 30 minutes.
Standardization	• Not standardized. Revised CHART was developed with additional "cognitive independence" scale to increase applicability to stroke population.
Reliability	
Test-Retest	• Dijkers (1991) found subscale coefficients to be in excellent range (r=0.80 to 0.95), as well as the coefficient for the total score (r=0.93).
Internal Consistency	• Not reported.

continued

Table 8-7 (continued)

CRAIG HANDICAP ASSESSMENT AND REPORTING TECHNIQUE (CHART)

Validity

Content
- Based on ICIDH (WHO, 1980)—Ensured domain of handicap areas are covered in full, without overlap with impairment and disability.

Construct
- Distinguished between groups (i.e., based on culture, age, education, injury level, time since injury); however, the authors recommend that group differences should be interpreted with caution (Hall, Dijkers, Whiteneck, Brooks, & Stuart Krause, 1998).
- Rasch analysis supported underlying structure and linearity of CHART.

Criterion
- Concordance of CHART scores with therapist ratings of high vs low handicap.

Overall Utility

Research
- Useful for measuring community reintegration of broad populations such as SCI clients.
- Useful in rehabilitation program evaluation.

Clinical
- May be useful for measuring change in performance (before vs after intervention), although does not appear to have been specifically tested for this.

Strengths
- Focuses on objective, observable criteria to limit interpreter bias.
- Normative data has been established with large sample sizes.
- Views occupation in a manner similar to occupational therapy perspective.

Weaknesses
- The CHART has a ceiling effect, particularly for the SCI population.
- Economic self-sufficiency scale is based on US income, limiting international interpretation.
- Large percentage of incomplete data for the economic self-sufficiency subscale in large studies, which impacts total scores reported in research.
- Reliance on total scores may mask important differences at the subscale level.

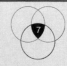

Table 8-8

World Health Organization— Disability Schedule II (WHO-DAS II)

Source	World Health Organization
Important References	Chwastiak, L. A., & Von Korff, M. (2003). Evaluation of the World Health Organization Disability Assessment Schedule (WHO-DAS II) in a primary care setting. *Journal of Clinical Epidemiology, 56(6),* 507-514.
	World Health Organization. (2001). *International Classification of Functioning, Disability and Health.* Geneva, Switzerland: World Health Organization.
Purpose	• To assess a person's general level of disability, in accordance with the ICIDH-2.
Type of Client	• Adults aged 18 and older, across a wide spectrum of cultures and diagnoses.
Clinical Utility	
Format	• Reflects six domains of functioning in daily life: 1) communication, 2) physical mobility, 3) self-care, 4) interpersonal interactions, 5) domestic responsibilities and work, and 6) participation in society.
	• Scoring: Produces scores for each domain, as well as a total score. Scores range from 0 to 100, with higher scores reflecting greater disability.
Procedures	• Interview format. Can be administered in person or over the phone.
Completion Time	• 12 item versions: 5 minutes.
	• 36 item versions: 20 minutes
Standardization	• Has been translated into 15 languages.
Reliability	
Test-Retest	• Not reported.
Internal Consistency	• Excellent. Cronbach's alpha=0.95 for the total score and ranged from 0.65 (self-care) to 0.91 (work and household) for each domain
Validity	
Content	• Initial draft containing 89 items was site-tested in 19 countries. Measure was then decreased to 36 items based on the results of these studies, and a 12 item screening tool was developed.
Convergent	• In 2 samples (people with depression and people with low back pain) Total WHO-DAS II scores correlated moderately with composite scores from the SF-36 (r= -0.72). Strong correlations were found between WHO-DAS II subscales, and subscales of SF-36 that reflect the same ICIDH-2 dimensions for both the psychiatric condition and the physical condition.
Criterion	• Not reported.
Overall Utility	
Research	• Measure clinical outcomes and treatment effectiveness.
	• Identify level of disability in a sample.
Clinical	• Identify needs.
	• Development of treatment plans.
	• Track functioning over time.
	• Measure clinical outcomes and treatment effectiveness.
Strengths	• Conceptually linked to the ICIDH-2.
	• Cross-cultural measurement of disability.
	• Has been shown to be responsive to change.
Weaknesses	• Potential for ceiling effect limits responsiveness to change for people with mild to moderate impairments or disabilities.

Table 8-9

PERSONAL CARE PARTICIPATION ASSESSMENT AND RESOURCE TOOL (PC-PART), FORMERLY THE HART

Source	The PART Group, PO BOX 1039 G, Greythorn 3104, Australia, (fax) +61 3 9816 4404, (e-mail) PARTGroup@bigpond.com.
Important References	Vertesi, A., Darzins, P., Edwards, M., Lowe, S., & McEvoy, E. (2000). Development of the Handicap Assessment and Resource Tool (HART). *Canadian Journal of Occupational Therapy, 67,* 120-127.
	Smith, R., Darzins, P., Steel, C., Murray, K., Osborne, D., & Gilsenan, B. (2001). *Outcome Measures in Rehabilitation. Report to the Department of Human Services.* Retrieved April 6, 2005 from http://www.health.vic.gov.au/subacute/outcome_phase1.pdf.
	Darzins, P., Bremner, F., & Smith, R. (2002). *Outcome Measures in Rehabilitation Phase 2. Report to the Department of Human Services.* Retrieved April 6, 2005 from http://www.health.vic.gov.au/subacute/outcomefinal.pdf.
	Darzins, P. (2003). *Section 10.8. The Handicap Assessment and Resource Tool (HART) and the ICF, in ICF Australian User Guide, Version 1.0.* Retrieved April 6, 2005 from http://www.aihw.gov.au/publications/dis/icfaugv1/modules/ugmod_108.pdf.
	Barbara, A., & Whiteford, G. (2005). The clinical utility of the Handicap Assessment and Resource Tool: An investigation of its use with the aged in hospital. *Australian Occupational Therapy Journal,* in press.
Purpose	• To assess what people can do alone, or get done for them, regarding personal care in their usual environments with the usual available help.
	• To comprehensively assess and record personal care participation—the minimum set of survival tasks for living in a given setting.
Type of Client	• Adults of any age, and also suitable for older youths. Can assess people with cognitive impairment or limited insight as well as the cognitively intact. Can assess people who cannot communicate.
Clinical Utility	
Format	• The PC-PART consists of full colour work sheets and a bi-fold summary sheet.
	• The worksheets guide the assessment and record the assessment.
	• The summary sheet gives an easily overviewed summary, risk assessment and plan.
	• Contains 43 items in 7 domains: Clothing (5), Hygiene (8), Nutrition (8), Mobility (9), Safety (6), Residence (5), and Supports (2). Items are categorized as either "OK by self", OK with help," or "Not OK."
	• In addition the risk in each item is categorized as "high", "medium," or "low."
Procedures	• Administration: Each item is assessed by asking a single question of the person being assessed and, separately, of a key informant. If the given answers agree, the item can be scored. If the person being assessed and the key informant disagree, then the item is scored by either direct observation or from assessing a standard task (that is to be done with the usually available help). Key informants can be interviewed by telephone.
	• Self-administered for people who are motivated, cognitively intact and who have good insight. This is only done at the clinician's discretion. There are no reliability studies of this. Self-administering the PC-PART can be used as screening checklist.

continued

Table 8-9 (continued)

PERSONAL CARE PARTICIPATION ASSESSMENT AND RESOURCE TOOL (PC-PART), FORMERLY THE HART

	• Scoring: The PC-PART does not provide an overall participation score. It lists personal care participation items and displays performance on these. This helps users to determine for which items or domains help is needed or is being provided.
	• Users can note change and infer improvement or deterioration. If users ignore the underlying construct of participation they can simply treat the scores as continuous variables with interval characteristics—this crude summation is discouraged for individuals, but if appropriately interpreted may be valid for aggregate data.
Completion Time	• Initial assessments take about 40 minutes, including explanation, data collection, and documentation. Assessment of complex situations takes longer, especially if multiple key informants are needed.
	• Comprehensive assessment of personal care participation, including documentation of findings, using the PC-PART is faster than equivalent non-structured assessment.
Standardization	• Manual provides comprehensive instructions—experienced clinicians can successfully use it without training or extensive reference to the manual.
Reliability	
Test-Retest	• A prior version of the PC-PART (2000) showed good test-retest reliability, with kappa scores in each domain ranging from a low of 0.63 to 1.0.
Inter-Rater	• Comparison between two pairs of experienced occupational therapists—kappa scores ranged from 0.63 to 1.0.
	• The current version is undergoing reliability testing—results expected by mid 2005.
Internal Consistency	• No data available.
Validity	
Content	• Items were created by a clinician driven item-generation process, compared to an extensive literature review, reviewed by a group of experts, and then collated into an initial draft. Early drafts of the PC-PART were piloted with small samples. Subsequently, testing occurred with numerous samples including, developmentally disabled youths, adults with acquired brain injury, psychiatric hospital patients and older adults. Testing has been done in urban and rural settings, and in culturally and linguistically diverse groups. Testing was done in Canada and Australia.
Construct	• PC-PART data patterns matched clinical outcomes of rehabilitation and geriatric management and evaluation patients in consecutive case series in two units.
Criterion	• No data available.
Overall Utility	
Research	• Can be used to examine and compare personal-care participation patterns of patients, including changes over time.
	• Can be used as an outcome measure for both in-patient and out-patient rehabilitation.
Clinical	• Provides useful information to clinicians and patients about the presence of personal-care participation restrictions that threaten survival.
	• Can be used to assess the need for interventions, the effectiveness of interventions and the efficiency of interventions.

continued

Table 8-9 (continued)

PERSONAL CARE PARTICIPATION ASSESSMENT AND RESOURCE TOOL (PC-PART), FORMERLY THE HART

Strengths	• Helps assessors to consider whether improvements in body structure or function or in activity are likely to eliminate participation restriction and whether environmental modification will be required. • Found to be acceptable to clinicians. • Found to be superior to the SMAF in large scale testing in numerous rehabilitation and aged care services. • Theoretically based on the WHO-ICIDH and subsequently on the WHO-ICF. • Measures just personal care participation—the tasks necessary for survival. • User-friendly for clinicians and time efficient. • Comprehensive, hence no critical survival items missed. • Written in common language, hence is easy to administer. Wording deals well with potentially embarrassing items. Acceptable to patients. • Two instructional videos are available: "HART" and the "ICF," and "How to use the PC-PART in rehabilitation."
Weaknesses	• Looks longer and more daunting than it is. • Only measures one small component of health status. Users who do not appreciate this are disappointed by its narrow focus. • Additional psychometric testing is required to develop a valid approach to summation of scores within and across domains.

Editors' Notes for Chapter 9

Mine the Gold

Development and education specialists address play as the milieu for children's growth and skill development. When combined with occupational therapy knowledge about both the meaning of play and the components of performance, there is substantial evidence from the literature to guide our thinking.

Become Systematic

Observation of play can be entertaining and informative. Children can shift play emphasis very quickly, so without a systematic data gathering method, documentation can be dependent on a particular therapist's focus for that day.

Use Evidence in Practice

Evidence about play suggests that when we use systematic documentation about aspects of play, we can design and structure more effective interventions.

Make Occupational Therapy Contribution Explicit

Play is a major life occupation for children. Occupational therapists need to participate in play assessment to inform families and team members of our interest and expertise in the meaning of play performance.

Engage in Occupation-Based, Client-Centered Practice

Measuring play enables occupational therapist's to focus their expertise on the complexity of performance within meaningful occupation. The occupational therapist can also capture performance component skills and liabilities as the child needs to use them, rather than in isolation.

CHAPTER

9

MEASURING PLAY PERFORMANCE

Anita C. Bundy, ScD, OTR, FAOTA

INTRODUCTION

Societal values regarding the worth of play depend on our beliefs about what play is, what it looks like, and what purpose it serves. Play is a primary occupation. However, much of our knowledge and actions about play come into conflict with culturally held beliefs about the best way to use our time. To provide optimal intervention to young children and their caregivers, we must resolve these conflicts within ourselves and help others to do so as well.

WHAT IS PLAY? (FROM THE PERSPECTIVE OF OCCUPATIONAL THERAPY ASSESSMENT)

There is little agreement and much ambiguity about virtually every aspect of play, from its definition, to its purpose, to the ways in which it manifests itself (Sutton-Smith, 1997). The only thing clear about play is that it is a multifaceted and complex phenomenon. For the purposes of assessment in occupational therapy, play is comprised of five factors. These are:

1. What the player does.
2. Why the player enjoys chosen play activities.
3. How the player approaches play (and other activity).
4. The player's capacity to play.
5. The relative supportiveness of the environment.

When doing play assessment, occupational therapists must be aware of the factor(s) addressed by the assessment(s) they have chosen. To do a complete evaluation, a therapist should consider each of the five factors. Of

course, it may not always be necessary or possible to evaluate each factor for every child. In that case, therapists must choose assessments that reflect the factors of greatest interest (Table 9-1).

WHY MEASURE PLAY?

Play is the primary occupation of children. Play is also an important source of skill development and acculturation. In short, there is no more important way in which children spend their time. While occupational therapists who work with children have focused historically on the skills and capacities underlying play (and function in general), a new era of professional awareness and accountability is causing therapists to "move up the hierarchy" and focus their assessment on occupations their clients need and want to do in their daily lives. Clearly, play fits that description.

ISSUES RELATED TO MEASURING PLAY

While occupational therapists claim play as a primary occupation, culturally held beliefs often interfere with their valuing it. Is play really as important as self-care, school, or, in fact, any childhood occupation? Clinicians are not alone in undervaluing play. In the United States, third party payers may confuse play with diversion, which is not reimbursable. The educational system, the largest employer of American therapists who work with children, may not find play to be educationally relevant. Parents may feel children with disabilities cannot afford to "waste time" when they are so far behind their peers developmentally or when they are needed to help out at home or in the family business.

Table 9-1

ASSESSMENTS BY FACTORS

Assessment	Factors What Player Does	Why Player Enjoys Activity	How Player Approaches Play	Capacity of Player	Support From Environment
Play History			2		2
Pediatric Interest Profiles	1				
Assess of Ludic Behaviors	1		1	1	2
Pediatric Activity Card Sort	1				
Test of Playfulness (TOP)			1		
Child Behaviors Inventory of Playfulness			1		
Revised Knox Preschool Play Scale	2			1	
Transdisciplinary Play-Based Assessment				1	
Child-Initiated Pretend Play Assessment (CHIPPA)	2				
Test of Environmental Supportiveness		2			1
Home Observation for Measurement of the Environment					1

1=Address one or more play factors without penalizing children for disabilities not directly related to the factor
2=Commonly used by occupational therapists in clinical practice or research.

Even if a therapist wanted to evaluate play for its own sake, few assessments exist (Bundy, 1993; Morrison & Metzger, 2001). Moreover, evaluation of all the factors related to play requires a test battery. Since no such battery currently exists, therapists must choose assessments carefully to be certain that they reflect the factors particularly relevant to the child. The inclusion of the word "play" in the title of an assessment does not mean that assessment will provide a complete, or even a valid, evaluation of play.

Perhaps, in part, because of the lack of valid and reliable tools, therapists often resort to informal assessment based on unstructured observation of a child's play. This approach may yield valuable information to the experienced examiner who is cognizant of play's many facets. However, as play is very complex, formal measures provide the structure needed by most examiners to conduct and interpret the results of assessment in the most thor-

ough and efficient way possible. Optimal intervention depends on quality interpretation of assessment data.

REVIEW OF RECOMMENDED MEASURES

The assessments reviewed in this chapter (see Tables 9-2 to 9-9) represent four of the five play-related factors. While each assessment has been "assigned" to a factor, some reflect more than one. Recommended assessments pertaining to both primary and secondary factors are shown in Table 9-1. Assessments were selected because they met at least one of the following criteria. They: 1) address one or more play factors without penalizing children for disabilities not directly related to the factor, or 2) are commonly used by occupational therapists in clinical practice or research.

Table 9-2

PLAY HISTORY

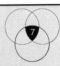

Play Factors (Primary, Secondary)	What the player does (environmental supportiveness, how the player approaches play).
Sources	Behnke, C., & Fetkovich, M. M. (1984). Examining the reliability and validity of the Play History. *American Journal of Occupational Therapy, 38*, 94-100.
	Bryze, K. (1997). Narrative contributions to the Play History. In L. D. Parham & L. S. Fazio (Eds.), *Play in occupational therapy for children* (pp. 23-34). St. Louis: C. V. Mosby.
	Takata, N. (1974). Play as a prescription. In M. Reilly (Ed.), *Play as exploratory learning* (pp. 209-246). Beverly Hills, CA: Sage.
Purpose	• Examination of children's play experiences and opportunities through the eyes of caregivers and across development.
	• Can be used for understanding children better and for intervention planning.
Type of Client	• Children (infancy through mid-adolescence) for whom play is a concern. Can be used across diagnoses.
Most Relevant Service Settings	• Home.
Clinical Utility	
Format	• Administered through a semi-structured interview with a parent or other caregiver.
Procedures	• Comprised of two information-gathering sections: previous play experiences and actual play examination. These are designed to capture the form (play style) and content of children's play over time.
	• The Play History is recorded on a taxonomy of play development that includes five epochs (sensorimotor, symbolic, and simple constructive; dramatic; complex constructive; pre-game; and recreation) Each epoch is divided into four elements (materials, actions, people, setting). Examiners describe each element as evidence for or against and encouragement or discouragement from caregivers. The examiner then interprets the data and develops a plan for intervention if needed.
Completion Time	• Not specified. As a lot of information is gathered, the assessment can be rather time-consuming, especially when gathering data about older children.
Standardization	• In order to retain the richness of the data, Takata has emphasized the need for flexibility in gathering data using the Play History.
Reliability	
Internal Consistency	• Not reported.
Test-Retest	• At 3-week intervals, the overall coefficient was 0.77 with category coefficients ranging from 0.41 to 0.78.
Inter-Rater	• Using videotaped interviews, overall inter-rater reliability was 0.91. Category coefficients ranged from 0.58 to 0.85. Reliability was higher with typically developing children than with children with disabilities (Behnke & Fetkovich, 1984).
Intra-Rater	• Not reported.
Validity	
Content	• Based on extensive literature review. However, the literature (particularly that on which the descriptions of the play epochs are based) is primarily theory, rather than research-based.
	• Investigations of adolescents (e.g., Csikszentmihalyi & Larson, 1984) suggest that content validity of some epochs may be in question.

continued

Table 9-2 (continued)

PLAY HISTORY

Convergent	• When correlated with the Minnesota Child Development Inventory, the coefficient for typically developing children was 0.97 and for children with disabilities, 0.70. Average correlation between epoch scores and age was 0.85 (0.94 for typically developing children; 0.79 for children with disabilities).
Construct	• No evidence presented.
Strengths	• Currently, the only assessment that enables examiners to explore play over time.
	• Examiners unfamiliar with play development may find this tool particularly useful.
Weaknesses	• Limited evaluation of reliability and validity.
	• Some information contained in the play epochs may be outdated.

ASSESSING WHAT THE PLAYER DOES (PLAY ACTIVITY)

Players choose to be involved in many different kinds of activities. These activities can be considered to be play if they meet three criteria. They are relatively intrinsically motivated, internally controlled, and free of some of the constraints of reality (Bundy, 2002; Neumann, 1971). When an activity is intrinsically motivating, it is done for its own sake, for the pure pleasure of doing it rather than for any external reward. An activity is internally controlled when players are in charge of their actions and some aspects of the activity's outcome. When an activity is free of some of the constraints of reality, players can leave behind some of the rules and expectations of objective reality; they are free to pretend to be someone else or to tease and joke playfully and engage in benign mischief (Bundy, 2002; Neumann, 1971). Four assessments are reviewed: the Play History (Bryze, 1997; Takata, 1974), the Pediatric Interest Profiles (Henry, 2000), the Assessment of Ludic Behaviors (ALB) (Ferland, 1997), and the Pediatric Activity Card Sort (Mandich et al., 2004); the latter is a broad assessment covering more than just play. In addition to these three assessments, Bryze (1997) argued compellingly for the use of narrative methodology in gathering information related to play interests and activities. See Chapter 5 for a discussion of narrative methodology.

ASSESSING WHY THE PLAYER ENJOYS AN ACTIVITY

Intrinsic motivation is an important characteristic of play (Rubin, Fein, & Vandenberg, 1983). Understanding the source of a player's motivation to engage in a particular activity (the benefits he or she derives from it) can be particularly helpful when, for example, a client's goal is to increase his or her repertoire of enjoyable play activities. Unfortunately, this play factor is relatively elusive and difficult to evaluate. Not surprisingly, there are no standardized assessments available reflecting this play factor. A lack of assessments, however, does not negate the importance of this play factor. Therapists are encouraged to glean information about the source of a player's motivation through observation of a child playing and interview of caregivers and children. Much can be learned about a child's motivation in the context of other play assessments: Play History, Pediatric Interest Profiles, Pediatric Activity Card Sort (PACS), Assessment of Ludic Behavior (ALB), Revised Knox Preschool Play Scale (PPS-R) (Knox, 1997), Test of Playfulness (ToP) (Bundy, 1997), and Test of Environmental Supportiveness (TOES) (Bronson & Bundy, 2001). When gathering information about a child's motivation, the therapist first identifies activities from which a child gains particular pleasure, then the therapist examines those activities for underlying patterns suggestive of motivation (e.g., mastery, social interaction, sensation).

ASSESSING HOW A PLAYER APPROACHES PLAY (AND OCCUPATIONS IN GENERAL)

More important than the play activities in which a child engages may be the manner in which that child approaches play (Bundy, 1993). This disposition to play is termed *playfulness* (Barnett, 1990; Lieberman, 1977). Playfulness reflects the same traits characteristic of a play transaction: intrinsic motivation, internal control, and freedom from some constraints of reality. While playfulness may be observed in play, it is not specific to play and may be seen in an individual's approach to any activity. Two assessments of playfulness that show promise for use by occupational therapists are reviewed here: the ToP (Bundy, 1997) and the Child Behaviors Inventory of Playfulness (CBIP)

Table 9-3

PEDIATRIC INTEREST PROFILES: SURVEY OF PLAY FOR CHILDREN AND ADOLESCENTS*

Play Factors **(Primary, Secondary)**	What the player does.
Source	Therapy Skill Builders, 555 Academic Court, San Antonio, TX, 78204-2498, (phone) 800-211-8378, (fax) 800-232-1223.
Important References	Henry, A. D. (1998). Development of a measure of adolescent leisure interests. *American Journal of Occupational Therapy*, *52*, 531-539.
Purpose	• Provide an easy way to gain a profile of a child's play interests.
Type of Client	• Children and adolescents between 6 and 21 years of age regardless of type of disability.
Most Relevant Service Settings	• Easily used in most any setting.
Clinical Utility	
Format	• Paper-and-pencil checklist format. • Can be administered individually or in a small group setting.
Procedures	• Children/adolescents respond to questions regarding interest, participation, enjoyment, etc., in leisure/play activities typical of peers. • KPS and PPS use drawings to represent activities.
Completion Time	• Approximately 15 minutes (for KPS) to 30 minutes (for ALIP).
Standardization	• Each test consists of standard choices to which the child/adolescent responds.
Reliability	
Internal Consistency	• ALIP—Cronbach's alpha ranged from 0.59 to 0.80 for subscale scores and was 0.93 for total scores for questions regarding level of interest in activities (n=88 adolescents with various disabilities).
Inter-Rater	• Not reported.
Intra-Rater	• Not reported.
Test-Retest	• KPS—Pearson Product Moment coefficients ranged from 0.45 to 0.91 for total scores (n=31 children without disabilities). • PPS—Not reported. • ALIP—Pearson Product Moment coefficients ranged from 0.61 to 0.85 for total scores (n=28 adolescents without disabilities). • ALIP—Pearson Product Moment coefficients ranged from 0.62 to 0.78 for total scores (n=88 adolescents with various disabilities).
Validity	
Content	• Items for all three versions developed from interviews and preliminary surveys of children or adolescents in the targeted age range.
Convergent	• Not reported.
Construct	• ALIP—Question regarding level of enjoyment in activities was shown to discriminate among adolescents with and without disabilities.
Strengths	• The only assessments specifically devoted to developing a profile of play interests from the perspective of children and adolescents. • Require minimal examiner training.
Weaknesses	• Activities seem most relevant to North American children.

*Comprised of three assessments: the Kids Play Survey (KPS) (6 to 9 years), Pre-Teen Play Survey (PPS) (9 to 12 years), and Adolescent Leisure Interest Profile (ALIP) (12 to 21 years).

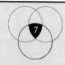

Table 9-4

ASSESSMENT OF LUDIC BEHAVIORS (ALB)*

Play Factors (Primary, Secondary)	What the player does; how the player approaches play; capacity to play, (environmental supportiveness).
Source	Ferland, F. (1997). *Play, Children with physical disabilities and occupational therapy.* Ottawa, Ontario, Canada: University of Ottawa.
Purpose	• Although not explicitly stated, the primary purposes of the ALB appear to be to understand children's play and for intervention planning. The ALB also provides a profile of attitude, interests, and abilities that could also serve as a measure of progress.
Type of Client	• Preschool-aged children with physical disabilities with or without cognitive impairments.
Most Relevant Service Settings	• OT clinical settings are specified, although any supportive play setting likely could support the observation.
Clinical Utility	
Format	• Parent Interview portion: A structured interview is administered prior to observing the child in play. The interview consists of eight questions regarding the child's interests and preferences, ludic attitude, communication with and by the child, and available play materials as well as background information and a schedule of typical weekly activities.
	• The observational portion: Occurs during child's free play. Scores are awarded in five areas: 1) general level of interest in the environment, 2) ludic interests in actions and use of space and objects, 3) ludic abilities with regard to actions and use of space and objects, 4) ludic attitude, and 5) communication of needs and feelings. Each item is scored on a 3-point (0 to 2) scale.
Procedures	• Ideally, the interview portion of the ALB is conducted with both parents.
	• The examiner creates a playful environment, rich with opportunities and freedom. The examiner scores the ALB as the child plays. Toward the end of the session, if items have not been observed, the examiner initiates an activity that includes those items and encourages the child to get involved.
Completion Time	• Assumed to be approximately 1 hour for each part (observation and interview).
	• Additional time is required for interpretation and intervention planning.
Standardization	• Items for both portions are standard and described completely in Ferland's book.
Reliability	• No evidence of reliability is reported.
Validity	
Content	• Both instruments were developed to conform to the Ludic Model, which was based on the results of an extensive 2-year qualitative study.
	• Various versions of both instruments have been reviewed by three groups of occupational therapist experts who made suggestions that led to improved clarity and completeness of the instruments.
Convergent	• Not reported.
Construct	• Not reported.
Strengths	• A comprehensive assessment of play; it reflects three play factors directly and at least one more indirectly.
	• Reflects an articulated theory of play.
Weaknesses	• Lacks statistical evidence for validity or reliability, thus results must be viewed with caution.
	• Only intended for use with children with physical disabilities.

*Two parts: Observation-based assessment and parent interview.

Table 9-5

PEDIATRIC ACTIVITY CARD SORT (PACS)

Play Factors	What the player does.
Source	Canadian Occupational Therapy Association, CAOT publications ACE, Canadian Association of Occupational Therapists, CTTC Building, 3400-1125 Colonel By Drive, Ottawa, Ontario, Canada, K1S 5R1, (Web) www.caot.org.
Important References	Several master's projects have been conducted regarding this measure. For more information, contact: A. Mandich in the Department of Occupational Therapy at the University of Western Ontario, London, Ontario, Canada.
Purpose	• Measures child's level of occupational engagement in a range of activities (including play) and participation at a particular point in time.
	• Can be used to initiate goal setting for occupational therapy intervention.
Type of Client	• Children between the ages of 6 to 12 years of age with various diagnoses and physical disabilities (e.g., developmental coordination disorder (DCD), Asperger's Syndrome, etc.)
Most Relevant Service Settings	• Schools, pediatric facilities, or private practice; also as a research instrument to explore occupational engagement.
Clinical Utility	
Format	• Consists of cards (depicting personal care, school/productivity, hobbies/social activities), and sports and a scoring sheet.
Procedures	• Administered by occupational therapists or certified occupational therapy assistants to either children or their parents. Examiners show cards and ask whether (and how frequently) children engage in activities depicted. Children identify their five most important activities and five activities they want to do.
Completion Time	• Can be administered in 15 to 20 minutes. More time may be required for elaboration of activities.
Standardization	• Criterion referenced.
Reliability	• Studies are currently being conducted.
Validity	
Content	• Activities were identified initially through observation and experiences of the authors with children, literature search, and review of existing occupational therapy assessments.
	• Five steps were taken for instrument validation: first, item validation was undertaken with 13 children between the ages of 6 to 12 years (McClenaghan, 1999); second, parents corroborated their children's (n=11) reports (Bowman, 1999). Next, the instrument was shown to be sensitive to age (Horn & Williams, 2000). Finally, the PACs was shown to detect differences in occupational profile between children with DCD and typically-developing children (n=10; ages 6-10) (Liston, 2002).
Strengths	• Occupation-based assessment supporting a client-centered approach.
	• Photographs are appealing to children.
	• Good tool for research.
Weaknesses	• New instrument; limited evidence for reliability or validity.

Table 9-6

TEST OF PLAYFULNESS (ToP) VERSION 4

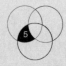

Play Factors (Primary, Secondary)	How the player approaches play.
Source	Currently available primarily for research purposes by contacting the author: Anita Bundy, ScD, OTR, School of Occupation and Leisure Sciences, University of Sydney, PO Box 170, Lidcombe NSW, Australia, (e-mail) a.bundy@fhs.usyd.edu.au.
Important References	Bundy, A. C. (1997). Play and playfulness: What to look for. In L. D. Parham & L. S. Fazio (Eds.), *Play in occupational therapy for children* (pp. 52-66). St. Louis: C.V. Mosby.
	Bundy, A. C., Nelson, L., Metzger, M., & Bingaman, K. (2001). Reliability and validity of a test of playfulness. *Occupational Therapy Journal of Research, 21,* 276-292.
	Okimoto, A. M., Bundy, A. C., & Hanzlik, J. R. (2003). Playfulness in children with and without disability: Measurement and intervention. In C. Royeen (Ed.), *Pediatric issues in occupational therapy.* Bethesda, MD: American Occupational Therapy Association, 254-267.
	Hess, L., & Bundy, A. C. (2003). The association between playfulness and coping in adolescents. *Physical and Occupational Therapy in Pediatrics, 23,* 5-17.
	Harkness, L., & Bundy, A. C. (2001). Playfulness and children with physical disabilities. *Occupational Therapy Journal of Research, 21,* 73-89.
	Leipold, E., & Bundy, A. C. (2000). Playfulness and children with ADHD. *Occupational Therapy Journal of Research,* 61-79.
	Reed, C., Dunbar, S., & Bundy, A. C. (2000). The effect of inclusive programming on the playfulness of preschoolers with and without autism. *Physical and Occupational Therapy in Pediatrics, 19,* 73-91.
Purpose	• Designed to capture four elements of playfulness in children: intrinsic motivation, internal control, freedom from some constraints of reality, and framing (the ability to give and read cues).
Type of Client	• All children, infants through adolescents, regardless of disability for whom play and playfulness are concerns.
Most Relevant Service Settings	• Any setting that supports free play although natural play settings (e.g., home, neighborhood, school) are preferred.
Clinical Utility	
Format	• Twenty-nine-item observational assessment. Each item is scored on a 4-point scale (0 to 3) reflecting extent, intensity, or skill.
Procedures	• Administered during 15- to 20-minute free play sessions. Ideally, the ToP is given in an environment familiar to the child with familiar toys and playmates. Raters are urged to administer the ToP in more than one setting (e.g., indoors and outdoors) and to refrain from interaction with the child unless the child's safety is threatened.
Completion Time	• Twenty to 30 minutes (including scoring time) for each setting.
	• Interpretation requires additional time.
Standardization	• Data have been collected on children 3 months through 18 years (majority on children 3 to 10 years) in the United States, Canada, Central America, South Africa, and Australia. Also has been used widely in Scandinavia.
	• Items are standard and described completely in the manual. Version 2 of the ToP is described in Parham & Fazio's (1997) book.

continued

Table 9-6 (continued)

TEST OF PLAYFULNESS (ToP) VERSION 4

Reliability	• Detailed information on the reliability of Versions 1 and 2 of the ToP are available in Bundy et al. (2001).
	• Version 4 (reported below unless otherwise indicated) comprises several new items; evidence for reliability.
Internal Consistency	• Cronbach's alpha equivalent near 1.00.
Inter-Rater	• Data from 95% of raters (n~300) demonstrate goodness of fit to the Rasch model.
Intra-Rater	• Not reported.
Test-Retest	• Currently being addressed; not yet published.
Validity	
Content	• Based on a thorough review of the literature.
Convergent	• Correlation of Version 3 with the Children's Playfulness Scale (Barnett, 1990) was moderate at 0.46.
Construct	• Using Rasch analysis, 28 of 29 items have been shown to have acceptable goodness of fit statistics and, therefore, to conform to the expectations of the measurement model.
Strengths	• Easy to administer by raters familiar with minimal training.
	• Requires no special test equipment.
	• Seems to be sensitive to the effects of intervention.
	• Guidelines provided in Bundy (1997) enable examiners to interpret observations as the basis for intervention planning.
	• Large data base (n~2000 observations).
Weaknesses	• Not yet available commercially.
	• Does not yield a standard score except in the context of research where the author provides this to the researcher.

(Rogers, Impara, Frary, et al., 1998). In addition, the reader is referred to the ALB (Ferland, 1997), described earlier, as it also is an assessment of the way children approach play.

ASSESSING A PLAYER'S CAPACITY TO PLAY

Until recently, most assessments of play have focussed on players' capacity for play (i.e., performance components) and skill development derived from play. While underlying capacity and skill development are important, they reflect only one factor related to play. Three assessments administered in the context of play are reviewed: the PPS-R (Knox, 1997), the Transdisciplinary Play-Based Assessment (2nd edition; TPBA) (Linder, in press), and the Child-Initiated Pretend Play Assessment (CHIPPA; Stagnitti, 2003). The latter examines cognition in the context of pretend play. In addition, the reader is referred to the ALB (Ferland, 1997) as it also is an assessment of the abilities children use in play. However, it is important to note that there are a myriad of assessments that one might use to assess children's underlying skills. The advantage of assessments such as those reviewed here is that they allow the examiner to see what skills a child actually uses in play. Thus, it is important to ensure that play is the context for the assessment. Setting up the environment in a manner conducive to play is an important factor in evaluation of underlying skills conducted in the play context. Such environments include familiar playmates and toys, adults who are minimally intrusive, an implicit agreement between players and caregivers that children can use toys in whatever manner they see fit, and scheduling that reduces the likelihood that a child is tired, hungry, or sick (Rubin et al., 1983).

ASSESSING THE SUPPORTIVENESS OF THE PLAY ENVIRONMENT

Play represents a transaction between a player and the environment. Thus, if we are to do a thorough evaluation of play, we need to include investigation of the relative

Table 9-7

CHILD BEHAVIORS INVENTORY OF PLAYFULNESS (CBIP)

Play Factors **(Primary, Secondary)**	How the player approaches play.
Source	Rogers, C. S., Impara, J. C., Frary, R. B. et al. (1998). Measuring playfulness: Development of the Child Behaviors Inventory of Playfulness. In S. Reifel (Ed.), *Play & culture studies* (Vol. 1, pp. 121-136). Greenwich, CT: Ablex.
Purpose	• Constructed as a brief trait-rating instrument suitable for use with parents and teachers who have received no specialized training.
Type of Client	• Piloted on a sample of 892 children attending preschool through fourth grade. • Presumably, all children were typically developing. However, the CBIP appears suitable for older children and for children with disabilities.
Most Relevant Service Settings	• Useful in virtually any setting in which adults are available to fill it out.
Clinical Utility	
Format	• The CBIP is a 28-item caregiver questionnaire that assesses two factors: playfulness and externality. • Each item is rated on a 5-point scale (1 to 5).
Procedures	• Parents or teachers rate the child's behaviors on the scale.
Completion Time	• Not specified. Presumed to be approximately 15 minutes.
Standardization	• The CBIP is a survey instrument. No manual is available. However, the items are very clearly stated.
Reliability	
Internal Consistency	• Cronbach's alpha coefficients ranged from 0.81 to 0.94 for items related to playfulness and from 0.62 to 0.72 for items related to externality.
Inter-Rater	• Correlation coefficients ranged from 0.12 to 0.60 for playfulness and from 0.11 to 0.57 for externality, depending on the sample. Teachers attained higher correlations than did parents.
Intra-Rater	• Not reported.
Test-Retest	• Not reported.
Validity	
Content	• Original items were developed by noted play experts. • A second panel of experts evaluated the original pool of items. The current items reflect agreement by the second panel.
Convergent	• The CBIP was correlated with the Behavioral Style Questionnaire, on which lower scores reflect "easier" temperament traits. Coefficients for mothers rating both scales ranged from -0.41 to 0.02 for playfulness and -0.04 to 0.49 on externality. Coefficients for fathers ranged from -0.49 to 0.19 on playfulness and from -0.18 to 0.28 on externality. • The CBIP was also correlated with the Matthews Youth Test for Health (MYTH-Form 0) (Matthews & Angulo, 1980). The correlation between playfulness and impatience-aggression was 0.10 and between playfulness and competitiveness was 0.59. The coefficients for externality were 0.29 with impatience-aggression and -0.15 with competitiveness.

continued

Table 9-7 (continued)

CHILD BEHAVIORS INVENTORY OF PLAYFULNESS (CBIP)

Construct	• The results of the CBIP were correlated with an observation of playfulness. The coefficient for playfulness with dependent behaviors was -0.42 and with pretense ranged from 0.15 to 0.41. The coefficient for externality with dependent behaviors was 0.43 and with pretense ranged from 0.10 to 0.22.
Strengths	• Good means for obtaining information from parents and teachers about playfulness of children in preschool through fourth grade.
	• Probably most useful for gathering descriptive information and for research purposes.
Weaknesses	• Reliability between raters is questionable so information must be used with caution or gathered from multiple sources.
	• Although item means and subscale means are provided, there is little basis for making meaningful judgments regarding overall scores of individual children.

supportiveness of the environment. Environmental assessment should address both its human and non-human aspects. Review of relevant literature suggests caregivers, playmates, objects, space, and qualities of the sensory environment are critical aspects for inclusion in an assessment of environmental supportiveness for play. Unfortunately, few assessments exist that include all important aspects and have been found to be psychometrically sound. Two assessments are reviewed: the TOES (Bundy, 1999) and the Home Observation for Measurement of the Environment (HOME) (Bradley et al., 2000; Bradley, Caldwell, & Corwyn 2003; Caldwell & Bradley, 1984). While it shows promise, the TOES is in a relatively early stage of development. Various versions of the HOME are designed for children 0 to 15 years; they focus on the family-based and home-based childcare settings. However, the HOME is a broad assessment and contains only a few items directly related to play.

RECOMMENDATIONS AND FUTURE DIRECTIONS

Play may be the most important occupation in which children engage. Thus, occupational therapists should include play assessments in their evaluation repertoire routinely. Further, play is among the most complex of childhood activities. Thus, occupational therapists must evaluate all relevant factors related to play when play is a concern for their young clients. At present, no batteries of play scales exist to facilitate its thorough evaluation. Thus, therapists will need to choose among assessments representing the various play factors to glean the information they desire. Finally, since play often is undervalued by caregivers, therapists have an important responsibility to educate others about the many benefits of play including, but not limited to, skill development.

Given the importance and relative complexity of play, there are fewer than necessary valid and reliable assessments available for use by occupational therapists. Thus, we also have a responsibility to continue to develop and test play-related assessments.

REFERENCES

Barnett, L. A. (1990). Playfulness: Definition, design, and measurement. *Play and Culture, 3,* 319-336.

Behnke, C., & Fetkovich, M. M. (1984). Examining the reliability and validity of the Play History. *American Journal of Occupational Therapy, 38,* 94-100.

Bledsoe, N. P., & Shepherd, J. (1982). A study of reliability and validity of a preschool play scale. *American Journal of Occupational Therapy, 36,* 783-788.

Bowman, K. (1999). *Development of an activity card sort for children: Do parental reports on an activity card sort reflect similar results as their children?* Unpublished master's project, University of Western Ontario, London, Canada.

Bradley, R. H. (2000). Deceived by omission: The difficulty of matching measurement and theory when assessing the home environment. *Journal Research on Adolescence, 10,* 307-314.

Bradley, R. H. (1994). The HOME Inventory: Review and reflections. In H. Reese (Ed.), *Advances in child development and behavior* (pp. 241-288). San Diego, CA: Academic.

Bradley, R. H., & Caldwell, B. M. (1979). Home observation for measurement of the environment: A revision of the preschool scale. *American Journal of Mental Deficiency, 84,* 235-244.

Bradley, R. H., Caldwell, B. M., & Corwyn, R. F. (2003). The Child Care HOME Inventoried: Assessing the quality of family child care homes. *Early Childhood Research Quarterly, 18,* 294-309.

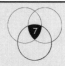

Table 9-8

REVISED KNOX PRESCHOOL PLAY SCALE (PPS-R)

Play Factors (Primary, Secondary)	Player's capacity to play, (what the player does in play).
Source	Knox, S. (1997). Development and current use of the Knox Preschool Play Scale. In L. D. Parham & L. S. Fazio (Eds.), *Play in occupational therapy for children* (pp. 35-51). St. Louis: C. V. Mosby.
Important References	Bledsoe, N. P., & Shepherd, J. (1982). A study of reliability and validity of a preschool play scale. *American Journal of Occupational Therapy, 36,* 783-788.
	Harrison, H., & Kielhofner, G. (1986). Examining the reliability and validity of the Preschool Play Scale with handicapped children. *American Journal of Occupational Therapy, 40,* 167-173.
	Knox, S. (1974). A play scale. In M. Reilly (Ed.), *Play as exploratory learning* (pp. 247-266). Beverly Hills, CA: Sage.
	Bundy, A. C. (1989). A comparison of the play skills of normal boys and boys with sensory integrative dysfunction. *Occupational Therapy Journal of Research, 9,* 84-100.
	Clifford, J. M., & Bundy, A. C. (1989). Play preference and play performance in normal preschoolers and preschoolers with sensory integrative dysfunction. *Occupational Therapy Journal of Research, 9,* 202-217.
Purpose	• Provides a developmental description of a child's underlying capacities for play. • Can be used either as a "diagnostic" tool or to measure effectiveness of intervention. • Also provides some limited information about a child's play interests.
Type of Client	• Children aged 0 to 6.
Most Relevant Service Settings	• Preschools, childcare centers, homes, and other settings where natural play environments are available
Clinical Utility	
Format	• An observational assessment administered both indoors and outdoors. • A child's behavior is observed as it reflects four play dimensions: Space management, material management, imitation, and participation. Dimensions are scored in 6-month increments up to age 3 and in yearly increments thereafter.
Procedures	• As children play in familiar settings with suitable playthings and playmates present, examiners score the children's behavior on items reflecting each dimension. Dimension scores are determined by averaging the item scores. An overall score is calculated by averaging dimension scores
Completion Time	• Two 30-minute observations, one indoors and one outdoors.
Standardization	• Not standardized. It is administered in familiar environments.
Reliability	• All reliability and validity information is based on the version of the PPS described by Bledsoe & Shepherd (1982) and a study completed by Harrison & Kielhofner (1986).
Internal Consistency	• Not reported.
Inter-Rater	• Coefficients ranged from r=0.88 to 0.996; p=0.0001 (higher with typically developing children than with children with disabilities).
Intra-Rater	• Not reported.
Test-Retest	• Correlation coefficients range from r=0.91 to 0.965; p=0.0001.

continued

Table 9-8 (continued)	
REVISED KNOX PRESCHOOL PLAY SCALE (PPS-R)	

Validity

Content
- All versions of the PPS have been based on thorough review of literature.

Convergent
- Correlation coefficients with Lunzer's Scale of Organization of Play Behavior ranged from r=0.59 to 0.64 (Hulme & Luzner, 1966).
- With Parten's Social Play Hierarchy (Parten 1932), they ranged from 0.60 to 0.64.
- With chronological age, they ranged from 0.74 to 0.95. In most cases, correlations were higher for typically developing children than for children with disabilities.

Construct
- Not reported.

Strengths
- Especially good for children whose underlying capacities cannot be evaluated easily with standardized testing.

Weaknesses
- Cannot serve as a sole measure of play.

Bradley, R.H., Corwyn, R. F., Caldwell, B. M., Whiteside-Mansell, Wasserman, G. A., & Mink, I. T. (2000). Measuring the home environments of children in early adolescence. *Journal of Research on Adolescence, 10,* 247-288.

Bronson, M., & Bundy, A. C. (2001). A correlational study of the Test of Playfulness and the Test of Environmental Supportiveness. *Occupational Therapy Journal of Research, 21,* 223-240.

Bryze, K. (1997). Narrative contributions to the Play History. In L. D. Parham & L. S. Fazio (Eds.), *Play in occupational therapy for children* (pp. 23-34). St. Louis: C. V. Mosby.

Bundy, A. C. (1989). A comparison of the play skills of normal boys and boys with sensory integrative dysfunction. *Occupational Therapy Journal of Research, 9,* 84-100.

Bundy, A. C. (1993). Assessment of play and leisure: Delineation of the problem. *American Journal of Occupational Therapy, 47,* 217-224.

Bundy, A. C. (1999). *Test of environmental supportiveness.* Ft. Collins, CO: Colorado State University.

Bundy, A. C. (1997). Play and playfulness: What to look for. In L. D. Parham & L. S. Fazio (Eds.), *Play in Occupational Therapy for Children.* St. Louis: C. V. Mosby.

Bundy, A. C., Nelson, L., Metzger, M., & Bingaman, K. (2001).Reliability and validity of a test of playfulness. *Occupational Therapy Journal of Research, 21,* 276-292.

Bundy, A. C. (2002). Play theory and sensory integration. In A. C. Bundy, S. J. Lane, E. A. Murray (Eds.), *Sensory integration: Theory and practice* (2nd ed.). Philadelphia: F. A. Davis.

Caldwell, B. M., & Bradley, R. H. (1984). *Administration manual: Home observation for measurement of the environment* (rev. ed.). Little Rock, AR: University of Arkansas at Little Rock.

Clifford, J. M., & Bundy, A. C. (1989). Play preference and play performance in normal preschoolers and preschoolers with sensory integrative dysfunction. *Occupational Therapy Journal of Research, 9,* 202-217.

Csikszentmihalyi, M., & Larson, R. (1984). *Being adolescent: Conflict and growth in the teenage years.* New York: Basic.

Ferland, F. (1997). *Play, children with physical disabilities and occupational therapy.* Ottawa, Ontario: University of Ottawa.

Friedli, C. (1994). *Transdisciplinary play-based assessment: A study of reliability and validity.* Doctoral dissertation. University of Colorado, Denver.

Harrison, H., & Kielhofner, G. (1986). Examining the reliability and validity of the Preschool Play Scale with handicapped children. *American Journal of Occupational Therapy, 40,* 167-173.

Harkness, L., & Bundy, A. C. (2001). Playfulness and children with physical disabilities. *Occupational Therapy Journal of Research, 21,* 73-89.

Henry, A. D. (1998). Development of a measure of adolescent leisure interests. *American Journal of Occupational Therapy, 52,* 531-539.

Henry, A. (2000). *Pediatric interest profiles.* San Antonio: Therapy Skill Builders.

Hess, L. & Bundy, A. C. (2003). The association between playfulness and coping in adolescents. *Physical and Occupational Therapy in Pediatrics, 23,* 5-17

Horn, S. & Williams, M. (2000). *Development and piloting of the Pediatric Occupational Card Sort (POCS): Stage II.* Unpublished master's thesis, University of Western Ontario, London, Ontario, Canada.

Hulme, I. & Luzner, E. (1966). Play, language, and reasoning in subnormal children. *Journal of Child Psychology, 7,* 107-123.

Knox, S. (1974). A play scale. In M. Reilly (Ed.), *Play as exploratory learning* (pp. 247-266). Beverly Hills, CA: Sage.

Knox, S. (1997). Development and current use of the Knox Preschool Play Scale. In L. D. Parham & L. S. Fazio (Eds.), *Play in occupational therapy for children* (pp. 35-51). St. Louis: C. V. Mosby.

Table 9-9

CHILD-INITIATED PRETEND PLAY ASSESSMENT (ChIPPA)

Play factors **(Primary, Secondary)**	Player's capacity to play, (what the player does in play).
Sources	Stagnitti, K. (2003). *The development of a child-initiated assessment of pretend play.* Doctoral thesis, LaTrobe University, Melbourne Australia. For training or research use, contact the author: karen.stagnitti@deakin.edu.au.
Important References	Stagnitti, K. (1998). *Learn to play: A practical program to improve a child's imaginative play skills.* Melbourne: Co-ordinates Therapy.
	Stagnitti, K. & Unsworth, C. (2000). The importance of pretend play to child development: An occupational therapy perspective. *British Journal of Occupational Therapy, 63,* 121-127.
	Stagnitti, K., Unsworth, C. A. & Rodger, S. (2000). Development of an assessment to identify play behaviours that discriminate between the play of typical preschoolers and preschoolers with pre-academic problems. *Canadian Journal of Occupational Therapy, 67,* 291-303.
	Stagnitti, K., & Unsworth, C. (2004). The test-retest reliability of the Child-Initiated Pretend Play Assessment. *American Journal of Occupational Therapy, 58,* 93-99.
Purpose	• Measures the quality of children's spontaneous pretend play.
Type of Client	• Children aged 3 years to 7 years for whom pretend play is a concern (e.g., children with autism spectrum disorder, developmental delay, emotional distress, and learning problems).
Most Relevant Service Settings	• Early intervention program, hospital and community settings.
Clinical utility	
Format	• Observational assessment with a total of three items (i.e., percentage of elaborate play actions, number of object substitutions, and number of imitated actions) scored in two 15 minute sessions (conventional imaginative play using conventional toys and symbolic play using unstructured objects); combined scores also are calculated.
Procedures	• Rater should be a professional trained to work with children. Elaborate play actions are scored by calculating the percentage of the child's actions that meet specified criteria. Number of object substitutions is the number of objects used as something else. Number of imitated items is the number of times the child imitates an action previously modeled by the examiner. Inexperienced raters may need to videotape the play for later scoring.
Completion Time	• For 3-year-olds, administration and recording time is 18 minutes; for 4- to 7-year-olds 30 minutes. Scoring requires an additional 5 to 10 minutes.
Standardization	• Standard scoring instructions appear in the unpublished manual.
Reliability	
Internal Consistency	• Not reported.
Inter-Rater	• Percentage of elaborate play action scores were 0.96 or 0.98 (kappa), number of object substitutions were 1.00 or 0.97 (kappa), and number of imitated actions ranged from 0.98 to 1.00 (kappa) (Stagnitti, Unsworth, & Rodger, 2000).
	• Inter-rater reliability studies have yet to be completed without the use of videotapes.
Intra-Rater	• Not reported.

continued

Table 9-9 (continued)

CHILD-INITIATED PRETEND PLAY ASSESSMENT (CHIPPA)

Test-Retest	• With children 4 to 5 years (n=38; including four with developmental delay), elaborate play ranged from r=0.73 to 0.85, number of object substitutions for symbolic play r=0.56, and for the conventional imaginative and symbolic play r=0.57. The remaining items were not normally distributed. Wilcoxon Matched-Pairs Signed-Ranks test were non-significant (p=0.35 to 0.97); percentage of agreement ranged from 63% to 84% (Stagnitti & Unsworth, 2004).

Validity

Content	• Expert review suggested that the ChIPPA has moderate to high content validity (Stagnitti, 2002a).
	• Play materials were tested for gender neutrality and developmental sensitivity (Stagnitti, Rodger, & Clarke, 1997).
Convergent	• The ChIPPA has been compared with the Miller Assessment for Preschoolers (Miller, 1982) and Lieberman's Playfulness Scale. The former is a measure of pre-academic ability and the latter a measure of playfulness.
	• Correlations between the ChIPPA and the Miller ranged from -0.09 to 0.4 with positive significant relationships between all sub-tests of the Miller and elaborate play scores. Number of object substitutions was positively and significantly related to the co-ordination, visual perception, and complex tasks sub-tests of the Miller. Correlation between Lieberman's Playfulness Scale and number of object substitutions was statistically significant at 0.4 (Stagnitti, 2002a).
Construct	• Not reported.

Strengths

• Covers the area of pretend play comprehensively; assesses both conventional imaginative and symbolic play.

• Suitable as a measure in research or clinical practice—has established psychometric properties.

• Allows the assessment of cognitive skills in the context of spontaneous play activity.

• Has been shown to distinguish between typically developing children and children with occupational performance difficulties in play.

Weaknesses

• Scoring is complicated, requires considerable practice, and intense concentration by the rater.

• Cannot serve as a sole measure of play.

• Inter-rater reliability in clinical situations is yet to be established.

Leipold, E., & Bundy, A. C. (2000). Playfulness and Children with ADHD. *Occupational Therapy Journal of Research,* 61-79.

Lieberman, J. (1977). *Playfulness: Its relationship to imagination and creativity.* New York: Academic Press.

Linder, T. W. (in press). *Transdisciplinary play-based assessment: A functional approach to working with young children* (Rev. ed.). Baltimore: Paul H. Brookes.

Liston. (2002). *The Pediatric Activity Card Sort: A comparison of occupational profiles for children with developmental coordination disorder and their typically developing peers.* Unpublished master's project, University of Western Ontario, London, Ontario, Canada.

Mandich, A., Polatajko, H., & Baum, C. (2003). *Occupation-based assessment in children: The Pediatric Activity Card Sort [Abstract]. CAOT Conference Proceedings* (p. 45). Winnipeg, Canada: MB.

Matthews, K. A., & Angulo, J. (1980). Measurement of the Type A behavior pattern in children: Assessment of children's competitiveness, impatience-anger, and aggression. *Child Development, 51,* 466-475.

McClenaghan, K.. (1999). *Development of the Pediatric Activity Card Sort: Stage one.* Unpublished master's project, University of Western Ontario, London, Ontario, Canada.

Miller, L. (1982). *Miller Assessment for Preschoolers.* Littleton, CO: Foundation for Knowledge in Child Development.

Table 9-10

TRANSDISCIPLINARY PLAY-BASED ASSESSMENT (TPBA) 2ND ED.

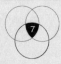

Play Factors (Primary, Secondary)	Player's capacity to play.
Source	Linder, T. W. (in press). *Transdisciplinary Play-Based Assessment: A functional approach to working with young children* (Rev. ed.). Baltimore: Paul H. Brookes.
Important References	Friedli, C. (1994). Transdisciplinary play-based assessment: A study of reliability and validity. Doctoral dissertation. University of Colorado, Denver. Myers, C. L., McBride, S. L., & Peterson, C. (1996). Transdisciplinary, play-based assessment in early childhood special education: An examination of social validity. *Topics in Early Childhood Special Education, 16,* 102-127.
Purpose	• To assess underlying developmental skills, learning style, interaction patterns, and other behaviors in children.
Type of Client	• Any child functioning between birth and 6 years of age for whom development is a concern.
Most Relevant Service Settings	• Community and early childhood settings with inter- or transdisciplinary teams.
Clinical Utility	
Format	• Observational assessment administered by a team (including parents). Examiners are encouraged to be flexible in order to meet the needs of the child. The TPBA is organized into four domains of development: cognitive, sensorimotor, emotional-social, and communication and language. Summary forms provide options for identifying most frequently observed strengths (or present performance), concerns, and areas of "readiness" (or next steps) for intervention in relation to observation guideline questions. • Detailed age tables enable observers to determine the developmental level of observed behaviors across each of the subcategories of each of the four domains.
Procedures	• Parents complete developmental questionnaires about their child's functioning at home. Then, a team observes the child for 1 to 1.5 hours during play activities with a play facilitator, parents, and if possible a peer or sibling. The play session comprises six aspects depending on the needs of the child: 1) unstructured facilitation, 2) structured facilitation, 3) child-child interaction, 4) parent-child interaction, 5) motor play, and 6) snack. Generally, the play session is videotaped. • During the observation (and later review of videotape), team members complete worksheets. Team discussion is an important part of the TPBA process. Following the observation, a brief post-session meeting is held. A second brief meeting is held in preparation for a later program planning meeting. Following the program planning meeting, a formal report is written.
Completion Time	• The TBPA is a lengthy process, including a 60- to 90-minute observation. No time is specified and clearly it varies from child to child.
Standardization	• Criterion-referenced.
Reliability	• Reports below are based on the first version. Additional work with the revised edition is in progress.
Internal Consistency	• Not reported.
Inter-Rater	• Good as reported by Friedli (1994).
Intra-Rater	• Good as reported by Friedli (1994).
Test-Retest	• Not reported.

continued

Table 9-10 (continued)

TRANSDISCIPLINARY PLAY-BASED ASSESSMENT (TPBA) 2ND ED.

Validity	• Reports below are based on the first version. Additional work with the revised edition is in progress.
Content	• Based on a thorough review of literature; item content supported by a panel of experts across the U.S.
Convergent	• Friedli (1994) compared results with those from the Batelle Developmental Inventory with favorable findings. Additional work is underway with the new version.
Construct	• Not reported.
Strengths	• Children's abilities are assessed in one play session in a non-threatening context that fosters their best performance.
	• Reports were found to be completed within required U.S. federal timelines more frequently (Myers, McBride, & Peterson, 1996).
	• Team functioning is fostered through the administration and interpretation process.
	• Families are integrally involved in a meaningful way.
Weaknesses	• Relatively little statistically based evidence for reliability or validity.
	• Cannot be used as a sole measure of play.
Final Word	• The TPBA is a kind way to assess the skills children use in play (and other occupations). The new edition is considerably more comprehensive than earlier versions.
	• Work is underway to support its validity and reliability. The TPBA fosters a cohesive team, including parents as important members.

Morrison, C.D., & Metzger, P. (2001). Play. In J. Case-Smith (Ed.), *Occupational therapy for children*. St. Louis: Mosby, pp. 528-544.

Myers, C. L., McBride, S. L., & Peterson, C. (1996). Transdisciplinary, play-based assessment in early childhood special education: An examination of social validity. *Topics in Early Childhood Special Education, 16,* 102-127.

Neumann, E. A. (1971). *The elements of play*. New York: MSS Information.

Okimoto, A. M., Bundy, A. C., & Hanzlik, J. R. (2003). Playfulness in children with and without disability: Measurement and intervention. In C. Royeen (Ed.), *Pediatric issues in occupational therapy*. Bethesda, MD: American Occupational Therapy Association, 254-267.

Parham, L. D., & Fazio, L. S. (Eds) (1997). *Play in occupational therapy for children*. St. Louis: C. V. Mosby.

Parten, M. (1932). Social participation among preschool children. *Journal of Abnormal Social Psychology, 27,* 243-249.

Reed, C., Dunbar, S., & Bundy, A. C. (2000). The effect of inclusive programming on the playfulness of preschoolers with and without autism. *Physical and Occupational Therapy in Pediatrics, 19,* 73-91.,

Rogers, C. S., Impara, J. C., Frary, R. B., et al. (1998). Measuring playfulness: Development of the child behaviors inventory of playfulness. In S. Reifel (Ed.), *Play & culture studies* (Vol. 1, pp. 121-136). Greenwich, CT: Ablex.

Rubin, K., Fein, G. G., & Vandenberg, B. (1983). Play. In P. H. Mussen (Ed.), *Handbook of child psychology: Socialization, personality, and social development* (Vol. 4, pp. 693-774). New York: Wiley.

Stagnitti, K. (1998). *Learn to play: A practical program to improve a child's imaginative play skills*. Melbourne: Co-ordinates Therapy.

Stagnitti, K. (2002). *The development of a child-initiated assessment of pretend play*. Vol. 1. Unpublished doctor of philosophy thesis, LaTrobe University, Melbourne, Australia.

Stagnitti, K., & Unsworth, C. (2000). The importance of pretend play to child development: An occupational therapy perspective. *British Journal of Occupational Therapy, 63,* 121-127.

Stagnitti, K., Unsworth, C. A. & Rodger, S. (2000). Development of an assessment to identify play behaviours that discriminate between the play of typical preschoolers and preschoolers with pre-academic problems. *Canadian Journal of Occupational Therapy, 67,* 291-303.

Stagnitti, K., & Unsworth, C. (2004). The test-retest reliability of the Child-Initiated Pretend Play Assessment. *American Journal of Occupational Therapy, 58,* 93-99.

Sutton-Smith, B. (1997). *The ambiguity of play*. Cambridge, MA: Harvard.

Takata, N. (1974). Play as a prescription. In M. Reilly (Ed.), *Play as exploratory learning* (pp. 209-246). Beverly Hills, CA: Sage.

Table 9-11

TEST OF ENVIRONMENTAL SUPPORTIVENESS (TOES)

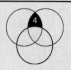

Play factors (Primary, Secondary)	Supportiveness of environment (Why player enjoys activity).
Source	Currently available primarily for research purposes by contacting the author: Anita Bundy, ScD, OTR, School of Occupation and Leisure Sciences, University of Sydney, PO Box 170, Lidcombe NSW, Australia, (fax) 61 2 9351 9166 (e-mail) a.bundy@fhs.usyd.edu.au.
Important References	Bronson, M., & Bundy, A. C. (2001). A correlational study of the Test of Playfulness and the Test of Environmental Supportiveness. *Occupational Therapy Journal of Research, 21*, 223-240.
Purpose	• Developed as a companion tool to the ToP to explore the ways in which a child's playfulness is affected by the environment.
	• It provides a basis for intervention planning and consultation with caregivers.
Type of Client	• Designed for use with younger children and adolescents (age range 1.5 to 15 yrs) when concerns are present about the supportiveness of the environment for play.
Most Relevant Service Settings	• Home, preschool, other community-based settings, early childhood centers.
Clinical Utility	
Format	• Seventeen-item observational assessment scored on a +2 to -2 scale.
	• Contains items concerning caregivers, playmates (of varying ages), play objects, space, and quality of the sensory environment.
Procedures	• The TOES is scored by an unobtrusive observer following a 15- to 20-minute free play session in an environment in which the child usually plays.
Completion Time	• Five to 10 minutes for scoring following the observation.
Standardization	• The manual delineates recommended procedures and carefully describes each item. Data have been collected on children between 1.5 and 15 years, typically developing and with varying disabilities, in the United States, Canada, Central America, and to a lesser extent, Scandinavia and Australia.
Reliability	• Reliability of the TOES has been tested primarily in very supportive environments. Thus, the levels of separation of the normative data are quite small. While the author assumes this to be an artifact of a small sample size, further research is necessary.
Internal Consistency	• Cronbach's alpha equivalent for items=0.99.
Inter-Rater	• Using Rasch analysis, data from 100% of raters (n~25) demonstrate goodness of fit to the measurement model.
Intra-Rater	• Not reported.
Test-retest	• Not reported.
Validity	
Content	• Developed based on a thorough review of related literature with input from a panel of experts.
Convergent	• Not reported.
Construct	• Using Rasch analysis, 16 of 17 items have been shown to have acceptable goodness of fit statistics and, therefore, to conform to the expectations of the measurement model.
	• Data from 95% of children tested (both typically developing and with various disabilities) demonstrated goodness of fit to the Rasch model.

continued

Table 9-11 (continued)

TEST OF ENVIRONMENTAL SUPPORTIVENESS (TOES)

Validity

   Content
- Developed based on a thorough review of related literature with input from a panel of experts.

   Convergent
- Not reported.

   Construct
- Using Rasch analysis, 16 of 17 items have been shown to have acceptable goodness of fit statistics and, therefore, to conform to the expectations of the measurement model.
- Data from 95% of children tested (both typically developing and with various disabilities) demonstrated goodness of fit to the Rasch model.

Strengths
- Sets play in the context of children's motivations; thus the assessment of environmental supportiveness is individualized.
- Easy to use; requires no special equipment, and minimal rater training.
- Provides a good basis for consultation with caregivers regarding the play environment.

Weaknesses
- Not yet available commercially.
- Does not yield a standard score except in the context of research where the author provides this to the researcher.

Table 9-12

HOME OBSERVATION FOR MEASUREMENT OF THE ENVIRONMENT (HOME)

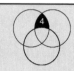

Play Factors (Primary, Secondary)	Supportiveness of environment.
Several Versions	• Standard (for use in children's homes: Infant/Toddler, Early Childhood, Middle Childhood, and Early Adolescence)
	• Child Care: Infant/Toddler and Early Childhood
	• Comprehensive (includes Standard, Childcare, and Disability Adapted versions).
Source	Available from Home Inventory LLC Distribution Center, c/o Lorraine Coulson, 2627 Winsor Drive, Eau Claire, Wisconsin, 54703, (phone/fax) 715-835-4393, (e-mail) lrcoulson@ualr.edu (email). Information also available from authors: Dr. Robert Bradley (rhbradley@ualr.edu) and Dr. Bettye M. Caldwell (BMCaldwell@ualr.edu).
Important References	Bradley, R. H. (1994). The HOME Inventory: Review and reflections. In H. Reese (Ed.), *Advances in child development and behavior* (pp. 241-288). San Diego, CA: Academic.
	Bradley, R. H. (2000). Deceived by omission: The difficulty of matching measurement and theory when assessing the home environment. *Journal Research on Adolescence, 10,* 307-314.
	Bradley, R. H., & Caldwell, B. M. (1979). Home observation for measurement of the environment: A revision of the preschool scale. *American Journal of Mental Deficiency, 84,* 235-244.
	Bradley, R. H., Caldwell, B. M., & Corwyn, R. F. (2003). The Child Care HOME Inventories: Assessing the quality of family child care homes. *Early Childhood Research Quarterly, 18,* 294-309.
	Bradley, R. H., Corwyn, R. F., Caldwell, B. M., Whiteside-Mansell, L., Wasserman, G. A., & Mink, I. T. (2000). Measuring the home environments of children in early adolescence. *Journal of Research on Adolescence, 10,* 247-288.
Purpose	• The various versions of the HOME are designed to investigate the quantity and quality of stimulation support and structure of the family home and home-based childcare facilities for young children. Although not direct measures of play, several items examine play-related issues (e.g., presence of toys and games; time out doors for play).
Type of Client	• Both Infant and Toddler scales (family and child care based) can be used to with children from birth to 3 years; both Early Childhood scales with 3 to 6 year olds; the Middle Childhood scale (family based) with 6 to 10 year olds; and the Early Adolescent scale (family-based), with 10 to 15 year olds. The HOME has been used with children of varying socioeconomic and ethnic origins.
Most Relevant Service Settings	• Home and family-based child care.
Clinical Utility	
Format	• Checklist based on observation and interview. The family-based Infant and Toddler scale comprises 45 items divided into six subscales, the child-care version 43 items and six subscales. The family-based Early and Middle Childhood scales consist of 55 items and eight subscales, the childcare version of the early childhood scale comprises 58 items and eight subscales. The Early Adolescent family-based version consists of 60 items and seven subscales.

continued

Table 9-12 (continued)

HOME OBSERVATION FOR MEASUREMENT OF THE ENVIRONMENT (HOME)

Procedures	• Information is gathered during observation at the home and interview with a parent or childcare provider.
Completion Time	• Approximately 1 hour.
Standardization	• Items are described in the manuals.
Reliability	
Internal Consistency	• Previously reported as >0.80 for total scores; coefficients for subscales range from 0.30 to 0.80. However, Bradley et al. (2003) noted that they no longer report internal consistency estimates as such reliability estimates assume effect indicators and the HOME Inventories are composed of cause indicators.
Inter-Rater	• Percentage of agreement at least 85%; coefficients (Kappa, intraclass, Pearson) >0.80.
Intra-Rater	• Not reported.
Test-Retest	• Infant/Toddler family-based scale examined at 6-, 12-, and 24-month age levels; subscale coefficients ranged from 0.24 to 0.07. Early Childhood scale: subscale coefficients ranged from 0.05 to 0.70. Others are unknown.
Validity	
Content	• All versions based on careful literature review.
Convergent	• Extensive studies positively correlating HOME total and subscale scores with measures of child development, health, and well-being. Maternal and paternal education also positively correlates with subscale scores for young children. For adolescents, HOME scores together with SES predicted such variables as self-efficacy and conscientious or task-oriented behavior; the exact variables differed by ethnic group. The childcare versions of the HOME are positively related to the Observational Record of the Caregiving Environment (ORCE) and the PROFILE. Family-based versions of the HOME discriminate between supportive and "at-risk" homes for young children.
Construct	• Research seems to corroborate the scale structure of the HOME (Bradley, 1994). Bradley has offered in depth reflection on the difficulty of establishing construct validity with the HOME.
Strengths	• Easy to use, requires no special equipment, and minimal examiner training.
	• Applied to a wide age span.
	• Perhaps the only assessment of home-based childcare settings.
Weaknesses	• Items related to supportiveness of the environment for play must be teased out from the others.
	• May not work well in families with all backgrounds.
	• Standard scales may not work with children who have significant disabilities since relevance of some objects and the needs of some children may differ widely from those described. Disability-adapted version may work better.
Final word	• An easy to use assessment of multiple aspects of both family- and child-care based home environments. Since play is an important activity occurring in these environments, several items pertain to supportiveness for play. May not be useful for children with significant limitations.

Editors' Notes for Chapter 10

Mine The Gold

Work is a central construct underlying productivity and one of the key domains of occupational therapy practice. It is a professional and practice imperative that occupational therapists embrace a client-centered, systematic way with which to approach the measurement and analysis of client skills and abilities to engage in work roles.

Become Systematic

It is important for therapist to use a theoretical framework to facilitate systematic, comprehensive, and balanced assessments of work performance. The Person-Environment-Occupation (PEO) model of occupational performance within a client-centered approach is a useful framework to employ.

Using Evidence in Practice

Conclusions made following assessment of work performance are used to make critical decisions that seriously influence the lives of injured workers. Therefore, it is essential that therapists make such determinations based on evidence directed by clinical reasoning, and also to be able to communicate about and explain the bases for these determinations.

Engage in Occupation-Based Assessments of Occupational Performance

Occupational therapists are in a position to make a unique contribution to measuring work performance by engaging in occupation-based assessments of occupational performance. Occupational therapists possess the knowledge base, understanding and appreciation, creativity and negotiation skills to ameliorate the gap between the worker's impairment or disability and his or her functioning within the workplace.

CHAPTER 10

MEASURING WORK PERFORMANCE FROM AN OCCUPATIONAL PERFORMANCE PERSPECTIVE

Sue Baptiste, MHSc, OT Reg. (Ont.), FCAOT; Susan Strong, MSc, OT Reg. (Ont.); and Brianna MacGuire, MScOT, OT Reg. (Ont.)

SETTING THE CONTEXT

Work is a central construct underlying productivity, and one of the key domains of occupational therapy practice. Although individuals engage with their world in many different ways, it is through work that much of life's meaning is actualized. Therefore a professional and practice imperative for occupational therapists is to embrace a client-centered, systematic way with which to approach the measurement and analysis of client skills and abilities to engage in work roles. For the purposes of this chapter "work" is defined as the occupations in which individuals engage in order to participate in their communities and for which they are remunerated or rewarded in some way. Remuneration or reward can be in the form of payment, as in paid work, or in satisfaction or sense of achievement, as in voluntary occupations.

The Person-Environment-Occupation (PEO) model was selected to examine work and its measurement because of its relevance to occupation-centered practice, and the value of its overarching view of people engaged in doing within their own life circumstances. It is critically important to reflect within worker and workplace evaluation a balanced view of all three interconnecting elements. Examining the worker's abilities without a context in which to place them represents an incomplete approach to assessment and treatment in occupational therapy, in fact in rehabilitation more broadly. Therefore, the importance of viewing work within the context of the person engaged in occupations within the relevant environment best facilitates the emergence of occupation-centered, client-centered service.

The PEO Model (Figure 10-1) works in congruence with other foundational models that underlie occupational therapy practice (CAOT, 1997). This approach to practice provides therapists with a tool to help them analyze and understand problems in the occupational performance of their clients, expands options for planning of interventions and evaluation, and assists in the clear communication to others of what is occupational therapy practice in occupational settings.

The involvement of occupational therapists in the evaluation of work performance is one part of a very complex whole evaluation system. There are links to vocational counseling, workplace adaptation and ergonomics—the process of measurement of work performance does not stand alone and can involve many sectors of society and often many clients at the same time. The central clients are the workers themselves. However, in many situations, depending on the therapist's role, other players are simultaneously clients of the occupational therapist. Occupational therapists can be hired for consultation or onsite provision of service working in a myriad of roles involving evaluation of work performance such as clinical occupational therapists, third part assessors, return-to-work coordinators, disability management consultants, and vocational case managers or specialists (Gowan & Strong, 2003). The participation of therapists at worksites is expanding as therapists move out of the traditional hospital or clinic-based service structures. In many of these roles, the therapist provides service to not only a worker or group of workers but multiple players in the workplace-compensation-health care system (e.g., occupational health and human resource personnel, management, labor, adjudicators, nurse case managers, health care providers, legal personnel). The therapist's provision of services takes place within organizations that possess unique cultures and subcultures with formal and informal rules. The therapist must have an understanding of each organization's culture and each service user's expectations in order for evaluations of work performance to be relevant and used by the organization.

After reading this chapter, the reader will have:

- Explored the complex field of work performance evaluation within an occupation-centered framework

- Become familiar with the relationships between the worker, the job, and the workplace and the importance of viewing work performance evaluation—and practice in general—in this comprehensive manner

- Gained an understanding of potential models for approaching work performance evaluation

- Begun the process of defining a personal approach to work performance evaluation that celebrates the unique view of the occupational therapy discipline

There are definite links to other chapters in this book, given the complex connections between the individual, his work and his workplace. Most specifically, links will be observed between chapters examining the measurement of the environment (Chapter 17) and of client-centered practice (Chapter 6). In order to clarify the context for considering the measurement of work performance, it is helpful to provide some definitions of terms that will be used in this chapter. In the field of vocational evaluation some terms are used interchangeably thus 'muddying' their meaning. Table 10-1 outlines commonly used terms, their definitions, and what aspects of the PEO Model are examined by the identified practice. Note, only some terms encompass all aspects of the PEO model, a necessary requirement to fully measure occupational performance. Table 10-2 provides and overview of common factors considered in vocational rehabilitation framed within the PEO elements of the model.

WHAT ARE WE MEASURING?

Work performance and the assessment of it, is viewed as the complex task of observing and testing worker skills and abilities in the context of the desired job and workplace in which the worker intends to work. The aim is to provide information for vocational rehabilitation, return to work planning and/or disability management practices. Work performance evaluations are not to be confused with performance appraisals conducted by employers to determine the extent an employee's performance matched an organization's standards for purposes of promotion/demotion or employee development.

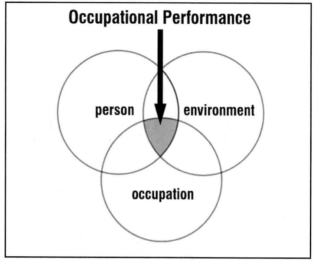

Figure 10-1. The Person-Environment-Occupation (PEO) Model. (Reprinted with permission from Law, M., et al. [1996]. The person-environment-occupation model: A transactive approach to occupational performance. *Canadian Journal of Occupational Therapy,* 63[1], 9-23.)

Historically, evaluations focused primarily on the individual, often reduced to the physical functioning of a body part and the elemental motions or basic task elements of a job. Today, explorations of measurement and work performance entail a detailed review of ways in which personal, environmental and occupational elements can be evaluated through a lens of occupation-centered practice. Assessment of work performance requires the assessment to shift focus from an assessment of components to an assessment of PEO relationships. Work performance assessments examine the individual with respect to their role as worker with all that that entails and their ability to carry out the duties within a given position at a workplace. For example, it is not sufficient that a worker be able to perform the physical components of his particular job; he must also be able to engage in the necessary relationships and communications at work. Similarly, this worker must be able to maintain his personal life outside of work, and thus must be assisted in developing the necessary stamina, habits, and coping strategies that will make this integrated effort successful. This is in contrast to the narrow evaluations of old, and has profound implications for assessment approaches and the selection of measures.

In Figure 10-2, Innes (2001) illustrated a typology of individual functional levels and job requirement levels and their relationships with the types of work-related assessments. The diagram is useful in communicating relationships and for the selection of measures appropriate to the functional level needing to be assessed. For example, a person can be assessed in their role as cabinet maker working

Table 10-1

TERMS APPLIED TO THE PEO MODEL

Term	*Definition*	*P-E-O Fit*
Vocational Rehabilitation	The network of services, programs, and the professionals who work within these structures that address the needs of injured workers for their eventual return to employment.	P + E + O
Vocational Assessment	The process of determining the abilities of injured workers and the feasibility of returning to the work place. By identifying the barriers to working, vocational assessment begins the process of rehabilitation planning.	P + E + O
Functional Capacity Evaluation (FCE), Functional Abilities Evaluation (FAE), Functional Assessment (FA) for Injured Workers	These types of vocational assessment (FCE, FAE, FA) are somewhat interchangeable depending on geographic location. These assessments involve a process of assessing an individual's physical and functional abilities related to a person's ability to work.	P + O
Work Place Evaluation	A type of vocational assessment that takes place in the work place. It may include all or components of a FCE and a work trial.	P + E + O
Work Site Analysis	Involves the detailed examination, appraisal, and evaluation of the worksite to which a particular worker is returning or, from a more general perspective, the examination of a workplace to identify risk factors for injury and adherence to safe, healthy work practices.	E
Job Demands Analysis	Provides an in-depth analysis and profile of a job's physical, emotional, and cognitive demands. It can be a general resource to the work place as well as a valuable tool to assist in the determination of job scope and attributes for the purpose of placing or returning employees to that work place. A Physical Demands Analysis only examines the physical components of a job.	O
Ergonomic Analysis	A broad generic term referring to a spectrum of work analysis. It involves the identification of work demands and risks for injury from both a person and work systems perspective. Bohr (1998) believes ergonomic assessments are an appropriate match for client-centered approaches because of the flexibility to select tools appropriate for the situation from many types of assessments including biomechanical analysis, physiological assessments, and psychological demands analysis.	O + E
Transferrable Skills Analysis	Identifies a worker's characteristics, abilities, and skills that have been developed during performance of any past occupations that can be applied to successfully perform at work in the current marketplace. They are used to make vocational disability determinations for disability insurers and for assessing damages in civil litigation.	P

Figure 10-2. Typology of individual functional levels and job requirement level. (Adapted from Innes, E., & Straker, L. [1998]. A clinician's guide to work-related assessments: 2 design problems. *Work*, 11(2), 202.)

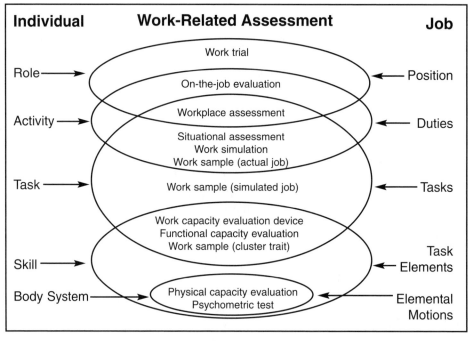

in a position as supervisor using a work trial, on-the-job evaluation or workplace-based assessment. This approach would be in keeping with a work performance assessment framed by the PEO model (Table 10-2). Another assessor may choose to assess the same person at the level of activity (e.g., ability to make a table), testing all the activities the worker must perform within his or her duties or responsibilities. This can be accomplished by on-the-job evaluations, workplace-based assessment or removed from the actual work setting by situational assessments, work simulations and use of work samples involving performance of actual job activities (e.g., build an actual table using tools he or she would normally us at the workplace). Another assessor may choose to use only work samples that simulate a job or evaluate one or two tasks (e.g., take measurements), and the worker's ability to perform at the level of tasks. This approach is somewhat removed from the full work and workplace context and not in keeping with a work performance assessment framed by the PEO model. Many of the commercially available assessments and work capacity evaluation devices primarily measure the person at the level of skill or body system such that only elemental motions (e.g., body position, strength, range of motion), and task elements (e.g., lift wood from floor to workbench, hit nail with hammer) are evaluated; an approach that is several steps removed from the full work and workplace context. It is for this very reason that assessors will use work capacity evaluation devices as a screen and proceed to use work samples, work simulations, and when at all possible, to bring in the full context, situational assessments, and workplace-based assessments.

Approaches to work and work ability that focus on the

elemental motions, task elements, in other words the component level of jobs will not be found in this chapter. Many of the existing standardized tools are framed at a component level (e.g., strength testing) rather than at the level of occupation. Component level measures do not fit with the focus of this chapter; this is a reminder to occupational therapy practitioners that component-based practice does not readily allow for the application of an occupation-centered approach to assessment and intervention. The reader is directed to publications elsewhere for review of components of work assessment (Pratt,1997; Jacobs & Bettencourt, 1999), listing of work-related assessments (Jacobs, 1991), or for an understanding of the step-by-step process of work assessment (Rice & Luster, 2002). The emphasis in the chapter is assessment of work at the level of occupational performance.

CLIENT-CENTERED ASSESSMENTS OF OCCUPATIONAL PERFORMANCE

Occupation-centered practice is exemplified through the application of the model of person-environment-occupation. Also, this model fits impeccably well with the underlying principles of client-centered practice. Clients should be seen as central to the whole process of work performance measurement. The client should be included from the beginning as an active participant in providing information, giving feedback regarding the results of the evaluation and receiving a copy pf the final report.

Strong and Shaw (1999) illustrate such an application in their work applying a client-centered framework to working with clients using an ergonomic base for assess-

Table 10-2

EXAMPLES OF PEO FACTORS OFTEN CONSIDERED IN VOCATIONAL REHABILITATION

Person-Based Factors	*Environmental Factors*	*Occupational Factors*
Primary/secondary diagnosis	Interior/exterior work	Lifting
Date of injury	Hot/cold working conditions	Carrying
Time off work	Humidity/dryness	Pushing/pulling
Medications	Vapor fumes	Gripping
Contraindications	Ventilation	Sitting
Pain	Noise	Standing
IADL functioning	Proximity to moving objects	Walking
Resting heart rate/blood pressure	Hazardous machines	Running
Posture	Radiant/thermal energy	Jumping/climbing
Weight/height	Congested work site	Reaching
Coordination/balance	Unstable footing	Twisting/rotating
Movement characteristics	Vibration/jarring (whole or part of body)	Bending/stooping
Range of motion		Crouching/kneeling
Strength (agonists/antagonists)	Stairs	Crawling
Muscle tone/spasms	Wet/slippery surface	Balancing (static/dynamic)
Atrophy/edema		Keyboarding/fine finger dexterity
Neurological reflexes		Driving
		Interaction with public
		Sudden/unpredictable movement
		Shovelling
		Work pace
Hearing	Traveling	Tools/equipment used
Vision	Degree of self-supervision required	Protective equipment required
Visual perceptual tactile	Degree of supervision exercised	Required training, certification, and licensing
	Deadline pressures	Attention to detail required
	Need to work cooperatively with others	Multi-tasking
	Exposure to emotional situations	
	Exposure to confrontational situations	
Reading literacy		
Writing literacy		
Numerical skills		
Communication		
Memory		
Computer literacy		

ment and intervention. As they identify, the PEO model is of particular value when therapists need to determine the barriers facing the resolution of ergonomic issues, when defining performance components ad conditions within the environment, determining the resources brought to the circumstance by the client, and when moving from planning to engagement in intervention and evaluating the results of the intervention.

MEASUREMENT OF THE OCCUPATION IN WORK PERFORMANCE ASSESSMENT

Measurement of the occupation or job is essential for assessment of occupational performance. While there are those who conduct work assessments by assessing only the client, when taking a client-centered, occupation-based approach to assessment and intervention there is little disagreement of the necessity to include assessment of a job in a real work context. This means assessing the demands of the work role: the duties or responsibilities and the related activities the person must carry out related to a given position. Other key elements of work role include: whether working alone or with others; the degree of autonomy within the role description; expectations of others, be they co-workers or supervisors; and so on. Findings from measurement of the occupation are fundamental for the validity of the assessment protocol during assessment of the person, and necessary to ensure interpretation of findings are meaningful.

In practice, measurement focuses on a particular or designated job when a worker has a job to return to, perhaps with modifications or accommodations, or is being assessed for suitability of performing a new job. When a worker does not have a job offer or particular job to return to, the assessor still must evaluate a potential job or job type from which to make a comparison of a worker's abilities, and make recommendations for rehabilitation and/or return to work planning. There are several methods for obtaining information about work for assessment, including job descriptions, descriptions of job types (e.g., National Occupational Classification, Dictionary of Occupational Titles), and direct observation while performing a job demands analysis.

Occupational analysis is a key tool from any occupational therapist's basic tool kit that has ready applicability to this area of practice. Our training in occupational analysis tells us that we must examine all relevant aspects of the person, environment and occupation in order to facilitate occupational performance. A detailed overview of this method is beyond the scope of this chapter, but an excellent resource for a renewed understanding of occupational analysis includes *Task Analysis: An Individual and Population Approach* (Watson & Wilson, 2003) and is highly recommended reading. *Work performance* and the assessment of it is viewed as the complex task of observing

and testing worker skills and abilities in the context of the desired job and workplace to which the worker is to be returned.

Job Descriptions

Most workplaces have written job descriptions for every position within their organizations that define the functions of the job. There is no standard format. Most include responsibilities, essential and nonessential tasks, whether the tasks are occasionally or regularly part of the job. Job descriptions are generic descriptions that lack important details about how a position has been implemented within a particular job by a specific person. They can be relied upon to give a general outline of responsibilities and tasks that must be reviewed with a worker and supervisor for further information.

National Occupational Classification and Dictionary of Occupational Titles

Both of these resources provide a general understanding of the scope of jobs and potential demands of job types. The Dictionary of Occupational Titles (DOT) (U.S. Department of Labor, 1991) is a large compendium of job described according to 20 physical demands of work developed by the government of the United States. In the Revised Classification of Jobs (Miller et al., 1980) the DOT classification was expanded to describe the demands of work by intensity and frequency. However descriptions are broad (e.g., sedentary/light/medium/heavy/very heavy; constantly/frequently/occasionally/never) and difficult to apply. Job types have been analyzed and described according to demands related to data, person, and things. This resource is used widely by job seekers, employers, educational/training institutions, and researchers, to detail the tasks performed, the educational requirements and generic skills needed for more than 12,000 types of American jobs (http://www.wave.et/upg/immigration/ dot_index.html).

Another more recent compendium of analyzed jobs is the National Occupational Classification (NOC) (2001), a publication of the Canadian Government, which contains the classification structure and descriptions of over 500 occupational groupings representative of the Canadian labor market (http://www23.hrdc.gc.ca/2001/e/generic/welcome.shtml). The NOC has attempted to expand the job descriptions beyond the education/training requirements; worker functions related to data, people, things and physical job demands (body position, limb co-ordination, strength, vision, hearing) to include some environmental conditions (location, hazards, discomforts), labor market conditions, aptitudes, and interests. The NOC database can be searched using inexpensive software.

It still remains necessary to assess the demands of a particular job directly because many particular jobs vary from these compendiums (Lechner, 1998). Also, most workers in a position must perform additional duties and activities not considered within one job.

Job Demands Analysis

A job demands analysis (JDA) is the cornerstone of understanding the key elements of any specific job prior to returning a worker to the workplace. Although JDAs have become an expected component of every assessment, they are criticized for the inconsistent quality of information (Functional Assessment Network, 2003). These assessments are performed by individuals with a variety of training and there is no industry standard format. There are many published lists of the necessary elements to be evaluated during a JDA and how (Jacobs & Bettencourt, 1999). It is important to consult the people who perform the job, as they are the ones who ultimately know the job's demands and review a draft JDA with worker(s) and supervisor(s).

An excellent example of such a tool is that developed for the City of Toronto. The task of redeveloping a Physical Demands Analysis (PDA) tool was undertaken at the time when seven smaller municipalities amalgamated to create a mega-city. The idea of a PDA was defined specifically as a document and process that outlines the physical demands of a series of tasks or a particular job. The information gleaned from completing this process is then used in identifying any intervention or treatment goals, planning the treatment, identifying the point at which a worker is ready to return to work, and if there are any needs for accommodation or adaptation of the job or workplace. A literature review was completed from which key elements were distilled that would provide an enhanced approach to JDA for the new municipality. These elements informed the addition of several components to the existing PDA tool, thus requiring that it be renamed as a JDA. These included: definitions for behavioral and cognitive demands and ratings; the creation of subcategories to provide more details for some demands; and the facilitation of links across other components of the return to work process, such as the Job Match System. All forms are on-line and are readily accessed by all partners in the work assessment and return to work model. The resulting tools are all available within the City's Integrated Disability and Safety Management system. The process of developing a detailed and explicit return to work process for the new city is well articulated in internally generated reports (Raybould, McIlwain, Hardy, & Byers, 2002). The authors underline the overall success of the new tool, as stated by disability management staff and external service providers, as being due to the manner in which more specific and detailed information is provided concerning job demands (p. 5). Other essential components of this standardized JDA model include: rating scales, lists of categories, a direct link to the functional ability assessment,

notes on a job matching function, and a clear synopsis of conclusions. Perhaps the most compelling elements of this approach to developing a system such as this is its comprehensiveness, the use of guidelines to operationally define most items, and the fact that it is computerized and directly linked with the functional assessment process in totality.

The City of Toronto's JDA is one of the few that examines the emotional and cognitive demands of jobs. Another way to obtain information about emotional and cognitive demands is by questionnaires or interview. Therapists can ask workers in a work group to complete simple questions about comfort levels and job demands. A well-standardized, easy to use tool for examining the social and psychological characteristics of jobs is the Job Content Questionnaire (Karasek, 1985) (Table 10-5) based on Karasek's Demand/Control Model of job strain.

IADL Performance and Work Measurement

Assessment and measurement of client abilities in IADL occupations do not have a direct link to return to work, although the indirect link is clear. Often the potential is great for a client's broader experience of living to be a rich context for developing higher tolerance in functional areas and in general tasks of daily living. Therefore, consideration should be given for the manner in which these elements of a client's life are identified, measured and interventions planned. As previously mentioned, the effort expended in managing and coping with one's everyday occupations (associated with self-care and home management) can have particular effects on the ability of workers to return to work and to stay working. Occupational therapists are particularly invested in facilitating their clients to return to a well-balanced lifestyle that includes self-care, work, leisure and rest. To simply ascertain a worker's ability to do his job cannot be construed as a statement of his readiness to return to the workplace. Therefore, it is essential that the total output of energy and effort expended by a client is examined to provide the information necessary for the clinician to provide a realistic appraisal of work. Altogether, a worker's experiences performing IADL can create an ideal environment within which he/she can prepare for returning to the work place and within which a baseline for tolerance to occupational performance can be determined.

MEASUREMENT OF THE ENVIRONMENT IN WORK PERFORMANCE ASSESSMENT

Already in this book, the reader will have seen, and potentially read, a chapter focused on environment (Chapter 17) and the many rich ways to assess its impact on occupation. The intent is to not repeat the information here but highlight a few elements significant to work assessment.

There have been radical shifts within the working environments of many societal sectors over the past two decades. Expectations of security and loyalty have been greatly altered and, at the least, shaken from traditional models and ways of doing business. Consequently, there has been a heightened awareness developing concerning the impact of environmental factors on the interface between the worker and what they do. More and more attention is being paid to seeking input around workers' sense of the importance of environmental elements in supporting them at work. The Work Environment Scale (WES) has been a consistent tool with which such questions have been, and are being, considered and is well worth studying. In their study of nurses' perceptions of their work environment, Avallone and Gibbon (1998) found by using the WES that approximately three-quarters of the respondent sample were satisfied with their work environment, with distinct differences between the three units under study. Exploring a different question but still within the discipline of nursing, Thomas (1992) reported on a study that addressed the perceptions of qualified nurses and auxiliary nursing staff concerning the work environment. Her findings were centered upon differences between employee satisfaction within different work settings, but not between different employment categories. Both studies support the importance of considering the cultural elements of work environments when determining the "fit" between worker and job, between worker and worker, and between worker and supervisor. More specifically, Schaefer and Moos (1996) examined the relationships between work stressors and work climate, together with job morale and functioning. Their findings would indicate that more positive work climates were directly linked to reports of higher morale related to work and role. Stressors related to relationships and workload had clear relationships to lower job satisfaction, additional job-related distress, depression and physical symptoms. Cohesive relationships between workers were predictive of a heightened intent to stay in the job (p.63).

Often the environment is viewed as under the purview of ergonomists and input from the occupational therapy perspective can be minimized or absent. Biomechanics is at the basis of ergonomics (Jacobs & Bettencourt, 1999) and therefore can present a more focused approach to return to work than that offered by occupational therapists. Therein, perhaps, lies the importance of the two disciplines working collaboratively and with respect towards their differing views of the worker and the workplace. Occupational therapists offer an understanding of the worker and the workplace from the microscopic level to the job itself.

There are different methods and sources to obtain information about the work environment. The assessor can record structured observations using Work-Site Analysis forms, Risk Assessment forms, and videotaping (with permission) can assist. Worker's perceptions of the work environment can be sought by interview and questionnaires. An example of a standardized work environment questionnaire is The Work Environment Scale (Schaefer & Moos, 1996), which samples workers' perceptions of the workplace's social environment. With respect to relationships (coworker cohesion, supervisor support, worker's feelings of involvement), opportunities for personal growth (autonomy, task orientation, work pressure), and how the workplace system maintains itself and deals with change (clarity of communication/rules, managerial control, innovation, physical comfort). The Job Content Questionnaire (Karasek, 1985 not in the list) also taps social support, decision latitude together with job security. Worker's perceptions of social support in a broader sense, from family, friends, significant others, and the adequacy of the support can be obtained in the Multidimensional Scale of Perceived Social Support (Zimet et al., 1988) reviewed in the Environment Chapter.

MEASUREMENT OF THE PERSON IN WORK PERFORMANCE ASSESSMENT

The most unique contribution that occupational therapists can give to the enterprise of work performance evaluation is their knowledge of what impact illness or impairment has upon function and the potential emergence of disability. It is therefore essential that individuals be viewed from the level and perspective of the roles that they play. The ultimate outcomes of occupational therapy assessment and intervention within the work and vocational spheres should be viewed from this complex perspective. These outcomes are focused upon: the need to perform; to meet the demands of the job and the work environment through the utilization of skill, knowledge and experience; and also includes the recognition that personal satisfaction is key to a successful work life. Therapists are requested by various referral sources to perform work-related assessment for a myriad of reasons, but the final outcome should always reflect the perspective of the individual performing the job in the context within which the job is most usually performed. Occupational therapists bring their knowledge of the physical, mental, spiritual, and emotional elements of people to this arena and with that knowledge comes the ability to deal with concomitant emotional and cognitive issues that may impact on work performance.

The Role of Pain

The assessment of pain can be seen as residing at an impairment level and therefore may not have a central place in this discussion of occupation-centered practice.

However, pain tends to become an overarching issue that affects every aspect of a client's functioning, thus impacting upon the whole work experience. The physical self is most frequently compromised due to fear of re-injury or illustrated by measurable functional deficits. Mood level is a component that is greatly affected by pain, with the pervading attitudes or chosen coping strategies influencing work abilities and readiness to reenter the work place. Observing the worker in context is critical, in addition to using self-reports through which the worker can provide a baseline of activity/functional levels during a day or week. For the individual returning to work from an injury or illness, the self-report system should include commentary about differing pain levels. It is also very important to be aware of, and to include, worker self-report about the aftermath of the assessment itself. If the three or four assessments resulted in a severe increase in pain and reduction in physical mobility, then the results of the assessment are different from a circumstance where there were no such sequelae. Reports should include a client self-statement of the aftermath of the assessment within one to two days post-assessment (Innes & Straker, 2002a). This is not the place for a detailed analysis of the optimal ways to measure pain, but the reader is encouraged to explore frequently used pain measurement tools such as self-report diaries and pain level scales (Huskisson, 1974; Kerns, Turk, & Rudy, 1985; Melzack, 1975; Fairbank, Daies, Couper, & O'Brien, 1980; Chan, Goldman, Ilstrup, Kunselman, & O'Neil, 1993). It is also advantageous to be conversant with cognitive behavioral strategies of coping with pain to be able to advise and teach clients potential ways of managing their pain to facilitate and maximize their functional capacity.

Measurement of Maximal Effort

One of the perceived significant problems with evaluating someone's functional capacity and work readiness is the ability to determine the effort that is expended by the client during the assessment process. This issue has arisen from a pervasive attitude adopted by many report users towards questioning a worker's motivation and investment in returning to productive employment. How does one ensure that a client is expending maximum effort? This has proven to be a complex and daunting issue. Effort assessment has become known as the assessment of MVE or "maximum voluntary effort" testing (Niemayer, Matheson, & Carlton, 1989).

Over the past few years, many attempts have been made to develop technologies and techniques that will measure, in an objective fashion, the subjective construct of effort (Strong & Westmorland, 1996), but with little success. There are many competing potential reasons for a worker being assessed to exhibit inconsistent performance; it shows a faulty logic to assume that the sporadic performance outputs are due to attempts to mask real ability. Reasons include the fear of re-injury, anxiety at the thought of being in a test situation, tiredness, pain or poor physical fitness. Similarly, other reasons could include depression, some additional impairment yet to be determined, as well as the inability to understand directions (Blankenship, 1994; Hirsch et al., 1991; Matheson, 1988a; Niemeyer & Jacobs, 1989). With so many factors influencing the consistency of performance during testing, assessors have requested the development of guidelines that will steer their approach to assessment in a viable direction, and for the research. No study has demonstrated a relationship between a worker's level of co-operation during an assessment and a worker's level of effort expended at work or co-operation with the return to work process.

At the time of the functional assessment, the assessor is expected to engage with the worker in a therapeutic manner respecting his/her individuality. A professional rapport should be established through the use of interventions that are necessary to ensure that optimal performance can be facilitated. For example, time spent on alleviating any anxieties on the part of the worker is time very well spent. Similar attention should be paid to addressing the need for pain management strategies, correcting of unsafe body mechanics and the provision of helpful adaptations. The Reviewing the purpose of the FA, along with a transparent exchange concerning mutual expectations, is very important. Assurance should be given regarding the observation of any inconsistencies as the assessment progresses; if this were to occur, the assessor should assure the worker that they will be discussed as they arise and before any documentation is completed. When dealing with such inconsistencies in work performance, it is essential that they be discussed in a thoughtful and tactful way, giving the worker the chance to respond, and provide some insight or further information regarding his or her performance. The worker should be reassured of the centrality of his or her position within the assessment process. The assessment should be an accurate reflection of the worker and the worker's abilities on a day-to-day basis within the work context.

There is a critical need to obtain feedback from the worker in order to determine what the experience has been for him or her. To discount the input of the key player in the work performance evaluation is both short sighted and rooted in a purely physical model of practice. This is yet another example of why the PEO model is so essential. There should also be an opportunity to repeat the assessment as necessary and to ensure that the length of the assessment period itself is of sufficient length to allow for a realistic profile of work ability to be revealed. Through this type of strategy, it is therefore possible to develop a profile based on multiple methods, which, by definition, will present a more credible and encompassing picture of the worker in context. Without a doubt, a sound approach to determining the level of effort during assessment should be taken, with the inclusion of a rigorous and well developed interview protocol such as the Worker Role Interview (Velozo, Kielhofner, & Fisher, 1998) (Table 10-6).

Strong & Westmorland (1996), in their monograph addressing the dilemma of effort testing, conclude their work with this summary:

> "This issue of reliability and validity of ...approaches [to effort assessment] and how to make the subjective more objective still remains. Given the complexity of determining effort in relation to work and the plethora of measures, technologies and protocols currently employed, much more emphasis needs to be placed on: a) the theoretical basis of the constructs relevant to disability and work in order to guide practice; b) the standardization of practices; and c) the evaluation of such practices and their measures" (p. 72).

Despite the passage of time, the dilemma remains a key area for further research and one of supreme delicacy for occupational therapists involved in vocational evaluation.

Self-Perception of Performance

All too frequently, work assessment is focused upon the evaluation of physical components (Velozo & Innes). Strong and Rebeiro (2003) offer a well-articulated discussion of the need for an approach to work rehabilitation for clients with mental illness that incorporates a more integrated view of the person, the occupation and the environment. This framework was adapted from the work of Ochocka (1994) and Strong (1995) and defines "factors of success," thus facilitating the development of a measurement plan to match the framework components. This model introduces essential elements for assessment of attitude (of the worker, co-workers, supervisor, and employer), work culture (sense of safety, teamwork, responsiveness, flexibility, and chances for advancement) and job specifics (scope for challenge and variety balanced with routine and success experiences).

There is a growing body of knowledge and understanding related to the importance of a worker's sense of self-efficacy in the rehabilitation process. In fact, there are data that point to the fact that levels of self-efficacy predict the degree to which clients will adhere to treatment and rehabilitation program expectations and can be changed with appropriate input from therapist and others within the client's support system (Bandura, 1991; McAuley, Lox, & Duncan, 1993).

Williams and Myers have developed the Functional Abilities Confidence Scale (Williams & Myers, 1998b), which is a measure with potential for use by practitioners in identifying a client's initial level of confidence and then monitoring progress throughout a rehabilitation program. The measure explores the sense of comfort, ease and safety with which clients with low back pain approach their exercise and functional rehabilitation programs and is used in concert with the Resumption of Activities of Daily Living Scale (RADL) (Williams & Myers, 1998a). These measures are still in the process of testing, however preliminary findings would indicate that they show sound psychometric properties when used with clients who have problems with acute and chronic pain (Williams, Hapidou, & Cullen, 2003).

FUNCTIONAL CAPACITY EVALUATION: AN EXAMPLE OF PERSON-OCCUPATION MEASUREMENT

It is important for therapists to understand that work performance evaluation continues to be a growing area of exploration and inquiry. Specifically, evidence supporting client-centered work performance is still in the development stages. Much of what has been published to date is of a narrative and situational nature and existing research has varying levels of rigor.

A Functional Capacity Evaluation is a process which includes a sequence of tests that objectively assess an individual's ability to perform certain tasks in relation to activities of daily living (ADL) and/or work related tasks. The FCE findings are intended to be used together with other relevant information as part of a disability management practice to successful return a worker to work. The completion of a FCE can bring all the parties to the table to negotiate a shared understanding and collaboratively plan next steps. FCEs have been shown to be helpful for understanding an injured worker's abilities related to a job, determining work suitability or job modification, assisting with graduated return to work or rehabilitation planning and enabling workers to explore for them selves their own work abilities (Strong, Baptiste, Clarke, Cole, & Costa, 2004b). However, in practice, these assessments are sometimes used concurrently for multiple purposes, some of which are not supported by research (Strong et al., 2002).

There are many different approaches to FCEs. To date there are no empirical studies that compare one approach to another, and definitively demonstrate which is "the best". In a study of 23 assessment providers who varied in training, team composition and theoretical approach, qualitative and quantitative strategies were used to generate an in-depth understanding of the similarities and differences in assessment practices (Strong, Baptiste, Cole, Clarke, Costa, Shannon, Reardon, & Sinclair, 2004a). Assessment approaches were found to share common elements and variations that were described along continua of five dimensions: nature of assessor-evaluee interactions, fixed-flexible protocol delivery, efforts to contextualize, perceptions and use of evidence, and provider organizational environment.

In order to fill some of the gaps in knowledge and understanding about these issues, a recent comprehensive study documented FCE practices in southern Ontario. The study process followed a cohort of injured workers undergoing assessments, and also included interviews with the various players involved in administering FCEs and utilizing the results within the employer and compensation payment systems (Strong et al., 2002).

These approach dimensions can be used as a focus for appraising practices. The dimensions highlight the importance of: 1) on-going dialogue between the assessor and evaluee within a partnership; 2) flexible delivery of assessment protocol directed by clinical reasoning; 3) assessor making efforts to contextualize the assessment by considering work/workplace, clinical, and whole person factors during the assessment planning and analysis; 4) assessor's thinking critically and using an awareness of the assessment's limitations; 5) assessor's working in an environment that encourages assessor's to practice to the best of their abilities (Table 10-3).

Assessors employ a variety of assessment methods and obtain information from different sources. Directed by clinical reasoning, the assessor selects relevant tests from a battery of assessment methods including worker self report (interviews, disability questionnaires, perceptions of pain scales), clinical observation (musculoskeletal screen, quality of movement), standardized instruments (dynamometer, Minnesota Rate of Manipulation) and systems (Arcon, Blankenship, Ergos, Hanoon, Key, Isernhagen), functional tasks (painting, ADL), work sample (VALPAR Component Work Samples, and BTE Work Simulators), and work simulation tasks (box lifting). Some of these sampling systems have undergone extensive testing to support their reliability and validity, and can serve as one of multiple critical pieces in understanding a person's ability to perform work (Pratt, 1997).

The credibility of these assessments has been criticized. They take place in a political climate, with animosity between stakeholders amidst a vacuum of universal standards or guidelines. While an FCE can be an important piece in the puzzle of returning someone to a work role, assessors and employers are often working with very unclear boundaries and expectations. Often an FCE is expected to be a panacea and therefore the results of this evaluation are often applied inappropriately. There are unclear guidelines for what an FCE report should look like and therefore there are very unclear ideas or expectations for the appropriate measurement tools to employ in the process. To improve assessment practices, the Functional Assessment Network (FAN), a multistakeholder group with representatives from the whole assessment system of providers, users (in workplaces, compensation and health-

care sectors, and injured workers and representatives), gathered to come to consensus about the issues and take action (Strong et al., 2004c). After over a year of working together in small task groups, FAN developed educational materials, an algorithm for employers to guide employers' decisions about when to consider using FCEs, and guidelines for each stage of the FCE process (www.fhs.mcmaster.ca/rehab/faculty/research/wfu/wfuactivities.html).

These guidelines identify key activities, principles and performance criteria during initiation or the referral stage, FCE administration, generation of the opinion, writing of the report and use of the report's information. The performance criteria identify what FAN view as standards. For example:

- "Medical clearance is requested and obtained prior to proceeding…" (p. 6).
- "When an assessor is asked to determine whether a worker can perform a particular job, the assessor must have an understanding of the work and workplace demands for that particular job… The assessor should not rely solely on job descriptions and the NOC (National Occupational Classification) or DOT (Dictionary of Occupational Titles) to provide sufficient information about job demands" (p. 9).
- "It is insufficient to rely solely on standardized evaluation systems" (p.9).

It is critical for assessors to consider the limitations of the reliability and validity of using a standardized FCE when interpreting their findings from such assessments. These limitations include the psychometric properties of the tool being used, the fact that these evaluations happen at one point in time only, and that they provide a test situation that is out of the context of the worker in the role in the workplace (Strong et al., 2002). A therapist cannot solely rely on an FCE to determine a person's capability to perform work, as they are designed to measure generic physical skills, functional abilities, and not the unique performance demands of individual jobs.

Therapists will use strategies to work within the limitations of the FCEs to increase overall assessment rigor (Strong et al., 2004a). Current knowledge would suggest strongly that it is essential to complete the FA over 2 days or longer thereby allowing a comparison of information over time. There should be repeat testing, with the use of multiple methods for triangulation or comparison of information. The worker is a critical source of data when trying to understand the work experience and expectations. For example, the worker can inform the assessor of details of the typical work day, any difficulties experienced with work performance and other demands at work including the relationships within the workplace form co-workers to supervisors. Such contextual information should be obtained and used to adjust the protocol and then to

Table 10-3

COMMON ELEMENTS AND VARIATIONS IN ASSESSMENT APPROACHES

FA Approach Dimensions	Continuum	Rating Scales
Nature of assessor-evaluee interactions		
The extent and nature of the interaction between the assessor and worker during the assessment.	On-going dialogue between the assessor and evaluee partnership *to* one way communication, minimal/no interaction with only recordings of observations	4. Dialogue of information/thoughts/feelings: partnership and coaching for best performance. 3. Exchange of information (two-way communication). 2. Minimal interaction: restricted to provision of information, perhaps systematically part of the protocol (one-way communication). 1. No evidence of interaction: recordings of observations only.
Fixed or flexible protocol delivery		
The extent to which administration of the protocol varies between evaluees, based on clinical reasoning.	Flexible delivery of protocol, where the assessor plans an individualized assessment directed by understanding of the referral source's needs and the nature of the worker's injury/illness *to* a fixed protocol, requiring low clinical understanding and directed by tools/technology.	4. Flexible delivery of protocol based on clinical understanding. 3. More towards flexible delivery of protocol. 2. More tendency for fixed delivery of protocol and lower reliance on clinical understanding. 1. Fixed delivery of protocol and low reliance on clinical understanding.
Efforts to contextualize		
The extent to which contextual factors (re: work/workplace, clinical, and whole person) are reflected in the administration of the protocol, analysis, and interpretation.	The FA's planning and analysis consider the worker's individual circumstances to significant *to* gaps in the use/integration of this background information.	4. Fully or comprehensively contextualized FA (i.e., all three contexts considered during assessment, analysis and conclusions and/or recommendations). 3. Tendency towards complete contextualization, but not comprehensiveness. 2. Minimal contextualization, although occasionally observed. 1. No background information or significant gaps in background information.
Perceptions and use of evidence		
Assessors' familiarity and understanding of the best available evidence, and use of it with their training and experience when making decisions about each worker assessed.	Assessor is aware of and critically considers the most current available evidence in combination with their training and experience *to* limited evidence of critical thinking; significant gaps in evidence-based practices with decisions made based on historical practices.	4. Consumer of research and evidence-based practice (includes: critically selects, applies and interprets tools; reflective clinician). 3. Evidence of critical thinking. 2. Possesses some information: some reflection, unaware of issues/controversy. 1. No evidence of critical thinking, decisions based on historical practices.

continued

Table 10-3 (continued)

COMMON ELEMENTS AND VARIATIONS IN ASSESSMENT APPROACHES

FA Approach Dimensions	*Continuum*	*Rating Scales*
Provider organizational environment		
How the organization is structured with supports and resources to enable assessors to practice to the best of their abilities.	Assessors have ready access to a range of assessment modalities to tailor assessment, and actively seek and use multiple, varied supports/resources *to* limited access to resources; practice is restricted either due to lack of availability or the culture of the organization.	4 Multiple and varied resources and opportunities which assessors are actively seeking and using. 3. Varied resources and opportunities 2. Limited resources and opportunities. 1. Limited access to resources and opportunities (either due to unavailability or the culture of the organization).

Adapted with permission from Strong, S., et al. (2004a). FA approach dimensions rating scales. *Canadian Journal of Occupational Therapy*, 71(1), 13-23; and Strong, S., et al. (2002). Continuum of functional assessment approach dimensions. *Canadian Journal of Occupational Therapy*, 71(1), 13-23.

Table 10-4

PROGRESSION OF A FUNCTIONAL ASSESSMENT PROCESS

Step 1	Before a referral is sent, the worker completes a signed consent to identify who is to receive a copy of the report
Step 2	The physician completes a medical release to determine if the worker is able to participate in the FA activities
Step 3	Before the assessment, information is shared with the assessor about the work demands and work environment
Step 4	The testing is completed by trained professionals
Step 5	The location for the assessment is determined: FAs can be performed in many different settings (clinics, homes, workplaces) generally over a 2-day period
Step 6	The assessor/assessment team will complete a report that will provide: a professional opinion, recommendations, a summary of the worker's abilities, and limitations and barriers to returning to work
Step 7	A copy of the report should be provided to the worker

---

incorporate within the process of clinical reasoning and professional judgment that is employed during the analysis and interpretation of findings. The occupational therapist should balance the use of standardized measures with individualized measures, for example performing a work simulation and requesting a work-site-based assessment as a standard element of the overall assessment process. Also, findings should be viewed as capturing optimal performance (i.e., an overestimation of the person's abilities relative to working full time throughout the year and conclusions should be adjusted accordingly). Other frequently used tools with supportive evidence can be found in Tables 10-7, 10-10, and 10-11.

Connecting the Pieces

When approaching the measurement of work performance it is critical that practitioners refresh their knowledge and understanding of the basic principles of measurement. For example, it is essential that any tool should be used swith the population and for the purpose for which it was designed, and that any results stemming from applying the tool should not be taken out of context and should relate directly to the goal of the assessment. Also, normative data tables should be cited with caution when compiling assessment results for individual clients. The success of good assessment reporting lies with the use of clear and succinct clinical reasoning based on data triangulated from multiple sources.

While attention to measuring the functional capacity and overall ability of the individual is naturally central to the evaluation of work, this element cannot and should not be considered out of context—simply, the person doing something somewhere should remain the overarching agenda of occupation-centered practice. The practice area is fraught with complex challenges relative to the fit, or lack thereof, between the person, what is observable, what is measurable, and what is perceived or believed to be the individual's motivation and commitment to the tasks at hand. There is a distinct danger of making assumptions based on observation alone, therefore it is critical that practice is framed within an evidence-based approach. What remains is to define "evidence" in a manner that will be inclusive of many sources of information. An approach to work-related assessment that combines qualitative and quantitative data sets is becoming more the expectation and the norm. This approach has been suggested and reinforced throughout the most recent literature generated both from North America and Australia. (Strong & Westmorland,1996; Innes & Straker, 2002a; Strong et al., 2002). With this in mind, the tools chosen to be reviewed and recommended in this chapter are representative of the best evidence-based information as well as illustrative of a broad-based approach to data gathering and interpretation, utilizing multiple sources through varied means, from interview to observation of testing protocols.

The importance is unequivocal of having overarching frameworks to provide guidance and support to a process as complex as assessing for return to work. As occupational therapists engaged in assessing injured workers it is central to that endeavor that the central goal is one of return to work. To enable that process to become institutionalized and widely recognized, a framework for essential players, relationships, roles, expectations and outputs needs to be in place. WorkCover New South Wales has developed an integrated example of such a framework. Guidelines have been developed for the involvement of all sectors together with timelines and details of how the processes are expected to work The documentation provides many tools to assist everyone in "making it happen" (www.workcover. act.gov.au). Over the past 5 years, Strong et al (2002, 2004c) have focused on exploring the lived experience of injured workers, together with that of other players in the work assessment process, out of which has stemmed the McMaster Model (Figure 10-3) for a proposed model for functional assessment. This model provides an integrated approach for assessors through which it is clear that the functional assessment itself is part of a very complicated whole. This model was distilled from the conversations held at multiple focus groups involving all stakeholders in mixed groups. It was this model that FAN members used to create their assessment guidelines (FAN, 2003).

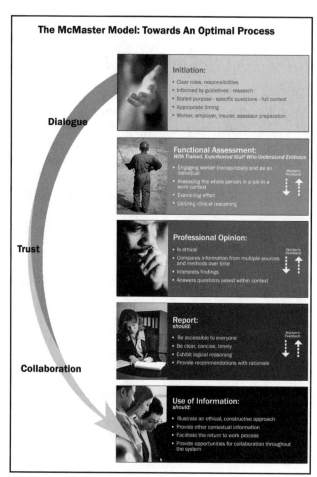

Figure 10-3. McMaster Model.

When implementing the person-environment-occupation framework as a basis for client-centered, occupation-centered practice, it can seem unwieldy and unnatural to try to un-bundle the pieces. In fact, it is the reverse. Perhaps one of the most unique features of the application of occupational therapy theory and practice to the endeavor of work performance assessment is the ability of occupational therapists to see the relationships between these three components through a different lens. Then, after exploring and examining these connections, to then present the unified picture back again to facilitate others' understanding of the complexities of such assessment and the implications to each worker. This is far from being an easy thing to do, but it is at the very crux of occupational therapy practice.

Perhaps one of the most important reasons for taking an occupation-based approach to practice is exactly that this is a chance for the philosophy of the occupational therapy profession to shine through. Once this approach has become familiar and is recognized as a key element by partners in the process, then by definition the approach is reinforced. In an arena where there are many players and several with similar skill sets, it is imperative that unique contributions are realized and supported to avoid duplication and to support collaborative practice.

Established attitudes can become obstacles to changing the manner in which practice can be manifested. Expectations from others for a more component-based assessment approach can be powerful. Also, working at the impairment and component level is sometimes much easier than to apply the multifaceted lens required by an occupation-centered focus.

SUMMARY

It is important to appreciate that work performance evaluation continues to be a growing area of exploration and inquiry. Specifically, evidence supporting client-centered work performance is still in the development stages. Much of what has been published to date is of a narrative and situational nature and existing research has varying levels of rigor.

"Research has tended to focus on characteristics of the worker and the assessment instruments, and has not dealt with the assessor or assessment protocol as a whole to date." (Strong et al., 2002).

Key components to be remembered are:

- Occupation is contextually defined; without connections to the work site, the work team and the worker, the occupation in and of itself means nothing.

- Measurement tools are only as good as the manner in which they are applied; through the application and use of tools that are credible, reliable and valid, practitioners can feel more assured that the process of assessment also gains some degree of credibility. However, without a marriage with sound clinical reasoning and critical thinking, assessment results remain uni-dimensional and lacking in relevance to individual workers and their futures.

- A client-centered approach relies upon an open, honest and respectful relationship being developed between the practitioner and the worker; it is therefore essential that this set of beliefs and values be carried forward into the complex world of vocational assessment and rehabilitation, encompassing everyone involved in the process.

- The PEO model provides an excellent framework from which to base an approach to the measurement of work performance.

REFERENCES

Avallone, I., & Gibbon, B. (1998) Nurses' perceptions of their work environment in a nursing development unit. *Journal of Advanced Nursing, 27,* 1193-1201

Bandura, A. (1991). Self-efficacy mechanisms in physiological activation and health-promoting behavior. In: Maddux. J. (ed). *Neurobiology of learning emotion and affect.* 4th ed. New York, NY: Raven press, ps. 229-269.

Biernacki, S. D. (1993). Reliability of the Worker Role Interview. *American Journal of Occupational Therapy, 47,* 797-803.

Blankenship, K. L. (1994). *The Blankenship System of Functional Capacity Evaluation: The procedure manual.* Macon, GA: The Blankenship Corp.

Bohr, P. C. (1998). Chapter 12: Work Analysis. In P.M. King (ed.), *Sourcebook of occupational rehabilitation* (pp.229-245). New York: Plenum Press.

CAOT. (1997). *Enabling occupation: A Canadian perspective.* Ottawa, Ontario: CAOT Publications ACE.

Carpenter, L., Baker, G. A., & Tyldesley, B. (2001).The use of the Canadian Occupational Performance Measure as an outcome of a pain management program. *Canadian Journal of Occupational Therapy, 68(1),*16-22.

Chan, C., Goldman, S., Ilstrup, D., Kunselman, A., & O'Neil, P. (1993). The pain drawing and Wadell's nonorganic physical signs in chronic low-back pain, *Spine, 18(13),* 1717-1722.

Cheng,Y., Luh, W., & Guo, Y. (2003). Reliability and validity of the Chinese version of the Job Content Questionnaire in Taiwanese workers. *International Journal of Behavioural Medicine, 10(1),* 15-30.

Ekbladh, E., Haglund, L., & Thorell, L. (2004). The Worker Role Interview: Preliminary data on the predictive validity of return to work of clients after an insurance medicine investigation. *Journal of Occupational Rehabilitation, 14(2),* 131-141.

Fairbank, J., Daies, J., Couper, J., & O'Brien, J. (1980). The Oswestry low back pain disability questionnaire. *Physiotherapy, 66,* 271-273.

FAN (2004). *Work Function Unit.* Available at www.fhs.mcmaster.ca/rehab/faculty/research/wfu/wfuactivites.html. Retrieved May 15, 2005.

Gern, A. (1993). *Validity of the Worker Role Interview.* Master's Thesis, University of Illinois at Chicago.

Gibson, L, & Strong, J. (2003). A conceptual framework of functional capacity evaluation for occupational therapy in work rehabilitation. *Australian Occupational Therapy Journal, 50,* 64-71.

Gowan, N., & Strong, S. (2002). The workplace: The expanding world of occupational therapy. *OT Now, Sept/Oct,* 9-14.

Hirsch, G., Beach, G., Cooke, C., Menard, M., & Locke, S. (1991). Relationship between performance on lumbar dynamometry and Waddell score in a population with low-back pain. *Spine, 16,* 1039-1043.

Innes, E. & Straker, L. (2002). Workplace assessments and functional capacity evaluations: Current practices of therapists in Australia. *Work, 18,* 51-66.

Innes, E. & Straker, L. (2002a). Workplace assessments and functional capacity evaluations: current practices of therapists in Australia. *Work, 18,* 51-66.

Innes, E. & Straker, L. (2002b). Strategies used when conducting work-relatedv assessments. *Work, 19,* 149-1656.

Innes, E. & Straker, L. (2003). Attributes of excellence in work-related assessments. *Work, 20,* 63-76.

Jacobs, K. (1991). *Occupational therapy: Work-related programs and assessments* (2nd ed.). Boston: Little, Brown.

Jacobs, K & Bettencourt, C. M. (1999). *Ergonomics For therapists.* (2nd Edition). Woburn, MA: Butterworth-Heinmann.

Karasek, R. A. (1985). *Job Content Questionnaire and user's guide.* Lowell, MA: University of Massachusetts Lowell, Dept. of Work Environment.

Karasek, R.A., & Theorell, T. (1990). *Healthy work: Stress, productivity and the reconstruction of working life.* New York: Basic Books.

Karasek, R., Brisson, C., Kawakami, N., Houtman, I., Bongers, P. & Amick, B. (1998). The Job Content Questionnaire (JCQ): An instrument for internationally comparative assessments of psychosocial job characteristics. *Journal of Occupational Health Psychology, 3(4),* 322-355.

Kerns, R., Turk, D., Rudy, T. (1985). The West Haven-Yale multidimensional pain inventory. *Pain, 34,* 217-230.

Kielhofner, G., Mallinson, T., Crawford, C., Nowak, M., Rigby, M., Henry, A., & Walens, D. (1998). *The Occupational Performance History Interview (Version 2.0) OPHI-II.* Chicago: Model of Human Occupation Clearinghouse.

Keilhofner, G., Henry, A. (1988). Development and investigation of the Occupational Performance History Interview. *American Journal of Occupational Therapy, 42(8),* 489-498.

Keilhofner, G., Mallinson, T., Forsyth, K., Lai, J. S. (2001). Psychometric properties of the second version of the Occupational Performance History Interview (OPHI-II). *American Journal of Occupational Therapy, 55(3),* 260-7.

Law, M., Cooper, B., Strong, S., Stewart, D., Rigby, P., & Letts, L. (1996). The Person-Environment-Occupation Model: A transactive approach to occupational performance. *Canadian Journal of Occupational Therapy, 63(1),* 9-23.

Lechner, D. E., Bradbury, S. F., & Bradley, L. (1998). Detecting sincerity of effort: A summary of methods and approaches. *Physical Therapy, 78(8),* 867-888.

Lin, F. L. (1994). *The Worker Role Interview: construct validity across diagnoses.* Master's Thesis, University of Illinois at Chicago.

Mallinson, T., Mahaffey, L., & Keilhofner, G. (1998). The Occupational Performance History Interview: Evidence for three underlying constructs of occupational adaptation. *Canadian Journal of Occupational Therapy, 65(4),* 219-228.

Matheson, L., Ogden, L., Violette, K., & Schultz, K. (1985). Work hardening: Occupational therapy in industrial rehabilitation. *American Journal of Occupational Therapy, 39(5),* 314-321.

Matheson, L. (1988). How do you know that he tried his best? The reliability crisis in industrial rehabilitation. *Industrial Rehabilitation Quarterly, 1(1),* 1-12.

McCauley, E., Lox. C., & Duncan, T. E. (1993). Long-term maintenance of exercise self-efficacy, and physiological change in older adults. *Journals of Gerontology, 48,* 218-224.

McColl, M. A., Paterson, M., Davies, D., Doubt, L., & Law, M. (2000). Validity and community utility of the Canadian Occupational Performance Measure. *Canadian Journal of Occupational Therapy, 67(1),*22-30.

Melzack, R. (1975). The McGill pain questionnaire: Major properties and scoring. *Pain,* 1, 277-299.

Miller, A. R., Trieman, D.J., Cain, P. S., & Roos P. A. (eds.). (1980). *Work, Jobs, and Occupations: A Critical Review of the Dictionary of Occupational Titles.* Final report to the U.S. Dept. of Labor from the Committee on Occupational Classification and Analysis. Washington, DC: National Academy Press

Moser, C. (Ed.) (2003). Study points to good practices for conducting and using FAs. *Back to Work, 7(5),* 1-2.

Niemeyer, L. O., & Jacobs, K. (1998). *Work hardening: State of the art.* Thorofare, NJ: SLACK Incorporated.

Niemeyer, L.O., Matheson, L. N., & Carlton, R. S. (1989). Testing consistency of effort: BTE work simulator. *Industrial Rehabilitation Quarterly, 2(1),* IRQ.

Ochocka, J., Roth, D., Lord, J., MacGillivary, H. (1994). *Workplaces that work.* Kilchener, Ontario: Centre for Research and Education.

Ostry, A.S., Marion, S. A., Demers, P.A., Hershler, R., Kelly, S., Teschke, K., & Hertzman, C. (2001). Measuring psychosocial job strain with the Job Content Questionnaire using experienced job evaluators. *American Journal of Industrial Medicine, 39(4),* 397-401.

Pratt, J. (1997). Work assessments. In J. Pratt & K. Jacobs (Eds.), *Work Practice. International Perspectives* (pp. 101-125). London: Butterworth-Hienemann.

Raybould, K., McIlwain, L., Hardy, C. & Byers, J. (2002). *Improving effectiveness of the Job Demands Analysis Tool at the city of Toronto.* Internal document, City of Toronto, Ontario.

Rice, V. J., & Luster, S. (2002). Restoring competence for the worker role. In C. A. Trombly & M. V. Radomski (Eds.), *Occupational therapy for physical dysfunction* (5th ed.). Baltimore, Maryland: Lippincott Williams & Wilkins.

Schaefer, J., & Moos, R. H. (1996). Effects of work stressors and work climate on long-term care staff's job morale and functioning. *Research in Nursing and Health, 19,* 63-73.

Storms, G., Casaer, S., De Wit, R., Van den Bergh, O., & Moens, G. (2001). A psychometric evaluation of a Dutch version of the Job Content Questionnaire and of a short direct questioning procedure. *Work & Stress, 15(2),* 131-143.

Strong, S. (1995). *An ethnographic study examining the experience of persons with persistent mental illness working at an affirmative business.* Master's thesis submitted to School of Graduate Studies, Master of Science, McMaster University, Hamilton, Ontario.

Strong, S. (2002). Functional Capacity Evaluations: The good, the bad, and the ugly. *OT Now,* January/February, 5-9.

Strong, S., & Shaw, L. (1999). A Client-Centered Framework For Therapists in Ergonomics. In K. Jacobs & C. M. Bettencourt, (Eds.), *Ergonomics For Therapists* (2nd Ed.). Woburn, MA: Butterworth-Heinmann.

Strong, S., Baptiste, S., Clarke, J., Cole, D., Costa, M., Reardon, R., Shannon, H. & Sinclair, S. (2002). *Assessment of a person's ability to function at work.* Research report. (WSIB Grant #980028). Hamilton, Ontario: Work Function Unit, School of Rehabilitation Science, McMaster University.

References concluded on page 172

Table 10-5

JOB CONTENT QUESTIONNAIRE (JCQ)

Source	Karasek, R.A (1985). *Job Content Questionnaire and user's guide*. Lowell: University of Massachusetts Lowell, Department of Work Environment.
Important References	Cheng, Y., Luh, W., & Guo, Y. (2003). Reliability and validity of the Chinese version of the Job Content Questionnaire in Taiwanese workers. *International Journal of Behavioural Medicine, 10(1)*, 15-30.
	Ostry, A. S., Marion, S. A., Demers, P. A., Hershler, R., Kelly, S., Teschke, K., & Hertzman, C. (2001). Measuring psychosocial job strain with the Job Content Questionnaire using experienced job evaluators. *American Journal of Industrial Medicine, 39(4)*, 397-401.
	Karasek, R. A., & Theorell, T. (1990). *Healthy work: stress, productivity and the reconstruction of working life*. New York: Basic Books.
	Karasek, R., Brisson, C., Kawakami, N., Houtman, I., Bongers, P., & Amick, B. (1998). The Job Content Questionnaire (JCQ): An instrument for internationally comparative assessments of psychosocial job characteristics. *Journal of Occupational Health Psychology, 3(4)*, 322-355.
	Storms, G., Casaer, S., De Wit, R., Van den Bergh, O., & Moens, G. (2001). A psychometric evaluation of a Dutch version of the Job Content Questionnaire and of a short direct questioning procedure. *Work & Stress, 15(2)*, 131-143.
Purpose	• Measure perceptions of social and psychological characteristics of jobs for assessments of work quality at both the level of the individual and system or organizational level.
Type of Client	• Individual workers.
	• Work organizations.
Clinical Utility	
Format	• Self-report instrument of 49 questions organized along five scales: 1) decision latitude, 2) psychological demands, 3) social support, 4) physical demands, 5) job insecurity
Procedure	• Rate statements about their jobs using a 4-point scale (1=fully agree/very unlikely; 4=fully disagree/very likely).
	• Scores are summed within five scales, and are often collapsed into dichotomous scores for interpretation of high & low.
	• Scores can be compared to national scale scores or norms from US and Sweden by sex, occupation, and industry (e.g., compare findings in a plant to national averages)
Completion Time	• 15 minutes
Standardization	• Manual with norms.
	• Has been translated in over a dozen languages. International board of researchers decides on policy and development issues.
	• Short direct-questioning format (subscales condensed to one question) validated in Holland as a potential screening tool.
Reliability	
Internal Consistency	• Cronbach's alpha were 0.71 and 0.76 with one notable item-to-total Pearson correlation of 0.21 for control subscale "repetitive work."
	• Psychological Demands scale has consistently scored lower than other scales (i.e., 0.57 to 0.67 in four different samples).

continued

Table 10-5 (continued)

JOB CONTENT QUESTIONNAIRE (JCQ)

Inter-Rater	• Group ICCs of modified version of JDQ ranged from 0.63 to 0.92.
Intra-Rater	• Modified version of JDQ was used to examine 54 jobs in a "typical" coastal sawmill in Canada. ICCs were in the fair to satisfactory range (0.54 to 0.75), for all scales except Psychological Demands, which had an ICC of 0.23.
Test-Retest	• Chinese version found Pearson's correlation coefficients in the moderate range (r=0.62 to 0.73), except for coworker support scale (r=0.36).
Validity	
Content	• Scales are based on Karasek's demand/control model of job strain development. Items derived statistically from survey data collected for the U.S. Department of Labor (1969, 1972, 1977). Core set of 27 questions developed on a pooled sample of 4,900 respondents.
	• To increase efficiency, utility and applicability, test has had multiple revisions.
Criterion	• Individual subscales of the Dutch version correlated significantly with 7 criterion variables, including a General Health Questionnaire.
Construct	• Karasek et al., (1998) established cross-national validity in United States, Canada, Netherlands, and Japan across wide occupational spectrum (16,601 participants), and ages; conditions in modern industrial nations are more consistent across national boundaries than across occupational groups; consistent ability to discriminate occupation
	• Items from multiple versions of JDA have factored consistently with theoretical constructs of the JDA.
	• Scores predictive of job-related illness development (e.g., psychological distress, coronary heart disease, musculoskeletal disease, reproductive disorders) in several countries (Karasek et al., 1998) and confirmed constructs of Karasek's demand/control model (Karasek & Theorell, 1990).
Strengths	• Well standardized for multiple cultures.
	• Can be self-administered with minimal assistance.
	• Has a theoretical basis that allows application in social policy and organizational change.
	• Used broadly in many different settings to both analyze effect of job characteristics on individual's relative risk of job-related illness development, and testing of social policy effect on worker group's activation, motivation and job satisfaction.
Weaknesses	• For comprehensive assessment of stress, would need to add measure of non-job-related stress. For coping with stress, would need to add personality scales.
	• Demand/control model does not account for cognitive appraisal of events.
	• Psychological Demands subscale consistently performs weaker than other subscales.
	• Organization-level job factors not included.
Final Word	• A well standardized tool with broad application and use.

Table 10-6

WORKER ROLE INTERVIEW

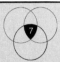

Source	Velozo, C. A., Kielhofner, G., & Fisher, G. (1998). *A user's guide to the Worker Role Interview. (Version 9.0)*. Chicago: Model of Human Occupation Clearing House, Department of Occupational Therapy, University of Illinois.
	AOTA Products, P.O. Box 3800, Forrester Center, WV, 25438, (phone) 887-404-AOTA.
Important References	Biernacki, S. D. (1993). Reliability of the Worker Role Interview. *American Journal of Occupational Therapy, 47*, 797-803.
	Ekbladh, E., Haglund, L., & Thorell, L. (2004). The Worker Role Interview: Preliminary data on the predictive validity of return to work of clients after an insurance medicine investigation. *Journal of Occupational Rehabilitation, 14(2)*, 131-141.
	Gern, A. (1993). *Validity of the Worker Role Interview.* Master's Thesis, University of Illinois at Chicago.
	Lin, F. L. (1994). *The Worker Role Interview: Construct validity across diagnoses.* Master's Thesis, University of Illinois at Chicago.
	Velozo, C. A., Kielhofner, G., Gern, A., Lin, F. L., Azhar, F., Lai, J. S., & Fisher, G. (1999). Worker Role Interview: Validation of a psychosocial work-related measure. *Journal of Occupational Rehabilitation, 9(3)*, 153-168.
Purpose	• Identify the psychosocial and environmental variables influencing a worker returning to work.
	• Intended to be used during initial assessment as part of a physical and/or work capacity assessment.
	• Facilitate rehab planning by offering worker's perceptions and information about worker's ability to adjust habits and routines, commitment to the worker role.
Type of Client	• Injured workers in vocational assessment/rehabilitation.
Clinical Utility	
Format	• Therapist rates on a four-point scale 17 factors that support and interfere with successful return-to-work.
	• The WRI has six content areas with the following subcontent areas or rated factors: 1) Personal Causation—personal assessment of abilities & limitations, expectations of job success, takes responsibility; 2) Values—commitment to work, work-related goals; 3) Interests—enjoys work, pursues interests consistent with work; 4) Roles—identifies with being a worker, appraises work expect expectations, influence of other roles; 5) Habits—work habits, daily routine, adapts routine to minimize difficulties; 6) Environment—physical setting, perception of family and peers, perception of boss, perception of coworkers.
Procedures	• Five steps: interview preparation, semi-structured interview (at start of initial assessment), the usual physical/work capacity assessment procedures used by the organization, scoring the WRI Rating Form (following initial assessment), rescoring WRI Rating Form (at discharge from treatment).
	• Therapist rates each subcontent area on a scale of 1 (strongly interferes with returning to job) to 4 (strongly supports client returning to job) giving brief comments in the margin to support each rating.
Completion Time	• 30 to 45 minutes for interview, plus observation of work capacity assessment

continued

Table 10-6 (continued)

WORKER ROLE INTERVIEW

Standardization	• WRI user's manual and videotape of interview administration available.
Reliability	
Internal Consistency	• Velozo et al. (1999) used Rasch Analysis to determine person separation reliability (analogous to Cronbach's alpha). They found that the WRI reliably differentiated injured workers based on ability levels.
Inter-Rater	• Biernacki (1993) computed for three raters (n= 30 adults in rehab for upper extremity injury): ICCs of six content areas ranged from 0.46 to 0.92 with a total value of 0.81. Suggests need for refinement in three areas (Values, Roles, Habits), potential improvement with training.
Intra-Rater	• Not reported.
Test-Retest	• High reliability. ICCs ranged from 0.86 to 0.94 with total value of 0.95.
Validity	
Content	• Items are based on the Model of Human Occupation (Kielhofner, 1995) and review of literature of factors impacting return to work.
Criterion	• Found evidence that the WRI discriminated between clients on psychosocial capacity for work.
	• Velozo et al. (1999) studied work-injured claimants and found that the WRI did not predict return to work.
	• Ekbladh, Haglund, & Thorell (2004) found that only 5 of 17 items predicted return to work for 48 injured workers; content area Personal Causation had the best predictive validity, while content areas values, interests and habits demonstrated no predictive validity.
Construct	• Velozo et al. (1999) conducted 2 studies with injured workers that found the WRI measures a uni-dimensional construct.
Strengths	• Has a theoretical basis.
	• Provides descriptive information about how a worker views self as a worker and work environment.
	• Facilitates understanding potential barriers to return to work and thereby facilitates rehab planning.
Weaknesses	• Suggested questions require re-organization for better flow and rephrasing to reduce reactivity.
	• Needs to be more broadly applied and tested in a variety of settings, therapists, and populations before used as an outcome measure.
Final Word	• One of the few tools available to assess psychosocial and environmental variables influencing a worker returning to work.

Table 10-7

OCCUPATIONAL PERFORMANCE HISTORY INTERVIEW II

Source	Kielhofner, G., Mallinson, T., Crawford, C., Nowak, M., Rigby, M., Henry, A., & Walens, D. (1998). *The Occupational Performance History Interview (Version 2.0)* OPHI-II. Chicago, Il: Model of Human Occupation Clearinghouse.
Important References	Keilhofner, G., & Henry, A. (1988). Development and Investigation of the Occupational Performance History Interview. *American Journal of Occupational Therapy*, 42(8), 489-498.
	Keilhofner, G., Mallinson, T., Forsyth, K., Lai, J. S. (2001). Psychometric Properties of the second version of the Occupational Performance History Interview (OPHI-II). *American Journal of Occupational Therapy*, 55(3), 260-7.
	Mallinson, T., Mahaffey, L., & Keilhofner, G. (1998). The Occupational Performance History Interview: Evidence for three underlying constructs of occupational adaptation. *Canadian Journal of Occupational Therapy*, 65(4), 219-228.
Purpose	• Designed to assess three constructs of occupational adaptation: occupational identity, occupational competence, and the impact of occupation behavior settings.
PEO Focus	• Person, environment, and occupation.
Type of Client	• Occupational therapy clients who are capable of responding to an in-depth interview.
Clinical Utility	
Format	• Semi-structured interview. Focuses on following thematic areas: 1) Occupational roles, 2) Daily routine, 3) Activity/occupational choices, 4) Critical life events, and 5) Occupational behavior settings. Can be administered as single, comprehensive interview, or as two shorter interviews (one focused on client, one focused on environment).
Procedures	• Interview administered by occupational therapist. It consists of 3 rating scales (Occupational Identity, Occupational Competence, Occupational Behavior Settings) and the Life History Narrative (qualitative data from interview).
Completion Time	• Takes approximately 1 hour.
Standardization	• Manual available from AOTA provides rating scales and suggests possible sequence and format of questions.
Reliability	
Internal Consistency	• Not reported.
Observer	• Rater separation statistics indicated that raters have the same degree of severity and leniency.
Test-retest	• Not reported, however data for original OPHI showed poor to adequate test-retest reliability (r=0.31 to 0.68).
Validity	
Content	• Using RASCH analysis methods, strong evidence that test items captured underlying traits. Low percentage of misfit statistics (8% to 9%) indicate validity across different subjects.
Criterion	• Not reported.
Construct	• Separation statistics indicate OPHI-II can detect meaningful differences between persons and levels of competence.

continued

Table 10-7 (continued)

OCCUPATIONAL PERFORMANCE HISTORY INTERVIEW II

Strengths	• OPHI-II can be readily learned through the manual, and used with a wide variety of clients. • Validity evidence is stronger than the original OPHI. • Based on well-known theory. • Intervention plan can be developed from assessment results.
Weaknesses	• Therapist, rather than client assigns the scores. • Presumes therapist familiarity with Model of Human Occupation. • Administration may be time consuming.
Final Word	• Client-centered assessment for establishment of clinical goals. Most appropriate when therapy can be structured to maximize knowledge of client's life history.

Strong. S., Baptiste, S., Cole, D., Clarke, J., Costa, M., Shannon, H., Reardon, R. & Sinclair, S. (2004a). Functional Assessment of Injured Workers: A profile of assessor practices. *Canadian Journal of Occupational Therapy, 1(71),* 13-23.

Strong, S., Baptiste, S., Clarke, J., Cole, D., & Costa, M. (2004b). Use of functional capacity evaluations in workplaces and the compensation system: A report on workers' and report users' perceptions. *Work: Journal of Assessment, Prevention and Rehabilitation, 23(1),* 67-77.

Strong, S., Baptiste, S., Polanyi, M., Clarke, J., Woodward, C., & Dobbins, M. (2004c). *Towards best practices of Functional Assessment: An innovative model for research dissemination.* Research Report. (WSIB Grant #01043) Hamilton, ON: Work Function Unit, School of Rehabilitation Science, McMaster University.

Strong, S., & Rebeiro, R. (2003). Creating supportive work environments for people with mental illness. In: L. Letts, P. Rigby, & D. Stewart (eds.). *Using environment to enable occupational performance.* Thorofare, NJ: SLACK Incorporated.

Strong, S., & Westmorland, M. (1996). *Determining claimant effort and maximum voluntary effort testing: A discussion paper.* Report for The Institute of Work & Health and the Ontario Insurance Commission. Work Function Unit, McMaster University, Hamilton, Ontario.

Thomas, L. (1992). Qualified nurse and nursing auxiliary perceptions of their work environment in primary, team and functional nursing wards. *Journal of Advanced Nursing. 17,* 373-382.

Velozo, C. A. (1993). Work evaluations: Critique of the state of the art of functional assessment of work. *American Journal of Occupational Therapy, 47,* 203-209.

Velozo, C. A., Kielhofner, G., Gern, A., Lin, F. L., Azhar, F., Lai, J. S., & Fisher, G. (1999). Worker Role Interview: Validation of a psychosocial work-related measure. *Journal of Occupational Rehabilitation, 9(3),* 153-168.

Watson, D. E. & Wilson, S. A. (2003). *Task analysis: An individual and population approach.* Bethesda: MD, AOTA Press.

Williams, R.& Myers, A. (1998a). A new approach to measuring recovery in injured workers with acute low back pain: resumption of activities of daily living scale. *Physical Therapy, 78(6),* 613-623.

Williams, R., & Myers, A. (1998b). Functional abilities confidence scale: a clinical measure for injured workers with acute low back pain. *Physical Therapy, 78(6),* 624-634.

Williams, R., Hapidou, E., & Cullen, K. (2003). Use of self-efficacy and resumption of activities of daily living scales in chronic pain. *Physiotherapy Canada, 55(2),* 87-95.

WorkCover. (1998). *Rehabilitation and Rehabilitation Providers: Guidelines for insurers, employers and rehabilitation providers.* WorkCover, New South Wales.

Wressle, E., Lindstrand, J., Neher, M., Marcusson, J., & Henriksson C. (2003). The Canadian Occupational Performance Measure as an outcome measure and team tool in a day treatment programme. *Disability and Rehabilitation, 25(10),* 497-506.

Table 10-8

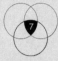

CANADIAN OCCUPATIONAL PERFORMANCE MEASURE (COPM)

Source	Law, M., Baptiste, S., Carswell, A., McColl, M. A., Polatajko, H., & Pollock, N. (1998). *The Canadian Occupational Performance Measure* (3rd ed.). Toronto: CAOT. (Web) ww.caot.ca
Important references	Wressle, E., Lindstrand, J., Neher, M., Marcusson, J., & Henriksson, C. (2003). The Canadian Occupational Performance Measure as an outcome measure and team tool in a day treatment programme. *Disability and Rehabilitation, 25(10)*, 497-506.
	McColl, M. A., Paterson, M., Davies, D., Doubt, L., & Law M. (2000). Validity and community utility of the Canadian Occupational Performance Measure. *Canadian Journal of Occupational Therapy, 67(1)*, 22-30.
	Carpenter, L., Baker, G. A., & Tyldesley, B. (2001). The use of the Canadian Occupational Performance Measure as an outcome of a pain management program. *Canadian Journal of Occupational Therapy, 68(1),* 16-22.
Purpose	• Developed to be compatible with the Canadian Guidelines for client-centered practice (CAOT, 1981, 1991). It offers a measure of occupational performance that is based on a client-centered approach to practice.
Type of Client	• All occupational therapy clients.
Clinical Utility	
Format	• Administered in three sections corresponding to self-care, productivity and leisure.
Procedures	• Semi-structured interview, focusing on problem identification. Client subjectively scores his or her performance and satisfaction with identified occupational performance issues.
Completion Time	• Average of 30 to 40 minutes
Standardization	• Administration manual available. There is also a videotape available of sample administrations with different age groups.
Reliability	
Internal Consistency	• 0.56 (Performance); 0.71 (Satisfaction) (Law et al., 1998).
Observer	• Not reported.
Test-Retest	• In the range of 0.80 for both subscales (Carswell et al., 2004).
Validity	
Content	• Based on the process of development (Law et al., 1998).
Criterion	• Based on relationships with a number of widely used measures and constructs (for
Construct	a review, see Carswell et al., 2004.)
Strengths	• Clients find COPM helpful in identifying their problems.
	• Therapists and other professionals find information helpful and unique.
	• Intensifies focus on occupational performance in therapy.
Weaknesses	• Requires good interviewing skills to administer.
	• Can be time consuming if interview focuses on problem parameters, instead of just on problem identification.
Final Word	• Efficient method of gaining client's perspective for treatment planning, for establishing treatment goals, and for measuring the effects of treatment.

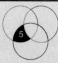

Table 10-9

VALPAR COMPONENT WORK SAMPLES (VCWS)

Source	VALPAR International Corporation, PO Box 5767, Tucson, Arizona, USA, 5703-5767
Important references	*Valpar Component Work Samples (VCWS) Manuals.* Tucson, AZ: VALPAR International Corporation.
Purpose	• Developed in order to assess task performance on simulated work tasks. The tasks have all been analyzed according to the *Dictionary of Occupational Titles.*
Type of Client	• Adolescents and adults for whom the worker role is pertinent.
Clinical Utility	
Format	• Consists of individual work samples that simulate task performance, (e.g., for repetitive assembly work). For each task, there is a complete analysis of the skills and attitudes required for worker to complete that task.
Procedures	• The client is instructed to perform each task according to a standard procedure, and then scored on timing and other characteristics.
Completion Time	• Tasks range from completion time of 20 to 90 minutes.
Standardization	• The VALPAR is a complete a standardized measure with specific manuals, instructions and scoring directions for each work sample.
	• Methods-Time-Measurement (MTM) methodology provides a time standard for the completion of the work sample. (MTM is standard representative of the time it would take for a well-trained worker to perform the task in a typical industrial set ting in an 8 hour work day).
	• MTM has also been used to establish normative data for the VALPAR Work samples related to Time percentiles and Time percent.
Reliability	
Internal Consistency	• Not reported.
Test-Retest	• Reliability values of 0.70 to 0.99.
Validity	
Content	• Many studies have been completed demonstrating high correspondence between items on the VALPAR Work Samples and required worker characteristics in the Dictionary of Occupational Titles.
Criterion	• Not reported.
Construct	• The VALPAR Work Samples are able to discriminate between workers employed or not employed in specific jobs.
Strengths	• Provides a comprehensive assessment of simulated job tasks.
	• The Samples have been well tested and scoring information for normative comparison is extensive.
Weaknesses	• Extensive cost.
	• Requires more psychometric testing for predictive validity of return to work.
Final Word	• Useful for assessment of person and occupation, but does not take into account unique environmental demands with each job.

Table 10-10

SPINAL FUNCTION SORT

Source	Employment Potential Improvement Corporation, P.O. Box 3897, Ballwin, MO, 63022.
Important references	Gibson, L., & Strong, J. (1996). The reliability and validity of a measure of perceived functional capacity for work in chronic back pain. *Journal of Occupational Rehab, 6(3)*, 159-175.
	Matheson, L., & Matheson, M. (1989). *PACT Spinal Function Sort*. Wildwood, MO: Employment Potential Improvement Corporation.
	Matheson, L., Matheson, M., & Grant, J. (1993). Development of a measure of perceived functional ability. *Journal of Occupational Rehabilitation, 3(1)*, 15-30.
	Matheson, L., Mooney, V., Grant, J., Leggett, S., & Kenny, K. (1996). Standardized evaluation of work capacity. *Journal of Back and Musculoskeletal Rehabilitation, 6(3)*, 249-264.
	Robinson, R. C., Kishino, N., Matheson, L., Woods, S., Hoffman, K., Unterberg, J., Pearson, C., Adams, L., &. Gatchel, R. J. (2003). Improvement in postoperative and nonoperative spinal patients on a self-report measure of disability: the Spinal Function Sort (SFS). *Journal of Occupational Rehabilitation, 13(2)*,107-13.
	Sufka, A., Hauger, B., Trenary, M., Bishop, B., Hagen, A., Lozon, R., & Martens, B. (1998). Centralization of low back pain and perceived functional outcome. *Journal of Orthopaedic & Sports Physical Therapy, 27(3)*, 205-212.
Purpose	• To evaluate self-perceived ability to perform frequently encountered physical work tasks
	• To compare the evaluee's perception of ability to perform these tasks with his or her perception of the tasks and demand levels that are required in his or her occupational role.
Type of Client	• Adolescents and adults for whom the worker role is pertinent.
Clinical Utility	
Format	• 50-item instrument organized in a test booklet, each item composed of a drawing of an adult of working age performing a work task. Two of the items have matched pairs in the instrument to allow checks on internal consistency.
Procedures	• Each evaluee is provided a test booklet, response sheet, and a pencil. The evaluee describes his or her ability to perform the task along a 5-point scale from "able" to "unable." The test is administered on an un-timed basis.
Completion Time	• 6 to 12 minutes.
Standardization	• Administration procedures were developed in six industrial rehabilitation clinics with 180 subjects.
	• Each drawing is accompanied by a simple task description presented in English, French, German, or Spanish. A tape recording of the task descriptions is provided for evaluees who are not functionally literate.
Reliability	
Internal Consistency	• Matheson et al. (1993) reported that the split-half reliability of the Spinal Function Sort was evaluated through a comparison of odd and even items, yielding a Spearman-Brown correlation of 0.983. Gibson & Strong (1996) reported a Cronbach's alpha of 0.98.
Test-Retest	• Matheson, et al (1993) performed separate studies for men and women based on the "Rating of Perceived Capacity." Pearson coefficients for a 3-day interval were 0.85 for 126 adult males and 0.82 for 84 adult females. Similar coefficients have been reported in other studies.

continued

Table 10-10 (continued)

SPINAL FUNCTION SORT

Validity

Content
- The test was constructed from a pool of more than 200 items. This initial set was administered to 105 subjects who were asked to "select those tasks that you perform on at least a weekly basis." From this set were culled items that were frequently endorsed.

Criterion
- Studied in a sample of 85 injured workers in a work hardening program (Townsend, 1996). Statistically significant and meaningful relationships were found between SFS scores and performance in a physical-demanding functional capacity evaluation and an inverse relationship was found between reports of pain and SFS scores.
- Was found to detect a significant improvement in Ratings of Perceived Capacity scores after a functional restoration program in postoperative and non-operative subjects with low back pain.

Construct
- Gibson & Strong (1996) describe a multi-trait, multi-method approach to establishing construct and discriminant validity. Among the scales used were the Work Re-Entry Questionnaire, Pain Disability Index, Self-Efficacy Scale, Pain Self-Efficacy Questionnaire, and Visual Analogue Scale. In each case the SFS correlated significantly and in the expected direction.

Strengths
- Is widely used across the world in rehabilitation settings.
- Has had extensive reliability and validity testing.
- Has shown good predictive ability for lift capacity and work disability in people with musculoskeletal impairments.

Weaknesses
- Paper and pencil format cannot replace value of observation of task performance.

Final Word
- Useful tool with good psychometric properties that can be incorporated as part of return to work process.

Table 10-11

FEASIBILITY EVALUATION CHECKLIST

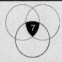

Source	Program in Occupational Therapy, Washington University School of Medicine, 4444 Forest Park Avenue, St. Louis, MO, 63108.
Important References	Matheson, L., Ogden, L., Violette, K., & Schultz, K. (1985). Work hardening: Occupational therapy in industrial rehabilitation. *American Journal of Occupational Therapy, 39(5)*, 314-321.
Purpose	• Designed to evaluate the presence of behavioral requirements all employers in the competitive labor market have of any employee. These include attendance, timeliness, workplace tolerance, and ability to accept supervision.
Type of Client	• Adolescents and adults for whom the worker role is pertinent.
Clinical Utility	
Format	• 21-item behavior rating scale. Each item is briefly described on the scale.
Procedures	• 21 factors in the FEC are measured by observation of the evaluee in an actual or simulated work environment, often in a sheltered workshop or at a therapeutic workstation. The work environment must be structured to approximate the temporal demands of work, requiring regular daily attendance and adherence to a set schedule.
Completion Time	• 3 minutes to 5 minutes.
Standardization	• The administration procedures were developed at the Work Preparation Center at Rancho Los Amigos Hospital in Downey, California.
Reliability	
Internal Consistency	• Not reported.
Test-Retest	• Matheson (1979) used a simple scoring system to identify the number of items that were rated "non-feasible" with 43 industrial rehabilitation clients. Over a 24-hour interval, the FEC demonstrated a reliability coefficient of 0.78.
Validity	
Content	• The items for the FEC were identified by employers and rehabilitation placement specialists in a survey conducted at Rancho as those that most often cause a return to work attempt by a disabled client to result in failure. Altogether, 53 items were identified. These were grouped and items that overlapped were consolidated to provide the current set of 21 items.
Criterion	• Not reported.
Construct	• Not reported.
Strengths	• Has been used in a wide variety of rehabilitation settings since its introduction.
	• Can be used by professional raters, para-professional raters, and for self-rating by clients.
Weaknesses	• Need to observe client for a full workday over multiple days in work environment or simulated work environment.
Final Word	• Can be used to evaluate first steps in the return to work process. Requires more validity testing.

Editors' Notes for Chapter 11

Mine the Gold

Rehabilitation professionals from several disciplines (e.g., nursing, occupational therapy, medicine, physical therapy) have long acknowledged the importance of basic activities of daily living (BADL) for characterizing recovery and habilitation.

Become Systematic

Use of BADL measures ensures that therapists remember to address all the relevant functions in each assessment. Since many of these measures use rating scales to characterize the level of dependence/independence, their use makes it easy to document changes in performance.

Use Evidence in Practice

Because these BADL measures have been used in many types of studies, we can offer clients and their families clear information about our ability to chart their recovery/habilitation as a routine aspect of intervention. This enables the client/family to participate in decisions about their own care.

Make Occupational Therapy Contribution Explicit

BADL have been a traditional aspect of occupational therapy practice. Using the measures in this chapter links our interest in the client's life with his or her need to care for him- or herself.

Engage in Occupation-Based, Client-Centered Practice

BADLs are a very personal part of everyone's daily routines. By measuring this aspect of performance, we acknowledge the person's need for taking care of self as central to the recovery/habilitation process.

MEASURING OCCUPATIONAL PERFORMANCE IN BASIC ACTIVITIES OF DAILY LIVING

Lori Letts, PhD, OT Reg. (Ont.) and Jackie Bosch, MSc, OT Reg. (Ont.)

WHAT ARE ACTIVITIES OF DAILY LIVING?

Occupational therapists, both in assessment and intervention, address the abilities of clients to independently manage their activities of daily living (ADL). ADL are often viewed as key areas for assessment and intervention since we understand them to be important foundations for participation in the community. ADL are one of three areas of occupation that is composed of activities of daily living, instrumental activities of daily living (IADL), education, work and play, and leisure and social participation (American Occupational Therapy Association [AOTA], 2002). Occupational therapists have a general understanding of what is meant by the term activities of daily living.

Despite its strong historical and current place in occupational therapy practice, the definitions used by therapists to describe ADL vary. Although occupational therapists have an understanding of the phrase as an umbrella term that relates to a person's basic self-care, there is no consistent definition apparent in the literature. For example, in the *Occupational Therapy Practice Framework* (AOTA, 2002, p. 620), the term activities of daily living is defined as "activities that are oriented toward taking care of one's own body". The glossary in the text by Christiansen and Baum (1997, p. 591) defines ADL as the "typical life tasks required for self-care and self-maintenance, such as grooming, bathing, eating, cleaning the house, and doing laundry." While some of those activities are the same as those in the *Occupational Therapy Practice Framework*, others would fall under IADL. Trombly (2002) describes ADL as universal tasks that a person undertakes to maintain health, while Spear and Crepeau (2003, p. 1025) define them as "activities involving taking care of oneself".

There is also variability in the terms used to describe ADL, including self-care, basic ADL, personal ADL, personal care, and function. Although there are differences in definitions, there is a common understanding of what we mean by ADL in those activities that people do to take care of themselves on a day-to-day basis. What is less consistent is which components of ADL should be included in any instruments that attempt to measure a client's abilities in daily living activities.

CHALLENGES OF ADL ASSESSMENT

Despite the variety of formal definitions, the profession of occupational therapy is confident in its overall understanding of the concept of ADL and use of that knowledge in everyday practice. However, ADL have historically been challenging to measure. It appears that part of the reason for that difficulty is related to the inconsistency and lack of agreement about which activities actually comprise ADL. If there is not a clear and consistent definition of the construct to be measured, establishing the appropriate content for an instrument is difficult. Ideally, assessments should be developed based on a defined concept, rather than having the instrument content determine our understanding of the concept (Unsworth, 1993). It appears that in measures of ADL, part of the challenge has been an inadequate articulation of the concept, so that instrument content development has varied. Even when instruments measure the same concept, they do so with varying definitions. This has been demonstrated clearly by Rogers,

Gwinn, and Holm (2001) in their comparison of the FIM, MDS, OASIS, and MDS-PAC.

Since ADL is a broad term that encompasses many tasks and activities, most instruments are developed by selecting specific activities that are representative of the entire construct. There are variations and debate as to which areas of ADL are most important. Importance can be influenced by whether one is looking at individual clients or groups of clients, the developmental stage of the population, the diagnosis, and lifestyles prior to the onset of difficulties.

ADL are measured by occupational therapists for different reasons (Law & Letts, 1989). If used as an outcome measure, an overall sense of the client's ability to perform in the area of ADL is sought. In clinical practice settings, clinicians may be interested in more detailed and descriptive information than might be available through an instrument focused on ADL as the outcome. For example, one item used to describe the client's ability to dress independently may not adequately represent the complexity of the dressing task, which parts are difficult and easy for the client, what kinds of cues or strategies can be effectively used to improve dressing skills, etc.

Despite the challenges associated with defining, and thus establishing measures of ADL, a number of instruments that focus on performance in ADL have been developed over the years. The earliest to be published may have been the Katz Index (Katz, Ford, Moskowitz, Jackson, & Jaffe, 1963) and the Barthel Index (BI) (Mahoney & Barthel, 1965). Many others have been developed since then. The challenge is to find the ADL instrument that meets the needs and criteria of different practice and research settings.

METHOD OF REVIEW OF ADL INSTRUMENTS

For this chapter, a list of potential measures to be reviewed was first generated based on general literature review, review articles that have examined ADL instruments, and personal resources. Eighty-three measures were on the initial list. This list was then reviewed with specific criteria for inclusion in this chapter, since the intent is to include the best measures available in the area, not all of the available instruments. The two authors independently considered the following criteria: clinical usefulness, current use for clinical or research purposes, existence of at least some reliability and validity testing, and availability of information about the instrument through a peer-reviewed publication. As well if the instrument included non-ADL items (e.g., instrumental activities were a substantial part of the instrument), an ADL subscale was required for the instrument to be included in this review. The two authors formulated decisions for inclusion by consensus. Instruments were eliminated if they had not

been cited in articles in the last 15 years, or if they were not currently used in practice settings. Some were eliminated if they were not used clinically and had no psychometric testing. One, the Klein Bell ADL assessment (Klein & Bell, 1982), was excluded since the authors could not find a current source for the measure. The final list of instruments includes 16 ADL assessments. Each instrument was then reviewed using criteria from the Outcome Measures Rating Form (CanChild, 1999), and information from that rating is summarized in Tables 11-1 through 11-15. A list of instruments considered and not included in the review is available from the authors.

CHOOSING AN APPROPRIATE ADL INSTRUMENT

When reviewing ADL instruments for use in occupational therapy practice, it is first useful to consider what general areas each of the instruments cover, or which client populations they have been designed for, as listed below. It may be useful to begin by considering whether it is important to have all clients rated on the same activities (activity-specific measures) or on activities that are deemed by the client as important or problematic for them (client-identified activities). This will help to further narrow down the choice. Following the name of each instrument, an "O" or "C" is included. This indicates whether the instrument was intended for use as an outcome measure (for evaluation), or more as an instrument to describe a person's abilities for design of a clinical intervention, or both. This list should provide initial direction in guiding selection of an appropriate instrument.

ADL Instruments with Client-Identified ADL Activities

- Canadian Occupational Performance Measure (COPM)—C, O (reviewed in detail in Chapter 6)
- Juvenile Arthritis Self-Report Index (JASI)—C, O
- Patient Specific Functional Scale (PSFS)—O

Activity Specific ADL Instruments

- Activities Scale for Kids (ASK)—C, O
- Arnadottir OT-ADL Neurobehavioral Evaluation (A-ONE)—C, O
- Arthritis Impact Measurement Scales (AIMS2)—O
- Barthel Index (BI)—O
- Child Health Questionnaire (CHQ)—O
- Functional Autonomy Measurement System (SMAF)—C, O
- Functional Independence Measure (FIM)/WeeFIM —O

- Health Assessment Questionnaire (HAQ)/Child Health Assessment Questionnaire (CHAQ)—O
- Juvenile Arthritis Functional Assessment Scale (JAFAS)/Juvenile Arthritis Functional Assessment Report (JAFAR)—O
- Juvenile Arthritis Self-Report Index (JASI)—C, O
- Katz Index of Activities of Daily Living—O
- Melville Nelson Self Care Assessment—C, O
- Pediatric Evaluation of Disability Inventory (PEDI)—C, O
- Physical Self-Maintenance Scale (PSMS)—O

ADL Instruments for Use With Adults With Physical Disabilities

- Arnadottir OT-ADL Neurobehavioral Evaluation (A-ONE)—C, O
- Arthritis Impact Measurement Scales (AIMS2)—O
- Barthel Index (BI)—O
- Functional Independence Measure (FIM)—O
- Health Assessment Questionnaire (HAQ)—O
- Katz Index of Activities of Daily Living—O

ADL Instruments Designed for Children

- Activities Scale for Kids (ASK)—C, O
- Child Health Questionnaire (CHQ)—O
- Functional Independence Measure for Children—O
- Juvenile Arthritis Functional Assessment Scale (JAFAS)/Juvenile Arthritis Functional Assessment Report (JAFAR)—O
- Juvenile Arthritis Self-Report Index (JASI)—C, O
- Pediatric Evaluation of Disability Inventory (PEDI)—C, O
- WeeFIM (see review of FIM)—O

ADL Instruments Designed for Older Adults

- Functional Autonomy Measurement System (SMAF)—C, O
- Melville Nelson Self Care Assessment—C, O
  - Physical Self-Maintenance Scale (PSMS)—O

ADL Instruments Designed for Specific Impairments

- Arnadottir OT-ADL Neurobehavioral Evaluation (A-ONE)—C, O

- Arthritis Impact Measurement Scales (AIMS2)—O
- Health Assessment Questionnaire (HAQ)/Child Health Assessment Questionnaire (CHAQ)—O
- Juvenile Arthritis Self-Report Index (JASI)—C, O
- Juvenile Arthritis Functional Assessment Scale (JAFAS)/Juvenile Arthritis Functional Assessment Report (JAFAR)—O

The review tables that follow provide more detailed information about the instruments that were considered among the best ADL measures available. The instruments are ordered alphabetically. For each instrument, details are provided about the purpose, format, procedures, and psychometric testing that have been completed on the instrument. Reliability, validity, and responsiveness to change are presented in a standard format, beginning with information about the population tested (including sample size where available), followed by the value and statistic used. In the final section of each table, strengths and weaknesses of the instrument or research related to it are summarized, and a final word is included to describe overall findings or usefulness of the instrument. Two or three important references are included in the tables, with further references available in the list at the chapter's end. This should assist occupational therapists in considering the applicability of the instrument to their practice settings.

DISCUSSION: ISSUES IN MEASUREMENT OF SELF-CARE

Is the construct of ADL being adequately measured in the current measures that are available? This is an important question to consider, since it influences whether or not new instruments should be developed to address some missing component of ADL that is not adequately measured, or the entire construct itself. Overall, it appears that, in fact, with the currently available instruments, clinicians should be able to locate one that adequately meets their needs for either clinical assessment or evaluation purposes. There is a range of instruments available, some of which can be used with a large group of clients, regardless of their types of disability or disease. There are also more specific instruments available to meet demands of instruments related to diagnostic groups. With the current status of evidence available, it might even be argued that the FIM/WeeFIM and Barthel Index have become "gold standards" in ADL outcome assessment, at least in the context of stroke rehabilitation, the setting within which most of the research has been conducted. Both have long histories of use in rehabilitation evaluations (the Barthel the longest of the two), with research conducted internationally to examine their psychometric properties and more information now emerging regarding their responsiveness to change. That is not to say, however, that the FIM and

Barthel are appropriate in all contexts. Depending on the intended use of an ADL assessment, the clinical population and the setting, other assessments reviewed here may be more appropriate.

A major difference among the instruments reviewed is related to the use of self-report vs. observation of performance in ADL. Although many occupational therapists using an ADL assessment to plan specific interventions want to observe their clients' performance, there are other times when self-report is also useful and more practical. Instruments like the BI, which have been tested for both uses, can be useful for outcome evaluation during rehabilitation as well as telephone follow-up. Taking this a step further, some measures (e.g., COPM and PSFS) are designed so that clients identify the activities to be measured. Although individually unique, the psychometric properties of these instruments are promising and align with principles of client-centered practice.

Another difference that can be noted amongst the instruments reviewed is the number of items. For example, the WeeFIM consists of 18 items, while the Pediatric Evaluation of Disability Inventory (PEDI) includes 197 functional performance items, and the COPM may include only one or two items under ADL. In comparing instruments to select an appropriate measure, this difference is an important consideration in relation to the purpose of collecting data. Both the COPM and the WeeFIM are designed more for outcome evaluation, to enable a clinician, client, or the team to compare occupational performance in ADL and other performance areas across points in time. In comparison, the PEDI, while it can also be used for outcome evaluation, provides much more detailed information that can be used to more directly influence intervention planning. Information can be gathered about a child's abilities, the amount of caregiver assistance provided, and the frequency with which task modifications are used. If the purpose of the assessment is not only to observe but to document the details of a child's performance in a descriptive format, an instrument like the PEDI would meet that need.

A question that remains unanswered is whether or not it is actually necessary for ADL instruments and, in turn, the clinicians who use them, to be attempting to measure the entire domain of ADL. There has been little research done to demonstrate the links in performance between one ADL task like feeding and that of dressing or bathing. Although many occupational therapists in practice feel a need to observe clients in all areas of ADL, is it necessary to document all of those areas? Could we not, through a sampling of specific activities, generalize to others? Some analyses are beginning to show promise in exploring the relationships between different aspects of ADL. Guttman scaling was used in the past (e.g., Katz and now the ADL staircase), and Rasch analysis is becoming more common

(e.g., PEDI, FIM). Both of these methods provide information about the hierarchical relationships amongst activities, so that it may in fact be possible to make assumptions about a client's ability to perform simple tasks if more difficult ones are accomplished. This area of research needs further exploration but may allow therapists and clients to more efficiently proceed through assessment of ADL.

One component of occupational performance that the instruments reviewed in this chapter do not address is the difference in performance that can occur across different environments. For example, occupational therapists know that there are times when clients can perform better in their home environments than in a rehabilitation setting. However, these variations, which may be related to the physical, social, or cultural environment, are not accounted for in the instruments. In fact, this is difficult to do in a standardized instrument. The COPM and the PSFS are both instruments that allow clients to describe their performance as it occurs in natural settings, and other self-report measures may also allow that consideration. An observation-based instrument that shows promise is the Enviro-FIM, which is described in Chapter 17 of this text, since it accounts for the person's performance in light of the environment in which the task is undertaken. As rehabilitation professionals continue to be more concerned about participation as well as activities, environmental influences on ADL performance will need to be built into or reflected in its assessment.

SUMMARY

In this chapter, a number of clinically relevant assessments of ADL have been systematically reviewed. They include instruments that would be useful to occupational therapists for clinical assessment or evaluation purposes. Although further research is needed related to the assessment of activities of daily living, there are a number of instruments from which occupational therapists can choose.

FUTURE RESEARCH DIRECTIONS

In this review and discussion, a number of areas of future research can be identified. The first of these is the need to continue to examine the sensitivity to change of ADL instruments, particularly those which are designed for evaluation. Although significantly more research has been conducted in this area since the first edition of this text, it is a property of instruments that continues to require further attention. In an evaluation, it is crucial to know the degree of change that will be reflected in the scores of an ADL instrument. As well, when an ADL score changes, clinicians using evaluative instruments need to be able to rely on research to tell them if a change in ADL score is meaningful clinically, or due to chance. There are a variety of methods to examine change scores in rehabilitation measures (Stratford, Binkley, & Riddle, 1996), and these approaches need to be applied to ADL instruments. As more research is conducted in this area, clinicians will also need guidance to help them interpret the results of research.

A second area for future research is the need to more closely examine clinical utility. Reliability and validity of instruments are vital pieces of information that should be used in selecting an appropriate measure. However, it is also necessary to know specific information about how an instrument can be used in different settings by different people. Clinical utility focuses on such factors, and although often information can be gleaned from manuals, a more systematic approach to examining the usefulness of instruments in a variety of clinical and research settings would make instrument selection easier and more streamlined.

A focus on client-centered assessment and environmental influences on ADL performance are also warranted. Of the instruments reviewed, the COPM, the PSFS, and Part 2 of the JASI are designed so that the client identifies the areas that will be measured. While occupational therapy practice has moved towards a client-centered model, our assessments of occupational performance do not often reflect that. Current instruments might be used differently, so that only applicable items are included in assessments, but research to explore how that might be done has not been undertaken. The ways in which environmental circumstances influence ADL measurement have also not been considered at great length in the literature, even though they clearly influence functional abilities.

Finally, occupational therapists need to systematically gather and share data on their clients' activities of daily living scores. Although ADL is frequently a major area of focus in practice, there is little literature available that discusses the effectiveness of ADL interventions. Only by documenting performance and change in ADL, will occupational therapy demonstrate that a focus on activities of daily living as one area of occupational performance is justified.

REFERENCES

Aitken, D. M., & Bohannon, R. W. (2001). Functional independence measure versus short form-36: Relative responsiveness and validity. *International Journal of Rehabilitation Research, 24(1)*, 65-68.

AOTA. (2002). Occupational therapy practice framework: Domain and process. *American Journal of Occupational Therapy, 56*, 609-639.

Arnadottir, G. (1990). *The brain and behavior: Assessing cortical dysfunction through activities of daily living (ADL)*. St. Louis: C. V. Mosby.

Asumussen, L., Olson, L. M., Grant, E. N., Landgraf, J. M., Fagan, J., & Weiss, K. B. (2000). Use of the Child Health Questionnaire in a sample of moderate and low-income inner-city children with asthma. *American Journal of Respirology and Critical Care Medicine, 162*, 1215-1221.

Baildam, E. M., Holt, P. J., Conway, S. C., & Morton, M. J. (1995). The association between physical function and psychological problems in children with juvenile chronic arthritis. *British Journal of Rheumatology, 34*, 470-477.

Berg, M., Jahnsen, R., Froslie, K. F., & Hussain, A. (2004). Reliability of the pediatric evaluation of disability inventory (PEDI). *Physical and Occupational Therapy in Pediatrics, 24(3)*, 61-77.

Berod, A. C., Klay, M., Santos-Eggimann, B., & Paccaud, F. (2000). Anxiety, depressive or cognitive disorders in rehabilitation patients: Effect on length of stay. *American Journal of Physical Medicine and Rehabilitation, 79*, 266-277.

Black, T. M., Soltis, T., & Bartlett, C. (1999). Using the functional independence measure instrument to predict stroke rehabilitation outcomes. *Rehabilitation Nursing, 24(3)*, 109-114.

Bourke-Taylor, H. (2003). Melbourne Assessment of Unilateral Upper Limb Function: Construct validity and correlation with the Pediatric Evaluation of Disability Inventory. *Developmental Medicine & Child Neurology, 45*, 92-96.

Boyd, A., & Dawson, D. R. (2000). The relationship between perceptual impairment and self-care status in a sample of elderly persons. *Physical and Occupational Therapy in Geriatrics, 17(4)*, 1-16.

Braun, S. L., & Granger, C. V. (1991). A practical approach to functional assessment in paediatrics. *Occupational Therapy Practice, 2(2)*, 46-51.

Brorsson, B., & Hulter-Asberg, K. (1984). Katz index of independence in ADL: Reliability and validity in short-term care. *Scandinavian Journal of Rehabilitation Medicine, 16*, 125-132.

Brown, G. T., & Wallen, M (2002). Functional assessment tools for paediatric clients with juvenile chronic arthritis: An update and review for occupational therapists. *Scandinavian Journal of Occupational Therapy, 9*, 23-34.

Bruce, B. & Fries, J. F. (2003). The Stanford Health Assessment Questionnaire: A review of its history, issues, progress and documentation. *Journal of Rheumatology, 30*, 167-78.

CanChild Centre for Childhood Disability Research. (1999). Outcome measures rating form guidelines. Retrieved August 1, 2004 from: http://bluewirecs.tzo.com/canchild/patches/measguid.pdf

Center for Rehabilitation Effectiveness. (n.d.). Pediatric Evaluation of Disability Inventory—Computer Adaptive Testing (PEDI-CAT). Retrieved August 31, 2004 from: http://www.bu.edu/cre/projects/PEDI-CAT.htm

Chatman, A. B., Hyams, S. P., Neel, J. M., Binkley, J. M., Stratford, P. W., Schomberg, A., & Stabler, M. (1997). The Patient-Specific Functional Scale: Measurement properties in patients with knee dysfunction. *Physical Therapy, 77*, 820-829.

Christiansen, C., & Baum, C. (Eds.). (1997). *Occupational therapy: Enabling function and well-being (2nd ed.)*. Thorofare, NJ: SLACK Incorporated.

Ciesla, J. R., Shi, L., Stoskopf, C. H., & Samuels, M. E. (1993). Reliability of Katz's activities of daily living scale when used in telephone interviews. *Evaluation and the Health Professions, 16*, 190-204.

Cohen, M. E., & Marino, R. J. (2000). The tools of disability outcomes research functional status measures. *Archives of Physical Medicine & Rehabilitation, 81(Suppl. 2)*, S21-S29.

Collin, C., Wade, D. T., Davies, S., & Horne, V. (1988). The Barthel ADL index: A reliability study. *International Disabilities Studies, 10*, 61-63.

Coulton, C. J., Zborowsky, E., Lipton, J., & Newman, A. J. (1987). Assessment of the reliability and validity of the arthritis impact measurement scales for children with juvenile arthritis. *Arthritis and Rheumatology, 30*, 819-24.

Custers, J. W., Van der Net, J., Hoijtink, H., Wassenberg-Severijnen, J. E., Vermeer, A., & Helders, Pl J. (2002). Discriminative validity of the Dutch Pediatric Evaluation of Disability Inventory. *Archives of Physical Medicine and Rehabilitation, 83*, 1437-1441.

Daving, Y., Andren, E., Nordholm, L., & Grimby, G. (2001). Reliability of an interview approach to the Functional Independence Measure. *Clinical Rehabilitation, 15(3)*, 301-310.

Desrosiers, J., Bravo, G., Hebert, R., & Dubuc, N. (1995). Reliability of the revised functional autonomy measurement system (SMAF) for epidemiological research. *Age and Aging, 24*, 402-406.

Desrosiers, J., Rochette, A., Noreau, L., Bravo, G., Hebert, R., & Boutin, C. (2003). Comparison of two functional independence scales with a participation measure in post-stroke rehabilitation. *Archives of Gerontology & Geriatrics, 37*, 157-172.

Deutsch, A., Braun, S., & Granger, C. (1996). The Functional Independence Measure (FIM Instrument) and the Functional Independence Measure for children (WeeFIM Instrument): Ten years of development. *Critical Reviews in Physical Rehabilitation Medicine, 8*, 267-281.

Dewing, J. (1992). A critique of the Barthel Index. *British Journal of Nursing, 1*, 325-329.

Dijkers, M. P., & Yavuzer, G. (1999). Short versions of the telephone motor Functional Independence Measure for use with persons with spinal cord injury. *Archives of Physical Medicine and Rehabilitation, 80*, 1477-1484.

Dumas, H. M., Haley, S. M., Fragala, M. A., & Steva, B. J. (2001). Self-care recovery of children with brain injury: Descriptive analysis using the Pediatric Evaluation of Disability Inventory (PEDI) functional classification levels. *Physical & Occupational Therapy in Pediatrics, 21*, 7-27.

Eakin, P. (1993). The Barthel Index: Confidence limits. *British Journal of Occupational Therapy, 56*, 184-185.

Edwards, M. M. (1990). The reliability and validity of self-report activities of daily living scales. *Canadian Journal of Occupational Therapy, 57*, 273-278.

Eilertsen, T. B., Kramer, A. M., Schlenker, R. E., & Hrincevich, C. A. (1998). Application of Functional Independence Measure-function related groups and resource utilization groups-version III systems across post acute settings. *Medical Care, 36*, 695-705.

Feldman, A. B., Haley, S. M., & Coryell, J. (1990). Concurrent and construct validity of the Pediatric Evaluation of Disability Inventory. *Physical Therapy, 70*, 602-610.

Feldman, B. M., Ayling-Campos, A., Luy, L., Stevens, D., Silverman, E. D., & Laxer, R. M. (1995). Measuring disability in juvenile dermatomyositis: Validity of the childhood health assessment questionnaire. *Journal of Rheumatology, 22*, 326-31.

Feldman, A. B., Haley, S. M., & Coryell, J. (1990). Concurrent and construct validity of the Pediatric Evaluation of Disability Inventory. *Physical Therapy, 70*, 602-610.

Finch, E. Brooks, D., Stratford, P., & Mayo, N. (2002). *Physical rehabilitation outcome measures: A guide to enhanced clinical decision making* (2nd. ed.). Toronto, ON: Canadian Physiotherapy Association.

Fortinsky, R. H., Granger, C. V., & Selzer, G. B. (1981). The use of functional assessment in understanding home care needs. *Medical Care, 19*, 489-497.

Fricke, J., & Unsworth, C. A. (1996). Inter-rater reliability of the original and modified Barthel Index and a comparison with the Functional Independence Measure. *Australian Occupational Therapy Journal, 43*, 22-29.

Gannotti, M. E., & Cruz, C. (2001). Content and construct validity of a Spanish translation of the Pediatric Evaluation of Disability Inventory for children living in Puerto Rico. *Physical & Occupational Therapy in Pediatrics, 20*, 7-24.

Gardarsdottir, S., & Kaplan, S. (2002). Validity of the Arnadottir OT-ADL neurobehavioral evaluation (A-ONE): Performance in activities of daily living and neurobehavioral impairments of persons with left and right hemisphere damage. *American Journal of Occupational Therapy, 56*, 499-508.

Gosman-Hedstrom, G., & Svensson, E. (2000). Parallel reliability of the functional independence measure and the Barthel ADL index. *Disability & Rehabilitation, 22*, 702-715.

Granger, C. V., Albrecht, G. L., & Hamilton, B. B. (1979). Outcome of comprehensive medical rehabilitation: Measurement by PULSES Profile and the Barthel Index. *Archives of Physical Medicine & Rehabilitation, 60(4)*, 145-153.

Granger, C. V., Cotter, A. C., Hamilton, B. B., & Feidler, R. C. (1993). Functional assessment scales: A study of persons after stroke. *Archives of Physical Medicine and Rehabilitation, 74*, 133-138.

Granger, C. V., Cotter, A. C., Hamilton, B. B., Fiedler, R. C., & Hens, M. M. (1990). Functional assessment scales: A study of persons with multiple sclerosis. *Archives of Physical Medicine & Rehabilitation, 71*, 870-875.

Granger, C. V., Dewis, L. S., Peters, N. C., Sherwood, C. C., & Barett, J. E. (1979). Stroke rehabilitation: Analysis of repeated Barthel index measures. *Archives of Physical Medicine & Rehabilitation, 60*, 14-17.

Granger, C. V., Divan, N., & Fiedler, R. C. (1995). Functional assessment scales: A study of persons after traumatic brain injury. *American Journal of Physical Medicine and Rehabilitation, 74*, 107-113.

Granger, C. V., & Hamilton, B. B. (1992). UDS Report: The uniform data system for medical rehabilitation report of first admissions for 1990. *American Journal of Physical Medicine and Rehabilitation, 71,* 108-113.

Granger, C. V., Hamilton, B. B., Linacre, J. M., Heinemann, A. W., & Wright, B. D. (1993). Performance profiles of the functional independence measure. *American Journal of Physical Medicine and Rehabilitation, 72,* 84-89.

Guillemin, F. (2000). Functional disability and quality-of-life assessment in clinical practice. *Rheumatology, 39(Suppl.),* 14-23.

Guillemin, F., Coste, J., Pouchot, J., Ghezail, M., Bregen, C., Sany, J., The French Quality of Life in Rheumatology Group. (1997). The AIMS2-SF: A short form of the Arthritis Impact Measurement Scales 2. *Arthritis & Rheumatism, 40,* 1267-1274.

Haavardsholm, E. A., Kvien, T. K., Uhlig, T., Smedstad, L. M., & Guillemin, F. (2000). A comparison of agreement and sensitivity to change between AIMS2 and a short form of AIMS2 (AIMS2-SF) in more than 1000 rheumatoid arthritis patients. *Journal of Rheumatology, 27,* 2810-2816.

Hagsten, B., Svensson, O., & Gardulf, A. (2004). Early individualized postoperative occupational therapy training in 100 patients improves ADL after hip fracture: A randomized trial. *Acta Orthopedics Scandinavia, 75,* 177-183.

Haley, S. M., Coster, W. J., Ludlow, L. H., Haltiwanger, J. T., & Andrellos, P. J. (1992). *Pediatric Evaluation of Disability Inventory (PEDI) Version 1.0: Development, standardization and administration manual.* Boston: Trustees of Boston University, Center for Rehabilitation Effectiveness.

Haley, S. M., Ludlow, L. H., & Coster, W. J. (1993). Pediatric Evaluation of Disability Inventory: Clinical interpretation of summary scores using Rasch rating scale methodology. *Physical Medicine and Rehabilitation Clinics of North America, 4,* 529-540.

Hall, K. M., Cohen, M. E., Wright, J., Call, M., & Werner, P. (1999). Characteristics of the Functional Independence Measure in traumatic spinal cord injury. *Archives of Physical Medicine and Rehabilitation, 80,* 1471-1476.

Hamilton, B. B., Laughlin, J. A., Fiedler, R. C., & Granger, C. V. (1994). Interrater reliability of the 7-level functional independence measure (FIM). *Scandinavian Journal of Rehabilitation Medicine, 26,* 115-119.

HealthAct. (2004). *Child Health Questionnaire.* Retrieved August 30, 2004 from: http://www.healthact.com.

Hebert, R., Carrier, R., & Bilodeau, A. (1988). The functional autonomy measurement system (SMAF): Description and validation of an instrument for the measurement of handicaps. *Age and Ageing, 17,* 293-302.

Hebert, R., Guilabult, J., Desrosiers, J., & Dubuc, N. (2001). The functional autonomy measurement system (SMAF): A clinical-based instrument for measuring disabilities and handicaps in older people. *Geriatrics Today: Journal of the Canadian Geriatrics Society, 4(3),* 141-147.

Hebert, R., Spiegelhalter, D. J., & Brayne, C. (1997). Setting the minimal metrically detectable change on disability rating scales. *Archives of Physical Medicine and Rehabilitation, 78,* 1305-1308.

Heinemann, A. W., Linacre, J. M., Wright, B. D., Hamilton, B. B., & Granger, C. V. (1993). Relationships between impairment and physical disability as measured by the functional independence measure. *Archives of Physical Medicine and Rehabilitation, 74,* 566-573.

Hermodsson, Y., & Ekdahl, C. (1999). Early planning of care and rehabilitation after amputation for vascular disease by means of Katz Index of Activities of Daily Living. *Scandinavian Journal of Caring Sciences, 13,* 234-239.

Hobart, J. C., & Thompson, A. J. (2001). The five item Barthel index. *Journal of Neurology, Neurosurgery, and Psychiatry, 71,* 225-230.

Hocking, C., Williams, M., Broad, J., & Baskett, J. (1999). Sensitivity of Shah, Vanclay and Cooper's modified Barthel Index. *Clinical Rehabilitation, 13,* 141-147.

Howe, S., Levinson, J., Shear, E., Hartner, S., McGirr, G., Schulte, M., & Lovell, D. (1991). Development of a disability measurement tool for juvenile rheumatoid arthritis: The Juvenile Arthritis Functional Assessment Report for Children and their Parents. *Arthritis and Rheumatism, 34,* 873-880.

Hsueh, I. P., Lin, J. H., Jeng, J. S., & Hsieh, C. L. (2002). Comparison of the psychometric characteristics of the functional independence measure, 5 item Barthel index, and 10 item Barthel index in patients with stroke. *Journal of Neurology, Neurosurgery & Psychiatry, 73,* 188-190.

Hulter-Asberg, K. H., & Nydevick, I. (1991). Early prognosis of stroke outcome by means of Katz index of activities of daily living. *Scandinavian Journal of Rehabilitation Medicine, 23,* 187-191.

Hulter-Asberg, K. H., & Sonn, U. (1988). The cumulative structure of personal and instrumental ADL: A study of elderly people in a health service district. *Scandinavian Journal of Rehabilitation Medicine, 21,* 171-177.

Iwarsson, S., & Isacsson, A. (1997). On scaling methodology and environmental influences in disability assessments: The cumulative structure of personal and instrumental ADL among older adults in a Swedish rural district. *Canadian Journal of Occupational Therapy, 64,* 240-251.

Iyer, L. V., Haley, S. M., Watkins, M. P., & Dumas, H. M. (2003). Establishing minimal clinically important differences for scores on the Pediatric Evaluation of Disability Inventory for inpatient rehabilitation. *Physical Therapy, 83,* 888-898.

Katz, S. K., Downs, T. D., Cash, H. R., & Grotz, R. C. (1970). Progress in development of the index of ADL. *The Gerontologist, 10,* 20-30.

Katz, S., Ford, A. B., Moskowitz, R. W., Jackson, B. A., & Jaffe, M. W. (1963). Studies of illness in the aged: The index of ADL: A standardized measure of biological and psychosocial function. *JAMA, 185(12),* 94-99.

Kidd, D., Stewart, G., Baldry, J., Johnson, J., Rossiter, D., Petruckevitch, A., & Thompson, A.J. (1995). The functional independence measure: A comparative validity and reliability study. *Disability and Rehabilitation, 17,* 10-14.

Klein, R. M., & Bell, B. (1982). Self-care skills: Behavioral measurement with Klein-Bell ADL Scale. *Archives of Physical Medicine and Rehabilitation, 63,* 335-338.

Korner-Bitensky, N., & Wood-Dauphinee, S. (1995). Barthel index information elicited over the telephone: Is it reliable? *American Journal of Physical Medicine and Rehabilitation, 74*, 9-18.

Krishnan, E., Sokka, T., Hakkinen, A., Hubert, H. & Hannonen, P. (2004). Normative values for the Health Assessment Questionnaire Disability Index. *Arthritis and Rheumatism, 50*, 953-960.

Kucukdeveci, A. A., Yavuzer, G., Elhan, A. H., Sonel, B., & Tennant, A. (2001). Adaptation of the Functional Independence Measure for use in Turkey. *Clinical Rehabilitation, 15(3)*, 311-319.

Kwon, S., Hartzema, A. G., Duncan, P. W., & Min-Lai, S. (2004). Disability measures in stroke: Relationship among the Barthel Index, the Functional Independence Measure, and the Modified Rankin Scale. *Stroke, 35*, 918-923.

Laake, K., Laake, P., Hylen Ranhoff, A., Sveen, U., Wyller, T.B., & Bautz-Holter, E. (1995). The Barthel activities of daily living index: Factor structure depends upon the category of patient. *Age and Ageing, 24*, 393-397.

Landgraf, J. M., Abetz, L., & Ware, J. E. (1996). *The Child Health Questionnaire (CHQ) User's Manual.* Boston: The Health Institute, New England Medical Center.

Landgraf J. M., Abetz L., & Ware J. E. (1999). *The CHQ User's Manual* (2nd printing). Boston: HealthAct.

Landgraf, J. M., Maunsell, E., Speechley, K. N., Bullinger, M., Campbell, S., Abetz, L., & Ware, J. E. (1998). Canadian-French, German, and UK versions of the Child Health Questionnaire: Methodology and preliminary item scaling results. *Quality of Life Research, 7*, 433-445.

Law, M., & Letts, L. (1989). A critical review of scales of activities of daily living. *American Journal of Occupational Therapy, 43*, 522-527.

Lawton, M. P. (1988). Scales to measure competence in everyday activities. *Psychopharmacology Bulletin, 24(4)*, 609-614.

Lawton, M. P., & Brody, E. M. (1969). Assessment of older people: Self-maintaining and instrumental activities of daily living. *The Gerontologist, 9*, 179-186.

Lineker, S. C., Badley, E. M., Hawker, G., & Wilkins, A. (2000). Determining sensitivity to change in outcome measures used to evaluate hydrotherapy exercise programs for people with rheumatic diseases. *Arthritis Care and Research, 13*, 62-65.

Loewen, S. C., & Anderson, B. A. (1988). Reliability of the modified motor assessment scale and the Barthel index. *Physical Therapy, 68*, 1077-1081.

Lovell, D. J., Howe, S., Shear, E., Hartner, S., McGirr, G., Schulte, M., & Levinson, J. (1989). Development of a disability measurement tool for juvenile arthritis: The Juvenile Arthritis Functional Assessment Scale. *Arthritis and Rheumatism, 32*, 1390-1395.

Mahoney, S. I., & Barthel, D. W. (1965). Functional evaluation: The Barthel index. *Maryland State Medical Journal, 14*, 61-65.

Marshall, S. C., Heisel, B., & Grinnell, D. (1999). Validity of the PULSES profile compared with the Functional Independence Measure for measuring disability in a stroke rehabilitation setting. *Archives of Physical Medicine & Rehabilitation, 80*, 760-765.

Mason, J. H., Meenan, R. F., & Anderson, J. J. (1992). Do self-reported arthritis symptom (RADAR) and health status (AIMS2) data provide duplicative or complementary information? *Arthritis Care and Research, 5*, 163-172.

McCarthy, M. L., Silberstein, C. E., Atkins, E. A., Harryman, S. E., Sponseller, P. D., & Hadley-Miller, N. A. (2002). Comparing reliability and validity of pediatric instruments for measuring health and well-being of children with spastic cerebral palsy. *Developmental Medicine & Child Neurology, 44*, 468-476.

McCusker, J., Bellavance, F., Cardin, S., & Belzile, E. (1999). Validity of an activities of daily living questionnaire among older patients in an emergency department. *Journal of Clinical Epidemiology, 52*, 1023-1030.

Meenan, R.F. (1990). *AIMS2 User's Guide and the AIMS2.* Boston: Boston University.

Meenan, R. F., Mason, J. H., Anderson, J. J., Guccione, A. A., & Kazis, L. E. (1992). The content and properties of a revised and expanded Arthritis Impact Measurement Scales health status questionnaire. *Arthritis and Rheumatism, 35*, 1-10.

Melville, L. L., Baltic, T. A., Bettcher, T. W., & Nelson, D. L. (2002). Patients' perspectives on the Self-Identified Goals Assessment. *American Journal of Occupational Therapy, 56*, 650-659.

Msall, M. E., DiGaudio, K. M., & Duffy, L. C. (1993). Use of functional assessment in children with developmental disabilities. *Physical Medicine and Rehabilitation Clinics of North American, 4*, 517-527.

Msall, M. E., DiGaudio, K., Duffy, L. C., LaForest, S., Braun, S., & Granger, C. V. (1994a). WeeFIM: Normative sample on an instrument for tracking functional independence in children. *Clinical Pediatrics, 33*, 431-438.

Msall, M. E., DiGaudio, K., Rogers, B. T., LaForest, S., Catanzaro, N. L., Campbell, T., Wilczenski, F., & Duffy, L. C. (1994b). The functional independence measure for children (WeeFIM): Conceptual basis and pilot use in children with developmental disabilities. *Clinical Pediatrics, 33*, 421-430.

Murdock, C. (1992a). A critical evaluation of the Barthel index, Part 1. *British Journal of Occupational Therapy, 55*, 109-111.

Murdock, C. (1992b). A critical evaluation of the Barthel index, Part 2. *British Journal of Occupational Therapy, 55*, 153-156.

Nelson, D. L., & Glass, L. M. (1999). Occupational therapists' involvement with the minimum data set in skilled nursing and intermediate care facilities. *American Journal of Occupational Therapy, 53*, 348-352.

Nelson, D. L., Melville, L. L., Wilkerson, J. D., Magness, R. A., Grech, J. L., & Rosenberg, J. A. (2002). Interrater reliability, concurrent validity, responsiveness and predictive validity of the Melville-Nelson Self-Care Assessment. *American Journal of Occupational Therapy, 56,* 51-59.

Nichols, D. S., & Case-Smith, J. (1996). Reliability and validity of the Pediatric Evaluation of Disability Inventory. Pediatric *Physical Therapy, 8,* 15-24.

Nordmark, E., Jarnlo, G., & Hagglund, G. (2000). Comparison of the Gross Motor Function Measure and Pediatric Evaluation of Disability Inventory in assessing motor function in children undergoing selective dorsal rhizotomy. *Developmental Medicine and Child Neurology, 42,* 245-252.

Oczkowski, W. J., & Barreca, S. (1993). The functional independence measure: Its use to identify rehabilitation needs in stroke survivors. *Archives of Physical Medicine and Rehabilitation, 74,* 1291-1294.

Ottenbacher, K. J., Msall, M. E., Lyon, N. R., Duffy, L. C., Granger, C. V., & Braun, S. (1997). Interrater agreement and stability of the functional independence measure for children (WeeFIM): Use in children with developmental disabilities. *Archives of Physical Medicine and Rehabilitation, 78,* 1309-1315.

Ottenbacher, K. J., Msall, M. E., Lyon, N., Duffy, L. C., Granger, C. V., & Braun, S. (1999). Measuring developmental and functional status in children with disabilities. *Developmental Medicine & Child Neurology, 41,* 186-194.

Ottenbacher, K. J., Msall, M. E., Lyon, N., Duffy, L. C., Ziviani, J., Granger, C. V., & Braun, S. (2000a). Functional assessment and care of children with neurodevelopmental disabilities. *American Journal of Physical Medicine and Rehabilitation, 79,* 114-123.

Ottenbacher, K. J., Msall, M. E., Lyon, N., Duffy, L. C., Ziviani, J., Granger, C. V., Braun, S., & Feidler, R. C. (2000b). The WeeFIM instrument: Its utility in detecting change in children with development disabilities. *Archives of Physical Medicine and Rehabilitation, 81,* 1317-1326.

Ottenbacher, K. J., Taylor, E. T., Msall, M. E., Braun, S., Lane, S. J., Granger, C. V., Lyons, N., & Duffy, L. C. (1996). The stability and equivalence reliability of the functional independence measure for children (WeeFIM). *Developmental Medicine and Child Neurology, 38,* 907-916.

Pencharz, J., Young, N. L., Owen, J. L., & Wright, J. G. (2001). Comparison of three outcomes instruments in children. *Journal of Pediatric Orthopedics, 21,* 425-432.

Pengel, L. H. M., Refshauge, K. M., & Maher, C. G. (2004). Responsiveness of pain, disability and physical impairment outcomes in patients with low back pain. *Spine, 29,* 879-883.

Pincus, T., Summey, J. A., Soraci Jr., S. A., Wallston, K. A., & Hummon, N. P. (1983). Assessment of patient satisfaction in activities of daily living using a modified Stanford Health Assessment Questionnaire. *Arthritis and Rheumatism, 26,* 1346-53.

Pinsonnault, E., Desrosiers, J., Dubuc, N., Kalfat, H., Colvez, A., & Delli-Colli, N. (2003). Functional autonomy measurement system: Development of a social subscale. *Archives of Gerontology & Geriatrics, 37,* 223-233.

Plint, A. C., Gaboury, I., Owen, J., & Young, N. L. (2003). Activities Scale for Kids: An analysis of normals. *Journal of Pediatric Orthopedics, 23,* 788-790.

Post, M. W., Visser-Meily, J. M., & Gispen, L. S. (2002). Measuring nursing needs of stroke patients in clinical rehabilitation: A comparison of validity and sensitivity to change between the Northwick Park Dependency Score and the Barthel Index. *Clinical Rehabilitation, 16,* 182-189.

Rai, G. S., Gluck, T., Wientjes, H. J. F. M., & Rai, S. G. S. (1996). The functional autonomy measurement system (SMAF): A measure of functional change with rehabilitation. *Archives of Gerontology and Geriatrics, 22,* 81-85.

Rai, G. S., Kiniorns, M., & Burns, W. (1999). New handicap scale for elderly in hospital. *Archives of Gerontology and Geriatrics, 28,* 99-104.

Ramey, D., Fries, J., & Singh, G., (1996). The Health Assessment Questionnaire 1995 – status and review. In B. Spilker (Ed.), *Quality of life and pharmacoeconomics in clinical trials* (2nd ed., pp227-37). Philadelphia: Lippincott-Raven.

Ramey, D. R., Raynauld, J-P., & Fries, J. F. (1992). The Health Assessment Questionnaire 1992: Status and review. *Arthritis Care and Research, 5,* 119-129.

Ravaud, J.-F., Delcey, M., & Yelnik, A. (1999). Construct validity of the Functional Independence Measure (FIM): Questioning the unidimensionality of the scale and the "value" of FIM scores. *Scandinavian Journal of Rehabilitation Medicine, 31,* 31-41.

Reid, D. T., Boschen, K., & Wright, V. (1993). Critique of the Pediatric Evaluation of Disability Inventory. *Physical and Occupational Therapy in Pediatrics, 13(4),* 57-93

Ren, X. S., Kazis, L., & Meenan, R. F. (1999). Short-form Arthritis Impact Measurement Scales 2: Tests of reliability and validity among patients with osteoarthritis. *Arthritis Care Research, 12,* 163-171.

Reuben, D. B., Valle, L. A., Hays, R. D., & Siu, A. L. (1995). Measuring physical function in community-dwelling older persons: A comparison of self-administered, interviewer-administered, and performance-based measures. *Journal of the American Geriatrics Society, 43,* 17-23.

Ripat, J., Etcheverry, E, Cooper, J., & Tate, R. (2001). A comparison of the Canadian Occupational Performance Measure and the Health Assessment Questionnaire. *Canadian Journal of Occupational Therapy, 68,* 247-253.

Robinson, R. F., Nahata, M. C., Hayes, J. R., Rennebohm, R., & Higgins, G. (2003). Quality-of-life measurements in juvenile rheumatoid arthritis patients treated with entracept. *Clinical Drug Investigation, 23,* 511-518.

Rockwood, K., Howlett, S., Stadnyk, K., Carver, D., Powell, C., & Stolee, P. (2003). Responsiveness of goal attainment scaling in a randomized controlled trial of comprehensive geriatric assessment. *Journal of Clinical Epidemiology, 56,* 736-743.

Rogers, J. C., Gwinn, S. M. G., & Holm, M. B. (2001). Comparing activities of daily living assessment instruments: FIM, MDS, OASIS, MDS-PAC. *Physical and Occupational Therapy in Geriatrics, 18(3),* 1-25.

Rubenstein, L. Z., Schairer, C., Wieland, G. D., & Kane, R. (1984). Systematic biases in functional status assessment of elderly adults: Effects of different data sources. *Journal of Gerontology, 39(6),* 686-691.

Rubio, K. B., & Van Deusen, J. (1995). Relation of perceptual and body image dysfunction to activities of daily living of persons after stroke. *American Journal of Occupational Therapy, 49,* 551-559.

Ruperto, N., Ravelli, A., Migliavacca, D., Viola, S., Pistorio, A., Duarte, C., & Martini, A. (1999). Responsiveness of clinical measures in children with oligoarticular juvenile arthritis. *Journal of Rheumatology, 26,* 1827-30.

Salaffi, F., Stancati, A., & Carotti, M. (2002). Responsiveness of health status measures and utility-based methods in patients with rheumatoid arthritis. *Clinical Rheumatology, 21,* 478-487.

Salbach, N. M., Mayo, N. E., Higgins, J., Ahmed, S., Finch, L. E., & Richards, C. L. (2001). Responsiveness and predictability of gait speed and other disability measures in acute stroke. *Archives of Physical Medicine and Rehabilitation, 82,* 1204-1212.

Sandstrom, R., Mokler, P. J., & Hoppe, K. M. (1998). Discharge destination and motor function outcome in severe stroke as measured by the functional independence measure / function-related group classification system. *Archives of Physical Medicine and Rehabilitation, 79,* 762-765.

Settle, C., & Holm, M. B. (1993). Program planning: The clinical utility of three activities of daily living assessment tools. *American Journal of Occupational Therapy, 47,* 911-918.

Shah, S., & Cooper, B. (1993). Commentary on "A critical evaluation of the Barthel index". *British Journal of Occupational Therapy, 56,* 70-72.

Shah, S., Vanclay, F., & Cooper, B. (1989). Improving the sensitivity of the Barthel Index for stroke rehabilitation. *Journal of Clinical Epidemiology, 42,* 703-709.

Sharrack, B., Hughes, R. A. C., Soudain, S., & Dunn, G. (1999). The psychometric properties of clinical rating scales used in multiple sclerosis. *Brain, 122(2)* 141-159.

Shinar, D., Gross, G. R., Bronstein, K. S., Licata-Gehr, E., Edent, D. T., Babrera, A. R., Fishman, I. G., Roth, A. A., Barwick, J. A., & Kunitz, S. C. (1987). Reliability of the ADL Scale and its use in telephone interview. *Archives of Physical Medicine & Rehabilitation, 68,* 723-728.

Shitosuka, W., Burton, G. U., Pedretti, L. W., & Llorens, L. A. (1992). An examination of performance scores on activities of daily living between elders and right and left cerebrovascular accident. *Physical and Occupational Therapy in Geriatrics, 10,* 47-57.

Singh, G., Athreya, B. H., Fries, J. F., & Goldsmith, D. P. (1994). Measurement of health status in children with juvenile rheumatoid arthritis. *Arthritis and Rheumatism, 37,* 1761-1769.

Sinoff, G., & Ore, L. (1997). The Barthel activities of daily living index: Self reporting versus actual performance in the old-old (> 75 years). *Journal of the American Geriatrics Society, 45,* 832-836.

Smith, R. O., Morrow, M. E., Heitman, J. K., Rardin, W. J., Powelson, J. L., & Von, T. (1986). The effects of introducing the Klein-Bell ADL Scale in rehabilitation service. *American Journal of Occupational Therapy, 40,* 420-424.

Spadaro, A., Riccieri, V., Sili Scavalli, A., Sensi, F., Fiore, D., Taccari, E., & Zoppini, A. (1996). Interleukin-6 and soluble interleukin-2 receptor in juvenile chronic arthritis: Correlations with clinical and laboratory parameters. *Revue du Rhumatisme* (English Edition), *63,* 153-158.

Spear, P. S., & Crepeau, E. B. (2003). Glossary. In E. B. Crepeau, E. S. Cohn, , & B. A. B. Schell (Eds.), *Willard & Spackman's Occupational Therapy* (10th ed., pp. 1025-1035). Philadelphia, PA: Lippincott, Williams & Wilkins.

Spector, W. K., Katz, S., Murphy, J. B., & Fulton, J. P. (1987). The hierarchical relationship between activities of daily living and instrumental activities of daily living. *Journal of Chronic Diseases, 40,* 481-489.

Sperle, P. A., Ottenbacher, K. J., Braun, S. L., Lane, S. J., & Nochajski, S. (1997). Equivalence reliability of the functional independence measure for children (WeeFIM) administration methods. *American Journal of Occupational Therapy, 51,* 35-41.

Stanford University School University of Medicine, Division of Immunology & Rheumatology. (2004). The Health Assessment Questionnaire. Retrieved August 31, 2004 from http://aramis.stanford.edu

Stratford, P. W., Binkley, J. M., & Riddle, D. L. (1996). Health status measures: Strategies and analytic methods for assessing change scores. *Physical Therapy, 76,* 1109-1123.

Stratford, P., Gill, C., Westaway, M., & Binkley, J. (1995). Assessing disability and change on individual patients: A report of a patient specific measure. *Physiotherapy Canada, 47,* 258-263.

Szende, A., Schramm, W., Flood, E., Larson, P., Gorina, E., Rentz, A.M., & Snyder, L. (2003). Health-related quality of life assessment in adult haemophilia patients: A systematic review and evaluation of instruments. *Haemophilia, 9,* 678-687.

Tennant, A., Kearns, S., Turner, F., Wyatt, S., Haigh, R., & Chamberlain, M. A. (2001). Measuring the function of children with juvenile arthritis. *Rheumatology, 40,* 1274-1278.

Timbeck, R. J., & Spaulding, S. J. (2003). Ability of the Functional Independence Measure to predict rehabilitation outcomes after stroke: A review of the literature. *Physical and Occupational Therapy in Geriatrics, 22(1),* 63-76.

Trombly, C. A. (2002). Restoring the role of independent person. In C. A. Trombly & M. V. Radomski (Eds.), *Occupational therapy for physical dysfunction* (5th ed., pp. 629-663). Philadelphia, PA: Lippincott Williams & Wilkins.

Tsai, P. Y., Yang, T. F., Chan, R. C., Huang, P. H., & Wong, T. T. (2002). Functional investigation in children with spina bifida — measured by the Pediatric Evaluation of Disability Inventory (PEDI). *Child's Nervous System, 18,* 48-53.

Uniform Data System for Medical Rehabilitation. (n.d.a). UDSMR International: Sites. Retrieved Sept. 1, 2004 from http://www.udsmr.org/

Uniform Data System for Medical Rehabilitation. (n.d.b). UDSMR Databases. Retrieved Sept. 1, 2004 from http://www.udsmr.org/

Unsworth, C. A. (1993). The concept of function. *British Journal of Occupational Therapy, 56,* 287-292.

Valach, L., Signer, S., Hartmeier, A., Hofer, K., & Steck, G. C. (2003). Chedoke-McMaster stroke assessment and modified Barthel Index self-assessment in patients with vascular brain damage. *International Journal of Rehabilitation Research, 26,* 93-99.

van der Net, J., Prakken, A. B., Helders, P. J., ten Berge, M., Van Herwaarden, M., Sinnema, G., De Wilde, E. J., Kuis, W. (1996). Correlates of disablement in polyarticular juvenile chronic arthritis: A cross sectional study. *British Journal of Rheumatology, 35,* 91-100.

van der Putten, J. J., Hobart, J. C., Freeman, J. A., & Thompson, A. J. (1999). Measuring change in disability after inpatient rehabilitation: Comparison of the responsiveness of the Barthel index and the Functional Independence Measure. *Journal of Neurology, Neurosurgery & Psychiatry, 66,* 480-484.

van Meeteren, N. L. U., Strato, I. H. M., van Veldhoven, N. H. M. J., de Kleijn, P., van den Berg, H. M., & Helders, P. J. M. (2000). The utility of the Dutch Arthritis Impact Measurement Scales 2 for assessing health status in individuals with haemophilia: A pilot study. *Haemophilia, 6,* 664-671.

Wade, D.T. (1988). Commentary: Measurement in rehabilitation. *Age and Ageing, 17,* 289-292.

Wade, D. T., & Collin, C. (1988). The Barthel ADL Index: A standard measure of physical disability? *International Disabilities Studies, 10,* 64-67.

Wallace, D., Duncan, P. W., & Lai, S. M. (2002). Comparison of the responsiveness of the Barthel Index and the motor component of the Functional Independence Measure in stroke: The impact of using different methods for measuring responsiveness. *Journal of Clinical Epidemiology, 55,* 922-928.

Wassenberg-Severijnen, J. E., Custers, J. W., Hox, J. J., Vermeer, A., & Helders, P. J. (2003). Reliability of the Dutch Pediatric Evaluation of Disability Inventory (PEDI). *Clinical Rehabilitation, 17,* 457-462.

Waters, E., Salmon, L., & Wake, M. (2000). The Parent-Form Child Health Questionnaire in Australia: Comparison of reliability, validity, structure and norms. *Journal of Pediatric Psychology, 25,* 381-391.

Westaway, M., Stratford, P., & Binkley, J. (1998). The Patient-Specific Functional Scale: Validation of its use in persons with neck dysfunction. *Journal of Orthopedic Sports Physical Therapy, 27,* 331-338.

WHO. (1980). *International classification of impairments, disabilities and handicaps.* Geneva: Author.

WHO. (2001). *International classification of functioning, disability and health.* Geneva: Author.

Wressle, E., Eeg-Ologsson, A.-M., Marcusson, J., & Henriksson, C. (2002). Improved client participation in the rehabilitation process using a client-centred goal formulation structure. *Journal of Rehabilitation Medicine, 34,* 5-11.

Wright, F. V., & Boschen, K. A. (1993). The Pediatric Evaluation of Disability Inventory: Validation of a new functional assessment outcome instrument. *Canadian Journal of Rehabilitation, 7,* 41-42.

Wright, F. V., Kimber, J. L., Law, M., Goldsmith, C., Crombie, V., & Dent, P. (1996). The Juvenile Arthritis Functional Status Index (JASI): A validation study. *Journal of Rheumatology, 23(6),* 1066-1079.

Wright, F. V., Law, M., Crombie, V., Goldsmith, C. H., & Dent, P. (1994). Development of a self-report functional status index for juvenile rheumatoid arthritis. *Journal of Rheumatology, 21(3),* 536-544.

Wright, J., Cross, J., & Lamb, S. (1998). Physiotherapy outcome measures for rehabilitation of elderly people: Responsiveness to change of the Rivermead Mobility Index and Barthel Index. *Physiotherapy, 84,* 216-221..

Young, N. L. (n. d.). *The Activities Scale for Kids (ASK) manual.* Toronto, ON: The Hospital for Sick Children.

Young, N. L., Williams, J. I., Yoshida, K. K., Wright, J. G. (2000). Measurement properties of the Activities Scale for Kids. *Journal of Clinical Epidemiology, 53,* 125-137.

Young, N. L., Yoshida, K. K., Williams, J. I., Bombardier, C., & Wright, J. G. (1995). The role of children in reporting their physical disability. *Archives of Physical Medicine and Rehabilitation, 76,* 913-918.

Ziviani, J., Ottenbacher, K. J., Shephard, K., Foreman, S., Astbury, W., & Ireland, P. (2001). Concurrent validity of the Functional Independence Measure for Children (WeeFIM) and the Pediatric Evaluation of Disabilities Inventory in children with developmental disabilities and acquired brain injuries. *Physical and Occupational Therapy in Pediatrics, 21,* 91-101.

Table 11-1

ACTIVITIES SCALE FOR KIDS (ASK)

Source	N. L. Young, Pediatric Outcomes Research Team, The Hospital for Sick Children, 555 University Avenue, Toronto, Ontario, Canada, M5G 1X8
Important References	Young, N. L. (n. d.). *The Activities Scale for Kids (ASK) manual.* Toronto, ON: The Hospital for Sick Children.
	Young, N. L., Williams, J. I., Yoshida, K. K., & Wright, J. G. (2000). Measurement properties of the Activities Scale for Kids. *Journal of Clinical Epidemiology, 53,* 125-137.
	Young, N. L., Yoshida, K. K., Williams, J. I., Bombardier, C., & Wright, J. G. (1995). The role of children in reporting their physical disability. *Archives of Physical Medicine and Rehabilitation, 76,* 913-918.
Purpose	• A child self-report measure of physical disability that can be used as an outcome measure.
Type of Client	• Children aged 5 to 15 years with musculoskeletal disorders without significant cognitive impairment.
Clinical Utility	
Format	• Includes 30 items—personal care (3 items), dressing (4), eating and drinking (1), miscellaneous (2), locomotion (7), stairs (1), play (2), transfers (5), and standing skills (5).
	• There are two versions that can be used: the ASKp (performance measure) asks what the child "did do" in the last week; the ASKc (capability measure) asks what the child "could do" during the last week.
	• Each item is rated on a 5-point ordinal scale. An aggregate score is achieved by summing the item ratings.
Procedures	• Performance and capability versions may be administered together or separately to a single child or a group of children.
	• Children under 9 years of age may need a parent to read the questions for them. A clinician should not assist the child.
Completion Time	• The manual states that it takes approximately 30 minutes to complete the ASK the first time, and as little as 10 minutes on subsequent administrations.
	• A study by Pencharz, Young, Owen, & Wright (2001) noted a mean time of 9 minutes (range of 5 to 12 minutes).
Standardization	• The manual is readily available from the author, and provides information about the instrument development, reliability, validity and administration.
Reliability	• Sample was drawn from rheumatology, orthopaedic and physical therapy clinics at children's rehabilitation hospitals in Ontario, Canada. Children with significant cognitive impairment were excluded.
Test-Retest	• N=18 (mailed questionnaire sent to 40, 28 returned the first and 18 returned the second). An ICC of 0.97 was observed for the ASKp and 0.98 for the ASKc (Young, Yoshida, Williams, Bombardier, & Wright, 1995).
Internal Consistency	• Correlation between items was 0.99 (Cronbach's α) (Young, n.d.).
Intra-Rater	• Children's and parents' scores were used to calculate intra-rater reliability (n=28); intra-class correlation coefficients (ICC) for child raters are reported to be 0.97 (ASKp) and 0.98 (ASKc), and for parent raters they are 0.94 (ASKp) and 0.95 (ASKc) (Young, n.d.).
Inter-Rater	• Children's scores were compared to those of their parents (n=28); ICCs were 0.96 (ASKp) and 0.98 (ASKc) (Young, n.d.).

continued

Table 11-1 (continued)

ACTIVITIES SCALE FOR KIDS (ASK)

Validity

Content
- Content validity was established through the instrument development process, which involved children, their parents, and expert review. Rasch analysis was also conducted to examine item characteristics.

Construct
- The ASK was compared to the Childhood Health Assessment Questionnaire (CHAQ) (the CHAQ is not the accepted standard method for measurement of function in this population and therefore this was not considered criterion testing). The ASKp demonstrated a Pearson correlation of 0.81 with the CHAQ, and the ASKc demonstrated a Pearson correlation of 0.82 (Young, Williams, Yoshida, & Wright, 2000).
- Demonstrated high (r≥0.78) and moderate (r≥0.49) correlations respectively to the Pediatric Outcomes Data Collection Instrument (PODCI) and the Child Health Questionnaire Parent form (CHQ-PF-28) (Pencharz et al., 2001).
- The ASK was also compared to similar and dissimilar constructs of the HUI3 and demonstrated a Spearman's correlation of 0.43 and -0.03 respectively (Young et al., 2000).
- It has also been shown that for children with no disability, scores on the ASK differ significantly from children with mild disability (p=0.005) (Plint, Gaboury, Owen, & Young, 2003). Furthermore, scores for children with severe or moderate disability differ significantly from the ASK scores of those with mild disability (p<0.001 for both) (Plint et al., 2003).

Criterion
- 24 children (n=24) from rehabilitation clinics were asked to attend a clinic visit in which they completed half the questionnaire. They then demonstrated the activities from the questionnaire for clinicians who rated their performance (only ASKc was used). The result was a Pearson's correlation of 0.92 and an intraclass correlation of 0.89 (Young et al., 2000).

Responsiveness to Change
- The ASK performance score demonstrated similar change scores to the CHAQ, however, the ASK-capability produced smaller change scores abilities (Young et al., 2000).

Strength
- The ASK is innovative in that it is based on child self-report and allows the user to decide if the focus is on performance, capability, or both.
- The development process was rigorous and the psychometrics have been extensively studied. The correlations between other functional status measures and health status measures is promising.

Weaknesses
- Development and testing have been focused on children with musculoskeletal disorders; further exploration of its use with children with other impairments would be beneficial.
- 18/30 performance questions can be marked not applicable and this would most likely apply to younger age ranges. It is unclear how this may affect change scores, since ASKp is the more sensitive measure to change.

Final Word
- Appears to be used more in research settings, probably because of the ease of administration, its strong psychometric properties as well as its ability to provide a method for examining both a child's capabilities and performance of functional tasks. It is unclear if the clinical community will follow suit.

Table 11-2

ARNADOTTIR OT-ADL NEUROBEHAVIORAL EVALUATION (A-ONE)

Source	Arnadottir, G. (1990). *The brain and behavior: Assessing cortical dysfunction through activities of daily living (ADL)*. St. Louis: C. V. Mosby.
Important References	Gardarsdottir, S., & Kaplan, S. (2002). Validity of the Arnadottir OT-ADL neurobehavioral evaluation (A-ONE): Performance in activities of daily living and neurobehavioral impairments of persons with left and right hemisphere damage. *American Journal of Occupational Therapy, 56,* 499-508.
	Rubio, K. B., & Van Deusen, J. (1995). Relation of perceptual and body image dysfunction to activities of daily living of persons after stroke. *American Journal of Occupational Therapy, 49,* 551-559.
Purpose	• Designed to detect neurobehavioral dysfunctions, as well as functional levels (via ADL assessment).
Type of Client	• Designed for people over 16 years who have central nervous system dysfunctions of cortical origin. It may be particularly useful with people with perceptual impairments (Rubio & Van Deusen, 1995).

Clinical Utility

Format
- The A-ONE is divided into two parts: Part I includes the functional independence scale (FIS) and the neurobehavioral impairment scale (NIS). The FIS includes dressing, grooming and hygiene, transfers and mobility, feeding, and communication. There are 22 items in this area, and each is rated on a 0 to 4 scale. The NIS has two subscales: the Neurobehavioral Specific Impairment Subscale (NSIS) and the Neurobehavioral Pervasive Impairment Subscale (NPIS). The NSIS includes ratings on 10 neurobehavioral items after each ADL task (e.g., ideational apraxia, perseveration, abnormal tone). The NPIS determines the presence or absence of other neurobehavioral impairments observed throughout the assessment.
- Part II of the A-ONE attempts to localize possible lesion sites by comparing neurobehavioral observations to a chart on lesion sites.

Procedures
- Part I should be completed after two or three observations of clients engaging in ADL tasks in their natural environment. Part II is completed after Part I and requires no further administration with the client.

Completion Time
- The manual states that Part I can be completed in approximately 25 minutes, although it may take longer to observe the person completing ADL tasks on three different occasions.

Standardization
- There are no standardized instructions, allowing clinicians to adapt the testing environment to meet clients' typical environments and use their own equipment. General guidelines are provided, and detailed information about scoring is included.
- A small normative sample of 79 people from Iceland is reported in the text, which included hospital staff volunteers and patients with acute, non-neurological problems.

Reliability

Internal Consistency
- Not reported in the studies reviewed.

Inter-Rater
- Part I average of 0.84 (Kappa scores), and Part II average of 0.76 (Kappa scores) (Arnadottir, 1990).

Test-Retest
- Part I values of 0.85 or higher (Spearmans' rank order correlation) when clients were tested 1 week apart (Arnadottir, 1990).

continued

Table 11-2 (continued)

ARNADOTTIR OT-ADL NEUROBEHAVIORAL EVALUATION (A-ONE)

Validity

Content
- Content validity was established in its development, which included comprehensive literature review and review by experts (Arnadottir, 1990).

Criterion
- Part I of the A-ONE was found to discriminate between people with and without central nervous system dysfunction.
- Part II was tested by comparing agreement in the lesion site based on the A-ONE compared to a CT scan and computerized mapping EEG (exact values not included in studies reviewed). The relationships showed moderate agreement, indicating that the different localization techniques might best be considered complementary (Arnadottir, 1990).

Construct
- Examined the differences in ADL performance and neurobehavioral impairment between persons with left and right hemisphere damage; only scores on 3 (comprehension, speech, and shave/makeup) of the 18 ADL items on the FIS discriminated between the two groups (as was expected). On the NSIS, 13 of 39 items discriminated between the two groups (Gardarsdottir & Kaplan, 2002).

Responsiveness to Change
- Not reported in the studies reviewed.

Strengths
- Grounded in occupational therapy theory since neurological deficits are considered in the context of occupational performance.
- Allows simultaneous assessment of ADL and neurobehavioral functions.

Weaknesses
- Requires training (40 hours) to purchase forms and use, which may limit its accessibility to clinicians.
- Part I would be strengthened by further validity testing and more study on its responsiveness to change.
- Rubio and Van Deusen (1995) suggest that further research is needed before Part II can be used with confidence.

Final Word
- Part I of the A-ONE would be useful to most clinicians working with clients with central nervous system impairments; Part II may be more useful for research but requires more work to establish its utility.

Table 11-3

ARTHRITIS IMPACT MEASUREMENT SCALES (AIMS)

Source	The AIMS2 can be downloaded from http://www.qolid.org/public/aims/cadre/cadre.html. Permission to be used must be obtained from Robert F. Meenan, MD, MPH, MBA, Dean School of Public Health, (email) rmeenan@bu.edu.
	The AIMS2-SF is an appendix to the Guillemin (2000) publication.
Important References	Guillemin, F. (2000). Functional disability and quality-of-life assessment in clinical practice. *Rheumatology, 39(Suppl),* 14-23.
	Mason, J. H., Meenan, R. F., & Anderson, J. J. (1992). Do self-reported arthritis symptom (RADAR) and health status (AIMS2) data provide duplicative or complementary information? *Arthritis Care and Research, 5,* 163-172.
	Meenan, R. F., Mason, J. H., Anderson, J. J., Guccione, A. A., & Kazis, L. E. (1992). The content and properties of a revised and expanded Arthritis Impact Measurement Scales Health Status Questionnaire. *Arthritis and Rheumatism, 35,* 1-10.
	Meenan, R. F. (1990). *AIMS2 User's Guide and the AIMS2.* Boston: Boston University.
Purpose	• Original AIMS—Designed to measure health status in individuals with rheumatic diseases.
	• Revised version (AIMS2)—Developed to improve the psychometric properties of the measure as well as incorporate client perception of performance into the assessment.
	• The AIMS2-SF—Shorter version of the AIMS2.
	• The CHAIMS was developed for use with children but did not demonstrate strong psychometric properties (Coulton, Zborowsky, Lipton, & Newman, 1987) and therefore will not be presented here.
Type of Client	• Adults with any type of rheumatic disease. It has also been used with clients with haemophilia (Szende et al., 2003; van Meeteren, 2000).
Clinical Utility	
Format	• AIMS2—12 subscales (57 items): mobility, walking and bending, hand and finger function, arm function, self-care tasks, household tasks, social activity, support from family and friends, arthritis pain, work, level of tension, and mood. There are four additional components: symptom, affect, social interaction, and role. In addition, satisfaction with health, impact of arthritis on health, areas of health most requiring improvement, and general questions on current health and expectations for the future are asked. Each section consists of four to five questions to total 78 questions (there are about 10 questions at the end that refer to demographic issues).
	• The majority of questions ask the respondents to rank their performance, ability, or feeling on a 5-point scale (the anchors of the scale vary with the questions being asked) (Meenan, 1990).
	• The AIMS2-SF uses 26 of the original 78 items from the AIMS (Guillemin et al., 1997).
Procedures	• Both the AIMS2 and the AIMS2-SF are designed to be self-administered.
Completion Time	• AIMS2: Approximately 20 minutes (Meenan, 1990).
	• AIMS2-SF: Approximately 5 minutes (Guillemin, 2000).
Standardization	• The manual notes that subjects should be given the questionnaire and asked to complete it, with no further instruction.

continued

Table 11-3 (continued)

ARTHRITIS IMPACT MEASUREMENT SCALES (AIMS)

Reliability

Internal Consistency
- AIMS2: for the 12 subscales results ranged from 0.72 to 0.91 (Cronbach's coefficient α) for subjects with rheumatoid arthritis and 0.74-0.96 for those with osteoarthritis (Meenan, Mason, Anderson, Guccione, & Kazis, 1992).
- AIMS2-SF: The social interaction component demonstrated a Cronbach's α of 0.32. The other four components ranged from 0.74-0.87 (Guillemin et al., 1997). Ren, Kazis, and Meenan (1999) (n=147 patients with osteoarthritis) also noted low internal consistency with social interaction (0.46, Cronbach's α) and scores ranging form 0.80 to 0.86 for affect, symptom and physical components.

Intra-Rater
- Not applicable.

Inter-Rater
- Not applicable.

Test-Retest
- AIMS2: results ranged from 0.78 to 0.94 (intra-class correlation coefficient) (Meenan et al., 1992). N=127, patients with rheumatoid arthritis starting methotrexate treatment: results ranged from 0.73 to 0.90 (intra-class correlation coefficient) (Guillemin et al., 1997).
- AIMS2-SF: Results ranged from 0.76 to 0.81 (intra-class correlation coefficient) (Guillemin et al., 1997).

Validity

Content
- AIMS2: Ninety-six percent of test respondents (n=24) felt that the test was comprehensive. (Meenan et al., 1992).

Criterion
- AIMS2: The AIMS2 physical function measures were moderately correlated with the Rapid Assessment of Disease Activity in Rheumatology (RADAR) measure (r=0.11 to 0.52) while the AIMS2 arthritis pain scale was strongly correlated with the RADAR total joint score (r=0.72 to 0.76) (Mason, Meenan, & Anderson, 1992). This indicates that the AIMS2 physical functioning scale may be measuring constructs not present in the RADAR.
- AIMS2-SF: n=1030 patients with rheumatoid arthritis: the AIMS2 and AIMS2-SF were both administered: Intraclass correlations were lowest for Role (0.62), but ≥0.85 for all remaining components (Haavardsholm, Kvien, Uhlig, Smedstad, & Guillemin, 2000).

Convergent
- Similar scores between AIMS2-SF and AIMS2. Physical, symptomatic and affect components demonstrated strongest correlations (0.24 to 0.59 AIMS2-SF; 0.14 to 0.60 AIMS2) (Guillemin et al., 1997).

Construct
- Significant differences in performance subscale scores between those subjects who reported the performance areas as a health status problem were found (p < 0.001) in all groups. In addition, subjects' responses were also dichotomized based on identification of the performance area as a priority.

Responsiveness to Change
- AIMS2: N=31, attending an arthritis hydrotherapy program: values obtained at baseline, 10 weeks and 3 months, and compared to other measures (SF-36, WOMAC, VAS), no change detected (Lineker, Badley, Hawker, & Wilkins, 2000). Another study (Salaffi, Stancati and Carotti, 2002) found that the Italian version of the AIMS2 was more responsive to change than the SF-36, as well as two other utility measures.
- AIMS2-SF: Both the studies by Haavardsholm et al (2000) and Guillemin et al. (1997) demonstrated similar results for the AIMS2-SF and AIMS2 in terms of responsiveness to change indicating that the AIMS2-SF is at least as sensitive as the AIMS2. They also indicated that the physical and symptom component of both scales are most sensitive to change.

continued

Table 11-3 (continued)

ARTHRITIS IMPACT MEASUREMENT SCALES (AIMS)

Strengths

AIMS2
- Considered an accepted standard method for measurement of health status for clients with rheumatoid arthritis
- Well established reliability and validity. Although responsiveness was not demonstrated in one study, others studies have indicated that the measure is sensitive to change.
- Incorporates client satisfaction and client priorities for improvement.
- Assesses how much of the difficulties being experienced are attributable to arthritis.
- It has been translated into many languages and list of the available languages and psychometric properties can be found at the AIMS2 web site listed under "Source."

AIMS2-SF
- All of the above and easier to administer.

Weaknesses

AIMS2 and AIMS2-SF
- The physical component includes both ADL and IADL.
- The instrument is meant to be a general information source so specific assessment would be required to determine the reason for the deficit.
- AIMS2 must be purchased.

Final Word
- The AIMS2 provides information on a client's level of occupational performance when occupational performance is being most affected by the disease progression of arthritis. As a specific ADL tool, further information would be required to clearly understand the problems identified. The AIMS2-SF has shown similar psychometric properties overall and for the physical component, when compared to the AIMS2 yet it takes about one-fourth of the time to administer.

Table 11-4

BARTHEL INDEX

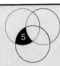

Source	Mahoney, S. I., & Barthel, D. W. (1965). Functional evaluation: The Barthel index. *Maryland State Medical Journal, 14*, 61-65.
	Note: The instrument is reviewed in a number of sources (Cohen & Marino, 2000; Dewing, 1992; Eakin, 1993; Finch, Brooks, Stratford & Mayo, 2002; Murdock, 1992a , 1992b; Shah & Cooper, 1993; Wade & Collin, 1988).
Important References	Collin, C., Wade, D. T., Davies, S., & Horne, V. (1988). The Barthel ADL index: A reliability study. *International Disabilities Studies, 10*, 61-63.
	Fricke, J., & Unsworth, C. A. (1996). Inter-rater reliability of the original and modified Barthel Index and a comparison with the Functional Independence Measure. *Australian Occupational Therapy Journal, 43*, 22-29.

Purpose
- To measure changes in functional status for clients undergoing inpatient rehabilitation.

Type of Client
- Adults with many diagnoses and physical disabilities (e.g., stroke). Used in rehabilitation, acute, and community settings.

Clinical Utility

Format
- Original Barthel (as cited in the Source) consists of 10 items (feeding, bathing, grooming, dressing, bowel control, bladder control, toilet transfers, chair/bed transfers, ambulation, and stair climbing).
- Scoring uses a 2- or 3-point ordinal scale. Scores for activities have been weighted, so final item scores range from 0 to 15. Total score on the assessment ranges from 0 to 100 in increments of 5. Many sources use a scoring system based on a total score of 20.
- Modified by Shah, Vanclay, and Cooper (1989) with a 5-point ordinal scale to be more sensitive to change.
- A five-item version (Hobart & Thompson, 2001) including transfers, bathing, toilet use, stairs, and mobility developed as an outcome measure that appears to be psychometrically equivalent to the 10-item measure.

Procedures
- Raters should be rehabilitation professionals. Rating is completed using information from records or following direct observation of functional performance.
- Telephone interview and self-report have both been explored (Korner-Bitensky & Wood-Dauphinee, 1995; Sinoff & Ore, 1997).

Completion Time
- Scoring takes 2 to 5 minutes, but observation can require about 1 hour.

Standardization
- No published manual available; scoring instructions included in original article. Guidelines used in different reliability and validity studies are not always provided.

Reliability
- Excellent.

Internal Consistency
- Original BI: Cronbach's coefficient α ranged from 0.87 to 0.95 for stroke and neurorehabilitation patients at admission and discharge. (Shah et al., 1989; Hobart & Thompson, 2001; Hsueh, Lin, Jeng, & Hsieh, 2002; Post, Visser-Meily, & Gispen, 2002)
- Modified BI: 0.90 (Shah et al., 1989)
- 5-item BI: Cronbach's coefficient α ranged from 0.71 to 0.88 (Hobart & Thompson, 2001; Hsueh, Lin, Jeng, & Hsieh, 2002)

continued

Table 11-4 (continued)

BARTHEL INDEX

- First stroke survivors referred for inpatient rehabilitation (n=258); original BI: 0.87 at admission and 0.92 at discharge (Cronbach's coefficient α) Modified BI: 0.90 at admission and 0.93 at discharge (Shah et al., 1989). Neurorehabilitation inpatients (n=418); 0.89 for original BI and 0.88 for 5-item version (Cronbach's coefficient α) (Hobart & Thompson, 2001). Stroke rehabilitation inpatients (n=118) in Taiwan; original BI: 0.84 on admission and 0.85 on discharge; 5-item BI: 0.71 on admission and 0.73 on discharge (Cronbach's α) (Hsueh, Lin, Jeng & Hsieh, 2002). Stroke rehabilitation inpatients (n=31); 0.87 to 0.95 (Cronbach's α) (Post, Visser-Meily, & Gispen, 2002).

Inter-Rater
- Individual items ranged from 0.71 to 1.00, with most above 0.85 (Spearman's rho correlation coefficients), and total scores were 0.99 or 1.00 (Pearson correlations coefficients) (Shinar, Gross, Bronstein, et al., 1987).
- Inpatients referred to occupational therapy (n=25): ranges from 0.57 to 0.85 for individual items (kappa) and an overall statistics of 0.975 (Intra-class correlation coefficient) (Fricke & Unsworth, 1996).

Intra-Rater
- Hospitalized patients with stroke (n=7): ranges from 0.84 to 0.97 for five different therapists (kappa) (Loewen & Anderson, 1988).

Validity

Content
- No specific method to ensure the content validity was reported. Laake, Laake, Hylen Ranhoff, Sveen, Wyller, & Bautz-Hoter (1995), using factor analysis, found a unidimensional score for stroke, but a two-factor structure for geriatric and hip fracture patients.
- In contrast, Valach et al. (2003) found a 3-factor structure for 147 post-stroke inpatients.

Convergent
- The Barthel has been compared to the Katz, the Kenny, the PULSES, and the FIM, all commonly accepted measures of ADL, and the correlations are generally good.
- Granger, Albrecht, and Hamilton (1979) report correlations with the PULSES to range from -0.74 to -0.90.
- Fricke & Unsworth (1996) report the BI correlated highly with the brief FIM, with ranges between 0.86 and 0.90 with different raters. Gosman-Hedstron & Svensson (2000) also found high concordance between the FIM and BI.
- Post et al. (2002) noted moderate to high correlations (r=0.34 to 0.94) when BI scores compared to the Northwick Park Dependency Score and a global dependency rating

Construct
- Individuals receiving scores of below 60 on the Barthel were dependent in self-care, and after stroke, people with scores greater than 45 were more likely to go home (Granger, Dewis, Peters, Sherwood, & Barrett, 1979). Initial scores predicted length of stay and rehabilitation outcome (Shah & Cooper, 1993). Granger et al. (1979) found initial scores post-stroke of over 40 were related to discharge home and over 60 to shorter stays.
- Fortinsky, Granger, & Seltzer (1981) found the score was strongly related to the number of tasks in which a person was independent. Kwon, Hartzema, Duncan, & Min-Lai (2004) examined the relationship between original BI scores and an indicator of level of disability (n=459 people on a stroke registry), and found that the BI differentiated all levels of disability except the two highest levels of function (demonstrating a potential ceiling effect).

continued

Table 11-4 (continued)

BARTHEL INDEX

	• Rehabilitation in-patients (n=127): 7 items of the BI predicted total scores on the Chedoke-McMaster Stroke assessment; total BI scores were predicted by three items of the same assessment (Valach et al., 2003).
	• Shinar et al. (1987) and Korner-Bitensky and Wood-Dauphinee (1995) found strong relationships between BI on self-report by telephone interview compared to observations on performance. Collin, Wade, Davies, and Horne (1988) found no systematic biases when comparing self-report, nurse report, and observation.
Responsiveness to Change	• Numerous studies have examined responsiveness to change using a variety of statistics including effect size and standardized response mean. Overall, the data on responsiveness to change is promising for the Barthel, although somewhat difficult to interpret since varying statistical methods have been used.
	• Effect sizes range from 0.37 (MS patients) to 0.95 (stroke patients) (Hobart & Thompson, 2001; Wright, Cross, & Lamb, 1998; van der Putten, Hobart, Freeman, & Thompson, 1999).
	• Standardized response mean: Stroke rehabilitation inpatients (n=118) in Taiwan: original BI and 5-item BI: 1.2 (Hsueh, Lin, Jeng, & Hsieh, 2002); first time stroke inpatients (n=50): 0.99 (Salbach, Mayo, Higgins, Ahmed, Finch, & Richards, 2001). Frail older adults (n= 265): 1.13 (standardized response mean); 0.46 (Norman's responsiveness statistic), indicating lower responsiveness than goal attainment scaling, but higher than other measures of function (Rockwood, Howlett, Standnyk, Carver, Powell, & Stolee, 2003)
	• Using five different approaches to examine responsiveness to change, the Modified BI was only slightly better than the original BI on most of the indicators (Hocking, Williams, Broad, & Baskett, 1999). When compared to the FIM on four statistical analyses of responsiveness, the BI was comparable for the entire sample and the FIM was slightly more sensitive for subjects who improved at least one level on the Rankin Index (Wallace, Duncan, & Lai , 2002).
	• People on a stroke registry who either improved or remained constant in function from 1 to 3 months post-stroke (n=372): a minimal clinically important change of one unit on the Modified Rankin index was 16 units on the BI, effect size=1.29 (Wallace et al., 2002)
Strengths	• Widely used and familiar to many.
	• Covers the areas of ADL comprehensively.
	• Used extensively in research.
	• Recent research suggests that the original and modified BI are responsive to change, especially for post-stroke inpatients.
Weaknesses	• Individual intervention plans may not be clear from examining the scores since not enough detail.
	• Adaptations have been made to items and scoring in the literature while still calling it the Barthel Index, so the literature must be read carefully.
	• Its ordinal scale has not been validated or shown to produce interval level measurements.
	• Potential ceiling and floor effects, especially for community-dwelling persons and diagnoses other than stroke.
Final Word	• The original Barthel is a reliable measure that can describe self-care status and has some predictive validity. It is useful for group evaluation, program evaluation, and in research.

Table 11-5

CHILD HEALTH QUESTIONNAIRE (CHQ)

Source	Available for a fee from HealthAct (www.healthact.com).
Important References	Landgraf, J. M., Abetz, L., & Ware J. E. (1999). *The CHQ user's manual* (2nd printing). Boston: HealthAct.
	Landgraf, J. M., Maunsell, E., Speechley, K. N., Bullinger, M., Campbell, S., Abetz, L., & Ware, J. E. (1998). Canadian-French, German, and UK versions of the Child Health Questionnaire: Methodology and preliminary item scaling results. *Quality of Life Research, 7*, 433-445.
Purpose	• The CHQ was designed to measure child and adolescent health in terms of physical and psychosocial functioning and well being (Landgraf et al., 1998).
Type of Client	• Designed for children 5 to 18 years old, regardless of diagnoses.
Clinical Utility	
Format	• The CHQ has both parent/proxy versions as well as self report.
	• There are two versions of the parent/proxy (CHQ-PF50, CHQ-PF28) form and these can be used with parents of children ranging from 5 to 18 years of age. The youth version (CHQ-CF87) is available for children 10 to 18 years of age who are able to respond themselves, but the authors are working on a shorter version and currently summary scores are not available, therefore the CHQ-CF87 will not be discussed here (HealthAct, 2004).
	• The CHQ-PF50 and CHQ-PF28 are most commonly sited in the literature and therefore will be presented here. The instrument is organized into 13 concepts, which includes a physical functioning concept that includes ADL items.
	• All questions are answered on a 4-point, ordinal scale.
Procedures	• The instrument can be self-administered by the parent or can be completed through interview. Self-administration is preferred.
	• Most questions are answered based on a 4-week recall. HealthAct offers a scoring and reporting service (for a fee) or you can purchase their scoring sheets and calculate the scores yourself but you need SPSS or SAS.
Completion Time	• The CHQ-PF50 can take 15 to 45 minutes to complete; CHQ-PF28 took an average of 10 minutes to complete (range 5 to 12) (Pencharz, Young, Owen, & Wright, 2001).
Standardization	• The manual that is provided with the purchase of the instrument is very comprehensive. It provides each of the forms of the instrument and includes instructions for self-administration and interview.
	• Norms for the summary scales are presented in the manual, based on responses of 391 parents of children 5 to 18 years of age sampled from the general U.S. population. Data from Waters, Salmon, & Wake (2000) indicate that the summary scores may actually be more useful for children with severe illness than for the general population.
	• Clinical profiles on parent responses are also presented from parents of children with asthma, attention deficit hyperactivity disorder, epilepsy, psychiatric diagnoses, and juvenile rheumatoid arthritis.
Reliability	
Internal Consistency	• CHQ-PF50: item-total correlations ranged from 0.19-0.92, (lower values are not unexpected since it is an ordinal scale); Cronbach's α ranged from 0.53-0.96, with a physical functioning component correlation of 0.91- 0.94 (Landgraf, Anetz, & Ware, 1996; Asumussen, Olson, Grant, Landgraf, Fagan, & Weiss, 2000; Waters, Salmon, & Wake, 2000).

continued

Table 11-5 (continued)

CHILD HEALTH QUESTIONNAIRE

	• McCarthy, Silberstein, Atkins, Harryman, Sponseller, & Hadley-Miller (2002) also report on Cronbach's α values for internal consistency that range from 0.80 to 0.94 for 5 of the concepts (n=147, children aged 3 to 10 years with spastic cerebral palsy), but it is unclear which of the parent forms (CHQ-PF50 or CHQ-PF28) was used.
Observer	• Not applicable.
Test-Retest	• CHQ-PF50; Intraclass coefficient (ICC) ranged from 0.37 to 0.84 with the physical functioning component correlation of 0.76 (Asmussen et al., 2000).
	• AUS CHQ-PF50: ICC for the overall group ranged from 0.08 to 0.77, however when the 25 children who had experienced a significant event in this time period were removed from the analysis, the ICC range was 0.49 to 0.78 (Waters et al., 2000).
Validity	
Content	• The developers used an extensive process to generate the items for the measure, including a review of the literature, existing measures, and use of experts in the field (Landgraf et al., 1996).
Discriminant	• The authors formulated hypotheses about the relative scores that would be expected in the general population and the clinical subgroups. For example, it was hypothesized that the general population would have the highest health ratings, and that the clinical group with epilepsy would have the lowest physical health ratings. All four of the hypotheses were supported (Landgraf et al., 1996).
	• CHQ-PF50, n=60, children with asthma aged 5 to 12 years; those with a lower symptom state scored higher on each of the items and summary scores (Asmussen et al., 2000).
	• Pencharz et al. (2001) also found that the CHQ-PF28 was able to discriminate between diagnoses, but noted that it was less able to do so then the Activities Scale for Kids (ASK) and the Pediatric Outcomes Data Collection Instrument (PODCI) (n=210 children aged 5 to 17 years with musculoskeletal disorders).
Construct	• Factor analysis confirmed that there is a two-dimensional higher order structure of physical and psychosocial dimensions of health (n=941, combined general population and specific condition groups). Validity was tested using the parent report forms only.
	• CHQ-PF28; n=210 children aged 5 to 17 years with musculoskeletal disorders, compared to the ASK ($r \geq 0.49$, Spearman rank correlation) and the PODCI ($r \geq 0.60$, Spearman rank correlation) (Pencharz et al., 2001).
Responsiveness to Change	• Not reported in the studies reviewed.
Strength	• Provides useful information about health from the perspective of children and parents.
	• Incorporates a broad definition of health that includes physical and psychosocial components.
	• Based on a sound conceptual framework and a rigorous psychometric testing.
Weaknesses	• The manual is very large and a bit difficult to navigate despite efforts to make it user-friendly.
	• The scoring and interpretation are complex.
	• The Australian group (Waters et al., 2000) could not replicate the summary scores for psychosocial and physical health in the general population casting some doubt on how to use the norms provided by the US group.
Final Word	• The CHQ would be most appealing to researchers wanting to incorporate considerations of health from the perspective of children and/or their parents. Further research on the child-completed version is needed.

Table 11-6

FUNCTIONAL AUTONOMY MEASUREMENT SYSTEM (SMAF)

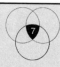

Source	Centre d'expertise, Institut universitaire de gériatrie de Sherbrooke, 375, rue Argyll, Sherbrooke, QC, Canada, J1J 3H5, (e-mail) smaf.iugs@ssss.gouv.qc.ca.
Important References	Desrosiers, J., Bravo, G., Hebert, R., & Dubuc, N. (1995). Reliability of the revised functional autonomy measurement system (SMAF) for epidemiological research. *Age and Aging, 24,* 402-406.
	Hebert, R., Carrier, R., & Bilodeau, A. (1988). The functional autonomy measurement system (SMAF): Description and validation of an instrument for the measurement of handicaps. *Age and Ageing, 17,* 293-302.
	Hebert, R., Spiegelhalter, D. J., & Brayne, C. (1997). Setting the minimal metrically detectable change on disability rating scales. *Archives of Physical Medicine and Rehabilitation, 78,* 1305-1308.
Purpose	• Designed to evaluate people's needs by measuring levels of disability and handicap. It considers not only the person's abilities and disabilities, but also the resources available to overcome the disabilities, and the stability of those resources.
Type of Client	• Designed for use with older adults in rehabilitation. Most studies have focused on people over 65, although one had a subsample under 65.
Clinical Utility	
Format	• Organized into five sections: ADL (7 items), mobility (6 items), communication (3 items), mental functions (5 items) and instrumental ADL (IADL) (8 items).
	• Each item has a 4-point scale used to rate the level of independence. In the ADL, mobility, and IADL items, a 0.5 option was added in the revised version, to indicate that a task can be done independently but with some difficulty (Desrosiers, Bravo, Hebert, & Dubuc, 1995).
	• A shorter version without the IADL and outside mobility items is used for people living in institutional settings. The SMAF is available in English, French, Dutch, and Spanish. Some work has been undertaken to develop a social functioning component to the SMAF (Pinsonnault, et al., 2003).
Procedures	• Completed based on interview and, in some cases, observation of the client completing the activities (decided by the rater). Research has been done with nurses, social workers, and occupational therapists completing it.
	• Once disability is rated, questions are considered related to whether or not the person has resources available to overcome the disability. Resources can be in the form of formal or informal help from people or assistive devices if these compensate for the disability. If the resources are available, the handicap score is 0.
	• The stability in future weeks of the resources is then considered. Scores are obtained by summing the items and can range from 0 (complete independence) to -87.
Completion Time	• In the studies completed, the instrument required about 40 minutes to complete.
Standardization	• A manual is available from the Sherbrooke University Geriatric Institute (Hebert, Guilabult, Desrosiers, & Dubuc, 2001). The forms include the assessment scale itself and an autonomy profile form (on which disability scores are totaled and can be monitored over a number of times).
	• The forms are fairly self-explanatory if the articles describing the instrument are first reviewed.
Reliability	
Internal Consistency	• Not reported in the studies reviewed.

continued

Table 11-6 (continued)

FUNCTIONAL AUTONOMY MEASUREMENT SYSTEM (SMAF)

Inter-Rater	• People over 65 living in a range of residential settings for elderly people in Quebec (n=45): mean Cohen's weighted Kappa ranged from 0.61 to 0.81 with a mean of 0.68; ADL items were 0.81 (Kappa) and 0.95 (ICC) (Desrosiers et al., 1995). Inpatients in acute/rehabilitation unit (n=94) with a slightly modified version of the SMAF: Kappas ranged from 0.74 to 0.86 between three raters (Rai, Kiniorns, et al., 1996).
Test-Retest	• People over 65 living in residential settings for elderly people in Quebec (n=45): mean Kappa of 0.73 (ranging from 0.59 to -0.74), and ICCs of 0.95 (ranging from 0.78 to 0.96). ADL items were 0.74 (Kappa) and 0.96 (ICC) (Desrosiers et al., 1995).

Validity

Content	• Developed based on literature review of other measures and the judgment of the developers, and was linked to the WHO International Classification of Impairment, Disability and Handicap (WHO, 1980).
	• It is not yet clear how the SMAF concepts of disability and handicap will conceptually link to the new WHO International Classification of Function, Disability and Health (ICF) (WHO, 2001).
Criterion	• Inpatients post CVA on an intensive functional rehabilitation program (n=132): FIM and SMAF total scores were highly correlated (0.93 to 0.95 at four points in time) (Desrosiers et al., 2003).
	• Day hospital patients (n=27) and acute medical inpatients (n=29): modified SMAF total scores correlated with a new handicap scale 0.77 for inpatients and 0.64 for day hospital patients (Rai et al., 1999).
	• Older adults visiting emergency departments (n=221): OARS ADL and SMAF ADL: 0.63 (Spearman correlations) (McCusker, Bellavance, Cardin, & Belzile, 1999).
Construct	• Residents of a long term care facility (n=99): SMAF ADL scores correlated with the required amount of nursing care, r=0.89 (Hebert et al., 1988).
	• Inpatients on an acute rehabilitation unit (n=94): significant changes in SMAF scores were noted between admission and discharge (Rai et al., 1996).
	• Inpatients (mostly older adults) admitted for treatment-rehabilitation with anxiety, depression or cognitive disorders (n=1385): gains of 5 points on the SMAF ADL score reduced the mean length of stay by a factor of 0.87 (independent effect) (Berod, Klay, Santos-Eggimann, & Paccaud, 2000).

Responsiveness to Change	• Two methods were used to identify the minimal metrically detectable change (i.e., change in score is not due to measurement error). They found that a change of SMAF score of 5 represented that level of change (Hebert, Spiegelhalter, & Brayne, 1997).
	• Inpatients post-CVA on an intensive functional rehabilitation program (n=132): Standardized response means of the ADL category was 0.88 (compared to 0.77 for the FIM self-care and sphincter control categories), and was 1.20 for the total score (compared to 0.97 for the FIM total) (Desroseirs et al., 2003).
Strengths	• Incorporates considerations of environmental resources and their stability, which is very useful for discharge planning or identifying service needs in community settings.
	• Can be administered by a multidisciplinary team.
	• It is one of the few instruments in which developers have worked to identify a significant change in score.
Weaknesses	• Further evidence of its use across different rehabilitation populations (particularly younger groups) is needed.
Final Word	• Provides very useful information, especially for discharge planning or identifying service needs in community settings in work with older adults.

Table 11-7

FUNCTIONAL INDEPENDENCE MEASURE (FIM) & WEEFIM

Source	Uniform Data System for Medical Rehabilitation, 232 Parker Hall, 3435 Main Street, Buffalo, NY 14214-3007. http://www.udsmr.org/
	Note: The FIM and WeeFIM have been extensively researched. Not all research could be included in this review table. A complete bibliography on each is available through the Web site above.
Important References	Deutsch, A., Braun, S., & Granger, C. (1996). The Functional Independence Measure (FIM Instrument) and the Functional Independence Measure for children (WeeFIM Instrument): Ten years of development. *Critical Reviews in Physical Rehabilitation Medicine, 8*, 267-281.
	Ottenbacher, K. J., Msall, M. E., Lyon, N., Duffy, L. C., Ziviani, J., Granger, C. V., Braun, S., & Feidler, R. C. (2000b). The WeeFIM instrument: Its utility in detecting change in children with development disabilities. *Archives of Physical Medicine and Rehabilitation, 81*, 1317-1326.
	Wallace, D., Duncan, P. W., & Lai , S. M. (2002). Comparison of the responsiveness of the Barthel Index and the motor component of the Functional Independence Measure in stroke: The impact of using different methods for measuring responsiveness. *Journal of Clinical Epidemiology, 55*, 922-928.
Purpose	• The FIM and WeeFIM are part of the Uniform Data System for Medical Rehabilitation (UDSMR).
	• The FIM was designed to measure the degree of disability being experienced, changes over time, and the effectiveness of rehabilitation.
	• The WeeFIM was designed with similar purposes for children receiving rehabilitation services.
	• Both measure severity of disability defined in terms of the need for assistance.
Type of Client	• FIM: Can be used with any rehabilitation client 7 years of age and older.
	• WeeFIM: designed for children from 6 months to 7 years.
Clinical Utility	
Format	• The FIM and WeeFIM have 18 items in six areas: self-care, sphincter control, mobility, locomotion, communication, and social cognition.
	• Each item is rated on a 7-point scale, from total assist to complete independence. Total scores range from 18 to 126.
	• FIM data can be described in terms of motor and cognitive subscales.
Procedures	• Both can be completed based on observations made by a clinician of any discipline, based on the client's usual rather than best performance. If observations are not possible, data can be collected through interview or medical record review.
	• A short version of the FIM (motor items) was successfully tested for telephone administration for follow up with clients discharged from spinal cord injury rehabilitation (Dijkers & Yavuzer, 1999).
Completion Time	• The instruments can be easily completed in 15 minutes. The observations required to complete the forms may require more time.
Standardization	• The manual (guide for the *Uniform Data Set for Medical Rehabilitation*) is available from the publisher.
	• Training for both the FIM and WeeFIM are required, with self-study of the manual, viewing videotapes, attendance at workshops, and a certification process with model case studies. Sites using the FIM must be licensed. Users subscribe annually to the UDSMR (with fees being ~$2575 for the FIM and ~$4000 for the WeeFIM).

continued

Table 11-7 (continued)

FUNCTIONAL INDEPENDENCE MEASURE (FIM) & WEEFIM

	• Adaptations or translations have been reported, and international sites using the FIM include: Australia, Canada, Chile, Finland, Hong Kong, Iceland, Italy, Mexico, Norway, South Africa, Spain, and Sweden (UDSMR).
	• Although there are no norms for the FIM, there are performance profiles (Granger, Hamilton, Linacre, Heinemann, & Wright, 1993), and articles on function-related and resource utilization groups (Eilertsen, Kramer, Schlenker, & Hrincevich, 1998; Sandstrom, Mokler, & Hoppe, 1998).
	• Norms for the WeeFIM were compiled based on 417 children with no developmental delay (Msall et al., 1994a).
Reliability	• Reliability of the FIM and WeeFIM are both excellent, with studies conducted to evaluate internal consistency, inter-rater and intra-rater or test-retest reliability, and results consistently high.
Internal Consistency	• FIM: neurorehabilitation inpatients (n=149): $\alpha=0.95$ for total FIM, 0.94 for motor component and 0.89 for cognitive component (Hobart et al., 2001).
	• FIM: stroke inpatients (n=118): Cronbach's $\alpha=0.88$ at admission and 0.91 at discharge for the motor subscale (Hsueh, Lin, Jeng, & Hsieh, 2002).
	• WeeFIM: children who had been preterm infants (n=149): 0.90 (Cronbach's α) (Msall, DiGaudio, & Duffy, 1993).
Inter-Rater	• FIM: ICC=0.96 for total scores, and ranged from 0.88 to 0.94 for items. Reliability was higher in a subset of 24 facilities with more training (Granger & Hamilton, 1992; Hamilton, Laughlin, Fiedler, & Granger, 1994).
	• FIM: Mean Kappa for items ranged from over 0.40 to 0.56 (social interaction items were lowest), and ICC was 0.92 for the summary motor items (Daving, Andren, Nordholm, & Grimby, 2001).
	• WeeFIM: Pearson r ranged from 0.74 to 0.96 (Msall, DiGaudio, & Duffy, 1993). also tested between raters with short and long delay; ICC for short was 0.97 (items ranged from 0.82 to 0.94), and for long delay was 0.94 (items ranged from 0.73 to 0.90) (Ottenbacher, Msall, Lyon, Duffy, Granger, & Braun, 1997).
	• WeeFIM: Children receiving inpatient and outpatient rehabilitation (n=20): 0.93 (ICC) for self-care, and ranged from 0.82 to 0.94 on the other subscales (Ziviani, Ottenbacher, Shephard, Foreman, Astbury, & Ireland, 2001).
Intra-Rater	• FIM: patients of an MS research clinic (n=35): self care items kappas ranged from 0.55 to 0.78, with ICC for total FIM of 0.94 (Sharrack, Hughes, Soudain, & Dunn,1999).
Test-Retest	• FIM: not reported in studies reviewed.
	• WeeFIM: ICC for total score = 0.98 (items ranged from 0.91 to 0.99) (Ottenbacher et al., 1996; Ottenbacher et al., 1997).
	• WeeFIM: Pearson r values ranged from 0.83 to 0.99 (Msall et al., 1993).
Validity	• Across numerous explorations of validity of the FIM and WeeFIM, both instruments consistently have results suggesting good validity.
Content	• Both were developed based on judgmental and statistical methods.
	• FIM: Rasch analysis on 27,699 rehabilitation patient FIM scores demonstrated two main constructs: motor (13 items) and cognitive (5 items) (Heinemann, Linacre, Wright, Hamilton, & Granger, 1993). FIM: Ravaud, Delcey, and Yelnik (1999), criticize the use of a summary score for the FIM because it is not based on a unidemensional construct.

continued

Table 11-7 (continued)

FUNCTIONAL INDEPENDENCE MEASURE (FIM) & WEEFIM

Convergent

- WeeFIM: well children (n=170), Rasch analysis confirmed the same two scales as the FIM, motor and cognitive (Msall et al., 1993).
- FIM: compared to the Barthel, FIM (motor) scores; Kappa=0.92 at admission and 0.88 at discharge (Kidd et al., 1995).
- Total FIM and total PULSES correlations were -0.82 at admission and -0.88 at discharge (Marshall, Heisel, & Grinnell, 1999).
- WeeFIM: compared to PEDI subscales; WeeFIM self care score Spearman correlation coefficients were 0.94 for self-care functional scale and 0.96 self-care caregiver assistance (Ziviani et al., 2001).
- WeeFIM total scores correlation was 0.92 (Spearman) with the total on the Battelle Developmental Inventory and 0.89 with the Vineland Adaptive Behavior Scales (Ottenbacher et al., 1999)

Predictive

- FIM: Admission motor FIM scores were the most significant predictors of motor status at discharge; admission functional status was consistently related to discharge functional status and length of stay, although the strength of the associations varied across impairment groups (Heinemann et al., 1994).
- The strongest predictor of discharge location was admission FIM scores (Oczkowski & Barreca, 1993); scores of over 80 were associated with likely discharge to home rather than a skilled nursing facility (Black, Soltis, & Bartlett, 1999).
- Timbeck & Spaulding (2003) conducted a review and concluded that FIM admission scores can predict discharge FIM scores, outcome disability and discharge location.
- WeeFIM: scores were significantly related to the amount of effort required to provide assistance to the child (0.69 to 0.96) and the time given to assist (0.40 to 0.88) (Msall et al., 1994b).

Construct

- FIM: scores were found to be linked to time required for help in ADL each day in patients with MS (Granger, Cotter, Hamilton, Fiedler, & Hens, 1990), stroke (Granger, Cotter, Hamilton, & Feidler, 1993), and post-traumatic brain injury (Granger, Divan, & Fiedler, 1995).
- Orthopedic inpatients: FIM self-care and total scores were significantly correlated with PT and OT visits and units as well as length of stay (Aitken & Bohannon, 2001). Kwon et al. (2004) found that the motor-FIM differentiated between three levels of disability (demonstrating a potential ceiling effect).
- WeeFIM: strong correlations were found between item scores and age (Braun & Granger, 1991); FIM scores were able to distinguish children with major impairments and no impairments and were related to parents' perceptions of the children's health status (Msall et al., 1993).
- Compared to a parent-report measure of the amount of assistance required, WeeFIM total scores had correlation of 0.91 and self-care correlation of 0.83. WeeFIM total scores were the major predictor of amount of assistance provided when included in a multiple regression analysis (Ottenbacher et al., 2000a).

Responsiveness to Change

- Research has been published focusing on the ability of the FIM to detect clinically important change, and to detect change in populations that are expected to change. The results indicate that the FIM and WeeFIM can be useful as an outcome measure, particularly with a post-stroke population.

continued

Table 11-7 (continued)

FUNCTIONAL INDEPENDENCE MEASURE (FIM) & WEEFIM

- A minimal clinically important change of one unit on the Modified Rankin index was 11 units on the FIM, effect size =1.29 (Wallace et al., 2002).
- When compared to the Barthel Index on four statistical analyses of responsiveness, the FIM was comparable for the entire sample and slightly more sensitive for subjects who improved at least one level on the Rankin Index (Wallace et al., 2002).
- Other studies that have examined the responsiveness of the FIM found effect sizes of 0.30 for patients with MS, 0.82 for patients with stroke (n=283) (van der Putten, Hobart, Freeman, & Thompson, 1999), and 1.62 for self care in orthopedic inpatients (n=28) (Aitken & Bohannon, 2001).
- Standardized response mean for the FIM self-care and sphincter control categories was 0.77, and 0.97 for the total score (both slightly smaller than the SMAF) (Desroseirs et al., 2003).
- WeeFIM: using five statistical analyses to examine responsiveness, the authors report that the WeeFIM was responsive to change (e.g., effect size was 0.62, standardized response mean = 1.31) (Ottenbacher et al., 2000b).

Strengths
- Excellent inter-rater reliability, construct validity and emerging information about responsiveness to change for both the FIM and WeeFIM.
- Used throughout the United States and other countries for outcome evaluation.
- Can be used in a variety of rehabilitation settings with all types of patients, and can be rated by many team members.

Weaknesses
- A ceiling effect on the cognition items may be observed in clients with SCI (Hall, Cohen, Wright, Call, & Werner, 1999) and other client groups with minimal cognitive impairment, and some ceiling and floor effects may be noted with the WeeFIM.
- Cost may be a barrier to accessing the instruments in some settings.

Final Word
- For rehabilitation settings interested in program evaluation, the FIM and WeeFIM are excellent tools. Recent research exploring their responsiveness to change has strengthened them further as evaluative instruments. Since they are widely known, used, and have very good psychometric properties, they should be considered first as outcome measures in rehabilitation.

Table 11-8

HEALTH ASSESSMENT QUESTIONNAIRE (HAQ)/ CHILDREN'S HEALTH ASSESSMENT QUESTIONNAIRE (CHAQ)

Source

HAQ: The questionnaire and manual (HAQ-PAK) can be found at http://aramis.stanford.edu

CHAQ: The questionnaire can be found as a figure (Figure 1) in Singh, Athreya, Fries, & Goldsmith, 1994.

Important References

HAQ:

Bruce, B., & Fries, J.F. (2003). The Stanford Health Assessment Questionnaire: A review of its history, issues, progress and documentation. *Journal of Rheumatology, 30*, 167-78.

Stanford University School University of Medicine, Division of Immunology & Rheumatology. (2004). *The Health Assessment Questionnaire.* Retrieved August *31*, 2004 from http://aramis.stanford.edu

CHAQ:

Singh, G., Athreya, B. H., Fries, J. F., & Goldsmith, D. P. (1994). Measurement of health status in children with juvenile rheumatoid arthritis. *Arthritis & Rheumatism, 37*, 1761-9.

Purpose

- HAQ: To obtain a personal assessment of the functional status of those with rheumatic diseases, but it could also be used as a generic functional measure with some adaptation (that would not affect the psychometric properties) (Stanford, 2004).

- CHAQ: To measure functional status in children with juvenile rheumatoid arthritis, ages 1 to 19 years (Singh, Athreya, Fries, & Goldsmith, 1994).

Type of Client

- HAQ: Although originally designed for study of adults with rheumatic diseases, the authors (Stanford, 2004) note that it has been used with different diagnoses and people and therefore should be considered a general health questionnaire (although some adaptations may be required).

- CHAQ: Used with clients having wide range of rheumatic diagnoses as well as dermatomyositis and spina bifida (Bruce & Fries, 2003).

Clinical Utility

Format

- HAQ Full version: Assesses five dimensions of health (disability, discomfort, drug side effects, dollar costs, and death)

- HAQ Disability Index (HAQ-DI): Shorter version, 20 questions in 8 categories; dressing, arising, eating, hygiene, walking, reaching, grip, and outside activity) and the discomfort index (which includes the Visual Analog Scale (VAS) Pain Scale and the VAS Patient Global).

- Other versions of the HAQ include: MHAQ (Modified HAQ; 8 items for the 8 sub categories of the HAQ-DI, perceived patient satisfaction and perceived degree of difficulty), RA-HAQ (Rheumatoid Arthritis HAQ; 8 questions, 3/8 differ from MHAQ. It has never been used clinically), HAQ-20 (uses all 20 of HAQ-DI questions, but scoring differs from HAQ), DHAQ (Difficult HAQ; does not include assistive devices in scoring) (Pincus, Summey, Soraci, Wallston, & Hummon, 1983; Wolfe, 2001).

- While the MHAQ has been used both in research and clinically, there is debate about its psychometric properties. The HAQ-20 and DHAQ are scoring variations of the HAQ and have not been reported on widely (Wolfe, 2001). Therefore of all noted, only the HAQ will be discussed.

continued

Table 11-8 (continued)

HEALTH ASSESSMENT QUESTIONNAIRE (HAQ)/ CHILDREN'S HEALTH ASSESSMENT QUESTIONNAIRE (CHAQ)

	• CHAQ: Similar to the HAQ-DI in the 8 categories but the authors have modified the questions within the categories slightly to ensure there are relevant questions for all age groups (Singh et al., 1994) It also includes the VAS Pain and VAS Global scales.
Procedures	• HAQ: Usually self-administered but can be given face-to-face or by telephone interview. Scoring is described in detail in the manual and although it is not simple, clear instructions are provided (Stanford, 2004).
	• CHAQ: Parent proxy or self-administered.
Completion Time	• HAQ: Full version 20 to 30 minutes; shorter version (HAQ-DI and the HAQ Pain Scale) approximately 5 minutes (Ramey, Fries, & Singh, 1996; Stanford, 2004).
	• CHAQ: Less than 10 minutes to complete (Singh et al., 1994).
Standardization	• HAQ: Krishnan, Sokka, Hakkinen, Hubert, & Hannonen (2004) established general population norms on a sample of 1,530 Finnish adults.
	• CHAQ: Not discussed in articles reviewed.
Reliability	
	• HAQ: The Ramey et al. (1996) review as well as the Bruce & Fries (2003) review together provide a comprehensive list of the over 350 studies that have been completed reviewing the issues of reliability, validity and responsiveness to change for the HAQ and CHAQ. The measures have been studied with a variety of populations. Therefore the data presented for these tools will not always specify sample sizes or populations as ranges are given from data from all studies.
Internal Consistency	• HAQ: Not discussed in articles reviewed.
	• CHAQ: n=72 children who had juvenile rheumatoid arthritis (JRA). Cronbach's α (overall) was 0.941 (Singh et al., 1994).
Intra-Rater	• Not applicable since the measure is self report.
Inter-Rater	• Not applicable since the measure is self report.
Test-Retest	• HAQ: Correlations range from 0.87 to 0.99 (Ramey, Raynauld, & Fries, 1992; Ramey et al., 1996; Bruce & Fries, 2003).
	• CHAQ: n=13 children with JRA. Spearman's correlation coefficient of 0.79 ($p<0.002$) (Singh et al., 1994). Feldman, Alyling-Campos, Luy, Stevens, Silverman, and Laxer (1995) demonstrated an intraclass correlation of 0.87 in 37 children with juvenile dermatomyositis.
Validity	
Content	• HAQ-DI: The original measure developed in 1978 was reviewed by expert panels then tested in studies of both subjective and objective assessment. There is expert consensus that the test possesses both face and content validity (Ramey et al., 1992; Ramey et al., 1996; Bruce & Fries, 2003).
	• CHAQ: Initially determined by 7 rheumatologists and 8 health care professionals including occupational and physical therapists (Singh et al., 1994).
Construct, Convergent	• HAQ: Demonstrated in many studies (Ramey et al., 1996; Bruce, & Fries, 2003).
	• CHAQ: n=72 children who had juvenile rheumatoid arthritis (JRA), compared to Steinbrocker functional class, physical symptoms (joint count stiffness) and physician's assessment, values ranged from (Kendall's tau b) 0.54 to 0.77 all significant at the $p<0.0001$ level. N=37 children with JDM, compared to disease severity Spearman's correlation was 0.71 ($p<0.002$), compared with proximal muscle strength rs= -0.57 ($p<0.002$), shoulder abduction rs=0.051 ($p<0.01$), knee extension rs=-0.40 ($p=0.05$) and grip strength rs=-0.079 ($p<0.20$).

continued

Table 11-8 (continued)

HEALTH ASSESSMENT QUESTIONNAIRE (HAQ)/
CHILDREN'S HEALTH ASSESSMENT QUESTIONNAIRE (CHAQ)

Criterion	• HAQ-DI: Has been widely studied and significantly correlated (0.71 to 0.95) with a wide variety of measures, including disease specific, generic health status, biochemical markers, and measures of self report.
	• Pearson product moment correlations were used to compare total performance scales on the Canadian Occupational Performance Measure with the HAQ-DI. These were not significantly correlated (-0.37), however when only those activities that were identified on the HAQ were included the correlations increased to -0.52 at the category level and -0.67 at the activity level (Ripat, Etcheverry, Cooper, & Tate, 2001).
	• CHAQ: No criterion measure is available to compare with.
Responsiveness to Change	• HAQ: The responsiveness to change has been well documented and the studies indicate that the measure is responsive to change (Bruce & Fries, 2003; Krishnan, et al., 2004; Ramey et al., 1996; Ramey et al., 1992). As well, evidence exists for the minimal clinically important difference ranging from 0.10 to 0.22 (Bruce & Fries, 2003).
	• CHAQ: Brown & Wallen (2002) studies are inconclusive as a study by Ruperto, Ravelli, Migliavacca, Viola, Postorio, Duarte, and Martini (1999) in children with juvenile chronic arthritis did not demonstrate responsiveness when compared with physician and parent global assessments, articular variables and laboratory indicators. Conversely, both Singh et al. (1994) and Feldman et al. (1995) did demonstrate responsiveness.
Strengths	HAQ: • Widely used in research as well as clinical practice, and the subscale of the HAQ. • DI has been included in many clinical studies. • Extensive development process and excellent psychometric properties • Validated translations available in 60 languages. CHAQ: • Thorough development and strong psychometric properties across a few different diagnostic groups. • Thorough validation of translations with more than 25 languages available
Weaknesses	• HAQ: It is a generic health status instrument and therefore additional information is needed to determine reasons for functional deficit. • CHAQ: Responsiveness to change has not been established.
Final Word	• HAQ: A really good functional status measure that is applicable to those with rheumatic conditions as well as those without. • CHAQ: This tool is simple to use and does provide reliable and valid results. Its use as an outcome measure is questionable because of the varying results in testing in terms of responsiveness to change.

Table 11-9

JUVENILE ARTHRITIS FUNCTIONAL ASSESSMENT REPORT (JAFAR)/ JUVENILE ARTHRITIS FUNCTIONAL ASSESSMENT SCALE (JAFAS)

Source	JAFAR-C and the JAFAS can be found free, online at: http://www.mrw.inter science.wiley.com/suppmat/0004-3591:1/suppmat/49_5S/v49_5S.5.html
Important References	JAFAR:
	Howe, S., Levinson, J., Shear, E., Hartner, S., McGirr, G., Schulte, M., & Lovell, D. (1991). Development of a disability measurement tool for juvenile rheumatoid arthritis: The Juvenile Arthritis Functional Assessment Report for Children and their Parents. *Arthritis & Rheumatism, 34*, 873-880.
	JAFAS:
	Lovell, D.J., Howe, S., Shear, E., Hartner, S., McGirr, G., Schulte, M., & Levinson, J. (1989). Development of a disability measurement tool for juvenile arthritis: The Juvenile Arthritis Functional Assessment Scale (JAFAS). *Arthritis & Rheumatism, 32*, 1390-1395.
Purpose	• The purpose of both is to measure disability due to JRA.
Type of Client	• JAFAR and JAFAS: Children with JRA age 7 to 18 years.
Clinical Utility	
Format	• JAFAR: There is a child report (JAFAR-C) and parent report version (JAFAR-P) both of which contain the same 23 questions in which either the child or parent reports on a 3 point scale as to whether the child is always, sometimes or almost never able to complete the functional task.
	• JAFAS: Ten functional tasks that the child is asked to perform in front of an observer. Time to task completion is considered in the scoring.
Procedures	• JAFAR C: Administered by a health professional using simple instructions. JAFAR P: Self-administered.
	• JAFAS: Therapist administered with specific standardized procedures as well as equipment.
Completion Time	• JAFAR C or P: 5 minutes to complete and 3 minutes to score. JAFAS: 10 minutes to complete.
Standardization	• JAFAR: Not discussed in the articles reviewed.
	• JAFAS: Specific procedures for administration available. No norms discussed in articles reviewed.
Reliability	
Internal Consistency	• JAFAR-C: Cronbach's α ranged from 0.83 to 0.85 (Howe et al., 1991; Tennant, Kearns, Turner, Wyatt, Haigh, & Chamberlain, 2001).
	• JAFAR-P: Cronbach's α ranged from 0.81 to 0.96 (Howe et al., 1991; Tennant et al., 2001; and Lovell et al., 1989).
Observer	• JAFAR C & P: Not applicable.
	• JAFAS: Inter-rater: n=21 children, aged 5 to 16 years with JRA, Kappa values for each question ranged from 0.07 to 1.00 (Tennant et al., 2001).
Test-Retest	• JAFAR C & P: Not reported in articles reviewed.
	• JAFAS: Not reported in articles reviewed.
Validity	
Content	• JAFAR C & P: Developed by the same panel of experts who developed the JAFAS. Item selection was done based on work done on JAFAS.

continued

Table 11-9 (continued)

Juvenile Arthritis Functional Assessment Report (JAFAR)/ Juvenile Arthritis Functional Assessment Scale (JAFAS)

	• JAFAS: Content was initially taken from the Arthritis Impact Measurement Scale (AIMS), Health Assessment Questionnaire (HAQ) and the McMaster Health Index (Lovell et al., 1989). An expert panel chose items and pilot tested prior to development of final test.
Convergent	• JAFAR C & P: n=72 (children) and n=70 (parents), correlations with a visual analog pain scale were 0.57 (Pearson's correlation coefficient (PCC) and 0.61 respectively (Howe et al., 1991); several other studies in comparable populations demonstrated similar results with JAFAR-C & P when compared to joint counts and bio chemical markers (Baildam, Holt, Conway & Morton, 1995; Spadaro. Riccierie, Sili, Scallia, Sensi, Fiore, Taccari, & Zoppini, 1996; van der Net, Prakken, Helders et al., 1996).
	• JAFAS: n=71 children with JRA, compared to number of involved joints, correlation of 0.40, compared to Steinbrocker functional class 0.59, compared to disease activity status, -0.32. The authors note the direction of these correlations were as expected (Lovell et al., 1989).
Construct	• JAFAR C & P: n=72 children, n=70 parents compared to JAFAS scores; JAFAR-C, 0.69 (PCC); JAFAR-P, 0.69 (Howe et al., 1991).
	• JAFAS: n=52, children 5 to 16 years of age with JRA, compared to the Physician's Global Assessment of Disease activity, JAFAR- C, 0.36, JAFAR-P, 0.34 and compared with joint count JAFAR-C, 0.29, JAFAR-P, 0.30 (Tennant et al., 2001).
Sensitivity to Change	• In a study comparing the JAFAR-C, JAFAR-P and JAFAS to the Children's Health Assessment Questionnaire (CHAQ), British authors noted that the CHAQ demonstrated an effect size of almost twice that of the other measures (Tennant et al., 2001).
	• Robinson, Nahata, Hayes, Rennebohm, & Higgins (2003) noted similar change scores between the CHAQ and the JAFAR in a sample of 21 children with JRA.
Strengths	• The JAFAR C & P as well as the JAFAS have undergone rigorous psychometric testing and demonstrate good reliability and validity.
	• All three are easy to administer however the JAFAR C & P do take less and time and do not require special equipment.
	• The JAFAR C & P are being used in research.
Weaknesses	• The authors note that the JAFAS should be considered as a separate measure to either of JAFARs, however they used the JAFAS as the comparator for construct validity, indicating that they are measuring similar constructs.
	• Special equipment is required to administer the JAFAS.
Final Word	• Although similar in construct since it is easier to administer, takes less time to complete, and provides the same information, the JAFAR C or P would seem to be the measure of choice. Just watch for future research regarding responsiveness as there is some doubt about this.

Table 11-10

JUVENILE ARTHRITIS SELF-REPORT INDEX (JASI)

Source	Wright, F. V., Law, M., Crombie, V., Goldsmith, C., Dent, P., & Shore, A. (1992). *The JASI*. Available from V. Wright, Arthritis and Orthopedic Program, Bloorview-MacMillan Centre, 350 Rumsey Road, Toronto, Ontario, Canada, M4G 1R8.
Important References	Wright, F. V., Kimber, J. L., Law, M., Goldsmith, C., Crombie, V., & Dent, P. (1996). The Juvenile Arthritis Functional Status Index (JASI): A validation study. *Journal of Rheumatology, 23(6)*, 1066-1079.
	Wright, F. V., Law, M., Crombie, V., Goldsmith, C. H., & Dent, P. (1994). Development of a self-report functional status index for juvenile rheumatoid arthritis. *Journal of Rheumatology, 21(3)*, 536-544.
Purpose	• Designed as a self-report measure of daily living and mobility activities of school-aged children with JRA.
Type of Client	• Tested with children from 8 years of age and up (Wright et al.,1996). It is designed for school-aged children and adolescents with JRA.
Clinical Utility	
Format	• The JASI is divided into two parts. In Part 1, children are asked to rate their performance on 94 items in five categories: self-care, domestic, mobility, school, and extracurricular. Each item is rated on a 7-point ordinal scale. In Part 2, the children identify and rate their performance on activities of most importance to them.
Procedures	• The instructions are reviewed with the child, and sample items are administered. If the child can understand the ratings and read the questions, he or she can complete it independently. If there are difficulties with reading, the administrator reads the items to the child.
Completion Time	• Administration time ranges from 30 to 45 minutes.
Standardization	• There is no manual that accompanies the instrument.
Reliability	
Internal Consistency	• Not reported in studies reviewed.
Observer	• Not reported in studies reviewed.
Test-Retest	• Part 1: ICC=0.99 at 2 to 3 weeks and 0.98 for a sub-group of 11 subjects at 3 months.
	• Part 2: Short-term reliability was 0.57 (weighted Kappa) after 2 to 3 weeks (Wright et al., 1996).
Validity	
Content	• Content validity was established through the instrument development process, which incorporated the use of experts including clinicians, children, parents, and teachers (Wright et al., 1994).
Convergent	• Not reported in studies reviewed.
Construct	• JASI scores were correlated with a number of measures used in pediatrics with a sample of 36 children with JRA: joint pain (r=-0.15), arthritis status (r=0.24); active joint count (r=-0.51); morning stiffness (r=-0.62); Bruininks subtest 8 (r+0.55 with n=30); grip strength (r=0.60); presence of hip synovitis (r=-0.62); hip flexion contracture (r=-0.65); timed walk (r=-0.66); Keitel upper extremity score (r=-0.72); ACR functional rating (r=-0.75); timed run (r=-0.79); total Keitel index (r=-0.89); Keitel lower extremity score (r=-0.91). Only the relationship to pain was less than expected (Wright et al., 1996).

continued

Table 11-10 (continued)

JUVENILE ARTHRITIS SELF-REPORT INDEX (JASI)

	• Comparisons were also made between self-report by children and observational scores completed by clinicians (n=430) for 60 of the items on the JASI that could be observed. Mean weighted Kappa score was 0.66 (indicating fair to good agreement); and further analysis indicated that there was not a strong bias for children to rate their performance higher than the clinicians.
Responsiveness to Change	• Children with JRA (n=430) were asked to rate the amount of change in their ability that they had experienced since initial testing, and these ratings were compared to actual performance ratings on retest. There was agreement of 57% between the two rating schemes at 2 to 3 weeks, and 53% at 3 months (n=411).
	• In examinations of the Standard Error of the Mean (SEM), the authors noted that the JASI is more sensitive to change for children with more severe involvement of JRA than children with mild involvement (Wright et al., 1996).
Strengths	• The JASI is innovative in its use of self-report.
	• Useful for treatment planning with priorities identified by the child in Part 2.
Weaknesses	• Further reliability and validity research is needed, particularly for Part 2 of the JASI.
	• More information about sensitivity to change is needed before it can be used confidently to evaluate outcomes.
Final Word	• For anyone working with children with JRA, the JASI is useful as an initial assessment to assist in treatment planning. It can contribute to client-centered practice since the children report their abilities in a variety of daily activities.

Table 11-11

KATZ INDEX OF ACTIVITIES OF DAILY LIVING

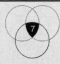

Source	Katz, S., Ford, A. B., Moskowitz, R. W., Jackson, B. A., & Jaffe, M. W. (1963). Studies of illness in the aged: The index of ADL: A standardized measure of biological and psychosocial function. *JAMA, 185(12),* 94-99.
Important References	Brorsson, B., & Hulter-Asberg, K. (1984). Katz index of independence in ADL: Reliability and validity in short-term care. *Scandinavian Journal of Rehabilitation Medicine, 16,* 125-132.
	Hulter-Asberg, K. H., & Sonn, U. (1988). The cumulative structure of personal and instrumental ADL: A study of elderly people in a health service district. *Scandinavian Journal of Rehabilitation Medicine, 21,* 171-177.
Purpose	• Designed to describe levels of function, to predict future function and level of care, and to evaluate programs.
Type of Client	• Developed from observations of older adults after hip fractures, but has been used with adults with musculoskeletal and neurological impairments, and with community-dwelling older adults.
Clinical Utility	
Format	• The original form includes 6 items that cover feeding, continence, transfer, toileting, dressing, and bathing.
	• Each item is rated on a 3-point scale (independence, receives assistance, dependent), which is converted to an independent/dependent rating (with the "receives assistance" falling under independent for some items and dependent for others).
	• A summary letter score on a Guttman scale, based on a hierarchy of the order in which ADL skills are lost and regained, is then used to indicate the types of ADL skills with which the person has difficulty.
	• With community-dwelling older adults, efforts have been made to add IADL items to the Katz, so that it is more sensitive to the types of difficulties that people have in daily living (Hulter-Asberg & Sonn, 1988; Iwarsson & Isacsson, 1997; Spector, Katz, Murphy, & Fulton, 1987).
Procedures	• The instrument was originally developed so that scoring was based on the 2-week period prior to the evaluation and can be administered based on interview and/or observation of some components.
	• A 5-item version (omitting continence) has been tested as a telephone interview (Ciesla, Shi, Stoskopf, & Samuels, 1993).
Completion Time	• Since the instrument administration is not standardized, it is difficult to estimate how long it would require. A 2-week observation is recommended prior to completion.
Standardization	• There are no formal instructions to administer and no manual. Information is included about the ratings in a number of the original journal articles.
Reliability	
Internal Consistency	• Random sample of South Carolina residents (n=6,472): using a 5-item telephone instrument, a Kuder-Richardson 20 statistic of 0.87 (Ciesla et al., 1993).
	• Frail elderly persons (n=83) with the urinary continence item deleted: Cronbach's α: 0.56 (Reuben, Valle, Hays, & Siu, 1995).
Inter-Rater	• Examined based on the number of differences between raters, and, in all cases, the inter-observer variability was low (Brorsson & Hulter-Asberg, 1984).
Test-Retest	• Not reported in the studies reviewed.

continued

Table 11-11 (continued)

KATZ INDEX OF ACTIVITIES OF DAILY LIVING

Validity

Content
- Content covers the main areas of ADL most commonly cited, although the authors do not justify item selection.
- The Guttman scaling was originally based on developmental and anthropological hierarchies. A very high percentage (~96%) of subjects could be classified by the index (Katz et al., 1963).
- Brorsson and Hulter-Asberg (1984) report coefficients of scalability ranging from 0.74 to 0.88.

Construct
- Compared to the amount of assistance required from a non-family attendant, there was a significant difference between those rated more independent than those less independent (Katz, Downs, Cash, & Grotz, 1970).
- Hypotheses have also been tested related to the order of recovery and these generally followed the scaling.
- Katz ratings were found to predict length of stay in hospital, type of discharge, actual residence 1-year post assessment and mortality in clients in acute care (Brorsson & Hulter-Asberg, 1984). Scores were also predictive of discharge location, length of stay in rehabilitation, and mortality (Hulter-Asberg & Nydevik, 1991; Hermodsson & Ekdahl, 1999)

Responsiveness to Change
- Not reported in the studies reviewed.

Strengths
- Quick to complete and easy to score.
- Considering its brevity, reliability and validity are good.
- Adaptations to add IADL may make the instrument more useful in community settings.

Weaknesses
- 2-week observations before scoring are unrealistic in many settings.
- May be less useful for planning individual intervention plans since its brevity makes it difficult to identify specific areas for intervention (Settle & Holm, 1993).
- No information on responsiveness to change cited.

Final Word
- The Katz can be used to examine the levels of function in inpatient programs that meets the needs of people with varying disabilities, especially for older adults anticipated to be in care for a long period.
- Comparisons were also made between self-report by children and observational scores completed by clinicians (n=430) for 60 of the items on the JASI that could be observed. Mean weighted Kappa score was 0.66 (indicating fair to good agreement); and further analysis indicated that there was not a strong bias for children to rate their performance higher than the clinicians.

Table 11-12

MELVILLE NELSON SELF-CARE ASSESSMENT (SCA)

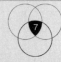

Source	The instrument is part of the Link-Nelson Occupational Therapy Evaluation for Skilled Nursing Facilities and is available from http://www.mco.edu/allh/ot/melville/sca.html.
Important References	Nelson, D. L., Melville, L. L., Wilkerson, J. D., Magness, R. A., Grech, J. L., & Rosenberg, J. A. (2002). Interrater reliability, concurrent validity, responsiveness and predictive validity of the Melville-Nelson Self-Care Assessment. *American Journal of Occupational Therapy, 56*, 51-59.
Purpose	• Provides an objective measure of self-care performance and support.
Type of Client	• Designed for use with patients in subacute and skilled nursing facilities.

Clinical Utility

Format
- Observational measure that is part of the Melville-Nelson Occupational Therapy Evaluation System for Skilled Nursing Facilities (SNF) and Subacute Rehabilitation, which also includes demographics and history information and the Self-Identified Goal Assessment (Melville, Baltic, Bettcher, & Nelson, 2002).
- Each of the seven sections (bed mobility, transfers, dressing, eating, toilet use, personal hygiene and bathing) is rated on self-performance and the support needed. For self-performance, each occupation is broken into sub-occupations (e.g., eating is broken into finger food, utensil and drink). For each sub-occupation, four tasks are considered within it (e.g., finger food is broken into grasp, to mouth, open mouth, and in mouth).
- Higher scores on self-performance indicate that more assistance is needed. A total score can also be calculated (maximum total is 140).
- For each of the seven self-care tasks, a single support score is also rated depending on the type of support needed (e.g., from no setup or physical help to two-person physical help required). A total support score is not calculated.

Procedures
- Observation of each of the self-care occupations is required to rate the SCA.
- Any items which are not applicable to the client are not scored, so scores reflect only applicable items (although it is not clear how this not-applicable status is indicated on the form).

Completion Time
- Administration time not described in the research reviewed. Observation of all components is required, which could take anywhere from 1 to 3 hours, depending on the client.

Standardization
- There is no manual and no norms.

Reliability

Internal Consistency
- Not reported in the studies reviewed.

Inter-Rater
- Patients receiving subacute rehabilitation (n=68), eight raters in four teams (one certified OT and one OT graduate student in each): ICC for total self-performance was 0.94, and for specific individual areas ranged from 0.77 to 0.98. For support, the ICCs ranged from 0.57 to 0.89 (Nelson et al., 2002).

Intra-Rater
- Not reported in studies reviewed.

Test-Retest
- Not reported in studies reviewed.

Validity

Content
- The content of the SCA follows the Minimum Data Set intentionally to ease administration for occupational therapists already completing the MDS for reimbursement purposes.

continued

Table 11-12 (continued)

MELVILLE NELSON SELF-CARE ASSESSMENT (SCA)

Convergent
- Patients receiving subacute rehabilitation (n=68): Total SCA self-performance scores were correlated with the FIM (Spearman rank order correlation (rho) with total FIM was -0.85) and Klein Bell (rho=-0.085).
- Correlations for the seven sub-scales of the SCA were also correlated with the relevant items from the FIM and Klein-Bell and all were statistically significant correlations. Correlations between SCA support scores and FIM and Klein Bell components were similar (Nelson et al., 2002).

Construct
- In a sample of 40 patients receiving subacute rehabilitation, discharge total self-performance SCA was correlated with caregiving time in home, FIM scores, and Klein Bell scores (Nelson et al., 2002).

Responsiveness to Change
- Responsiveness to change was examined by examining effect sizes (two different statistics) for a sample of 68 patients receiving subacute rehabilitation evaluated at admission and discharge. Eleven of 15 variables on the SCA showed significant change from admission to discharge. Effect sizes varied depending on how they were calculated, but were generally high for transfers, dressing and toileting, and lower for eating, personal hygiene, and bathing (Nelson et al., 2002).

Strengths
- Consistency with the MDS items makes completion of the SCA straightforward for clinicians in settings requiring the MDS, and should facilitate team communication.
- Observation of details within each sub-occupation provides clinicians with rich information for intervention planning.

Weaknesses
- Although the SCA is part of the Melville Nelson Occupational Therapy System for Skilled Nursing Facilities and Subacute Rehabilitation, it is not clear how the SCA relates to those other components, or how the three components should be used together.
- A ceiling effect was noted for discharge scores on the SCA, which is hypothesized to be related to the inclusion of the MDS items only, which tend to focus on basic rather than more complex ADL activities.

Final Word
- The SCA appears to offer occupational therapists working in SNFs and subacute rehabilitation an observation-based ADL assessment with enough detail to generate intervention plans. Further research is required on its psychometric properties. Information on its responsiveness suggests that it will be most useful for patients who are expected to have long stays with many self-care issues.

Table 11-13

PATIENT SPECIFIC FUNCTION SCALE (PSFS)

Source	Stratford, P., Gill, C., Westaway, M., & Binkley, J. (1995). Assessing disability and change on individual patients: A report of a patient specific measure. *Physiotherapy Canada, 47*, 258-263.
Important References	As above.
Purpose	• To provide a standardized measure for assessing the client's problems.
Type of Client	• Other than having the cognitive ability to identify current problems, the measure was designed to be used with any diagnosis.
Clinical Utility	
Format	• Therapist administered.
Procedures	• The therapist asks the client to identify up to five important activities that they are unable to or are having difficulty to perform. Clients then rate the difficulty on an 11-point scale.
	• Individual item as well as an activity summary score can be used.
Completion Time	• Approximately 4 minutes to clients with orthopedic conditions (Chatman, Hyams, Neel, Binkley, Stratford, Schomberg, & Stabler, 1997).
Standardization	• Specific wording for eliciting the response from the client is provided.
Reliability	
Internal Consistency	• N=38 adults with knee dysfunction, coefficient α, 0.97 (Chatman et al., 1997).
Inter Observer	• Not applicable.
Test-Retest	• N=63 adults with low back pain, intraclass correlation (ICC) for activity summary scores = 0.97 (Stratford et al., 1995).
	• N=31 adults with cervical dysfunction, ICC=0.91 for individual activities (Westaway, Stratford, & Binkley, 1998).
	• N=38 adults with knee dysfunction, ICC for item, R-0,84, ICC for activity summary, R=0.87 (Chatman et al., 1997).
Validity	• Note that the items identified by the client may or may not match those items contained in standardized assessments, thus negatively affecting construct validity.
Content	• Most important items are identified by the client.
Criterion	• Not addressed in studies reviewed.
Construct	• N=63 adults with low back pain, compared to the Roland-Morris Questionnaire (RMQ), r=0.59 to 0.74 (Stratford et al., 1995); n=31.
	• Adults with cervical dysfunction, r=0.74 to 0.80.
	• N=38 adults with knee dysfunction, compared to the SF-36 physical function domain, Pearson coefficients at baseline, 0.34, at follow-up 0.49 (Chatman et al., 1997).
Responsiveness to Change	• Pengel, Refshauge, and Maher (2004) found that the PSFS is more responsive to change compared with the RMQ and a pain scale (visual analog), while Westaway et al., (1998) demonstrated correlations with change in the neck disability index ranging from 0.79 to 0.81 for the first three activities.
Strengths	• This assessment is easy to use.
	• Reliability, validity and responsiveness to change have been demonstrated.
	• Client-centred approach to determining functional deficits.

continued

Table 11-13 (continued)

PATIENT SPECIFIC FUNCTION SCALE (PSFS)

Weaknesses	• The client must agree to participate in the process.
	• May still need more specific instruments to identify specifics of problems.
	• All psychometric testing done on a quite healthy adult orthopedic population.
Final Word	• This measure has promise both clinically and for research since it is brief and simple and seems to be demonstrating reasonable psychometric properties.

Table 11-14

PEDIATRIC EVALUATION OF DISABILITY INVENTORY (PEDI)

Source	Center for Rehabilitation Effectiveness, Boston University, 635 Commonwealth Avenue, Boston, MA, 02215, (phone) 617-358-0175, (fax) 612-353-7500, (e-mail) smhaley@bu.edu, (Web) http://www.bu.edu/cre/pedi/
Important References	Feldman, A. B., Haley, S. M., & Coryell, J. (1990). Concurrent and construct validity of the Pediatric Evaluation of Disability Inventory. *Physical Therapy, 70,* 602-610.
	Haley, S. M., Coster, W. J., Ludlow, L. H., Haltiwanger, J. T., & Andrellos, P. J. (1992). *Pediatric Evaluation of Disability Inventory (PEDI) Version 1.0: Development, standardization and administration manual.* Boston, MA: Trustees of Boston University, Center for Rehabilitation Effectiveness.
	Iyer, L. V., Haley, S. M., Watkins, M. P., & Dumas, H. M. (2003). Establishing minimal clinically important differences for scores on the Pediatric Evaluation of Disability Inventory for inpatient rehabilitation. *Physical Therapy, 83,* 888-898.
Purpose	• Designed for three purposes: to describe a child's functional status; for program evaluation of inpatient, outpatient, and school-based programs; and to monitor change in individuals or groups of children with functional disabilities.
Type of Client	• Designed for children between 6 months and 7.5 years (or older if their functional development is significantly delayed). It can be used with many diagnostic groups.
Clinical Utility	
Format	• Organized into three measurement dimensions: functional skills, caregiver assistance, and modifications. Each of these is organized into self-care, mobility, and social function.
	• The functional skills measure is organized hierarchically based on the order in which skills are typically achieved by children. Each item is scored on a capable/not capable dichotomous scale.
	• The caregiver assistance scale explores the amount of assistance the child requires in task areas that are more general than the specific items in the functional skills area. Each item is rated on a 6-item scale from total assistance to independence.
	• The modifications scale allows consideration of the frequency that modifications (either typical modifications used by children, or specific modifications used by children with disabilities) are used.
Procedures	• Either parents or professionals (health or educational) can complete the instrument. Parents can typically complete the functional skills component independently, as long as someone familiar with the PEDI reviews it with them afterward.
	• The caregiver assistance and modifications scales are more demanding to understand and may best be completed with structured interview with parents.
	• There is a computer program available to assist with scoring or it can be scored manually. Raw scores, normative standard scores, or scaled scores can be used.
	• It is possible to use only specific components of the instrument if appropriate for the child. Research indicates the self-care classification system seemed to reflect clinically important changes in skills between admission and discharge from an inpatient rehabilitation setting (Dumas, Haley, Fragala, & Steva, 2001).
Completion Time	• It can take 45 to 60 minutes to complete the instrument by interviewing parents; 20 to 30 minutes if a professional is completing it based on observations of the child.

continued

Table 11-14 (continued)

PEDIATRIC EVALUATION OF DISABILITY INVENTORY (PEDI)

Standardization
- The manual for the PEDI (Haley et al., 1992) is comprehensive. Norms are included based on a sample of 412 children from the northeastern United States. Clinical interpretation of scores is discussed by Haley, Ludlow, & Coster (1993).
- A computerized version of the PEDI has been developed and initial testing undertaken (Center for Rehabilitation Effectiveness, n.d.). Dutch, Norwegian, Spanish and Swedish versions are described in the literature with some psychometric testing done on most of the translations (Berg, Jahnsen, Frøslie, & Hussain, 2004; Custers et al., 2002; Gannotti & Cruz, 2001; Nordmark, Jarnlo, & Hagglund, 2000; Wassenberg-Severijen, Custers, Hox, Vermeer, & Helders, 2003).

Reliability
- Overall, the reliability of the PEDI is excellent. A number of studies have been undertaken by the developers as well as others, although the sample sizes tend to be small.

Internal Consistency
- Using the normative sample (n=412), Cronbach's α ranged from 0.95 to 0.99 (Haley et al., 1992).

Inter-Rater
- Intra-class correlation coefficients ranged from 0.96 to 0.99 for caregiver assistance scales (Haley et al., 1992).
- Children with disabilities (n=12); intra-class correlation coefficients ranged from 0.84 to 1.00 for caregiver assistance and modifications scales (Sundberg, 1992 as cited in Reid, Boschen, & Wright, 1993). Children with disabilities attending a rehabilitation day program (n=24);
- Comparison of responses from parent and rehabilitation team members; intra-class correlation coefficients ranged from 0.74 to 0.96, except the social function modifications scale (0.30) (Haley et al., 1992).
- Children receiving inpatient or outpatient rehabilitation (n=41): 0.83 (ICC) for self-care, and and 0.89 for self-care caregiver assistance (Ziviani et al., 2001).
- Children receiving occupational or physical therapy in the midwest United States (n=17); comparing parent and therapist ratings; intra-class correlation coefficients ranged from 0.2 to 0.93 for functional skill scales; 0.15 to 0.95 on the caregiver assistance scales (in both cases most were over 0.6) (Nichols & Case-Smith, 1996).

Intra-Rater
- Children receiving occupational or physical therapy in the Midwest United States (n=23); two interviews conducted by the same interviewer 1 week apart; intra-class correlation coefficients ranged from 0.67 to 1.00 on the functional skill scales, and 0.68 to 0.90 for the caregiver assistance scale (Nichols & Case-Smith, 1996).

Test-Retest
- Children with varying severities of cerebral palsy aged 3 to 7 years (n=21); four respondents (primary caregiver, classroom teacher, occupational therapist, and physical therapist) rated the child on two occasions 3 weeks apart; intra-class correlation coefficients all over 0.95 for total scores and above 0.80 for the three domains (Wright & Boschen, 1993).

Validity
- The validity of the PEDI overall is quite strong, with a mix of studies conducted by the developers and others.

Content
- When the instrument was developed, the content was evaluated by expert ratings of 31 people who reviewed its content. As well, Rasch modeling has been used to validate the content in terms of the developmental sequence of the tasks involved (Haley et al., 1992).

continued

Table 11-14 (continued)

PEDIATRIC EVALUATION OF DISABILITY INVENTORY (PEDI)

Convergent	• PEDI scores have been compared to a number of other developmental instruments with positive results, including the Battelle Developmental Inventory Screening Test (results ranged from 0.62 to 0.97) (Feldman, Haley, & Coryell, 1990), the WeeFIM (results ranged from 0.80 to 0.97) (Schultz as cited in Reid et al., 1993) and from 0.76 to 0.94 (spearman correlations) when PEDI self care scores were compared to WeeFIM subscales (Ziviani et al., 2001), the Gross Motor Function Measure (0.75 to 0.85) (Wright & Boschen, 1993), and the Peabody Developmental Motor Scales (0.24 to 0.95) (Nichols & Case-Smith, 1996).
Construct	• The developers examined the relationship between age and PEDI scores and found support for the hypothesis that scores increased with age. These data were also used to support hypotheses about the ability of the PEDI to differentiate between functional skills and caregiver assistance as separate constructs (Haley et al., 1992).
	• Children with spina bifida (n=63): PEDI scaled scores on ADL correlated with parent ratings of ADL independence (Tsai, Yang, Chan, Huang, & Wong, 2002).
	• Children with CP seen at a paediatric therapy centre (n=18): PEDI scores were correlated with the Melbourne Assessment of Unilateral Upper Limb Function with r=0.939 for the PEDI self-care component (Bourke-Taylor, 2003).
Responsiveness to Change	• PEDI scores were compared across time in two clinical samples. The scores changed in the expected direction in the two clinical groups, providing an indication of the PEDI's responsiveness (Haley et al., 1992).
	• Children with spastic diplegia undergoing selective dorsal rhizotomy (n=18): Scaled scores on the functional and caregiver assessment scales changed significantly between preoperative and 6 and 12 months postoperative assessments (normative scores did not change significantly) (Nordmark et al., 2000).
	• Children discharged from inpatient rehabilitation (n=53): In a sample of 53 children discharged from inpatient rehabilitation, a change of 11 points in the scaled score was estimated to be the minimal clinically important difference (Iyer, Haley, Watkins, & Dumas, 2003).
Strengths	• Well-developed and standardized instrument.
	• Appears to comprehensively evaluate function in young children.
	• Could be used to develop individual program plans, as well as program evaluation.
Weaknesses	• A ceiling effect may occur in some instances in ADL function for children with minimal impairment (Dumas et al., 2001).
Final Word	• Overall, the PEDI appears to be an excellent tool to evaluate ADL as one component of function-and taps into both the capacity to complete tasks, as well as the amount of assistance and types of modifications used to enable function. Recent information about the minimal clinically important difference provides useful information for clinical and evaluative purposes.

Table 11-15

PHYSICAL SELF-MAINTENANCE SCALE (PSMS)

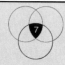

Source	Lawton, M. P., & Brody, E. M. (1969). Assessment of older people: Self-maintaining and instrumental activities of daily living. *The Gerontologist, 9*, 179-186.
Important References	Edwards, M. M. (1990). The reliability and validity of self-report activities of daily living scales. *Canadian Journal of Occupational Therapy, 57*, 273-278.
	Rubenstein, L. Z., Schairer, C., Wieland, G. D., & Kane, R. (1984). Systematic biases in functional status assessment of elderly adults: Effects of different data sources. *Journal of Gerontology, 39(6)*, 686-691.
Purpose	• Designed to measure basic self-care skills.
Type of Client	• Designed for use with older clients (over 60 years).

Clinical Utility

Format
- Consists of six items: toileting, feeding, dressing, grooming, physical ambulation, and bathing. In its original format, there are four levels of independence noted, but the person is scored 1 for independence and 0 if he or she requires other assistance. However, many users have adopted a 4-point rating scale.

Procedures
- The instrument can be administered based on observation or self-report. However, Settle and Holm (1993) note that without observation, the clinical usefulness of the PSMS is diminished for individual program planning.

Completion Time
- 20 to 30 minutes.

Standardization
- There are no formal instructions and no manual.
- Although not norms, Lawton (1988) cites mean scores on the PSMS as 20.61 for a sample of 253 community residents, 20.77 for a sample of 173 older adults living in public housing, 19.26 for 99 people receiving in-home services and 18.51 for 65 people on institutional waiting lists. These data are based on 7 items (transferring and getting outside were added and grooming removed) rated on a 3-point scale for each item.

Reliability

Internal Consistency
- Adults over 60 years from a variety of institutional and community service provider agencies (n=265): reproducibility coefficient of 0.96 reported (Lawton & Brody, 1969).

Observer (Inter-Rater)
- Patients over 60 with various self-care deficits (n=36); correlation of 0.87 (Pearson r) (Lawton & Brody, 1969).
- Patients on a geriatric assessment or reactivation unit over 65 (n=30); 0.96 (ICCs) (Edwards, 1990).
- Community dwelling and institutionalized older adults (n=76): 92% agreement (Boyd & Dawson, 2000)

Test-Retest
- Patients (impaired and non-impaired) (n=44); correlation of 0.91 (Pearson r) (Lawton & Brody, 1969).
- Patients on a geriatric assessment or reactivation unit over 65 (n=30), 1 week between ratings: 0.56 (ICCs) (Edwards [1990] notes that changes in status may have changed in some subjects in 1 week).

Validity

Content
- The items included in the PSMS were derived from literature review and primarily the Langley-Porter Neuropsychiatric Institute ADL Scale. It covers the main areas of personal ADL.

continued

Table 11-15 (continued)

PHYSICAL SELF-MAINTENANCE SCALE (PSMS)

Criterion	• Not reported in the studies reviewed.
Construct	• Edwards (1990) found that the PSMS distinguished between seniors discharged home vs those discharged to institutional settings.
	• In two studies (Edwards, 1990; Rubenstein et al., 1984), significantly different scores were noted for self-report vs direct observation, indicating that the two methods of data collection cannot be used interchangeably.
Convergent	• The PSMS has been examined in terms of its relationship to a number of other instruments. Geriatric inpatients (n=180): Lawton & Brody IADL Scale (r=0.61); physicians' ratings of physical capacity (r=0.62); mental status questionnaire (r=0.38), and a behavior and adjustment rating scale (r=0.38) (Lawton & Brody, 1969).
	• Patients on a geriatric assessment or reactivation unit over 65 (n=30): the mini--mental status exam (r=0.19), the FIM (r=0.70), the geriatric depression scale (r=0.25) (Edwards, 1990).
	• Community dwelling and institutionalized older adults (n=76): OSOT perceptual assessment r=0.435 and MMSE r=0.246 (Spearman Correlation), demonstrating a relationship between perceptual and (to a lesser extent) cognitive status and ADL performance (Boyd & Dawson, 2000).
Responsiveness to Change	• Frail older adults (n= 265): responsiveness of the PSMS discussed compared to goal attainment scaling, the Barthel, and IADL measure and a quality of life index. Statistics on the responsiveness of the total PSMS are not provided; the PSMS is more responsive than the Barthel on three of four indicators of responsiveness (Rockwood, et al., 2003).
Strengths	• Brief and flexible use, covers major areas of ADL.
	• Adequate reliability and validity.
	• For individual program planning, it would be best to use it with observation of task performance (since there are not enough items or detail within the items to give a therapist direction for intervention).
Weaknesses	• There is not enough information about its responsiveness to change, which limits its usefulness in evaluation.
Final Word	• The PSMS is a useful instrument that covers basic self-care skills in older adults and can be used at individual or group levels for description and evaluation.

Editors' Notes for Chapter 12

Mine the Gold

Occupational therapy practice has embraced basic activities of daily living (BADL). However, people, those we serve, define themselves not only with regard to their ability to perform self-care—but also by their participation in activities that are instrumental to their daily lives. Instrumental activities of daily living (IADL) are activities that sustain independence, require a higher level of physical and cognitive competency than BADL and include paying bills, preparing meals, housekeeping, driving, enjoying the garden, going to church, taking care of pets, and other related activities. These important activities are based on the needs and want of individuals and reflect cultural and personal preferences.

Become Systematic

By using IADL measures it is possible to characterize the level of functioning that a person is able to participate in and learn of those activities that are important to the person and his or her family. Instrumental activities require cognitive, physiological, psychological, and neurobehavioral capacities and can be the central focus of a rehabilitation plan.

Use Evidence in Practice

IADL measurement should command a central position in occupational therapy practice. By recording the activities the person wants and needs to do to retain independence, it will be possible to make recommendations to the client, to the family, and to agencies about the person's capacity.

Make Occupational Therapy Contribution Explicit

People's activities occur in a context; ideally, measurement of IADL capacity should occur in the specific environment where the activity typically is performed. Many IADL occur as part of rituals and routines and, if so, these must be observed, as testing out of context may unnecessarily limit the person's performance.

Engage in Occupation-Based, Client-Centered Practice

Occupation—the tasks, activities, and roles that the person defines as meaningful—are characterized in IADL. By focusing therapy goals on what the person wants and needs to do, an occupational therapy program meets the objective of client-centered practice. Also, of importance is that IADL are linked to life satisfaction and quality of life.

MEASURING PERFORMANCE IN INSTRUMENTAL ACTIVITIES OF DAILY LIVING

Laura N. Gitlin, PhD

WHAT ARE INSTRUMENTAL ACTIVITIES OF DAILY LIVING?

This chapter discusses Instrumental Activities of Daily Living (IADL) and their measurement, an important but frequently overlooked aspect of a comprehensive functional assessment for youths as well as young and older adults with cognitive, psychiatric, and/or physical impairment.

Lawton & Brody (1969) initially delineated IADL in 1969. Whereas Activities of Daily Living (ADL) refer to life-sustaining and basic self-care practices (e.g., feeding, dressing, bathing), Lawton & Brody suggested that IADL represent a secondary set of tasks essential to independent community living. They identified eight activities that reflect the core of this construct: managing money, using the telephone, taking medication, traveling, shopping, preparing meals, doing laundry, and housekeeping. Today, the centrality of IADL to quality of life and general well-being of individuals with disability is widely recognized. There is, however, no consensus as to the specific activities that are necessary for independent community living. Thus, although the eight activities first identified by Lawton & Brody remain central to this construct, there is wide variation in the number and type of activities that are included in more recently developed IADL measures (Gitlin, in press).

In a review of functional measures, Barer & Nouri (1989) categorized IADL items as representing three types of activities: getting about (e.g., using transportation, walking outside, getting into/out of cars, driving), house-hold-based activities (e.g., laundry, meal and snack preparation, housework), and other leisure-oriented activities (e.g., gardening, driving). Regardless of the specific items that are included in IADL measures, the activities they represent share important characteristics.

One important characteristic is that IADL represent activities within the disability and social limitation levels of the Nagi model of disablement (1979) and the disability and participation levels of the proposed revision of the International Classification of Impairments, Disabilities and Handicaps (ICIDH) (WHO, 1998). Deficits in IADL therefore reflect a combination of an underlying impairment (e.g., motor, psychiatric, cognitive), functional limitation (e.g., judgment, problem-solving), and the physical and social context of performance. Thus, to assess IADL status, it is important to understand both the context of performance as well as the underlying impairment in order to develop an appropriate treatment plan.

Another important characteristic is that IADL represent multi-step activities that are complex to perform. Performance can occur either inside or outside the home and requires the use of objects that are external to the individual, such as a telephone or other special instruments or tools. Independent performance requires a high level of social, physical, and mental skills such as judgment, initiation, sequencing, and problem-solving.

Furthermore, motivation, as well as personal preference and lifestyle choices, strongly influence performance capabilities. Some IADL tasks are gender and culturally specific, such as housekeeping, meal preparation, or financial management. For example, older men often report dependency in housekeeping or meal preparation because of long-standing behavioral preferences to disengage from these activities. Older women also tend to be dependent in money management due to their role history, as opposed to the consequence of a physical or cognitive deficit. Therefore, ratings of performance along these and other IADL items may suggest deficits, when in actuality it is the influence of personal preference or the physical and social environment that contributes to IADL behaviors.

In summary, the performance of IADL requires a much higher level of competency than that required for successful participation in ADL. It stands to reason that IADL represent one of the first performance domains affected by a disabling condition. Recent research has shown a hierarchical structure of dependency onset among individuals with chronic illness and physical disability. This population tends to experience ambulation difficulties initially, then IADL deficits, and lastly, ADL deficits in a somewhat sequential, overlapping order (Dunlop, Hughes, & Manheim, 1997). However, the underlying pattern of dependency or decline among the items traditionally included in IADL measures is not known. Decline in the ability to perform IADL may not occur progressively or follow a particular sequence or predictable order. That is, there does not appear to be a linear trend such that individuals experience a decline in successive fashion from one IADL activity to the next. Since each IADL requires different mental and physical functions, deficits can reflect an underlying motor or cognitive impairment, or a combination.

CLINICAL UTILITY OF IADL ASSESSMENT

Whereas the assessment of ADL is a routine component of occupational therapy (Law & Letts, 1989), that is not the case for IADL status. IADL assessments are still not well-recognized and tend to be used with less frequency in treatment (Wolf, 1997). However, consideration of IADL status is an important component of a comprehensive health assessment and clinical tool to guide treatment planning and therapeutic decision-making, especially for people with physical, psychiatric, or cognitive impairments (Gromak & Waskel, 1989). Disability represents a major adverse outcome of both aging and chronic illness that can impact performance of activities essential to independent community living. Deficits in IADL performance, in turn, have been shown to predict poor future health and functional status. Specifically, research suggests that IADL deficits are associated with age, risk of decline in ADL, comorbidity, hospitalization, and mortality (Kovar & Lawton, 1994).

Who specifically should be assessed for IADL status? The assessment of IADL status is particularly critical for older people, especially those with one or more chronic conditions (Andresen, Rothenberg, & Zimmer, 1997). The National Institutes of Health recommends the assessment of both ADL and IADL status as critical elements of a comprehensive geriatric assessment. Of utmost importance is the assessment of IADL status of older people with chronic illness following an acute hospital episode. This group, in particular, has been shown to experience reduced functional capacity and be at high risk of further functional decline (Hirsch, Sommers, Olsen, Mullen, & Winograd, 1990).

The assessment of IADL status is also very important for persons with mental illness and patients with traumatic brain injury who are preparing to return to community living (Rogers, Holm, Goldstein, McCue, & Nussbaum, 1994). In addition, an IADL assessment provides meaningful information when working with individuals who have Alzheimer's disease or a related disorder, or for those who experience a change in cognitive status. Research has shown that deficits in four IADL, in particular, are correlated with cognitive impairment. These performance areas include telephone use, transportation use, taking medication, and managing finances (Barberger-Gateau et al., 1992). Consequently, assessing IADL status is critical for the provision of individualized quality care for both young and old clinical populations with disability and for individuals in which a change in cognitive status is suspected.

Likewise, it is important to recognize for whom an IADL assessment is not relevant. The traditional IADL items and response options offered on most measures do not adequately differentiate among individuals without impairment or well populations. There is a ceiling effect in that IADL items cannot discriminate among groups, such as the well elderly or young and middle-aged adults with intact competence in daily living. A more useful approach with these populations is to assess what is sometimes referred to as "extended function," or higher order cognitive and motor abilities, such as leisure activity participation, exercise, driving, balance, and endurance.

CONSIDERATIONS IN MEASURING IADL

There is little consensus in the clinical and research communities as to how to assess IADL and rate performance capabilities. Although there are a number of standardized measures available for use by health professionals and researchers, each tool approaches measurement differently. On what basis then should a tool be selected? There are seven basic considerations in choosing an appropriate measure of IADL status. These are summarized in Table 12-1.

Table 12-1

SUMMARY OF SEVEN MEASUREMENT CONSIDERATIONS

Aspects to Consider	*Factors*
Purpose	• Discharge planning • Eligibility for services • Evaluation of treatment outcomes • Survey research • Evaluation in effectiveness studies
Population	• Age • Cognitive status • Cultural background
Psychometric properties	• Manualized • Known reliability • Known validity • Sensitivity to change
Information source	• Self-report • Proxy • Observation • Chart extraction
Item selection	• Congruence of items with treatment • Global, task-oriented, or process-type items • Cultural familiarity with test items
Response set	• Dependence vs difficulty • Capability vs actual performance
Client-centered vs standard	• Personal preference in selection of task performance vs gold standard approach

Purpose

Foremost in choosing a measure is to determine the specific purpose of the IADL assessment. An IADL assessment may be used to inform discharge planning, determine eligibility for a health or human service program, evaluate outcomes of a therapeutic intervention, describe populations in survey research, or evaluate treatment effectiveness in intervention studies. With regard to the clinical context, if the purpose of assessment is to inform discharge planning, then an approach that accounts for client preferences, safety of performance, and availability of social support is important. The issue of safe performance, especially with regard to independent travel, meal preparation, and medication taking, is perhaps chief among the performance concerns of therapists in developing a plan for discharge. The Performance Assessment of Self-Care Skills (PASS-Clinic or Home versions; see review of tool) for example is one of the few assessments that include a rating for safety and adequacy of performance in addition to determining level of independence.

Conversely, if the purpose is to determine eligibility for services, then an assessment that provides a rating of dependency level is appropriate. Dependency in an IADL is frequently used to identify individuals at risk and in need of specialized home care. The Caregiver Assessment of Function and Upset (CAFU, see review of tool) is an example of a measure that asks caregivers to rate the level of dependence on IADL tasks of their family member with dementia along a 7-point scale. Still another approach to measuring IADL status is required if the purpose of the assessment is to evaluate therapeutic outcomes. In this case, a measure that includes items that are relevant to the content of treatment and rates performance using a response set that is sensitive to change is preferable. For example, a measure that rates level of performance difficulty along a 3-point scale (1=no difficulty, 2=some difficult, 3=cannot do at all) may not adequately detect some

Table 12-2

SUMMARY OF MAJOR STRENGTHS AND LIMITATIONS OF SOURCES OF INFORMATION

Source of Information	Strength	Limitation
Self-report	• Ease of administration • Face-to-face, by telephone,	• Individuals rate themselves more independent than proxies
Proxy	• Useful with the cognitively impaired and very disabled	• Families report more disability than patient • Factors that influence family ratings are unknown
Performance-based	• Useful with cognitively impaired • Most objective measure	• Unclear how to interpret item incompletion • Unclear role of motivation • Requires trained tester and/or special props making broad application difficult
Medical records	• Low cost • Nurse documentation better than physicians	• Document may not be standardized • Low agreement between OT, nurse, and self-report ratings

of the small but important changes in IADL performance following an occupational therapy intervention that improves caregiver set-up and cueing techniques. Finally, if the purpose of the assessment is to describe population trends in IADL status in epidemiological or other survey-type research, then a measure that yields gross ratings, such as the response set in the previous example, may be adequate.

Population

The choice of an IADL measure will also depend, in part, on the population. Person-based characteristics such as age, cognitive status, and cultural background may affect the approach to obtaining information about IADL status and the specific items that may be amenable to assessment. For example, reliance on self-report of IADL status for individuals with severe psychiatric or cognitive impairment may not yield reliable ratings, or young adults may not have experience with financial or household management. The use of a standard measure that includes these items would therefore provide an inconclusive understanding of actual IADL performance and potential capabilities.

Psychometric Properties

Another consideration in choosing an IADL measure is whether the tool conforms to standards of measurement. It is important that the IADL assessment is manualized such that adequate instructions are provided to standardize its delivery. Standardization is important in order to ensure a

uniform approach so that derived ratings reflect real performance and not the biases or personal therapeutic styles of raters. Furthermore, as discussed in Chapters 2 and 3, it is preferable to use an assessment with known inter-rater reliability and test-retest reliability than a homegrown approach or a measure that lacks adequate psychometric properties. This ensures that the measure yields ratings that are invariant over time and across environmental contexts and raters. Also, using an assessment that has content, discriminatory, and construct validity is essential to ensure its ecological validity and adequacy. If the purpose of an assessment is to evaluate the effectiveness of occupational therapy treatment, then a measure with tested sensitivity to detect changes in IADL status would be important to select.

Thus, an IADL assessment should be chosen that is standardized and has adequate reliability and validity in order to minimize false positives and negatives and sensitivity to change. This is essential in order to ensure cost-effective and appropriate service provision (DePoy & Gitlin, 2005).

Source

Yet another consideration in measuring IADL status is the source from which evaluative judgments about a person's capabilities are obtained. There are four basic sources of information about IADL status: self-report, proxy, direct observation, or medical chart extraction. Each source has its strengths and limitations, as summarized in Table 12-2.

Self-Report

Self-report involves asking a client to rate him- or herself with regard to either the level of difficulty or dependence in each IADL. This approach can be conducted face-to-face, through a mail survey, or over the telephone. It does not require the expertise of a therapist to complete the assessment and is a quick, relatively simple, and cost-effective approach to obtaining IADL status. This approach is most useful in research, but it can also be used for clinical purposes. However, dependence on self-report does have its limitations. Clients tend to overestimate their abilities, underestimate their level of dependence, and are often unaware of their engagement in unsafe IADL practices. Also, little is known about the factors that influence self-ratings. Recent research shows that a low sense of personal mastery and depressive symptomatology may lead to the underestimation of performance capabilities (Kempen, Steverink, Ormel, & Deeg, 1996). It remains unclear as to the other factors that may effect self-ratings.

Proxy

The use of proxies is another source of IADL information. This approach involves asking a close family member or health professional to rate an individual's IADL status using a standard measure. As in self-report, ratings from a proxy can be derived in a face-to-face interview, telephone interview, or a mail survey. This approach provides helpful information, especially about patients who are cognitively or severely physically impaired and who may be unable to self-report their performance with accuracy. However, it is unclear as to the factors that influence the ratings of a proxy. A growing body of research on the relationship between proxy and self-report suggests that ratings from proxies can be biased. A recent study showed that the more burden a family caregiver feels, the greater likelihood that he or she will exaggerate the level of disability, compared with self-ratings by the older person (Long, Sudha, & Mutran, 1998).

Direct Observation

A typical self-report or proxy measure of IADL status yields a global rating of capability. It does not inform the clinician as to the specific aspects of an activity that may be difficult or, conversely, easy for a client to perform. In contrast, measures that use direct observation of real-time performance are task-oriented. That is, the performance of each step or component of an activity is observed and rated for its successful completion along a number of dimensions, including the time for activity completion and the need for and amount of verbal and/or tactile cueing. This enables the clinician to make a judgment as to the particular aspects of an activity that can and cannot be performed independently. Thus, a more accurate representation of strengths and deficits can be discerned.

Performance-based measures offer a more precise diagnostic tool to guide intervention and are especially useful with psychiatric and cognitively impaired patients.

Nevertheless, this approach does have several limitations. First, performance-based measures need to be administered by highly trained raters and thus are more costly to administer. Second, the assessment process typically requires special set-up or stations in a clinic (e.g., use of the cafeteria) or home setting that may not be feasible to implement. Third, this approach can be time-consuming even though only a few select IADL areas are observed. Another concern is that observing an individual simulate an activity in a clinical setting may still not provide an objective assessment of how an individual performs in his or her own environmental context. There is little research to date from which to determine whether a simulated context is ecologically valid or that ratings derived in the clinic reflect real-life performance. The environment, however, appears to have a clear effect on performance. One recent study of 20 persons with severe mental illness showed inconsistent performance across assessment sites and found a trend toward false positives. That is, some participants who were judged to be independent on the IADL assessment performed in a simulated setting were unable to perform the same tasks in their natural environment (Brown, Moore, Hemman, & Yunek, 1996). Another study with 20 older adults living in the community found that process skill abilities (e.g., ability to initiate and sequence) were affected by the environment more so than motor skills (e.g., ability to grasp, reach, or bend). Older people tended to perform process skills significantly better in their homes than in the clinic (Park, Fisher, & Velozo, 1993). These studies support the viewpoint that IADL assessments need to be conducted within the actual context in which performance occurs. The findings are consistent with clinical perspectives previously expressed in occupational therapy that emphasize the impact of environmental factors on occupational performance (Dunn, Brown, & McGuigan, 1994).

Finally, most performance-based measures include the observation of only a few areas of IADL status. However, it remains unclear as to whether ratings derived from the observation of one activity can be generalized to performance areas that are not observed.

The interest in performance-based measures is relatively recent. More research is required to understand what is actually being measured by this approach, the factors that influence discrepancies between self-report and direct observation, and the validity of ratings derived in simulated settings.

Chart Extraction

Another common source of IADL information is recordings in medical charts. This of course is an inexpensive, relatively easy approach from which to derive an assessment of IADL status. However, studies have shown differences among health professionals, and particularly between occupational therapists and nurses, as to how each profession rates IADL and ADL status of patients. Also, documentation may not be consistently recorded in charts or only select IADL may be notated. Finally, it is usually unclear whether medical chart ratings reflect scores derived from a standard assessment or reflect anecdotal comments or casual clinical observations.

Item Selection

Another consideration in selecting a measure is evaluating whether the items included in the tool are adequate for the purpose of the assessment. Three different approaches to item selection can be found in IADL measures. One approach is to include items in the measure that reflect broad activities as exemplified by the eight traditional items in Lawton's and Brody's (1969) IADL scale. Other more recently developed measures have used the same approach but include additional activities, such as leisure, work, or play. In this approach, individuals are assessed as to their level of difficulty or dependency in performing each activity. This approach to item inclusion yields a global score of performance. Measures do not account for personal preference, motivation, cultural background, or performance along specific components of the activity.

Another more clinically useful approach is task-oriented. A task-oriented approach, as exemplified by the Performance Assessment of Self-Care Skills (PASS) (1994) by Rogers et al., assesses the ability to perform each component of a complex activity. For example, a few sub-tasks involved in telephone use include looking up a telephone number, recognizing telephone signals, and dialing a number. An assessment of performance of each of these components yields an understanding of the aspects of telephone use an individual can accomplish independently, with cueing or set-up, or is unable to complete independently. This provides more detailed and precise information for treatment planning and implementation. Measures that use a task-oriented approach tend to be performance-based.

Another more recent approach to item inclusion is to focus on the underlying processes involved in performing an IADL. This approach observes clients simulating select activities, such as meal preparation in Baum and Edwards' (1994) Kitchen Task Assessment (KTA), as a means to explore underlying motor and cognitive processes involved in performance. This approach is also exemplified by Fisher's (1993, 1997) Assessment of Motor and Process Scale (AMPS). In this assessment, ratings are derived for the quality, effectiveness, and efficiency of motor and cognitive processing.

Response Set

Measures of IADL status use different response sets. One basic approach is to assess the level of dependency of the individual. Another is to assess the level of difficulty performing a task. These are distinct approaches that provide different types of information about a person's capabilities. Recent research suggests that assessments of level of difficulty yield substantially higher estimates of disability than scales that measure dependency (Kovar & Lawton, 1994; Gill & Kurland, 2003). Still other measures assess capability vs. actual abilities (e.g., "can do" vs "does"). This again is an important distinction that yields different understandings of a person's IADL status (Glass, 1998). Therefore, it is important to identify the specific type of ratings that reflect the purpose of the assessment and will yield clinically useful information.

Client-Centered vs Standard Approach

As discussed earlier, a distinguishing feature of IADL is the role of personal preference and lifestyle in shaping performance capability. An assessment of IADL status must be sensitive to a client's cultural background, motivations, and life choices. The relative benefits of a client-centered approach in occupational therapy as discussed in detail in Chapter 6 is relevant to a discussion of IADL measures as well. A client-centered approach seeks a detailed assessment of those areas of performance that are perceived by the client as important. Unfortunately, most existing IADL measures poorly account for personal preference and motivation. Also, they either exclude gender-biased items from the scale or overestimate dependence by their inclusion. More importantly, however, most assessments are evaluative and apply a gold standard of performance without accounting for the particular psychological, social, and physical environmental context.

SUMMARY OF SELECT IADL MEASURES

It is not possible to review the many published IADL scales within the scope of this chapter. Based on a systematic review of existing IADL measures, 12 were selected for discussion here. Measures were selected using the following criteria: 1) their potential utility for occupational therapy practice, 2) their inclusion of either components of an activity or at least two IADL, and 3) report on at least one aspect of their psychometric properties. Also, measures were selected to illustrate the range of approaches to item inclusion, source of information, and response sets. Of the 12 measures reviewed here, seven are designed specifically for use with patients with Alzheimer's disease or related disorders, and five are designed for use with a broad range of clinical populations, such as stroke patients and young and old adults with psychiatric or physical impairments or who are well.

Table 12-3 evaluates these measures along the seven measurement considerations discussed above. As shown, these scales are primarily for assessment purposes and most are relatively new and still in need of further psychometric testing.

Of the 12 measures, three reflect a global-item selection approach (Extended Activities of Daily Living Scale [EADL], IADL, and Canadian Occupational Performance Measure [COPM]); seven reflect a task-oriented approach to item selection (ADL Situational Test, Direct Assessment of Functional Abilities [DAFA], Caregiver Assessment of Function and Upset [CAFU], Direct Assessment of Functional Status [DAFS], PASS, Structured Assessment of Independent Living Skills [SAILS]), and the Test of Grocery Shopping Skills, and two reflect a process approach to item inclusion (e.g., KTA and AMPS). Furthermore, only two measures, the COPM and the AMPS, are client-centered and directly account for the influence of motivation, cultural background, and personal preferences in the design of the measure.

Measures for Persons With Dementia

Over the past decade, there has been an increased interest in developing adequate measures to evaluate persons with dementia. This is due primarily to three reasons. First, there are approximately 4.5 million Americans with the diagnosis of dementia, and this number is projected to increase exponentially as the baby boom generation advances in age (Brookmeyer, Gray, & Kraus, 1998). Second, as discussed earlier, decline in the performance of IADL has been shown to be an excellent indicator of cognitive impairment. Third, traditional IADL measures rely on self-report, an approach to assessment that yields overestimation of abilities among patients with dementia. Table 12-4 lists six relatively new measures of IADL status and their respective items for use with patients with Alzheimer's disease and related disorders. These measures also are summarized in Tables 12-6 through 12-9.

Each of the measures listed in Table 12-4 are performance-based except for the CAFU, but vary in the number of items that are assessed, the number and specific components of the tasks that are observed, time of administration, and psychometric properties. The CAFU is designed for use with family caregivers and provides a standardized approach by which clinicians can interview caregivers as to the level of assistance they are providing at home to their family member with dementia, as well as the caregivers reaction. While all of these measures as a whole are promising, they require more research to test their psychometric soundness. Also, these measures are designed for the purpose of assessment. They have not been evaluated for their sensitivity to detect change following an intervention.

The DAFS has been translated and administered to non-English-speaking patients, which gives it an added advantage. Both the ADL Situational Test and the KTA were developed by occupational therapists. These measures are advantageous to use because of their approach to the assessments of subtasks, which reflects the expertise in task analysis of occupational therapists. However, both require continued psychometric testing to fully evaluate their adequacy. The KTA has been criticized because of its exclusive focus on meal preparation and, specifically, the preparation of pudding. The issue of gender bias and the impact of previous exposure to pudding preparation on derived scores remain a concern. Of importance however, is that Baum & Edwards use the task of preparing pudding to examine fundamental cognitive processing skills such as initiation, organization, sequencing, safety, and judgment. These are critical components that underlie other IADL so that the level of support required by a dementia patient on this task may be transferable to other related performance domains. Nevertheless, transferability has not been tested empirically.

Measures for Physical Disability and Psychiatric Illness

Table 12-5 summarizes the items included in five IADL measures that can be used with individuals with physical, psychiatric, or cognitive impairments. These measures (except for the COPM) are also reviewed in Tables 12-6 through 12-13. As shown in Table 12-5, these measures vary with regard to the number and type of activities that are assessed. Of these measures, Lawton and Brody's (1969) IADL scale is perhaps the most widely used in both clinical and research communities and has the most extensive testing for its psychometric properties. Only the IADL and EADL scales have been used in research studies for repeated testing occasions.

The four other measures (PASS, COPM, AMPS, and Test of Grocery Shopping Skills) have been developed by occupational therapists and are relatively new. The PASS, a task-based scale, is quite extensive in that it assesses multiple components (independence, safety and quality and process of adequacy) of each activity included in the measure. Consequently, it is time-consuming to complete, although the amount of time varies by the client's level of competency.

The COPM has been discussed extensively in Chapter 6 and, thus, is only briefly mentioned here. There are three important advantages of the COPM as a measure of IADL status. First, it is one of the few assessments based in a client-centered framework. Second, it includes a wider range of performance areas than those typically included in other self-report and proxy measures, such as the IADL

Table 12-3

SUMMARY OF 12 IADL MEASURES AND THEIR CHARACTERISTICS

Scale	Population	Purpose	Psychometric Testing	Information Source	Type and # of IADL Domains	Response Set	Client Centered
ADL Situational Test[A]	Patients with dementia in	Assessment	Limited	Observation	Task-oriented K=4	0 (does not complete) to 4 (completes independently)	No
Assessment of Motor and Process Skills (AMPS)[A]	Range of populations	Assessment	Extensive	Observation	Process K=56 tasks	1=deficit 2=ineffective 3=questionable 4=competent	Yes
Canadian Occupational Performance Measure (COPM)[B]	Range of populations young and old	Assessment; treatment evaluation	Limited	Self-report; proxy	Global K=5	Performance • 1 (not able to do at all) to 10 (able to do extremely well) Satisfaction with performance • 1 (not satisfied at all) to 10 (extremely satisfied)	Yes
Direct Assessment of Functional Abilities (DAFA)[A] stages	Patients with dementia, mild to moderate	Assessment	Moderate	Observation	Task-oriented K=7	0 (independent functioning) to 3 (dependent functioning)	No
Direct Assessment of Functional Status (DAFS)[A]	Patients with dementia	Assessment	Moderate	Observation	Task-oriented K=5	Points given for each sub-task completed successfully	No
Extended Activities of Daily Living (EADL)[A]	Patients with stroke discharged from hospital	Assessment	Limited	Self-report; proxy	Global K=6	1 (unable to do) to 4 (does activity on own)	No

continued

Table 12-3 (continued)

SUMMARY OF 12 IADL MEASURES AND THEIR CHARACTERISTICS

Scale	Population	Purpose	Psychometric Testing	Information Source	Type and # of IADL Domains	Response Set	Client Centered
Instrumental Activities of (IADL)[A]	Range of population groups of elderly	Assessment	Extensive	Self-report	Global K=8	Varies by item (does activity, needs help, cannot do)	No
Kitchen Task Assessment (KTA)[A]	Patients with dementia at home	Assessment	Extensive	Observation	Process K=1	0=independent 1=required verbal cues 2=required physical 3=not capable	No
Performance Assessment of Self-Care (PASS)[A]	Geropsychiatry	Assessment	Limited	Observation	Task-oriented K=12	1 (normal performance) to 5 (maximum disability)	No
Structured Assessment of Independent Living Skills (SAILS)[A]	Patients with dementia	Assessment	Limited	Observation	Task-oriented K=6	0 (unable) to 3 (performs task)	No
Test of Grocery Shopping Skills	Persons with schizophrenia	Assessment;	Limited	Observation	Task-oriented K=1	Scored for accuracy, time, and efficiency	No
Caregiver Assessment of Function and Upset (CAFU)	Persons with dementia	Assessment of level of dependence, amount of caregiver assistance required; and caregiver level of upset	Moderate	Caregiver	Task-oriented K=8	1 (total dependence) to 7 (total independence)	No

A=Assessment is reviewed in this chapter; B=Assessment is reviewed in Chapter 6.

Table 12-4

IADL ASSESSMENTS FOR INDIVIDUALS WITH COGNITIVE IMPAIRMENT

IADL	Meal Prep	Finances	Telephone	Shopping	Travel	Laundry	Medication	Housekeeping	Other (Specify)
ADL Situational Test (Skurla et al., 1988)	X	X	X						
Direct Assessment of Functional Abilities (DAFA)* (Karagiozis et al., 1989)	X	X		X	X				X (Hobbies, awareness, reading)
Direct Assessment of Functional Status (DAFS)* (Loewenstein et al., 1989)	X	X	X	X					X (Preparing and mailing a letter)
Kitchen Task Assessment (KTA) (Baum et al., 1994)	X								
Structured Assessment of Independent Living Skills (SAILS)* (Mahurin et al., 1991)	X	X	X		X		X	X	X (Social interaction)
Caregiver Assessment of Function and Upset* (CAFU) (Gitlin et al., 2005)	X	X	X	X	X	X	X	X	X (Caregiver upset)

*Test also includes ADL items that are not reviewed here.

Table 12-5

IADL ASSESSMENTS FOR INDIVIDUALS WITH PHYSICAL, PSYCHIATRIC, OR COGNITIVE IMPAIRMENT

IADL	Meal Prep	Finances	Telephone	Shopping	Travel	Laundry	Medication	Housekeeping	Other (Specify)
Assessment of Motor and Process Skills (AMPS) (Fisher, 1991)	X	X	X	X	X	X	X	X	X (56 tasks possible to observe)
Canadian Occupational Performance Measure (COPM)* (Law et al., 1994)	X	X		X	X			X	X (Work: paid/unpaid, play, homework, leisure, socialization)
Extended Activities of Daily Living (EADL)* (Nouri et al., 1987)		X	X	X		X		X	X (Leisure, drive a car, socialization)
Instrumental Activities of Daily Living (IADL) (Lawton & Brody, 1969)	X	X	X	X	X	X	X	X	
Performance Assessment of Self-Care Skills (PASS)*	X	X	X	X		X	X		X (Safety, sew a button, prepare an envelope for mailing)

*Test also includes ADL items that are not reviewed here.

Table 12-6

ADL SITUATIONAL TEST

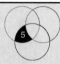

Source	Skurla, E., Rogers, J. C., & Sunderland, T. (1988). Direct Assessment of Activities of Daily Living in Alzheimer's disease. A controlled study. *Journal of the American Geriatrics Society, 36*, 97-103.
Purpose	• The ADL Situational Test is designed as a direct measure of functional performance in dementia patients.
Type of Client	• Dementia patients.
Clinical Utility	
Format	• The ADL Situational Test is completed by a health professional in a clinical setting. This is a direct measure of performance capacity
Procedures	• The test includes 4 tasks: dressing, meal preparation, purchasing, and telephone. Each task is broken down into subtasks (dressing=10 subtasks; meal prep=9; telephone=11; and purchasing=8.). Each task is set up in situations around a room. Specified visual, physical, and verbal prompting are used if patient cannot perform as required. Two scores are obtained for each item. Performance of each sub-task is scored 0 (does not complete) to 4 (completes task independently). Total score derived by adding ratings on each subtask. Maximum score for dressing=40; for meal prep=36; for telephone=44; for purchasing=32. Raw total score derived by dividing raw score by highest possible score to obtain percentage for each task. Second score was time required to complete each task.
Completion Time	• Completion time is variable and is based on individual performance capacity.
Reliability	• Not reported.
Validity	
Content	• The items on the ADL Situational Test were generated by four geriatric practitioners. Items appear to cover the domains that are problematic in dementia patients.
Criterion	• Not reported.
Construct	• The overall score on the ADL Situational Test was correlated with two mental status measures: the Short Portable Mental Status Questionnaire (r=40; p=0.14) and the Clinical Demential Rating Scale (n=9; r=0.05; p=0.03).
Overall Utility	• The ADL Situational Test is a performance-based measure. It is one of the few tests that examines subtasks of ADL and IADL. It thus provides a refined understanding of performance areas that are difficult for dementia patients. Nevertheless, the test has not been tested sufficiently for its psychometric properties.
	• The SFA was very carefully developed and appears to be a very practical and empirically robust measure. The scale was designed to reflect current models of function and special education legislation. It will help organize the input from a number of different sources into an assessment used to plan and evaluate interventions for school-aged children. The manual is informative and easy to read.
	• This is a new assessment with content that is well-referenced. However, as it is new, the scale itself is not yet referenced in any scholarly publications.

Table 12-7

ASSESSMENT OF MOTOR AND PROCESS SKILLS (AMPS)

Sources	Fisher, A. G. (1995). *Assessment of Motor and Process Skills*. Fort Collins, CO. Three Star Press.
	Fisher, A. G. (1993). The assessment of IADL motor skills: An application of many-faceted Rasch analysis. *American Journal of Occupational Therapy, 47,* 319-329.
Type of Client	• Younger and older adults
Clinical Utility	
Format	• The AMPS is administered by an occupational therapist who must be trained and calibrated in the use of this assessment. It is based on direct observation and provides evaluation of both motor and process skills.
Procedures	• The AMPS consists of 56 IADL tasks. Persons are observed performing two to three tasks of their choice. For each task, 15 motor and 20 process skills are evaluated. Each motor and process skill item is rated on a 4-point scale (1 [deficit] to 4 [competent skill]). A total of 36 discrete ratings are made in observation of a single IADL task.
Completion Time	• Varies by individual who must perform two to three IADL of their choice.
Reliability	
Internal Consistency	• A number of studies have tested the internal consistency of the AMPS and yield high Cronbach's alpha from r=0.74 to r=0.93.
Test-Retest	• Scores are high and range from r=0.70 to r=0.91 depending on test conditions and use of Rasch analysis.
Validity	
Content	• There are 56 tasks for the AMPS which have been refined and augmented based on testing with a wide range of cultural groups. The 16 motor and 20 process skills appear to be clinically valid. Both motor and process items represent a universal taxonomy of actions that can be observed during any performance task.
Construct	• A series of studies with persons with a wide range of conditions and ages has confirmed the validity of the AMPS. Testing has also established its validity with several other cultural groups.
Overall Utility	• The AMPS offers a standardized, contextual and culturally sensitive evaluation of IADL performance as well as the individual's underlying competency in motor and process skills. The AMPS can be used with clients with various conditions, with the young and old and with different cultural groups. It has extensive psychometric testing and continues to be evaluated for its properties and sensitivity to intervention and environmental factors. One potential barrier to its use is the need to undergo extensive training and a trial period for calibration.

and EADL. The inclusion of domains such as leisure, work (paid and unpaid), active recreation and play, and homework enable the occupational therapist to use this tool with a wide range of clinical populations and address a broad set of performance areas. Third, the COPM has been designed for use as an evaluation of post-treatment progress.

The AMPS represents an exciting new direction in the measurement of IADL status. It combines many positive features: it is process-based, involves direct observation,

and enables clients to select from a list of 56 IADL tasks in those areas of performance that are meaningful to them and for which they want to be evaluated. Limitations of the AMPS include the need for extensive training in its use and scoring and the amount of time for completing the assessment. Also, its use as a measure of treatment outcomes requires more evaluation.

The Test of Grocery Shopping Skills was developed and tested with persons with schizophrenia. It provides an observation-based evaluation with a natural environment.

Table 12-8

CAREGIVER ASSESSMENT OF FUNCTIONAL DEPENDENCE AND UPSET (CAFU)

Source	Gitlin, L. N., Roth, D. L., Burgio, L., et al. (2005). Caregiver appraisals of functional dependence in individuals with dementia and associated caregiver upset: Psychometric properties of a new scale and response patterns by caregiver-care recipient characteristics. *Journal of Aging and Health, 17(2),* 148-171 .
Purpose	• Assess level of dependence of individual with dementia and caregiver's reaction to providing assistance.
Type of Client	• Families caring for persons with dementia.
	• Used in rehabilitation, acute, home, and community settings.
Clinical Utility	
Format	• Eight IADL items (meal preparation, finances, telephone, shopping, travel, laundry, medications, housekeeping).
	• Scoring uses a 7-point interval scale for level of dependence (7=complete independence, 6=modified independence [needs extra time or assistive device], 5=supervision necessary, 4=minimal assistance, 3=moderate assistance, 2=almost total assistance, 1=totally dependent, unable to do); and a 5-point scale for caregiver upset (0=not at all, 1=a little, 2=moderately, 3=very much, 4=extremely).
	• Total IADL dependence score ranges from 8 to 56.
Procedures	• Caregivers rate level of dependence of family member for each task. If dependent, then caregiver asked their level of upset.
Completion Time	• Varies based on number of items of dependence but on average about 15 to 20 minutes.
Standardization	• Scoring instructions are in original article.
Reliability	• Excellent.
Internal Consistency	• Tested with 640 family caregivers of persons with dementia; For IADL dependence scale, Cronbach's coefficient alpha=0.80; for Upset with IADL dependence, Cronbach's coefficient alpha=0.84.
Inter-Rater	• Not reported.
Intra-Rater	• Not reported.
Test-Retest	• Not reported.
Validity	
Content	• Items reflect those used in well-established IADL scales.
Convergent	• Excellent convergent and discriminant validity was also obtained for both the functional capacity and upset measures.
Construct	• A two-factor structure for functional items was derived and excellent factorial validity obtained. Differential response patterns for level of dependence and caregiver upset was found for caregiver race, caregiver-care recipient relationship, and care recipient gender, but not for caregiver gender.
Overall Utility	• Systematic approach to obtain function ratings through proxy, covers the typical IADL areas along a 7-point response set, can be used for research or clinical purposes.
	• Adequate for diverse dementia caregiver population.
	• Useful in helping to derive diagnosis since change in IADL functioning part of the diagnostic process.
	• Further testing required to determine sensitivity to change.
	• Caregivers may over or underestimate dependence based on affective stance.
	• The CAFU is a new measure tested as part of a multi-site national randomized trial.
	• It provides a systematic approach to obtain dependence scores from family caregivers while also obtaining their reaction in order to plan for services.

Table 12-9

DIRECT ASSESSMENT OF FUNCTIONAL STATUS (DAFS)

Source	Loewenstein, D., Amigo, E., Duara, R., et al. (1989). A new scale for the assessment of functional status in Alzheimer's disease and related disorders. *Journal of Gerontology: Psychological Sciences, 44*, 114-121.
Purpose	• The DAFS was developed as a direct assessment of functional status.
Type of Client	• Patients with dementia.
Clinical Utility	
Format	• The DAFS can be administered in an outpatient setting and is based on direct observation of a patient's performance within each of seven functional domains.
Procedures	• The DAFS assesses time orientation (8 items, up to 16 points); communication skills (17 items, up to 17 points); financial abilities (21 items, up to 21 points); shopping subskills (8 items, up to 16 points); eating (5 items, up to 10 points); dressing behaviors (21 items, up to 13 points); and transportation (13 items, up to 13 points). A composite function score (maximum = 93 points) is derived from all scales except transportation.
Completion Time	• 30 to 35 minutes.
Reliability	
Internal Consistency	• Not reported.
Inter-Rater	• Inter-rater reliability calculated for 15 patients with dementia and 12 controls. Minimum of 85% agreement between raters. Kappas for subscales ranged from 0.911 to 1.000 (p <0.001).
Test-Retest	• For both patients and controls, highly stable ratings obtained over time for composite scale scores. In individual subscales, test-retest reliabilities ranged from 0.546 to 0.918 for patients with dementia and kappas ranged from 0.78 to 1.00.
Validity	
Content	• Items included in the DAFS derived from the literature and other IADL instruments.
Criterion	• The DAFS was compared to reported functional status at home using the Blessed Dementia Rating Scale (BDRS) (r= -0.66).
Construct	• Not reported.
Overall Utility	• The DAFS has excellent interrater and test-retest reliabilities and convergent and discriminative validity. The scale does not take a long time to complete and appears to be ecologically valid. The DAFS has also been translated and administered to

Further testing is required to determine its applicability to other populations.

SUMMARY

The activities that constitute IADL measures clearly reflect the domain of occupational therapy and its therapeutic interventions. The assessment of IADL status is an important component of occupational therapy treatment in acute, rehabilitation, home care, and community-based health care settings with both young and older persons with physical, psychiatric, or cognitive impairment.

The measures reviewed here are mostly designed for use in an initial assessment and may not be sensitive to detect change in IADL status following treatment. The EADL scale has been used to monitor IADL status over time in stroke patients for both clinical and research purposes. Only the COPM has been specifically designed to document progress following a therapeutic intervention for clinical purposes. Its application to the research context or specific procedures by which to quantify pre-post change needs to be further evaluated. Although performance-based measures may initially appear to offer a more objective, clinical picture of an individual, they should be used cautiously and as representing one aspect of IADL function.

The use of a standardized measure of IADL status provides a systematic approach to treatment planning and

---

Table 12-10

THE DIRECT ASSESSMENT OF FUNCTIONAL ABILITIES (DAFA): A COMPARISON TO AN INDIRECT MEASURE OF INSTRUMENTAL ACTIVITIES OF DAILY LIVING.

Source	Karagiozis, H., Gray, S., Sacco, J., Shapiro, M., Kawas, C. (1998). The Direct Assessment of Functional Abilities (DAFA): A comparison to an indirect measure of instrumental activities of daily living. *Gerontologist, 38,* 113-121.
Purpose	• The DAFA is designed as a direct performance measure of IADL status for a patient with dementia.
Type of Client	• Patients with dementia at mild to moderate stages.
Clinical Utility	
Format	• The DAFA is completed by a rater in a clinical setting using direct observation of performance in different locations in a clinic setting or in a test environment.
Procedures	• The DAFA includes 10 items representing 7 IADL domains. Scores for each item range from 0 (independent functioning) to 3 (depending functioning). Each item is scored by observing component parts of each task. An overall score for each item is the average of the component scores rounded to the nearest integer. The total score (0 to 30) is the sum of the integer scores for the 10 test items.
Completion Time	• Varies by subject with most severely demented taking up to 1.5 hours.
Reliability	
Internal Consistency	• Not reported.
Test-Retest	• Excellent test-retest reliability between visit 1 and visit 2 testing (n=43; r=0.95; p< 0.04) using both Pearson's correlation coefficient and intraclass correlation coefficient.
Validity	
Content	• The items on the DAFA were adapted from the Pfeffer Functional Activities Questionnaire (PFAQ), a self-report measure of IADL.
Criterion	• The DAFA was tested against the PFAQ. Demented subjects significantly overestimate their functional abilities and informants underestimate the subject's functional abilities. Subjects with greater cognitive impairment showed poorer judgment of their functional abilities.
Construct	• The DAFA was correlated with the Folstein Mini Mental Status Examination and the Clinical Dementia Rating Scale. Subject's accuracy (difference between observed and self-report functional scores) decreased with greater dementia severity.
Overall Utility	• This study showed that patients with dementia do not accurately report functional ability. The DAFA offers a standarized observational tool of IADL function in a clinical setting. It does take time to administer and special set up or use of different locations in a clinical setting (e.g., cafeteria, gift shop, exam room). Also, the scale was developed and tested on a very small sample and requires further psychometric testing.

---

evaluation of therapeutic outcomes. Overall, assessments recently developed by occupational therapists are promising but require continued psychometric testing and refinement. There is still a relative shortage of adequately tested IADL measures for use with clients with diverse physical and cognitive difficulties and which reflect the specific goals of occupational therapy practices. Nevertheless, the measures summarized here provide a uniform language and set of procedures that can enhance the rigor and systematic approach to assessment and treatment in occupational therapy.

Table 12-11

EXTENDED ACTIVITIES OF DAILY LIVING SCALE (EADL)

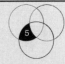

Source	Nouri, F. M., & Lincoln, N. B. (1987). An extended activities of living scale for stroke patients. *Clinical Rehabilitation 1*, 301-305.
Purpose	• The PASS is an overall assessment of functional independence for post-hospital follow-up and is designed for use as a mail survey.
Type of Client	• Stroke patients who are discharged home.
Clinical Utility	
Format	• The EADL is a self-report measure of 22 items representing 4 domains of daily living (mobility, kitchen, domestic and leisure.Items within each domain are rated from 1 (unable to do) to 4 (does activity on own). Items are scored within each domain.
Completion Time	• Not reported.
Reliability	
Internal Consistency	• High consistency obtained with a coefficient of reproducibility=0.85 to 0.86 and a coefficient of scalability 0.75 to 0.81.
Inter-Rater	• Not reported.
Test-Retest	• Not reported.
Validity	
Content	• The items on the EADL represent activities traditionally considered as IADL. Items appear to cover the activities that may be problematic for stroke patients.
Criterion	• Not reported.
Construct	• Not reported.
Overall Utility	• The EADL is a self-report or proxy test designed as a mail survey for stroke patients following hospitalization. It is easy to administer and can be used on repeated occasions to evaluate IADL status of stroke patients. Nevertheless, the test has not been tested sufficiently for its psychometric properties.

ACKNOWLEDGMENTS

The instruments reported here were identified as part of a larger funded project on functional assessments supported in part by grants from the National Institute on Aging awarded to the author (Enhancing Function in Frail Older Adults #R01 AG13687; Geriatric Leadership Award, # K07 AG00998).

REFERENCES

Andresen, E., Rothenberg, B., & Zimmer, J. G. (1997). Functional assessment. In E. Andresen, B. Rothenberg, & J. G. Zimmer (Eds.), *Assessing the health status of older adults* (pp. 1-40). New York: Springer.

Barberger-Gateau, P., Commenges, D., Gagnon, M., Letenneur, L., Sauvel, C., & Dartigues, J. F. (1992). Instrumental activities of daily living as a screening tool for cognitive impairment and dementia in elderly community dwellers. *Journal of American Geriatrics Society, 40*, 1129-1134.

Barer, D., & Nouri, F. (1989). Measurement activities of daily living. *Clinical Rehabilitation, 3*, 179-187.

Baum, C. M., & Edwards, D. (1993). Cognitive performance in senile dementia of the Alzheimer's type: The Kitchen Task Assessment. *American Journal of Occupational Therapy, 47(5)*, 431-436.

Brookmeyer, R., Gray, S., & Kraus, C. (1998). Projections of Alzheimer's disease in the United States and the public health impact of delaying disease onset. *American Journal of Public Health, 88*, 1337-1342.

Brown, C., Moore, W. P., Hemman, D., & Yunek, A. (1996). Influence of instrumental activities of daily living assessment method of judgments of independence. *American Journal of Occupational Therapy, 50(3)*, 202-206.

DePoy, E., & Gitlin, L. N. (2005). *Introduction to research: Understanding and applying multiple strategies*. (3rd ed.). St. Louis, Elsevier.

Dunlop, D. D., Hughes, S. L., & Manheim, L. M. (1997). Disability in activities of daily living: Patterns of change and a hierarchy of disability. *American Journal of Public Health, 87(3)*, 378-383.

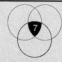

Table 12-12

KITCHEN TASK ASSESSMENT (KTA)

Source	Baum, C., & Edwards, D. F. (1994). Cognitive performance in senile dementia of the Alzheimer's type: The kitchen task assessment. *American Journal of Occupational Therapy, 47(5)*, 431-436.
Purpose	• The KTA is a functional measure of the level of cognitive support required by a person with Alzheimer's Disease to complete a cooking task successfully.
Type of Client	• Persons with Alzheimer's Disease living at home.
Clinical Utility	
Format	• The KTA is administered by an OT who observes these components in the course of observing making pudding: initiation, organization, performance of steps, sequencing, judgment/safety, and completion. The level of support required from tester is scored: 0 (independent); 1 (verbal cues); 2 (physical assistance); 3 (totally incapable). The higher the score, the more impaired the performance (total scores range from 0 to 18).
Completion Time	• Not reported.
Reliability	
Internal Consistency	• Cronbach alpha coefficients were high across all levels of dementia and ranged from 0.87 to 0.96.
Observer (Inter-Rater)	• Kendall's tau B was used to determine inter-rater reliability. Videotapes of 3 subjects were rated by 12 raters. The inter-rater reliability for the total score=0.85, range was 0.63 for safety to 1.0 for initiation.
Test-Retest	• Not reported.
Validity	
Content	• The KTA is a test of practical cognitive skills and measures processing skills of initiation, organization, sequencing, safety, and judgment.
Criterion	• Not reported.
Construct	• The relationship between subject's performance on the KTA and standard neuropsychological measures was highly significant. Analysis of variance of KTA scores across stages of dementia also yielded a significant F-ratio suggesting that performance of the KTA was affected by the progression of the disease.
Overall Utility	• Although the KTA involves observation of one activity, preparation of pudding, scores are derived for basic cognitive processes. As such, the KTA provides practical information to guide intervention. Because the activity observed involves meal preparation, it may be gender-biased. More research on its utility and predictive validity is necessary.

Dunn, W., Brown, C., & McGuigan, A. (1994). The ecology of human performance: A framework for considering the effect of content. *American Journal of Occupational Therapy, 48*, 595-607.

Fisher, A. G. (1993). The assessment of IADL motor skills: An application of many-faceted Rasch analysis. *American Journal of Occupational Therapy, 47*, 319-329.

Fisher, A. G. (1991). *Assessment of motor and process skills.* Fort Collins, CO: Three Star Press.

Fisher, A. G. (1997). Multifaceted measurement of daily life task performance: Conceptualizing a test of instrumental ADL and validating the addition of personal ADL tasks. *Physical Medicine and Rehabilitation: State of the Art Reviews, 11*, 289-303.

Gill, T. M., & Kurland, B. (2003). The burden and patterns of disability in activities of daily living among community-living older persons. *Journal of Gerontology: Medical Sciences, 58A(1)*, 70-75.

Gitlin, L., N., Roth, D. L., Burgio, L., et al. (2005). Caregiver appraisals of functional dependence in individuals with dementia and associated caregiver upset: Psychometric properties of a new scale and response patterns by caregiver-care recipient characteristics. *Journal of Aging and Health, 17.* 148-171 .

Table 12-13

PERFORMANCE ASSESSMENT OF SELF-CARE SKILLS (PASS)

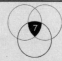

Sources	Rogers, J.C., Holm, M., Goldstein, G., McCue, M., & Nussbaum, P. (1984). Stability and change in functional assessment of patients with geropsychiatric disorders. *American Journal of Occupational Therapy, 48(10)*, 914-918.
	Rogers, J. C., & Holm, M. B. (1988). *Performance Assessment of Self-care Skills (3.1).* Pittsburgh, PA. Unpublished performance test.
	Holm, M. B. & Rogers, J. C. (1999). Performance Assessment of Self-care Skills. In: B. J. Hemphill-Pearson (Ed.). *Assessments in occupational therapy mental health: An integrative approach* (pp 117-123). Thorofare, NJ: SLACK Incorporated.
Purpose	• The PASS is a performance-based test to assess short-term functional change in elderly patients and to assist in discharge planning following hospitalization.
Type of Client	• Adults in clinic, hospital, or home and with a wide range of diagnoses, including the well population.
Clinical Utility	
Format	• For clinic and home versions, subjects are observed by an occupational therapist engaging in a daily living behavior. The PASS includes 26 task items, with criterion-referenced subtasks. The PASS-Clinic and PASS-HOME yields three scores; independence on each subtask, safety, and task adequacy.
Completion Time	• 1.5 to 3 hours.
Reliability	
Internal Consistency	• Not reported.
Inter-Rater)	• Agreement between five therapists participating in dyads rated 25 older adults from five diagnostic categories. Percent agreement ranged from 88% to 97% for each score (independence, safety, and task adequacy) and for both the clinic and home version.
Test-Retest	• Pass-clinic test-retest reliability was independence, r=0.92; Safety, 89% agreement, and Adequacy, r=0.82. For Pass-Home, test-retest reliability was independence, r=0.96; safety, 90% agreement; and adequacy, r=0.97.
Validity	
Content	• PASS items reflect common domains found in other ADL/IADL measures.
Criterion	• Not reported.
Construct	• PASS was found to correlate highly with neuropsychological variables.
Overall Utility	• The PASS-Clinic and PASS-HOME includes 18 IADL behaviors, which are not included on other measures. As a performance-based measure it is very promising, has been developed and tested for use in different settings and for a wide range of populations.

Gitlin, L. N. (in press). *Physical Function and the elderly: A comprehensive guide to its meaning and measurement.* Austin, TX: Pro Ed Press.

Glass, T. A. (1998). Conjugating the "tenses" of function: Discordance among hypothetical, experimental, and enacted function in older adults. *Gerontologist, 38,* 101-112.

Gromak, P. A., & Waskel, S. (1989). Functional assessment in the elderly: A literature review. *Physical & Occupational Therapy in Geriatrics, 7,* 1-12.

Hamera, E., & Brown, C. (2000). Developing a context-based performance measure for persons with schizophrenia: The test of grocery shopping skills. *American Journal of Occupational Therapy, 54,* 20-25.

Hirsch, C., Sommers, L., Olsen, A., Mullen, L., & Winograd, C. (1990). The natural history of functional morbidity in hospitalized older patients. *Journal of American Geriatrics Society, 38,* 1296-1303.

Table 12-14

STRUCTURED ASSESSMENT OF INDEPENDENT LIVING SKILLS (SAILS)

Source   Mahurin, R. K., DeBittignies, B. H., & Pirozzolo, F. J. (1991). Structured assessment of independent living skills: Preliminary report of a performance measure of functional abilities in dementia. *Journal of Gerontology: Psychological Sciences, 46,* 58-66.

Purpose   The PASS is designed as a direct measure of performance of daily activities.

Type of Client   Patients with dementia.

Clinical Utility

Format   • The SAILS is completed by a health professional in a clinical setting. It is a direct measure of performance.

Procedures   • The SAILS consists of 50 tasks. Each task is criterion-referenced with behaviorally anchored descriptions. Performance of each task is scored on a rating scale ranging from 0 to 3, with both time and accuracy contributing to the score. Each item yields a possible three points for a total maximum score of 150 points.

Completion Time • It takes approximately one hour to complete the SAILS.

Reliability

Internal Consistency • Not reported.

Inter-Rater   • Inter-rater reliability was extremely high (r=0.99).

Test-Retest   • Test-retest was high (total score: r=0.81).

Validity

Content   • Individual items of the SAILS were selected from a review of existing assessments. Items selected have theoretical relevance, practicality of implementing tasks in clinic setting and gradation of task difficulty.

Criterion   • Not reported.

Construct   • The SAILS was correlated with the MMSE, the Global Deterioration Scale, and the WAIS-R. Significant results were achieved at the 0.05 and 0.01 alpha levels.

Overall Utility • The SAILS is a performance-based measure for use in a clinic setting. It can be used with mild to severe dementia. Further research with larger numbers of subjects is required to establish its validity and generalizability to other settings and populations.

Karagiozis, H., Gray, S., Sacco, J., Shapiro, M., & Kawas, C. (1998). The Direct Assessment of Functional Abilities (DAFA): A comparison to an indirect measure of instrumental activities of daily living. *Gerontologist, 38,* 113-121.

Kempen, G., Steverink, N., Ormel, J., & Deeg, D. (1996). The assessment of ADL among frail elderly in an interview survey: Self-report versus performance-based tests and determinants of discrepancies. *Journal of Gerontology: Psychological Sciences, 51B,* 254-260.

Kovar, M. G., & Lawton, M. P. (1994). Functional disability: Activities and instrumental activities of daily living. In M. P. Lawton & J. A. Teresi (Eds.), *Annual review of gerontology and geriatrics* (pp. 57-75). New York: Springer.

Law, M., Baptiste, S., Carswell, A., McCall, M., Polatajko, H., & Pollock, M. (1994). *Canadian Occupational Performance Measure* (2nd ed.). Toronto, Ontario: Canadian Association of Occupational Therapists.

Law, M., & Letts, L. (1989). A critical review of scales of activities of daily living. *American Journal of Occupational Therapy, 43(8),* 522-528.

Lawton, M. P., & Brody, E. (1969). Assessment of older people: Self-maintaining and instrumental activities of daily living. *Gerontologist, 9,* 179-186.

Loewenstein, D., et al. (1989). A new scale for the assessment of functional status in Alzheimer's disease and related disorders. *Journal of Gerontology: Psychological Sciences, 44,* 114-121.

Long, K., Sudha, S., & Mutran, E. J. (1998). Elder-proxy agreement concerning the functional status and medical history of the older person: The impact of caregiver burden and depressive symptomology. *Journal of American Geriatrics Society, 46(9),* 1103-1111.

Mahurin, R. K., DeBittignies, B. H., & Pirozzolo, F. J. (1991). Structured assessment of independent living skills: Preliminary report of a performance measure of functional abilities in dementia. *Journal of Gerontology: Psychological Sciences, 46,* 58-66.

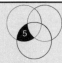

Table 12-15

TEST OF GROCERY SHOPPING SKILLS

Source	Hamera, E., & Brown, C. (2000). Developing a context-based performance measure for persons with schizophrenia: The Test of Grocery Shopping Skills. *American Journal of Occupational Therapy, 54*, 20-25.
Purpose	• The Test of Grocery Shopping Skills is designed as a direct performance measure of grocery shopping ability.
Type of Client	• Adolescents and adults.
Clinical Utility	
Format	• The Test of Grocery Shopping Skills is administered in a community grocery store and scored by a rater who observes performance. There are two forms of the measure designed for pretest/posttest purposes. The individual is given a list of 10 grocery items and instructed to locate the items at the lowest price.
Procedures	• The measure is scored in terms of accuracy (correct item and size at the lowest time).
Completion Time	• Varies by individual, with average of approximately 20 minutes for people with schizophrenia.
Reliability	
Inter-Rater	• For trained raters, inter-rater reliability was extremely strong at 0.99.
Test-Retest	• The two forms administered 3 weeks apart yielded reliability coefficients of 0.60 to 0.83.
Validity	
Content	• The measure was developed following observation and interview with people with severe mental illness to determine aspects of grocery shopping that were important and difficult.
Criterion	• Not reported.
Construct	• Correlations between the Test of Grocery Shopping Skills and the Test of Drug Store Shopping Skills ranged from 0.44 to 0.94. The Test of Grocery Shopping Skills discriminated performance between individuals with and without severe mental illness and was sensitive to change after a grocery shopping intervention.
Overall Utility	• The Test of Grocery Shopping Skills provides a direct performance assessment of a complex skill in the natural environment providing specific outcomes for both process and product. Psychometric properties have only been assessed with people with mental illness. The test is limited to only one aspect of community living.

Nagi, S. Z. (1979). The concept and measurement of disability. In E. D. Berkowitz (Ed.), *Disability policies and government programs* (pp. 1-15). New York: Praeger.

Nouri, F. M., & Lincoln, N. B. (1987). An extended activities of living scale for stroke patients. *Clinical Rehabilitation, 1,* 301-305.

Park, S., Fisher, A. G., & Velozo, C. A. (1993). Using the Assessment of Motor and Process Skills to compare performance between home and clinical settings. *American Journal of Occupational Therapy, 48,* 519-525.

Rogers, J. C., Holm, M. B., Goldstein, G., McCue, M., & Nussbaum, P. D. (1994). Stability and change in functional assessment of patients with geropsychiatric disorders. *American Journal of Occupational Therapy, 48(10),* 914-918.

Skurla, E., Rogers, J. C., & Sunderland, T. (1988). Direct assessment of activities of daily living in Alzheimer's disease. A controlled study. *Journal of the American Geriatrics Society, 36,* 97-103.

Wolf, H. (1997). Assessments of daily living and instrumental activities of daily living: Their use by community-based health service occupational therapists working in physical disability. *British Journal of Occupational Therapy, 60(8),* 359-364.

WHO. (1998). *International classification of impairment, activity and participation—ICIDH-2.* Geneva, Switzerland: Author.

Editors' Notes for Chapter 13

Mine the Gold

Recreation scholars and psychologists have provided much of the writing about the role of leisure in determining life satisfaction. Leisure activities provide individuals with a way to enact their interest and skills for the pleasure of doing so.

Become Systematic

Leisure and interest measures provide a structure for finding out the person's pattern and range of choices of these types of occupations. We can identify categories of skills and motivational factors that can be generalized to alternative life choices when original leisure options become too difficult.

Use Evidence in Practice

Leisure contributes to overall life satisfaction, well-being, and effective energy use. Persons who have a poor history of leisure use are at risk for decline when other aspects of performance deteriorate. Participation in leisure contributes to healthy outcomes and well-being.

Make Occupational Therapy Contribution Explicit

Leisure has a strong historic place in occupational therapy practice and the core philosophy of the profession. We demonstrate our emphasis on living a satisfying life by asking about and assessing participation in leisure occupations.

Engage in Occupation-Based, Client-Centered Practice

People need to see that we will continue to include aspects of their lives that are satisfying to them when they need professional services and care. A leisure focus illustrates our interest in reconstructing a full life with them.

13

Measuring Leisure Performance

Kate Connolly, PhD, MPA; Mary Law, PhD, OT Reg. (Ont.), FCAOT;
and Brianna MacGuire, MScOT, OT Reg (Ont.)

Leisure has played a significant role in society through the ages. Philosophers like Aristotle and Plato believed that the greatest good was happiness, and that in order to achieve a state of happiness, one must be free to experience unoccupied time. For Aristotle, leisure was time free from the demands of work; for Plato, leisure was a time for self-development, contemplation, and thought (Kelly, 1996).

Some of the current views of leisure reflect its multidisciplinary roots. Research into leisure is now commonly located in leisure studies, sociology, philosophy, history, psychology, and political studies. Csikszentmihalyi (1990) introduced the concept of "flow" into our current understanding of leisure, finding that when challenge and skill are matched, a state of mind is achieved where "consciousness is harmoniously ordered... and people are so involved in an activity that nothing else seems to matter" (pp 4-6). Murphy (1981) discussed a "holistic" concept of leisure, believing that elements of leisure can be expressed in all aspects of human experience and human behavior, be it work, play, school, religion, or other social spheres. By assuming a holistic approach, leisure activities are seen as being interchangeable between various spheres of daily living. As such, an individual considers multiple satisfactions when choosing leisure activities, satisfying a range of participant needs, preferences, and motives. In a sociological context, studies indicate that for adults, the informal and everyday experiences of their lives lie at the heart of their leisure experience (Kelly, 1996). These commonplace experiences could include, for example, time with family members and friends, enjoying the sunset while walking the dog, church involvements, and time involved with the various social relationships attached to work settings.

When compared to more traditional academic disciplines such as philosophy, history, and sociology, leisure as a field of scientific study is quite young. Current research into leisure reflects such social constructs as work and leisure, leisure and the life-cycle, leisure and gender, as well as more specific issues such as diversity, access, and inclusion. Of specific interest in this discussion are issues related to access and inclusion.

The importance of developing opportunities for people with limitations or disabilities to participate in community recreation programs has been well established. Research in leisure studies has identified both benefits to leisure participation, and barriers/constraints to leisure participation. The opportunity to develop social skills, a knowledge of community resources, a sense of belonging, a positive self concept, friendships, other social relationships, and a personally fulfilling way of life are some of the benefits that result from participation by people with disabilities in community settings (Lord, 1981; Schleien, Heyne, Rynders, & McAvoy, 1990; Schleien, Ray, & Green, 1997).

However, when constraints to leisure experiences exist, the role of the health care or therapeutic recreation practitioner is to assist the client negotiate their constraints to enable full access and participation in recreation activities. A key role for occupational therapists in this negotiation process is to identify ways in which either the environment or the resources attached to the activity can be adapted to meet the needs of the client, thus enabling participation in activities that lead to an enhanced quality of life.

CONSTRAINTS TO LEISURE

As mentioned, a key theoretical concept that is commonly discussed in the field of leisure is that of constraints. When Kelly (1996) discusses the concept of leisure, for example, he defines it as the use of time, rather than leisure as time. He goes on to suggest that leisure is relatively free from constraints and coercion, and that leisure is freely chosen.

Constraints are defined as those factors that intervene between the preference for an activity and the actual participation in it (Henderson, Bialeschki, Shaw, & Freysinger, 1989). Constraints include that which inhibits an individual spending more time on an activity, taking advantage of the leisure services available to the individual, or being able to achieve a desired level of satisfaction (Horna, 1994). Constraints can relate to such issues as role, gender, ethnicity, health status, class, and race—anything that creates a difficulty for an individual to accurately perceive if their choice of leisure is unconstrained.

CONSTRAINTS PERCEIVED BY INDIVIDUALS

Research into leisure constraints has identified the following as issues that impact a person's ability to participate in leisure activities: time commitments resulting from work and family demands; costs related to admission fees or equipment; facility limitations such as physical access; accessibility (which in this context refers to lack of transportation or opportunities near home); social isolation, if an activity where others are needed to participate; and personal reasons often related to the physical ability required to participate (Jackson, 1993). In some situations more closely related to occupational therapy, an ongoing experience of pain can also act as a constraint to leisure participation. For example, Strunin and Boden (2004) found that injured workers with occupational back injuries were limited or unable to participate in leisure activities with their spouses and their children as a result of high pain levels associated with their injuries. In addition to changed social roles such as being the household provider or homemaker, the inability to sit to play a game of cards with their spouse or throw a ball to their children was experienced as yet another loss in their quality of life.

Participants approach leisure activities with their own perceptions of both benefits and constraints. Dergance, Calmbach, Dhanda, Miles, Hazuda, and Mouton (2003) found that the sedentary elderly they studied experienced a lack of interest, self-discipline, enjoyment, knowledge, or good health that prevented them from participating in leisure time physical activity such as walking, swimming, or bicycling. While their perceptions of the benefits of leisure participation included decreased tension, depression, stress, and risk of disease, and increased self esteem, strength, and heart/ lung function, the majority of these elderly still chose to remain sedentary.

Women, in particular, experience (particular) constraints in their pursuit of leisure activities and this has been of interest to a number of feminist researchers in leisure studies. Shaw (1986) found that women, more than men, identified constraints to their leisure participation due to childcare responsibilities and household labor activities. In fact, many women lack the freedom to participate in leisure activities because of their social roles related to family, and the social expectations placed upon women by our society. Low paying jobs, little autonomy in the workplace, and lack of time due to family and childcare responsibilities all serve as constraints to leisure participation for women (Henderson, et al, Bialeschki, Shaw & Freysinger, 1996).

INSTITUTIONAL BARRIERS

In addition to perceived constraints to participation, institutional barriers to recreation exist that limit participation of people with disabilities in community recreation programs. Rather than any personal limitation, it is often the environment that is disabling for people with disabilities as they attempt to participate in community settings (Hahn, 1993; Crichton & Jongbloed, 1998). While all recreation participants can experience barriers such as a lack of financial resources, transportation, or skills, people with disabilities often experience these barriers in a more complex way. Barriers such as inaccessible facilities, lack of supportive staff, negative attitudes, and few efforts to reduce obstacles (e.g. special equipment, scheduling) are common in most community settings (Connolly & Law, 1999; Hutchison & McGill, 1992; Smith, Austin, & Kennedy, 1996). In addition, lack of friendship building programs or programs emphasizing competition create further barriers to participation, particularly for children with disabilities (Jones, 2003/2004).

Negotiating Constraints and Barriers

Of interest is that while some people accept their constraints and barriers and choose not to participate in recreation activities, many people successfully negotiate their constraints to allow them to engage in leisure services (Jackson, Crawford, & Godbey, 1993). Jackson and Ruck (1995) identified two kinds of constraint negotiation strategies—behavioral and cognitive, with behavioral strategies being the one more commonly adopted. For example, if lack of time is identified as a constraint to leisure participation, a negotiation strategy of a behavioral nature might be to budget or free up time from another activity so that some time could be devoted to the leisure endeavor. Likewise, if a lack of skills is identified as a constraint to leisure, some people mitigate this issue by acquiring the skills needed to participate through lessons or modifying the activity to match their skill level. Constraint negotiations of a cognitive level generally consist of accepting the constraint but participating anyways, or re-framing the goal to be that of simply having fun playing the sport, rather than winning the game.

In their work with clients, practitioners need to understand that leisure behavior and leisure satisfaction is influenced by four critical dimensions: that the participant perceives the choice to be theirs, commonly referred to as *perceived freedom* (Iso-Ahola, 1980; Mannell & Kleiber, 1997); that the participant feels a sense of personal motivation to participate, commonly referred to as *intrinsic motivation* (Iso-Ahola, 1980; Shaw, 1985); that the participant feels a sense of control over their lives and how they are functioning, often referred to as *self-efficacy* (Bandura, 1997); and finally, that the participant believes that he/she can influence or affect the outcome, commonly known as *personal causality* (Iso-Ahola, 1980). Participants with disabilities or limiting health issues often experience particular challenges to these primary dimensions of leisure in that they may not have the capability to successfully influence their proposed outcome or the self-efficacy needed to feel a sense of control over what they are doing and how they are functioning. In their investigations focusing on children with disabilities, Witt and Ellis (1984) found that while these children had participated in leisure activities and had developed skills in the activity, what had not been explored was how these children would define their level of success, their abilities, and their level of competence. As a result of this and other study into leisure, interest in concepts such as self-efficacy and personal causality have received increased attention by researchers. In regards to the role of the occupational therapist or therapeutic recreation practitioner, ensuring that the leisure options chosen by the participant addresses these four primary dimensions as closely as possible is an intervention goal (Stumbo & Peterson, 2004).

The Leisure Ability Model, as discussed by Stumbo and Peterson (2004), is one approach used to ensure that the client's needs are kept central to any activity choices made, and every effort is taken to adhere closely to the four dimensions related to leisure behavior and leisure satisfaction discussed above. The Leisure Ability Model identifies three program directions that can be taken to support clients in their leisure choices:

- *Functional Intervention.* Programs with this intent focus on the improvement of clients' physical, social, mental, and/or emotional behaviors.

- *Leisure Education.* Programs of this nature focus on assisting clients in learning new leisure skills, acquiring social skills, establishing awareness of self and leisure, and acquiring knowledge related to leisure resource utilization.

- *Recreation Participation.* Programs in this category provide individuals with the opportunity to engage in organized leisure activities and programs of their choice (p. 120).

As has been demonstrated in the discussion above, the benefits that people with limitations and disabilities can garner from leisure activities are numerous. Overcoming loneliness through the development of friendships and the increased perception of social support that results has generally been associated with leisure participation (Caldwell & Smith, 1988; Coleman & Iso-Ahola, 1993). Further, it has been suggested that perceived social support provides a coping mechanism for stressful life events (Coleman & Iso-Ahola, 1993). The benefits of leisure to health status is a growing area of research and investigation and correlations have been made between leisure participation, life satisfaction, and health. Iso-Ahola (1994) suggests the following model as developed from the literature:

leisure participation➤happiness/life satisfaction➤health

In closing, practitioners can use leisure as a tool to influence clients' health status in three ways: 1) as a tool to pursue or obtain health (e.g., the participation in exercise to address cardiovascular disease), 2) as a way of life (e.g., the pursuit of a lifestyle that promotes and is conducive to health), and 3) as possessing some qualities or characteristics pertinent or relative to health (e.g., sense of freedom, opportunities for social interaction, or the development of social supports) (Iso-Ahola, 1994). The suggestion that leisure brings about happiness, and happiness leads to health, demonstrates the critical importance of leisure as an intervention in the lives of clients.

The measures reviewed in this chapter focus on several aspects of assessing the leisure aspect of occupational performance, including assessment of interests, skills and abilities, and leisure participation.

REFERENCES

Bandura, A. (1997). *Self-efficacy: The exercise of control.* New York: Freeman.

Baum, C. M. & Edwards, D. (2001). *Activity Card Sort.* St. Louis, MO: Washington University at St. Louis.

Beard, J. G., & Ragheb, M. G. (1983). Measuring leisure motivation. *Journal of Leisure Research, 15(3)*, 219-228.

Bowman, K. (1999). *Development of an activity card sort for children: Do parental reports on an activity card sort reflect similar results as their children?* Unpublished master's project, University of Western Ontario, London, Ontario, Canada.

Burke, C., & Cooke, K. (2001). *Participation of children with DCD in activity: Is it really that important?* Unpublished master's project, University of Western Ontario, London, Ontario, Canada.

Caldwell, L., & Smith, E. (1988). Leisure: An overlooked component of health promotion. *Canadian Journal of Public Health, 79(April/May)*, 544-548.

Chang, Y., & Card, J. A. (1994). The reliability of the Leisure Diagnostic Battery Short Form Version B in assessing healthy, older individuals: A preliminary study. *Therapeutic Recreation Journal, 28,* 163-7.

Coleman, D., & Iso-Ahola, S. (1993). Leisure and health: The role of social support and self-determination. *Journal of Leisure Research, 25(2)*, 111-128.

Connolly, K. & Law, M. (1999). Collective voices: People with disabilities shaping municipal recreation access policy. *Journal of Leisurability, 26(1)*, 16-24.

Crichton, A., & Jongbloed, L. (1998). *Disability and social policy in Canada.* North York: Captus Press Inc.

Csikszentmihalyi, M. (1990). *Flow: The psychology of optimal experience.* New York: Harper & Row, Publishers, Inc.

Dergance, J., Calmbach, W., Dhanda, R., Miles, T., Hazuda, H., & Mouton, C. (2003). Barriers to and benefits of leisure time physical activity in the elderly: Differences across cultures. *Journal of the American Geriatrics Society, 51*, 863-868.

Di Bona, L. (2000). What are the benefits of leisure? An exploration using the Leisure Satisfaction Scale. *British Journal of Occupational Therapy, 63(2)*, 50-58.

Dijkers, M. (1991). Scoring CHART: Survey and sensitivity analysis. *Journal of the American Paraplegia Society, 14*, 85-86.

Ellis, G. D., & Witt, P. A. (1986). The Leisure Diagnostic Battery: Past, present and future. *Therapeutic Recreation Journal, 19,* 31-47.

Hahn, H. (1993). The potential impact of disability studies on political science (as well as vice versa). *Policy Studies Journal,* 21(4), 740-751.

Hall, K. M., Dijkers, M., Whiteneck, G., Brooks, C. A., & Stuart Krause, J. (1998). The Craig Handicap Assessment and Reporting Technique (CHART): Metric properties and scoring. *Topics in Spinal Cord Injury Rehabilitation,* 4(1), 16-30.

Henderson, K., Bialeschki, D., Shaw, S., & Freysinger, V. (1989). *A leisure of one's own: A feminist perspective on women's leisure.* State College, PA: Venture.

Henderson, K. A., Bialeschki, D., Shaw, S., & Freysinger, V. (1996). *Both gains and gaps: Feminist perspectives on women's leisure.* State College, PA: Venture.

Horn, S., & Williams, M. (2000). *Development and piloting of the pediatric occupational card sort (POCS): Stage II.* Unpublished master's thesis, University of Western Ontario, London, Ontario, Canada.

Horna, J. (1994). *The study of leisure.* Don Mills, ON: Oxford University Press.

Hutchison, P., & McGill, J. (1992). *Leisure, integration and community.* Concord: Leisurability Publications Inc.

Isa-Ahola, S. (1980). *The social psychology of leisure and recreation.* Dubuque, IA: Wm. C. Brown Company Publishers.

Iso-Ahola, S. (1994). Leisure lifestyle and health. In D. Compton & S. Iso-Ahola (Eds.), *Leisure and Mental Health* (pp. 42-60). Park City, UT: Family Development Resources, Inc.

Jackson, E. (1993). Recognizing patterns of leisure constraints: Results from alternative analyses. *Journal of Leisure Research, 25(2)*, 129-149.

Jackson, E. L., Crawford, D. W., & Godbey, G. (1993). Negotiation of leisure constraints. *Leisure Sciences 15*, 1-11.

Jackson, E. &, Rucks, V. (1995). Negotiation of leisure constraints by junior-high and high school students: An exploratory study. *Journal of Leisure Research, 27(1)*, 85-105.

Jones, D. (2003/2004). Denied from lots of places: Barriers to participation in community recreation programs encountered by children with disabilities in Maine: Perspectives of parents. *Leisure/Loisir, 28(1-2)*, 49-69.

Katz, N. (1988). Interest Checklist: A factor analytical study. *Occupational Therapy in Mental Health, 8(1)*, 45-55.

Katz, N., Karpin, H., Lak, A., Furman, T., Hartman-Maeir, A. (2003). Participation in occupational performance: Reliability and validity of the Activity Card Sort. *Occupational Therapy Journal of Research, 23(1)*, 10-17.

Kelly, J. (1996). *Leisure.* (3rd ed.). Boston: Allyn & Bacon.

King, G., Law, M., King, S., Hurley, P., Hanna, S., Kertoy, M., Rosenbaum, P., & Young, N. (in press). *Children's Assessment of Participation and Enjoyment (CAPE) and Preferences for Activities of Children (PAC).* San Antonio, TX: Harcourt Assessment, Inc.

King, G., Law, M., King, S., Rosenbaum, P., Kertoy, M., & Young, N. L. (2003). A conceptual model of the factors affecting the recreation and leisure participation of children with disabilities. *Physical and Occupational Therapy in Pediatrics, 23*, 63-90.

Kloseck, M., & Crilly, R. G. (1997). *Leisure Competence Measure: Adult version.* London, Ontario: Data System

Kloseck, M., Crilly, R. G., Ellis, G. D, & Lammers, E. (1996). Leisure Competence Measure: Development and reliability of a scale to measure functional outcomes in therapeutic recreation. *Therapeutic Recreation Journal, 30(1)*, 13-26.

Kloseck, M., Crilly, R. G., & Hutchinson-Troyer, L. (2001). Measuring therapeutic recreation outcomes in rehabilitation: Further testing of the Leisure Competence *Measure. Therapeutic Recreation Journal, 35(1)*, 31-42.

Klyczek, J. P., Bauer-Yox, N. & Fiedler, R. C. (1997). The Interest Checklist: A factor analysis. *American Journal of Occupational Therapy, 51(10)*, 815-23.

Liston, S. (2002). *The Pediatric Activity Card Sort: A comparison of occupational profiles for children with developmental coordination Disorder and their typically developing peer.* Unpublished master's project, University of Western Ontario, London, Ontario, Canada.

Lord, J. (1981). *Participation: expanding community and leisure experiences for people with severe handicaps.* Downsview: National Institute in Mental Retardation.

Table 13-1

LEISURE BOREDOM SCALE (LBS)

Source	Iso-Ahola, S. E., & Weissinger, E. (1990). Perceptions of boredom in leisure: Conceptualization, reliability and validity of the Leisure Boredom Scale. *Journal of Leisure Research, 22*, 1-17.
Important Reference	Wegner, L., Flisher, A. J., Muller, M., & Lombard C. (2002). Reliability of the Leisure Boredom Scale for use with high school learners in Cape Town, South Africa. *Journal of Leisure Research, 34(3)*, 340-51.
Purpose	• Designed to assess personal perceptions of boredom with available leisure opportunities. The need for the measure is based on theoretical constructs and research indicating that leisure boredom is associated with dissatisfaction and potential for destructive behavior.
Type of Client·	• Developed primarily for youth and young adults.
Clinical Utility	
Format	• Self-report format using 16 items scored on a 1 to 5 Likert scale. A higher score indicates greater boredom.
Completion Time	• Completion time is 10 minutes.
Standardization	• Used back-translation to create versions in Afrikaans and Xhosa for reliability study completed with adolescents in South Africa.
Reliability	
Test-Retest	• Study conducted in South Africa found concordance correlation coefficient (test-retest reliability of LBS as a whole) = 0.73 with 95% confidence interval (0.64 to 0.82).
	• Cohen's Kappa was moderate for 7 items (0.41 to 0.52) and within fair range for 2 items (0.32 to 0.38).
	• Observed agreement was preferred for 7 items (range: 38.8% to 66.6%).
Internal Consistency	• Three studies indicate Cronbach's alpha coefficients of 0.85, 0.88, and 0.86.
	• South African study found alpha coefficient ranged from 0.73 to 0.88.
Validity	
Content	• Used experts in leisure studies and students to jidge applicability of items for the questionnaire.
Construct	• Significant negative correlation between LBS and perceived social competence (-0.38) and self-as-entertainment (-0.49). Positive correlations between LBS and frequency (0.52) and depth (0.43) of boredom.
Criterion	• Significant negative correlations between LBS and Intrinsic Leisure Motivation Scale (-0.67) and Leisure Satisfaction Scale (-0.22).
Overall Utility	
Research	• May be useful in assessing whether leisure opportunities for youth and young adults (i.e., in recreation programs or in the community) are meeting the needs of this population.
Clinical	• Appears to be useful as a screening assessment to gather information about the nature of the leisure experiences for a young person.
Strengths	• Quick to administer.
	• Psychometric testing thus far supports its reliability and validity.
Weaknesses	• Further research regarding the predictive validity of the measure is required.

Table 13-2

LEISURE COMPETENCE MEASURE (LCM)

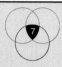

Source	Data System (Marita Kloseck), 9 Mount Pleasant Ave, London, ON, Canada, N6H 1C8
Important References	Kloseck, M., & Crilly, R. G. (1997). *Leisure Competence Measure: Adult version.* London, Ontario: Data System
	Kloseck, M., Crilly, R. G., Ellis, G.D & Lammers, E. (1996). Leisure Competence Measure: Development and reliability of a scale to measure functional outcomes in therapeutic recreation. *Therapeutic Recreation Journal, 30(1),* 13-26.
	Kloseck, M., Crilly, R.G., & Hutchinson-Troyer, L. (2001). Measuring therapeutic recreation outcomes in rehabilitation: Further testing of the Leisure Competence Measure. *Therapeutic Recreation Journal, 35(1),* 31-42.
Purpose	• Designed to summarize a leisure assessment process that gathers information about leisure functioning: it is also designed to evaluate changes in leisure functioning over time.
Types of Client	• Developed for and validated with an adult and older adult population.
Clinical Utility	
Format	• Eight subscales (leisure awareness, leisure attitude, leisure skills, cultural/social behaviors, interpersonal skills, community integration skills, social contact, community participation).
	• Scoring: Each item is rated on a 1 to 7 Likert scale (7=complete independence and 1=total dependence). Scaling is consistent with Functional Independence Measure. Change scores are determined by dividing the change in total LCM scores by the number of subscales.
Procedures	• Rated by service provider based on information obtained from observation, interview, records, and other team members.
Completion Time	• Approximately 1 hour for the assessment and 10 minutes for scoring.
Standardization	• Manual is available. No normative data.
.	• LCM has been modified based on feedback from practitioners and through research.
Reliability	
Test-Retest	• Not tested.
Inter-Rater	• Ranges from 0.71 to 0.91 for subscales and 0.91 for overall score. (Kloseck, Crilly, Ellis, & Lammers, 1996).
Internal Consistency	• Cronbach's alpha of 0.92. Has shown good to excellent internal consistency across a range of practice areas: spinal cord injury (a=0.70), traumatic brain injury (a=0.93), general neurological conditions (a=0.88), orthopedic conditions (a=0.90), and cerebrovascular accident (a=0.88) (Klosecke et al., 2002).
Validity	
Content	• Used 25 experts (recreation educators, recreation practitioners, physicians) to validate item selection.
Construct	• Correlations of the total score of the LCM are 0.54 with the Geriatric Depression Scale, 0.40 with the Mini-Mental Status Examination and 0.47 with the Life Satisfaction Index. Retrospective study of 640 clients of geriatric and rehabilitation units indicated that the LSM is sensitive to change over time.
	• Factor analysis (Kloseck et. al, 2002) revealed one factor that explained 58.9% of the variance.
Criterion	• Not tested.

continued

> ### Table 13-2 (continued)
> ## LEISURE COMPETENCE MEASURE (LCM)
>
> **Overall Utility**
> *Research*
> - Designed to have the potential for use internationally in databases of therapeutic recreation outcomes, across a variety of populations and settings.
>
> *Clinical*
> - Can be used as a standardized format for goal setting and intervention planning.
> - Can be used to monitor client's progress, or change in function.
>
> **Strengths**
> - Quick to administer.
> - Ability to detect change in various clinical populations.
> - Scaled to be consistent with Functional Independence Measure.
> - Theoretically based on WHO-ICF and Leisure Ability Model.
>
> **Weaknesses**
> - High potential for ceiling effect impacts ability to detect change, as large changes in one area may be diluted by no change in other areas.
> - Scale may be misinterpreted as nominal, when it is ordinal.
> - Requires further testing to establish validity and normative data.

Lysyk, M., Brown, G. T., Rodrigues, E., McNally, J., & Loo, K. (2002). Translation of the Leisure Satisfaction Scale into French: a validation study. *Occupational Therapy International, 9(1)*, 76-89.

Mann, W. C. & Talty, P. (1990). Leisure Activity Profile: Measuring use of leisure time by persons with alcoholism. *Occupational Therapy in Mental Health, 10(4)*, 31-41.

Mannell, R., & Kleiber, D. (1997). A social psychology of leisure. State College, PA: Venture.

Matsutsuyu, J. S. (1969). The Interest Checklist. *American Journal of Occupational Therapy, 23*, 323-328.

McClenaghan, K. (1999). *Development of the pediatric activity card sort: Stage one.* Master's project, University of Western Ontario, London, Ontario, Canada.

McParland, R. (1999). *Development of the activity card sort: Stimulus identification.* Master's project, University of Western Ontario, London, Ontario, Canada.

Murphy, J. (1981). *Concepts of leisure.* Englewood Cliffs, NJ: Prentice-Hall.

Peebles, J., McWilliams, L., Herchuk Norris, L., & Park, K. (1999). Population-specific norms and reliability of the leisure diagnostic battery in a sample of patients with chronic pain. *Therapeutic Recreation Journal, 33(3)*, 135-41.

Rintala, D., Hart, K., & Fuhrer, M. (1993). *Handicap and spinal cord injury: Levels and correlates of mobility, occupational and social integration.* Proceedings of American Spinal Injury Association Meeting.

Rogers, J. C., Weinstein, J. M., & Figone, J. J. (1978). The Interest Checklist: An empirical assessment. *American Journal of Occupational Therapy, 32*, 628-630.

Sachs, D., & Josman, N. (2003). The Activity Card Sort: A factor analysis. *Occupational Therapy Journal of Research, 23(4)*, 165-74.

Schleien, S., Heyne, L., Rynders, J., & McAvoy, L. (1990). Equity and excellence: Serving all children in community recreation. *Journal of Physical Education, Recreation and Dance, 61(8)*, 45-48.

Schleien, S. J., Ray, M. T., & Green, F. P. (1997). *Community recreation and people with disabilities: Strategies for inclusion.* (2nd ed.). Baltimore: Paul H. Brookes Publishing Co.

Shaw, S. (1985). The meaning of leisure in everyday life. *Leisure Sciences, 7*, 1-24.

Shaw, S. (1986). Leisure, recreation, or free time? Measuring time usage. *Journal of Leisure Research, 18*, 177-189.

Smith, R. W., Austin, D. R., & Kennedy, D. W. (1996). *Inclusive and special recreation: Opportunities for persons with disabilities.* (3rd ed.). Madison, WI: Brown & Benchmark Publishers.

Strunin, L., & Boden, L. (2004). Family consequences of chronic back pain. *Social Science & Medicine, 58(7)*, 1385-1393.

Stumbo, N., & Peterson, C. A. (2004). *Therapeutic recreation program design: Principles and procedures.* (4th. Ed.). San Francisco: Pearson Education, Inc.

Trottier, A. N., Brown, G. T., & Hobson, S. J. G. (2002). Reliability and validity of the Leisure Satisfaction Scale (LSS-short form) and the Adolescent Leisure Interest Profile (ALIP). *Occupational Therapy International, 9(2)*, 131-144.

Wegner, L., Flisher, A. J., Muller, M., & Lombard C. (2002). Reliability of the Leisure Boredom Scale for use with high school learners in Cape Town, South Africa. *Journal of Leisure Research, 34(3)*, 340-51.

Whiteneck, G. (1987). Outcome analysis in spinal cord injury rehabilitation. In M. Fuhrer (Ed.). *Rehabilitation outcomes: Analysis and measurement.* Baltimore: Paul H. Brooks.

Witt, P., & Ellis, G. (1984). The Leisure Diagnostic Battery: Measuring perceived freedom in leisure. *Society & Leisure, 7(1)*, 109-124.

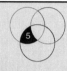

Table 13-3

LEISURE SATISFACTION QUESTIONNAIRE/ LEISURE SATISFACTION SCALE (LSS)

Source
Idyll Arbor Inc., 25119 SE 262nd St., P.O. Box 720, Ravensdale, WA, 98051-9763, (e-mail) Idyarbor@ix.netcom.com

Important References
Di Bona, L. (2000). What are the benefits of leisure? An exploration using the Leisure Satisfaction Scale. *British Journal of Occupational Therapy*, 63(2), 50-58.

Lysyk, M., Brown, G. T., Rodrigues, E., McNally, J., & Loo, K. (2002). Translation of the Leisure Satisfaction Scale into French: A validation study. *Occupational Therapy International*, 9(1), 76-89.

Trottier, A. N., Brown, G. T., & Hobson, S. J. G. (2002). Reliability and validity of the Leisure Satisfaction Scale (LSS-short form) and the Adolescent Leisure Interest Profile (ALIP). *Occupational Therapy International*, 9(2), 131-144.

Purpose
- To determine the extent to which a person believes their needs are satisfied through participation in leisure activities.

Type of Client
- Developed for use with the general population.

Clinical Utility

Format
- Original version: Self-report measure with 51 items scored on 5-point Likert-type scale, where 5 equals "almost always true for me" and 1 equals "almost never true for me."
- Short Form: 24-items (scored on the same scale) that are divided into 6 subscales: psychological scale (perception of freedom, enjoyment, involvement, and intellectual challenge while engaged in leisure activities), educational scale (belief that participation in leisure results in learning about self), social scale (degree to which leisure experiences provide rewarding social relationships), relaxation scale (degree to which leisure experiences reduce stress), physiological scale (degree to which leisure experiences contribute to physical fitness), and the aesthetic scale (perception of leisure experiences as pleasing and beautiful).

Procedures
- For the LSS-Short Form, respondents rate their satisfaction with leisure activities identified in the measure on a 5-point Likert scale.

Completion Time
- The short form of the LSS can be completed in 10 to 15 minutes.

Standardization
- Manual is available. French Canadian version has been standardized and correlated strongly (range of r=0.811 to 0.971) with the short version.

Reliability

Test-Retest
- Not tested.

Internal Consistency
- Internal consistency ranges from 0.86 to 0.92 with overall alpha coefficient of 0.96. The shortened version has an alpha reliability of 0.93.

Validity

Content
- Content validity was judged to be acceptable by 160 experts in the field of leisure.
- Di Bona (2000) found that perceived overall leisure satisfaction scores correlated with the total score of the LSS-Short form.

Construct:
- Not reported.

Criterion
- Not reported.

continued

Table 13-3 (continued)

LEISURE SATISFACTION QUESTIONNAIRE/
LEISURE SATISFACTION SCALE (LSS)

Overall Utility

Research
- Useful for examining the components of leisure activities that are needed for different populations in order for the activities to be beneficial.
- Could be incorporated into a needs review for program planning, or an evaluation of existing leisure programming.

Clinical
- The authors report the LSS can be useful for increasing a client's awareness of, and prioritizing activities he or she can do in his or her spare time.
- May be useful during initial assessment, intervention, and outcome evaluation.

Strengths
- Leisure Satisfaction Scale appears to be useful as an assessment of involvement in leisure activities.
- The LSS-Short Form can capture an individual's leisure patterns even in rural areas, where there may be a lack of typical facilities, programs, and transportation resources.
- Has been translated into French using established methodology for adapting existing outcome measures to be more culturally sensitive.

Weaknesses
- The original version requires more reliability and validity testing. This is particularly true for its ability to detect change if it is to be used at initial assessment, during treatment, and for outcome evaluation.
- The French Canadian version requires more testing with a variety of age and clinical diagnostic groups.

Table 13-4

ACTIVITY CARD SORT (ACS)

Source	Dr. Carolyn Baum, Program in Occupational Therapy, Box 8505, Washington University School of Medicine, 4444 Forest Park Blvd, St. Louis, MO, 63108
Important References	Baum, C. M., & Edwards, D. (2001). *Activity Card Sort.* St. Louis, MO: Washington University at St. Louis.
	Katz, N., Karpin, H., Lak, A., Furman, T., & Hartman-Maeir, A. (2003). Participation i occupational performance: Reliability and validity of the Activity Card Sort. *Occupational Therapy Journal of Rehabilitation, 23*(1), 10-17.
	Sachs, D., & Josman, N. (2003). The Activity Card Sort: A factor analysis. *Occupational Therapy Journal of Rehabilitation, 23*(4), 165-74.
Purpose	• Original version (older adult version) was designed to capture activity level of individuals with Alzheimer's Disease in instrumental, leisure and social activities; has been used with many different adult populations.
	• Institutional version can be used to establish functional treatment goals with a client.
	• Recovering version of ACS allows clinicians to record changes in activity patterns.
Type of Client	• Adults with and without cognitive loss.
Clinical Utility	
Format	• Can be performed with client, or with a parent or caregiver.
	• Has a Q-sort methodology (rank order procedure using piles or groups of objects). The client or his or her informant sorts photographs of people performing various activities into groups so that a general history of their participation in each activity can be obtained.
	• Photographs categorized into four domains: instrumental activities, low-demand leisure activities, high-demand leisure activities, and social activities. Clients do not group photographs according to these domains.
Procedures	• The client or his or her caregivers are asked to sort 80 photograph cards, one at a time, into groups. The groups vary, depending on the version of the tool being used.
	• In the healthy older adults version, cards are sorted into the following categories: 1) never done, 2) not done as an older adult, 3) do now, 4) do less, and 5) given up.
	• In the institutional version (hospital, rehab, long term care facility), the cards are sorted into two groups: 1) done prior to illness and 2) not done.
	• In the recovering version, the categories include 1) not done in the last 5 years, 2) gave up due to illness, 3) beginning to do again, and 4) do now.
	• Scoring: The sum total of current activities is divided by the sum total of previous activities. This provides a percent of retained activity level.
Completion Time	• Average completion time is 20 minutes. More time is required if the clinician asks probing questions about activities retained, lost, or desired.
Standardization	• The photographs can be tailored to the specific population of interest (i.e., different ages and cultures).
	• An Israeli version has been developed. Some pictures were removed and added from the original version of ACS. The final Israeli version is reported to have 88 pictures.

continued

Table 13-4 (continued)

ACTIVITY CARD SORT (ACS)

Reliability

Test-Retest
- Baum & Edwards (2001) reported a test-retest coefficient of 0.897 in a sample of 20 older adults living within the community.

Internal Consistency
- The Israeli version of the ACS had high internal consistency for IADL and social-cultural activities (a=0.82 and 0.80) and moderate internal consistency for low and high physical leisure activities (a=0.66 and 0.61) (Katz et al., 2003).

Validity

Content
- 2 content validity studies have been completed.
- The photographs were shown to an initial sample of 120 older adults, and then a second sample of 40 older adults (both samples were from the United States). After the sample provided feedback, 7 additional activities were added to the original ACS, to bring the total of the second edition of the ACS to 80.

Construct
- An Israeli study found the ACS differentiated well between healthy adults, healthy older adults, spouses or caregivers of individuals with Alzheimer's, individuals with multiple sclerosis and stroke survivors (1 year post-stroke) with regard to total retained activity level and individual activity areas (p<0.001) (Katz et al., 2003).
- Factor analysis of Israeli version of the ACS found young and older adults (n=184) classify activities into domains that are different than those suggested by the author. However, the authors in this study modified the scoring scale from the original version. This should be considered when using the tool in research for the purpose of examining the categorization and underlying dimensions of occupational performance (Katz et al., 2003).

Criterion
- A significant but moderate Pearson correlation coefficient was found between the Israeli version of the ACS category "doing now" and the number of hours a person reported being active on the Occupational Questionnaire (r=0.54).

Overall Utility

Research
- Useful for research directed at examining the occupational performance patterns of different age and diagnostic groups, as well as between genders.

Clinical
- Can be used as a guide for setting functional treatment goals with the client.
- The institutional version allows the therapist to create a pre-admission status for treatment planning and triggers ideas for intervention that include the person's prior experiences and interests.
- The recovering version allows clinicians to record changes in activity patterns, although the ability of the tool to detect change in performance has not been formally tested.

Strengths
- Allows client to describe how he or she engages in a variety of activities, but is also useful for individuals who have difficulties with speech or speaking English.
- The format is non-threatening, easy to understand and supports client-centered practice.
- Photographs can be modified based on the need of the population being assessed.

Weaknesses
- Has been adapted with minimal difficulty for a variety of populations, some cards from the original version suggest the focus is for a Christian population (i.e., reading the bible, going to church).
- Should not be the sole outcome measure used to establish treatment goals.
- The percentage score is somewhat arbitrary, as there is no standard for comparison.
- More research is necessary to determine whether the scores capture a change in behavior.

Table 13-5

PEDIATRIC ACTIVITY CARD SORT (PACS)

Source	Canadian Occupational Therapy Association, CAOT publications ACE, Canadian Association of Occupational Therapists, CTTC Building, 3400-1125 Colonel By Drive, Ottawa, Ontario, Canada, K1S 5R1, www.caot.org
Important References	Bowman, K. (1999). *Development of an activity card sort for children: Do parental reports on an activity card sort reflect similar results as their children?* Unpublished master's project, University of Western Ontario, London, Ontario, Canada.
	Burke, C., & Cooke, K. (2001). *Participation of children with DCD in activity: Is it really that important?* Unpublished master's project, University of Western Ontario, London, Ontario, Canada.
	Horn, S., & Williams, M. (2000). *Development and piloting of the pediatric occupational card sort (POCS): Stage II.* Unpublished master's thesis, University of Western Ontario, London, Ontario, Canada.
	Liston, S. (2002). *The Pediatric Activity Card Sort: A comparison of occupational profiles for children with developmental coordination Disorder and their typically developing peer.* Unpublished master's project, University of Western Ontario, London, Ontario, Canada.
	McClenaghan, K. (1999). *Development of the pediatric activity card sort: Stage one.* Master's project, University of Western Ontario, London, Ontario, Canada.
	McParland, R. (1999). *Development of the activity card sort: Stimulus identification.* Master's project, University of Western Ontario, London, Ontario, Canada.
Purpose	• Measures child's level of occupational engagement in a range of activities (including play) and participation at a particular point in time. Can be used to initiate goal setting for occupational therapy intervention.
Type of Client	• Children between the ages of 6 to 12 years of age with various diagnoses and physical disabilities (e.g., developmental coordination disorder (DCD), Asperger's Syndrome, etc.).
Clinical Utility	
Format	• Consists of cards (depicting personal care, school/productivity, hobbies/social activities, and sports) and a scoring sheet.
Procedures	• Administered by occupational therapists or certified occupational therapy assistants to either children or their parents. Examiners show cards and ask whether (and how frequently) children engage in activities depicted. Children identify their five most important activities and five activities they want to do.
Completion Time	• Can be administered in 15 to 20 minutes. More time may be required for elaboration of activities.
Standardization	• Criterion referenced.
Reliability	
Test-Retest	• Studies are currently being conducted.
Internal Consistency	• Studies are currently being conducted.
Validity	
Content	• Activities were identified initially through observation and experiences of the authors with children, literature search, and review of existing occupational therapy assessments.

continued

Table 13-5 (continued)

PEDIATRIC ACTIVITY CARD SORT (PACS)

- Five steps were taken for instrument validation: first, item validation was undertaken with 13 children between the ages of 6 to 12 years (McClenaghan, 1999); second, parents corroborated their children's (n=11) reports (Bowman, 1999). Next, the instrument was shown to be sensitive to age (Horn & Williams, 2000). Finally, the PACs was shown to detect differences in occupational profile between children with DCD and typically-developing children were explored with children (n=10; ages 6-10) (Liston, 2002).

Overall Utility

Research
- Can be used to explore occupational engagement.

Clinical
- Can be used in a variety of practice areas such as schools, pediatric facilities or private practice.

Strengths
- Occupation-based assessment supporting a client-centered approach.
- Photographs are appealing to children. Good tool for research.

Weaknesses
- New instrument; very limited evidence for reliability or validity.

Final Word
- The PACS is an occupational based pediatric self-report assessment tool that enables the therapist to focus intervention at the occupation level.

Table 13-6

PEDIATRIC INTEREST PROFILES: SURVEY OF PLAY FOR CHILDREN AND ADOLESCENTS

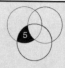

Source	Therapy Skill Builders, 555 Academic Court, San Antonio, TX, 78204-2498, (phone) 800-211-8378, (fax) 800-232-1223.
Important Reference	Henry, A. D. (1998). Development of a measure of adolescent leisure interests. *American Journal of Occupational Therapy, 52,* 531-539.
Purpose	• Provide an easy way to gain a profile of a child's play interests.
Type of Client	• Children and adolescents between 6 and 21 years of age regardless of type of disability.
Clinical Utility	
Format	• Comprised of three assessments: the Kids Play Survey (KPS) (6 to 9 years), Pre-Teen Play Survey (PPS) (9 to 12 years), and Adolescent Leisure Interest Profile (ALIP) (12 to 21 years).
Procedures	• Paper-and-pencil checklist format. Children/adolescents respond to questions regarding interest, participation, enjoyment, etc., in leisure/play activities typical of peers. KPS and PPS use drawings to represent activities. Can be administered individually or in a small group setting.
Completion Time	• Approximately 15 minutes (for KPS) to 30 minutes (for ALIP).
Standardization	• Each test consists of standard choices to which the child/adolescent responds.
Reliability	
Internal Consistency	• ALIP—Cronbach's alpha ranged from 0.59 to 0.80 for subscale scores and was 0.93 for total scores for questions regarding level of interest in activities (n=88 adolescents with various disabilities).
Test-Retest	• KPS—PPM coefficients ranged from 0.45 to 0.91 for total scores (n=31 children without disabilities).
	• PPS—not reported.
	• ALIP—PPM coefficients ranged from 0.61 to 0.85 for total scores (n=28 adolescents without disabilities).
	• ALIP—PPM coefficients ranged from 0.62 to 0.78 for total scores (n=88 adolescents with various disabilities).
Validity	
Content	• Items for all three versions developed from interviews and preliminary surveys of children or adolescents in the targeted age range.
Convergent	• Not reported.
Construct	• ALIP—question regarding level of enjoyment in activities was shown to discriminate among adolescents with and without disabilities.
Overall Utility	
Research	• Can be used with large population to gain general understanding of leisure patterns of children and youth.
Clinical	• Easily used in most settings.
	• Can be used to establish treatment goals.
Strengths	• The only assessments specifically devoted to developing a profile of play interests from the perspective of children and adolescents.
	• Require minimal examiner training.
Weaknesses	• Activities seem most relevant to North American children.
	• Relationship between measures not examined. Longitudinal study would be useful for predictive ability.

Table 13-7

INTEREST CHECKLIST AND ACTIVITY CHECKLIST

Important References
Katz, N. (1988). Interest Checklist: A factor analytical study. *Occupational Therapy in Mental Health, 8(1)*, 45-55.

Klyczek, J. P., Bauer-Yox, N., & Fiedler, R. C. (1997). The Interest Checklist: A factor analysis. *American Journal of Occupational Therapy, 51(10)*, 815-23.

Matsutsuyu, J. S. (1969). The Interest Checklist. *American Journal of Occupational Therapy, 23*, 323-328.

Rogers, J. C., Weinstein, J. M., & Figone, J. J. (1978). The Interest Checklist: An empirical assessment. *American Journal of Occupational Therapy, 32*, 628-630.

Purpose
- Primary purpose is to classify a person's level of interest in 80 different leisure activities. It has also been suggested that it can be used to determine if a person can express personal preferences, and discriminate between choices.
- The Activity Checklist can be used for the above purpose, as well as determining past and potential future activity interests.

Type of Client
- Developed for use within the general population (adolescent to adult). Note: Adolescent version is described elsewhere in this chapter.

Clinical Utility

Format
- The Interest Checklist originally developed by Matsutsuyu includes 80 items that can be classified into five categories: 1) Manual Skills, 2) Physical Sports, 3) Social Recreation, 4) ADL, and 5) Cultural/Educational.
- Katz revised the Interest Checklist and renamed the new version the Activity Checklist. It contains 60 of the original 80 items, which can be classified into four categories: 1) Sports and Physical Tasks, 2) Intellectual and Musical Tasks, 3) Social Tasks, and 4) Fine Manual Tasks and Homemaking.
- Both the Interest Checklist and the Activity Checklist have a self-report format.

Procedures
- For the Interest Checklist, the client indicates his or her level of interest for each item on a 3-point scale: no interest, casual interest or strong interest.
- For the Activity Checklist, the client completes the same 3-point scale as the Interest Checklist, as well as a 3-point scale for past performance of each item. The client is also asked to indicate yes or no for future performance.

Completion Time
- On average, the Interest Checklist can be completed in approximately 20 minutes.

Standardization
- Researchers have recommended and utilized various modifications of The Interest Checklist.
- Rogers et al. (1978) changed the rating scale to a 5-point Likert Scale (like very much, like, indifferent, dislike, and dislike very much).
- Katz (1988) changed "a few" items in the Physical Sports category so that the category would more closely reflect present day Israeli activities.

Reliability

Test-Retest
- Not reported.

Internal Consistency
- Not reported.

Validity

Content
- Interest Checklist items were selected by a panel of occupational therapists, based on empirical knowledge. The final 80 items selected met 2 criteria: 1) they were generally understood, and 2) they could be classified into one of the five theoretically defined categories identified by Matsutsuyu. Matsutsuyu does not describe how the five categories were developed.

continued

Table 13-7 (continued)

INTEREST CHECKLIST AND ACTIVITY CHECKLIST

Construct	• Three factor analysis studies have been completed on the Interest Checklist.
	• Rogers et al. (1978) found that only two of the five categories (Cultural/Educational and Physical Sports) were empirically independent; the assessment found significant differences between boys and girls in high school students aged 12 to 18 (n=143).
	• Katz (1988) found three of the five categories were empirically independent (Cultural/Educational, Physical Sports, and Social Recreation). She suggested a four-factor solution, whereby the remaining two categories (ADL and Manual Skills) be combined to form the fourth category (Fine manual tasks and homemaking). Katz found response differences between genders in a sample of 67 clients with psychiatric conditions.
	• Klyczek, Bauer-Yox, and Fiedler (1997) administered the Interest Checklist to students, working adults and retired older adults (n=367) and found 3 of the 5 categories were empirically independent for students and working adults and the social recreation was empirically independent for all three subject groups. They found that the Interest Checklist captured different patterns of interest in the five categories between study groups, depending on age or role.
Criterion	• Not reported.
Overall Utility	
Research	• Useful for determining differences in interest patterns between groups, particularly gender. However, additional research is necessary to assess the tool's ability to discriminate between populations with more varied characteristics (i.e., people with disabilities, age, etc.).
Clinical	• Useful for generating discussion about client's interests and determining activities to incorporate into therapy that are meaningful to the client.
Strengths	• Developed from six theoretical principles proposed by Matsutsuyu.
	• Encourages client-centered approach.
	• The addition of past performance and future interest scales to Katz's Activity Checklist provides the therapist with a broader context in which to view the client.
Weaknesses	• Minimal reliability testing.
	• Construct validity testing has produced mixed results (items have not clustered into consistent patterns).
	• Therefore, therapists may not be getting true picture of client interests.
	• Items need to be updated to reflect current activities.
	• Impact of gender and age on response patterns needs to be examined more closely.
	• Only assesses interest in activities; does not examine participation or enjoyment.

Table 13-8

CHILDREN'S ASSESSMENT OF PARTICIPATION AND ENJOYMENT (CAPE)

Source	Psychological Corporation, Skill Builders Division, 555 Academic Court, San Antonio, TX, 78204, (phone) 800-228-0752.
Important References	King, G., Law, M., King, S., Hurley, P., Hanna, S., Kertoy, M., Rosenbaum, P., & Young, N. (in press). *Children's Assessment of Participation and Enjoyment (CAPE) and Preferences for Activities of Children (PAC)*. San Antonio, TX: Harcourt Assessment, Inc.
	King, G., Law, M., King, S., Rosenbaum, P., Kertoy, M., & Young, N. L. (2003). A conceptual model of the factors affecting the recreation and leisure participation of children with disabilities. *Physical and Occupational Therapy in Pediatrics, 23*, 63-90.
Purpose	• To capture children/youth's participation in and enjoyment of day-to-day activities outside of mandated school activities.
Type of Client	• Children and youth aged 6 years to 21 years of age. It is not recommended for children or youth who do not understand the task of sorting and categorizing activities.

Clinical Utility

Format

- Contains 55 items that are divided into fve types of activity, or scales: Recreational (12 items), Active Physical (13 items), Social (10 items), Skill-Based (10 items), and Self-Improvement/Educational (10 items).

- Items can also be categorized into one of two domains: informal (40 items) or formal activities (15 items).

- The CAPE measures five dimensions of participation: diversity (number of activities, intensity (frequency-scale ranges from 0 to 7), with whom (seven possible responses), where (six possible responses) and enjoyment (scale ranges from 0 to 5).

Procedures

- Self-administered version: Children are asked to look at drawings of children performing 55 different activities and identify on a Likert-type scale if they have performed each activity in the last 4 months, how often, with whom they performed the activity and their level of enjoyment.

- Interviewer-assisted version: Phase 1—Child completes (alone or with parent) short questionnaire about whether they have performed each of the 55 activities in the past 4 months, and if so, how often. Phase 2—The interviewer asks the following questions for each activity the child has performed: who he or she performed the activity with?, where he or she performed the activity?, and how much he or she enjoyed the activity?.

- Scoring: The CAPE provides overall participation scores, scale scores and domain scores. From these scores, it can also provide 8 additional scores for each of the dimensions of interest.

Completion Time

- Self-administered version takes 20 to 30 minutes. Interview-assisted: Phase 1 generally takes 25 to 30 minutes to complete. Phase 2 takes an additional 20 to 30 minutes.

Standardization

- The CAPE can be self-administered, or interviewer-assisted. The manual provides comprehensive instructions, but training would be beneficial.

Reliability

Test-Retest

- For overall participation and formal and informal domains, ICCs for diversity and intensity scores ranged from 0.67 to 0.86, indicating adequate to good reliability. ICCs for enjoyment ranged from 0.12 (active physical activities) to 0.73 (recreational activities), indicating poor to good validity.

continued

Table 13-8 (continued)

CHILDREN'S ASSESSMENT OF PARTICIPATION AND ENJOYMENT (CAPE)

Internal Consistency	• Intensity scores for five scales (types of activities) ranged from 0.72 to 0.81 (good reliability). • Enjoyment scores had low reliability, except for recreational activities. • Cronbach's alpha was calculated for the domains and scales of the CAPE. Values ranged from poor to adequate: a=0.32 (Skill-based activities) to a=0.62 (social activities).
Validity	
Content	• Items were drawn from an extensive literature review, reviewed by a group of experts, and the initial draft of the CAPE was piloted with a small sample.
Construct	• Overall, domain and scale scores were compared with scores on measures of different constructs obtained from a longitudinal study of predictors of children's participation. There were small to moderate, but significant correlations between CAPE participation intensity and enjoyment scores and relevant outcome variables (r<0.01). • Comparisons between the CAPE intensity and enjoyment scores and the Preferences for the Activities of Children (PAC) preference scores were conducted. Correlations ranged from 0.22 to 0.61, which supported discriminant validity. • The CAPE was shown to discriminate between boys and girls for intensity and enjoyment as well as between children with and without disabilities and between age groups for intensity.
Criterion	• Significant relationships demonstrated between the CAPE and measures of family and child functioning.
Overall Utility	
Research	• Can be used to examine and compare the participation patterns of children and youth with or without disabilities, including changes over time. • It can be used as an outcome measure in a recreational program evaluation.
Clinical	• Provides useful information to a clinician about the type, intensity and enjoyment of activities their client has experienced. • Can be used to assess the effectiveness of intervention focused on improving the frequency, intensity, and/or enjoyment of participation of children in various extra-curricular activities.
Strengths	• Theoretically based on the WHO-ICF. It is a very comprehensive measure of participation. • User-friendly for children; captures the child's perspective of their own participation patterns. • Culturally sensitive. Pictures are gender-neutral, not culturally specific and include children with physical disabilities. • Different methods of administration allow for greater flexibility of use in clinical and research setting.
Weaknesses	• It is a complex tool that requires a solid understanding by the clinician prior to administration. • Additional psychometric testing is required to examine categorization of domain activities and scales.

Table 13-9

PREFERENCES FOR ACTIVITIES OF CHILDREN (PAC)

Source	Psychological Corporation, Skill Builders Division, 555 Academic Court, San Antonio, TX, 78204, (phone) 800-228-0752.
Important References	King, G., Law, M., King, S., Hurley, P., Hanna, S., Kertoy, M.,Rosenbaum, P., & Young, N. (in press). *Children's Assessment of Participation and Enjoyment (CAPE) and Preferences for Activities of Children (PAC)*. San Antonio, TX: Harcourt Assessment, Inc.
	King, G., Law, M., King, S., Rosenbaum, P., Kertoy, M. & Young, N. L. (2003). A conceptual model of the factors affecting the recreation and leisure participation of children with disabilities. *Physical and Occupational Therapy in Pediatrics, 23*, 63-90.

Purpose
- To assess the activity preferences of children and youth.

Type of Client
- Children and youth aged 6 years to 21 years of age. It is not recommended for children or youth who do not understand the task of sorting and categorizing activities.

Clinical Utility

Format
- Contains 55 items that are divided into 5 types of activity, or scales: Recreational (12 items), Active Physical (13 items), Social (10 items), Skill-based (10 items), and Self-improvement/Educational (10 items).
- Items can also be categorized into one of two domains: informal (40 items) or formal activities (15 items).

Procedures
- Self-administered version: Children are asked to look at drawings of children performing 55 different activities and record their preference for each activity by circling one of three facial expressions that correspond with their interest in the activity (I would not like to do at all, I would sort of like to do, I would really like to do).
- Interviewer-assisted version: The interviewer asks the child to sort the drawings into one of three piles using the same response options as in the self-administered version. A card containing enlarged facial expressions with corresponding written descriptions assists them in their sorting.

Completion Time
- Generally takes between 10 to 15 minutes to complete.

Standardization
- The PAC can be self-administered, or interviewer-assisted. The manual provides a script with administration instructions.

Reliability

Test-Retest
- Not reported.

Internal Consistency
- Cronbach's α was calculated for the domains and scales of the PAC. Domain values (formal/informal) were good (α=0.76 and 0.84), and values of α for the five scales ranged from 0.67 to 0.77, indicating fair to good reliability.

Validity

Content
- Items were drawn from an extensive literature review, reviewed by a group of experts, and the initial draft of the PAC was piloted with a small sample.

Construct
- There were small to moderate, but significant correlations between PAC preference scores and relevant outcome variables ($r<0.01$) from a longitudinal study of predictors of children's participation.
- Factor analyses were completed with two sets of data. Analysis revealed the presence of five factors, with 34.2 percent of the variance accounted for in the first analysis, and 36.1% of the variance accounted for in the second. The five factors provided support for the construct validity of the PAC.
- Comparisons between the PAC preference scores and CAPE intensity and enjoyment scores were conducted. Correlations ranged from 0.22 to 0.61, which supported concurrent validity.

continued

Table 13-9 (continued)

PREFERENCES FOR ACTIVITIES OF CHILDREN (PAC)

Criterion	• Not reported.
Overall Utility	
Research	• Can be used to examine and compare the participation preferences of children with and without disabilities.
	• It can be used as an outcome measure in a recreational program evaluation.
Clinical	• Provides activity options for children, and therefore can contribute to goal setting.
	• Provides options of activities with same underlying characteristics that can substitute for other activities (i.e., active physical activities, quiet leisure activities, etc.).
Strengths	• User-friendly for children & captures the child's perspective.
	• Culturally sensitive. Pictures are gender-neutral, include children with physical disabilities and of various cultural backgrounds.
	• Different methods of administration allow for greater flexibility of use in clinical and research setting.
	• Theoretically based on the WHO-ICF.
Weaknesses	• More reliability and validity testing needs to be conducted on this new measure.

Table 13-10

LEISURE ACTIVITY PROFILE (LAP)

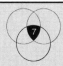

Source	Mann, W. C., & Talty, P. (1990). Leisure Activity Profile: Measuring use of leisure time by persons with alcoholism. *Occupational Therapy in Mental Health, 10(4)*, 31-41.
Purpose	• Measures the use of time spent by persons with alcoholism. It was designed to identify dysfunctional leisure activity patterns that are typically associated with high levels of alcohol consumption (Mann & Talty, 1990).
Type of Client	• Clients who have confirmed diagnosis of alcoholism.
Clinical Utility	
Format	• Consists of 38 items or activities, 19 typically associated with alcohol and 19 not typically associated with alcohol. Respondents identify how often they engage in each activity, if they do it alone or with others, whether they consume alcohol when performing the task; and their level of enjoyment for each activity.
	• Scoring: Raw frequency responses are translated into 5-point numerical scale.
Procedures	• Self report measure. Can also be administered by interview.
Completion Time	• Not reported.
Standardization	• Instructions are provided for interviewers.
Reliability	
Test-Retest	• Good test-retest results with a sample of 210 people without alcoholism (frequency of involvement, r=0.94; amount of alcohol consumption, r=0.90).
Internal Consistency	• Not reported.
Validity	
Content	• Test items were developed by asking 540 adult subjects to list 10 favorite leisure activities. From the 620 activities identified, the authors subjectively selected 19 assumed to be associated with alcohol consumption and 19 not associated with alcohol consumption.
	• Statistical relationship between activities and alcohol consumption has not been examined.
Construct	• Distinguished between 20 people with alcoholism and a sample of people without alcoholism regarding use of leisure time and activity participation (significance not reported).
Criterion	• Not reported.
Overall Utility	
Research	• Can be used to examine differing use of leisure time between people with and without alcoholism.
Clinical	• May be useful for identifying persons at risk for developing alcoholism, or breaking from sobriety (although has not been specifically tested for this).
	• May provide client and therapist with insight into behavior patterns that contribute to successful or unsuccessful sobriety. Provide direction for behavior modification.
Strengths	• Developed for a specific population. Has clinical and research implications.
Weaknesses	• Requires more validity and reliability testing with people who have alcoholism.
	• Needs to have normative data for people with and without alcoholism.

Table 13-11

CRAIG HANDICAP ASSESSMENT AND REPORTING TECHNIQUE (CHART)

Source	Whiteneck, G., Charlifue, S., Gerhart, K., Overholser, D., & Richardson, G. (1992). Quantifying handicap: A new measure of long-term rehabilitation outcomes. *Archives of Physical Medicine and Rehabilitation, 73*, 519-526.
Important References	Dijkers, M. (1991). Scoring CHART: Survey and sensitivity analysis. *Journal of the American Paraplegia Society, 14,* 85-86.
	Hall, K. M., Dijkers, M., Whiteneck, G., Brooks, C. A., & Stuart Krause, J. (1998). The Craig Handicap Assessment and Reporting Technique (CHART): Metric properties and scoring. *Topics in Spinal Cord Injury Rehabilitation, 4(1),* 16-30.
	Rintala, D., Hart, K., & Fuhrer, M. (1993). Handicap and spinal cord injury: Levels and correlates of mobility, occupational and social integration. *Proceedings of American Spinal Injury Association Meeting.*
	Whiteneck, G. (1987). Outcome analysis in spinal cord injury rehabilitation. In M. Fuhrer (Ed.). *Rehabilitation outcomes: Analysis and measurement.* Baltimore: Paul H. Brooks.
Purpose	• To measure the level of handicap experienced by an individual in a community setting.
Type of Client	• Designed for clients with spinal cord injuries. The Revised CHART has also been used in research for people with traumatic brain injury, stroke, multiple sclerosis, amputations, and burns.
Clinical Utility	
Format	• 27 questions belonging to five subscales: 1) physical independence, 2) mobility, 3) occupation, 4) social integration, and 5) economic self-sufficiency. There are two to seven items per subscale. Subscales correspond to 5 of 6 areas of handicap identified by ICIDH (WHO, 1980).
	• Scoring: Each subscale has a maximum score of 100 points, which corresponds to typical performance of average person without disability. High subscale and total scores indicate less handicap. The maximum economic self-sufficiency score corresponds to U.S. median income.
Procedures	• Self-report questionnaire that asks client to indicate time spent performing items. Can also be completed by caregiver as a proxy.
Completion Time	• Estimated to be 30 minutes.
Standardization	• Not standardized. Revised CHART was developed with additional "cognitive independence" scale to increase applicability to stroke population.
Reliability	
Test-Retest	• Dijkers (1991) found subscale coefficients to be in excellent range (0.80 to 0.95), as well as the coefficient for the total score (0.93).
Internal Consistency	• Not reported.
Validity	
Content	• Based on ICIDH (WHO, 1980)—ensured domain of handicap areas are covered in full, without overlap with impairment and disability.
Construct	• Distinguished between groups (i.e., based on culture, age, education, injury level, time since injury), however, the authors recommend that group differences should be interpreted with caution (Hall, Dijkers, Whiteneck, Brooks, & Stuart Krause, 1998).
	• Rasch analysis supported underlying structure and linearity of CHART.

continued

Table 13-11 (continued)

CRAIG HANDICAP ASSESSMENT AND REPORTING TECHNIQUE (CHART)

Criterion	• Concordance of CHART scores with therapist ratings of high vs low handicap.
Overall Utility	
Research	• Useful for measuring community reintegration of broad populations such as SCI clients.
	• Useful in rehabilitation program evaluation.
Clinical	• May be useful for measuring change in performance (before vs after intervention), although does not appear to have been specifically tested for this.
Strengths	• Focuses on objective, observable criteria to limit interpreter bias.
	• Normative data has been established with large sample sizes.
	• Views occupation in a manner similar to occupational therapy perspective.
Limitations	• The CHART has a ceiling effect, particularly for the SCI population.
	• Economic self-sufficiency scale is based on US income, limiting international interpretation.
	• Large percentage of incomplete data for the economic self-sufficiency subscale in large studies, which impacts total scores reported in research.
	• Reliance on total scores may mask important differences at the subscale level.

Table 13-12

LEISURE DIAGNOSTIC BATTERY

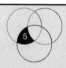

Source	Idyll Arbor, Inc., P.O. Box 720, Ravensdale, WA, 98051, (Web) www.idyllarbor.com.
Important References	Beard, J. G., & Ragheb, M. G. (1983). Measuring leisure motivation. *Journal of Leisure Research, 15(3)*, 219-228.
	Trottier, A. N., Brown, G. T., & Hobson, S. J. G. (2002). Reliability and validity of the Leisure Satisfaction Scale (LSS—short form) and the Adolescent Leisure Interest Profile (ALIP). *Occupational Therapy International, 9(2)*, 131-144.
Purpose	• To obtain a broad measure of a client's leisure aptitudes.
Type of Client	• Individuals who have: an adapted I.Q. of 80 and above, mental age of 12 years and older, Rancho Los Amigos Level of 7 and above, reality orientation level of mild to no orientation disability.
Clinical Utility	
Format	• The Leisure Diagnostic Battery is a combination of four separate assessments:
	Leisure Attitude Measure (LAM)—Reviews client's attitude toward leisure on three different component levels: 1) cognitive, 2) affective, and 3) behavioral.
	Leisure Interest Measure (LIM)—helps identify the degree to which a client is interested in each of the eight domains of leisure activities: 1) physical, 2) outdoor, 3) mechanical, 4) artistic, 5) service, 6) social, 7) cultural, and 8) reading.
	Leisure Motivation Scale (LMS)—Slightly modified version of Leisure Motivation Scale developed by Beard and Ragheb (1983). Measures client's motivation for participating in leisure activities. There is a Full Scale (48 items) and a Short Scale (32 items).
	Leisure Satisfaction Measure (LSM)—alternate version of Leisure Satisfaction Scale. Idyll Arbor developed this version with permission of original authors. Measures six subscales of satisfaction: 1) psychological, 2) educational, 3) social, 4) relaxation, 5) physiological, and 6) aesthetic.
Procedures	• LAM and LMS—Self report; recommended to be administered between fourth and seventh day of admission in inpatient setting.
	• LIM—Self-report; can be administered any time.
Completion Time	• LAM, LIM, and LMS: 5 to 25 minutes for client to complete 36 items, 29 items, and 48 items respectively; scoring <10 minutes.
	• LSM: 5 to 20 minutes to complete 24 items; scoring <10 minutes.
Standardization	• Instructions provided for administration and scoring for each assessment.
Reliability	
Test-Retest	• LAM, LIM, LMS—not reported
Internal Consistency	• LAM—Demonstrates good reliability for the total measure (a=0.94) and each component (cognitive a=0.91, affective a=0.93, and behavioral a=0.89).
	• LIM—Demonstrates good reliability for the total measure (a=0.87). The internal consistency of items within each domain was acceptable, however, the artistic domain demonstrated poor internal reliability.
	• LMS—Manual reports strong internal reliability and refers reader to Beard and Ragheb (1983). Full Scale is more reliable than Short Scale.
	• LSM—Alpha reliability coefficient for the overall score was very high (a=0.93).

continued

Table 13-12 (continued)

LEISURE DIAGNOSTIC BATTERY

Validity

Content
- LAM—The final version with 36 items was established after a literature review, expert reviews, empirical analysis, and factor analysis.
- LIM—The final version with 29 items was developed after a literature search, multiple expert reviews and empirical analyses.
- LMS—The manual reports strong content validity and refers reader to Beard and Ragheb (1983).
- LSM—The final version with 24 items was developed after a literature search, expert review, and field testing.

Construct
- LAM—Divergent validity was established in study that confirmed each question was placed correctly within each component.
- LIM and LMS—Not reported.
- LSM—Factor analysis showed that the psychological, educational, social and environmental subscales were clearly defined. The other two subscales were less clearly defined, but still within acceptable range.

Criterion
- LAM—Has been compared to 2 other leisure attitude scales (results not reported).
- LIM, LMS, and LSM—Not reported.

Overall Utility

Research
- Useful when trying to research multiple constructs of leisure participation.

Clinical
- LAM—Useful for determining if one or more areas are barriers to client's active participation in leisure activities.
- LIM—Can be used for goal setting and treatment planning.
- LMS—Can be used in treatment planning to encourage interest and participation.
- LSM—Useful in determining if recreation programming is meeting client's needs, and provides some direction to modify program as necessary.

Strengths
- Provides comprehensive assessment about a person's choices regarding leisure.
- Therapists gain four assessments

Weaknesses
- Reliability and validity data for each tool are summarized only very briefly with few statistical values, and are not referenced.
- Research required to examine the relationship between the tools, and the ability of all four (as a combination) to capture leisure from a broader perspective than existing measures.

Table 13-13

LEISURE DIAGNOSTIC BATTERY (LDB)

Source	LDB Project, Division of Recreation and Leisure Studies, North Texas University, Denton, TX, 76203.
Important References	Chang, Y., & Card, J. A. (1994). The reliability of the Leisure Diagnostic Battery Short Form Version B in assessing healthy, older individuals: A preliminary study. *Therapeutic Recreation Journal, 28*, 163-7.
	Ellis, G. D., & Witt, P. A. (1986). The Leisure Diagnostic Battery: Past, present and future. *Therapeutic Recreation Journal, 19*, 31-47.
	Peebles, J., McWilliams, L., Herchuk Norris, L., & Park, k. (1999). Population-specific norms and reliability of the leisure diagnostic battery in a sample of patients with chronic pain. *Therapeutic Recreation Journal, 33(3)*, 135-41.
	Witt, P. A., & Ellis, G. D. (1984). The Leisure Diagnostic Battery: Measuring perceived freedom in leisure. *Society and Leisure, 7*, 109-24.

Purpose
- The LDB was designed to assess an individual's perceived freedom in leisure, as well as perceived barriers to leisure participation.

Type of Client
- Originally developed for youth with disabilities. A version has been developed for adults and older adults.

Clinical Utility

Format
- Form A and Form C includes 95 items related to competence, control, needs depth, and playfulness; 24 items related to barriers; and 28 items related to knowledge.
- Form B is a short form of the LDB, including 25 items.
- Scoring: Form A and Form B have a 3-point scale. Form C has a 5-point scale. The mean sum of the five scales is considered an overall indicator of perceived freedom in leisure.

Procedures
- The LDB is a self-report measure.

Completion Time
- Version A and C takes 30 to 40 minutes. Version B takes 10 to 15 minutes.

Standardization
- Manual is available. Form A has been modified (wording less simplistic, rating scale changed from 3-point to 5-point scale) to create Form C, an adult version.

Reliability

Test-Retest
- Form A—Intra-class correlation coefficient of 0.72.

Internal Consistency
- Alpha coefficients of 0.83 to 0.94 for Form A and 0.89 to 0.94 for Form B.
- Form C—Alpha coefficients for the five scales ranged from 0.90 to 0.92. Alpha coefficient for the total score was 0.96.
- These values indicate that all forms of the LDB have excellent reliability.

Validity

Content
- Form A validated through factor analysis. Has not been completed for Form C.

Construct
- Form A—Moderate correlations between LDB and measures of barriers and knowledge regarding leisure. Correlation of 0.16 by gender. Has been found to be sensitive to change after a therapeutic recreation program.

Criterion
- Not reported.

Overall Utility

Research
- Can be used to examine/compare perceived freedom for and barriers to leisure activity for different populations.

Clinical
- Form C—Useful as an assessment and outcome measure for clients with chronic pain from musculoskeletal injuries.
- Not appropriate to measure treatment effectiveness, as playfulness scale appears to measure underlying personality characteristic.

continued

Table 13-13 (continued)

LEISURE DIAGNOSTIC BATTERY (LDB)

Strengths
- Has a theoretical basis.
- Normative data established for different populations.
- Measures more than one construct of leisure.

Weaknesses
- Requires more psychometric testing, particularly validity.
- Requires more testing on different adult populations.

Editors' Notes for Chapter 14

Mine the Gold

Social scientists have much information about the effect of role on a person's performance and life satisfaction. These constructs have informed the way in which occupational therapists include the concept of role in everyday practice.

Become Systematic

Provides structure for information that client provides about the roles that they fulfill in their daily life and any roles they are having difficulty in performing to their satisfaction.

Use Evidence in Practice

Gathering and using knowledge about how each person finds meaning through the roles in which they engage assists with the identification of therapy goals and facilitates active participation in the therapy process.

Make Occupational Therapy Contribution Explicit

Occupational therapists focus on how a person's roles support performance and facilitate changes in roles to improve performance and satisfaction.

Engage in Occupation-Based, Client-Centered Practice

Assessment and consideration of roles facilitates clients in achieving their goals related to occupational performance.

MEASUREMENT OF OCCUPATIONAL ROLE

Janice P. Burke, PhD, OTR/L, FAOTA and T. Brianna Lomba, OTS

ASSESSING OCCUPATIONAL ROLE

The profession of occupational therapy has long been committed to working with people to increase their participation in meaningful occupational roles. A significant body of literature exists in the theoretical domain of the field that attempts to carve out the construct of occupation and the related areas of occupational role (Fidler, 1991; Kielhofner & Burke, 1980; Matsutsuyu, 1971; Mosey, 1970; Reilly, 1962; Yerxa, Frank, Clark, et al., 1990). Similarly, practice-oriented materials and writings that fall into the category of professional guidelines address attention to the notion of occupational roles as the focus of occupational therapy intervention.

Given the professional orientation toward occupational roles, it is surprising to find little in the way of authentic, occupational therapy-based assessments for measuring the degree of function/dysfunction in occupational role performance. Of the seven occupational role assessments that were reviewed in this portion of the text, four were developed by occupational therapists (Tables 14-1 through 14-4). All four are representative of an era of theory development within occupational therapy that urged practitioners, scholars, and researchers to place their primary emphasis on occupation. The three assessments of the second group (Tables 14-5 through 14-7) were developed in the fields of social work and social science in an effort to understand how social performance is influenced by roles that are expected or enacted by an individual.

All of the assessments that were reviewed are in the beginning stages of development from a psychometric point of view. Each is more appropriate for assessment and intervention development and planning rather than a tool for measuring baseline behaviors that can be reassessed following a protocol of treatment.

REVIEW OF SELECTED ASSESSMENTS

Adolescent Role Assessment

This instrument was developed by Maureen Black as part of her master's thesis at the University of Southern California. Studying under the occupational behaviorist Dr. Mary Reilly, Black assembled a semi-structured interview that conceptualized the occupation role process in adolescence as a time in which an individual "develops and practices skills of occupational choice and eventually acquires the competence to enter adulthood and the larger society" (Black, 1976, p. 73). Black proposed this assessment as a method for historically reviewing an individual's skills as well as the preferences and choices that existed in the present. Following identification of needs and gaps, the therapist is able to develop an intervention plan to promote successful role enactment.

The Adolescent Role Assessment was derived from child and adolescent role-behavior literature. Most significantly, Black drew on the work of Eli Ginzburg, who developed the notion of occupational choice in adolescence as a preliminary and necessary series of three stages that must be successfully mastered in order to ensure adult occupational role performance.

Table 14-1

Adolescent Role Assessment

Source	Black, M. M. (1976). Adolescent Role Assessment. *American Journal of Occupational Therapy, 30(2)*, 73-79.
Important Reference	Huebner, R., Emery, L., & Shordike, A. (2002). The adolescent role assessment: Psychometric properties and theoretical usefulness. *American Journal of Occupational Therapy, 56* (2).
Purpose	• To assess past history and present organization of internalized roles. Provides a profile of the adolescent's role development within family, peer, and school situations.
Type of Client	• Adolescent, inpatient psychiatric setting; diagnoses include adjustment reaction, anorexia nervosa, school phobia, and depression.
Clinical Utility	
Format	• Interview covers 21 topics in six areas: childhood play, adolescent socialization in the family, school performance, peer interactions, occupational choice, and work.
Procedure	• Semi-structured interview with specific rating criteria.
Completion Time	• 30 minutes.
Reliability	
Internal Consistency	• A=0.75.
Inter-Rater	• Not reported.
Test-Retest	• R=0.91 on two small subsets of sample (n=0 40).
Validity	
Content	• Review of literature in human development, occupational choice, social psychology, and occupational behavior.
Criterion	• Not reported.
Construct	• Not reported.
Overall Utility	• Useful for developing rapport with an individual and identifying a profile of role important skills that are deficient. Clinically useful to guide treatment goals and plans. Further validation is needed.

The assessment was developed with a sample population of adolescents who were diagnosed with psychiatric problems, including adjustment reaction of adolescence, anorexia nervosa, school phobia, and depression. Subjects were in an inpatient psychiatric facility.

The semi-structure interview covers 21 topics in six areas: childhood play, adolescent socialization in the family, school performance, peer interactions, occupational choice, and work. Answers to questions yield both an objective rating (0 indicating marginal or borderline behavior, + indicating appropriate behavior, and − indicating inappropriate behavior) as well as qualitative information that can be used in treatment planning.

Black designed the Adolescent Role Assessment to be used as part of a battery of assessments to develop an occupational behavior profile of an individual's strengths and needs. Her concern was for collecting information about occupational role performance in order to provide a well-developed treatment plan.

Occupational Role History

This assessment tool is also part of the occupational behavior tradition that conceptualizes the developmental continuum of play and work, focusing on play as "the antecedent preparation area for work" (Florey & Michelman, 1982, p. 302). Like Black, Linda Florey and Shirley Michelman studied with Reilly and went on to work with individuals who had psychiatric difficulties. They maintained an orientation toward occupational roles, considering them to be a "developmental progression in the acquisition of role skills throughout the life cycle. Experiences in earlier roles have direct impact on skills and habits required for future roles" (Florey & Michelman, 1982, p. 303). Florey and Michelman conceptualized roles as much by social position as by tasks performed; therefore, the concept is expanded to include the child as player, the student, the worker, the volunteer, the homemaker, and the retiree as major occupational roles. The overriding

Table 14-2

OCCUPATIONAL ROLE HISTORY

Source	Florey, L. L., & Michelman, S. M. (1982). Occupational Role History: A screening tool for psychiatric occupational history. *American Journal of Occupational Therapy, 36(5)*, 301-308.
Purpose	• Screening tool for occupational role. Purpose is to identify 1) patterns of skills and patterns of dysfunction in past and current occupational roles, and 2) degree of balance or imbalance between leisure and occupational roles. Focus is on skills such as decision-making, problem-solving, and time management.
Type of Client	• Adult, acute psychiatric.
Clinical Utility	
Format	• Semi-structured interview screening tool.
Completion Time	• 30 minutes.
Reliability	
Internal Consistency	• Not reported.
Inter-Rater	• Not reported.
Test-Retest	• Not reported.
Validity	
Content	• Review of literature in occupation behavior, history taking, and occupational history.
Criterion	• Not reported.
Construct	• Not reported.
Overall Utility	• Useful for establishing treatment priorities in occupational role performance. Further validation is needed.

commonality among these roles is their meaning as vehicles for social involvement and productive participation.

In an effort to address the shortening lengths of hospital stays and the increased emphasis on acute care, Florey & Michelman designed the Occupational Role History, which builds on the work of occupational behaviorist Linda Moorhead's Occupational History. The Occupational Role History is a screening tool that uses a semi-structured interview format. The history looks at function in specific domains such as decision-making, problem-solving, and time management within roles of worker, student, homemaker, homemaker/student, homemaker/worker, and unspecified.

Information is collected in five areas:

1. Sequence and continuity of occupational roles and their components.

2. Identified preferences and satisfaction/dissatisfaction for interests, people, tasks, and environments.

3. The ability to acquire and keep "simultaneous occupational roles" (Florey & Michelman, 1982, p. 304).

4. Skills and problems.

5. Balance between roles that emphasize work, leisure, and maintenance.

Following administration of the assessment, data are interpreted to reflect patterns and skills that are functional, temporarily impaired (present in the past but disrupted in present), and dysfunctional. The authors demonstrated the utility of their assessment with case study examples.

Assessment of Occupational Functioning—Collaborative Version

The Assessment of Occupational Functioning—Collaborative Version (AOF-CV), created by Watts and Madigan in 1993, is the current version of the original Assessment of Occupational Functioning (AOF) developed in 1983 by Watts, Kielhofner, Bauer, Gregory, and Valentine. The AOF-CV was refined based on suggestions to improve communication across cultures and allow for self-administration with therapist follow-up. Both versions are based on the Model of Human Occupation (MOHO), an orientation that is closely associated with occupational behavior (Kielhofner & Burke, 1995). The model was developed by Gary Kielhofner and Janice Burke, who were

Table 14-3

ASSESSMENT OF OCCUPATIONAL FUNCTIONING —COLLABORATIVE VERSION

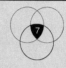

Source	Watts, J. H., & Madigan, J. M. (1993). Assessment of Occupational Functioning—Collaborative Version. (Available from author at the Virginia Commonwealth Department of Occupational Therapy Web site: http://www.sahp.vcu.edu/occu/html/assessment.htm).
Important References	Watts, J. H., Hinson, R., Madigan, M. J., McGuigan, P. M., & Newman, S. M. (1999). The Assessment of Occupational Functioning—Collaborative Version. In B. J. Hemphill-Pearson (Ed.), *Assessments in occupational therapy mental health: An integrative approach.* Thorofare, NJ: SLACK Incorporated.
	Watts, J. H., Brollier, C., Bauer, D., & Schmidt, W. (1988). A comparison of two evaluation instruments used with psychiatric patients in OT. *Occupational Therapy in Mental Health, 8(4),* 7-27.
Purpose	• To provide the therapist with information concerning the individual's values, personal causation, interests, roles, habits, and skills.
	• Yields qualitative as well as quantitative information coded to components of MOHO. Reveals person's overall occupational status prior to hospitalization or when a person is organizing their own time, and identifies areas requiring further assessment and treatment.
Type of Client	• Physically disabled and/or psychiatric populations in long-term, residential settings with elderly residents. Should only be used with patients who are capable of responding thoughtfully to an interview.
Clinical Utility	
Format	• Semi-structured interview and self-rating. Therapist or self-administration.
Completion Time	• 20 to 30 minutes as an interview, 12 minutes when self-administered with therapist follow-up for clarification. Use across cultures with collaborative administration for clarifying meanings of items.
Reliability	
Internal Consistency	• Current source uses existing reliability data from AOF, AOF revised.
	• N=83 (49 subjects from a geriatric center in a large state psychiatric hospital and long term physical disability facility; 34 subjects from the community with no disability).
	• Total score 0.78 with item coefficients lower.
	• Pearson product-moment correlations 0.70 to 0.90. Individual item coefficients range 0.48 to 0.94.
Test-Retest	• Intra-class correlation coefficients 0.78.
Validity	
Content	• Review of literature based on MOHO. Survey of experts from several English-speaking countries matched AOF-CV items to MOHO model components.
Concurrent	• Mixed; p<0.05 to 0.42 to -0.51; p<0.01 to 0.84. Concurrent validity has been established by comparing AOF and the OCAIRS using the Global Assessment Scale, and comparing the AOF with the Quality of Life Index.
Criterion	• Not reported.
Construct	• Not reported, referenced in unpublished studies.

continued

Table 14-3 (continued)

ASSESSMENT OF OCCUPATIONAL FUNCTIONING—COLLABORATIVE VERSION

Overall Utility	• Instrument will require further development to improve reliability and validity.
	• Designed as a brief screening tool and yields useful clinical information regarding descriptive information about individual and identification of problem areas, thus providing a starting point for understanding what is important to the individual and how the environment and specific circumstances supports and constrain occupational performance.
	• The AOF-CV can be used as a self-assessment with therapist follow-up. Patients gained useful insight from completing self-assessment; overall patients answered 89% of questions independently.

Table 14-4

SOCIAL PROBLEM QUESTIONNAIRE

Source	Corney, R. H., & Clare, A. W. (1985). The construction and testing of a self-report questionnaire to identify social problems. *Psychological Medicine, 15,* 637-649.
Important Reference	Piccinelli, M. (1997) Test-retest reliability of the Social Problem Questionnaire in primary care in Italy. *Social Psychiatry & Psychiatric Epidemiology, 32(2),* 57-62.
Purpose	• To screen individuals at risk for manifesting social maladjustment and/or dysfunction.
	• To obtain a reasonable estimate of the respondents' social and personal satisfaction.
Type of Client	• General practice patients, psychiatric outpatients, and social work clients, as well as the general population.
Clinical Utility	
Format	• 33-item self-report questionnaire covering 10 domains. A severity score and number of problems score is derived within each domain.
Completion Time	• 20 to 30 minutes.
Reliability	
Internal Consistency	• Comparison studies.
Inter-Rater	• Not reported.
Test-Retest	• CC=0.76 for severity score. Individual item coefficients range from 0.28 to 0.83.
	• ICC=0.62 for number of problems. Individual item coefficients range from 0.30 to 0.70.
	• R=0.77 for severity score. Individual item coefficients range from 0.30 to 0.84.
	• R=0.63 for number of problems. Individual item coefficients range from 0.29 to 0.74.
Validity	• Comparative studies with other questionnaires and between sample populations have been completed. Coefficients of agreement are available.
Content	• Derived from existing instruments. This assessment was adapted from the Social Maladjustment Schedule.
Criterion	• Not reported.
Construct	• Not reported.
Overall Utility	• Designed as research tool and/or clinical assessment and treatment planning tool. Further validation is needed.

	Table 14-5
	LIFE ROLE SALIENCE SCALE
Source	Amatea, E. S., Cross, E. G., Clark, J. E., & Bobby, C. L. (1986). Assessing the work and family role expectations of career-oriented men and women: The Life Roles Salience Scales. *Journal of Marriage and the Family, 48,* 831-838.
Purpose	• To assess the role expectations by measuring the personal importance attributed to participation in particular roles and the level of commitment of time resources to those roles.
Type of Client	• Men and women anticipating or currently engaged in occupational, marital, and parental life roles.
Clinical Utility	
Format	• Eight Likert-type attitudinal scales to assess four roles: occupational, marital, parental, and home care.
Completion Time	• Not reported
Reliability	
Internal Consistency	• Not reported.
Inter-Rater	• Not reported.
Test-Retest	• 0.79 or greater.
VALIDITY	
Content	• Derived from literature on social role theory, dual career stress and coping, career development, and marital and parental relationships.
Criterion	• Not reported.
Construct	• Reported as next step.
Overall Utility	• May be useful in research to further develop an understanding of occupational therapy and the attitudes that are influencing role performance relationship of stated value to time use.

also among Reilly's students. The model grew out of their efforts to identify a specific conceptual framework for guiding assessment and intervention in occupational therapy.

The AOF-CV, a semi-structured, self-report screening tool, assesses the structure of both the volitional and habitual subsystems of the individual through purposeful examination of personal causation, values, interest, roles, habits, and skills. The assessment consists of a recent employment work history, a 22-question interview, and a 5-point rating scale. The AOF-CV can be administered by the therapist as an interview, or through self-administration with therapist follow-up. Upon completion, the AOF-CV provides a vast array of qualitative information that may influence occupational performance. The instrument is recommended as an initial evaluation to identify where more evaluation is needed. The AOF-CV is for individuals who have physical and/or psychiatric disabilities and live in long-term residential settings.

Various studies have established validity and reliability of the AOF and the AOF-CV. The latest research on the

AOF-CV has examined content validity, terminology, and the usefulness of collaborative administration (Watts, Hinson, Madigan, McGuigan, & Newman, 1999).

ROLE CHECKLIST

The Role Checklist was developed by Frances Oakley as part of her master's thesis at the Medical College of Virginia (Oakley, 1982). The instrument serves to operationalize the construct of "role" put forth in the first edition of the Model of Human Occupation (MOHO) (Kielhofner & Burke, 1980). Role within MOHO is viewed as facilitating appropriate action and interaction with others. Roles organize behavior by influencing the manner and style of our interactions, defining certain tasks or performances associated with an enacted role, and partitioning daily and weekly cycles of activity to support the appropriate timing for enactment of selected roles (Dickerson, 1999, p.177).

The purpose of the Role Checklist is to obtain information about the types of roles people assume, value, and

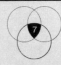

Table 14-6

PERSON IN ENVIRONMENT SYSTEM

Source	Williams, J. B. W., Karls, J. M., & Wandrei, K. (1989). The Person in Environment System for describing problems of social functioning. *Hospital and Community Psychiatry, 40(11)*, 1125-1127.
Purpose	• To provide a method for classifying problems in social functioning for identification and intervention on four factors: social role problems, environmental problems, mental disorders, and physical disorders.
Type of Client	• Individuals with mental health dysfunction.
Clinical Utility	
Format	• Classification-based rating scale completed by professional to code problems.
Completion Time	• Not reported.
Reliability	• In pilot testing.
Internal Consistency	• Not reported.
Inter-Rater	• Not reported.
Test-Retest	• Not reported.
Validity	• Planned for future.
Content	• Derived from 12-member task force of experts in social work.
Criterion	• Not reported.
Construct	• Not reported.
Overall Utility	• To classify problems in order to organize a treatment plan. Further validation is needed.

use to organize their daily lives. After a review of literature in social psychology, sociology, and occupational therapy a list of 20 roles were identified. Following feedback from students, faculty, and therapists, the instrument was narrowed down to include 10 roles, which include: student, worker, volunteer, caregiver, home maintainer, friend, family member, religious participant, hobbyist/amateur, and participant in organizations.

The self-report can be completed by the therapist after patient interview or by the patient independently. Part 1 of the assessment examines roles performed in the past, present, and anticipated future. Part 2 identifies the value ascribed to each of the roles, regardless of whether they have been or will be performed. Data collected from the checklist can assist the therapist in identifying potential problems with continuity of role performance. Role loss can also be assessed, as well as, the discrepancies between role performance and role value. This instrument is also useful for building rapport between the patient and therapist.

The Role Checklist can provide valuable role information about individuals from adolescence to older adulthood in a variety of settings and diagnostic categories. Current reliability and validity studies show satisfactory results; however, further research is needed in areas of reliability with specific patient populations, concurrent validity with other role assessments, and usefulness with diverse populations (Dickerson, 1999, p.189).

Three additional assessments are summarized in the tables accompanying this section. Using a social function orientation to role, the assessments inventory includes the kinds of skilled situations (social interactions, locating housing, managing finances) that produce problems or challenges for an individual. Assessments that can be used to inventory and identify problematic situations may be of assistance to occupational therapists who are seeking a method for identifying needs in a patient population.

REFERENCES

Amatea, E. S., Cross, E. G., Clark, J. E., & Bobby, C. L. (1986). Assessing the work and family role expectations of career-oriented men and women: The Life Role Salience Scales. *Journal of Marriage and the Family, 48*, 831-838.

Black, M. M. (1976). Adolescent Role Assessment. *American Journal of Occupational Therapy, 30(2)*, 73-79.

Corney, R. H., & Clare, A. W. (1985). The construction and testing of a self-report questionnaire to identify social problems. *Psychological Medicine, 15*, 637-649.

Table 14-7

ROLE CHECKLIST

Sources	Oakley, F., Kielhofner, G., Barris, R., & Reichler, R. (1986). The role checklist: Development and empirical assessment of reliability. *Occupational Therapy Journal of Research, 6*, 157-170.
	Dickerson, A. E. (1999). The role checklist. In B. J. Hemphill-Pearson (Ed), *Assessments in occupational therapy mental health: An integrative approach* (pp. 175-191). Thorofare, NJ: SLACK Incorporated.
Important Reference	Forsyth, K., & Keilhofner, G. (2003). Model of Human Occupation. In P. Kramer, J. Hinojosa, & C. B. Royeen (Eds.), *Perspectives in human occupation: Participation in Life* (pp. 45-86). Philadelphia, PA: Lippincott, Williams & Wilkins.
Purpose	• To obtain information about the types of roles people assume, value and use to organize their daily lives. The checklist is based on the Model of Human Occupation and is designed to identify the occupational behavior of patients.
Type of Client	• Across age groups from adolescent, adult, or geriatric populations with physical or psychosocial dysfunction.
Clinical Utility	
Format	• Two-part checklist based on client report of past, present, and future roles and the importance of each role to the client.
	• Checklist provides individual's view of their roles, how they have unfolded and been enacted over time, and the individual's value of the role.
	• Roles assessed include: student, worker, volunteer, caregiver, home maintainer, friend, family member, religious participant, hobbyist/amateur, and participant in organizations.
Completion Time	• 15 minutes.
Reliability	• Reliability supported by small homogeneous samples as reported by Dickerson (1999)in a summary review of unpublished data.
Internal Consistency	• Not reported.
Inter-Rater	• Not reported.
Test-Retest	• Part 1—Average percent agreement 87%, Part 2—Average percent agreement 79% on two subsets of sample (n=124).
Validity	
Content	• Review of literature in social psychology, sociology, and occupational therapy.
Concurrent	• Small homogeneous study established validity using Activity Configuration for identifying role participation as reported by Dickerson (1999) in a summary review of unpublished data.
Criterion	• Not reported.
Construct	• Not reported.
Overall Utility	• Assists therapist in gaining rapport and significant role information (current and past). No strong validity or reliability data for comparison. Useful for single case study and individual treatment planning.

Dickerson, A. E. (1999). The role checklist. In B. J. Hemphill-Pearson (Ed), *Assessments in occupational therapy mental health: An integrative approach* (pp.175-191).Thorofare, NJ: SLACK Incorporated.

Fidler, G. (1991). The challenge of change to occupational therapy practice. *Occupational Therapy in Mental Health, 11(1)*, 1-10.

Florey, L. L., & Michelman, S. M. (1982). Occupational Role History: A screening tool for psychiatric occupational history. *American Journal of Occupational Therapy, 36(5)*, 301-308.

Huebner, R., Emery, L., & Shordike, A. (2002). The adolescent role assessment: Psychometric properties and theoretical usefulness. *American Journal of Occupational Therapy, 56(2)*, 202-209.

Kielhofner, G., & Burke, J. P. (1980). A model of human occupation, part 1: Conceptual framework and content. *American Journal of Occupational Therapy, 9*, 572-581.

Matsutsuyu, J. (1971). Occupational behavior—A perspective on work and play. *American Journal of Occupational Therapy, 25*, 291.

Mosey, A. C. (1970). *Three frames of reference for mental health*. Thorofare, NJ: SLACK Incorporated.

Oakley, F. (1982). *The model of human occupation in psychiatry*. Unpublished master's degree project, Richmond, Va: Medical College of Virginia, Virginia Commonwealth University, Department of Occupational Therapy.

Oakley, F., Kielhofner, G., Barris, R., & Reichler, R. (1986). The role checklist: Development and empirical assessment of reliability. *Occupational Therapy Journal of Research, 6*, 157-170.

Piccinelli, M. (1997) Test-retest reliability of the Social Problem Questionnaire in primary care in Italy. *Social Psychiatry & Psychiatric Epidemiology, 32(2)*, 57-62.

Reilly, M. (1962). Occupational therapy can be one of the great ideas of 20th century medicine. *American Journal of Occupational Therapy, 25*, 243-246.

Watts, J. H., Brollier, C., Bauer, D., & Schmidt, W. (1988). A comparison of two evaluation instruments used with psychiatric patients in OT. Occupational Therapy in Mental Health, *8(4)*,7-27.

Watts, J. H., Hinson, R., Madigan, M. J., McGuigan, P. M., & Newman, S. M. (1999). The Assessment of Occupational Functioning—Collaborative Version. In B. J. Hemphill-Pearson (Ed.), *Assessments in occupational therapy mental health: An integrative approach* (pp. 193-203). Thorofare, NJ: SLACK Incorporated.

Watts, J. H., Kielhofner, G., Bauer, D. F., Gregory, M. D., & Valentine, D. B. (1986). The Assessment of Occupational Functioning: A screening tool for use in long-term care. *American Journal of Occupational Therapy, 40(4)*, 231-240.

Williams, J. B. W., Karls, J. M., & Wandrei, K. (1989). The person in environment system for describing problems of social functioning. *Hospital and Community Psychiatry, 40(11)*, 1125-1127.

Watts, J. H., & Madigan, J. M. (1993). Assessment of Occupational Functioning-Collaborative Version. Retrieved April 12, 2005 from http://www.sahp.vcu.edu/occu/html/assessment.htm).

Yerxa, E. J., Clark, F., Frank, G., et al. (1990). An introduction to occupational science, a foundation for occupational therapy for the 21st century. *Occupational Therapy in Health Care, 6*, 1-17.

Editors' Notes for Chapter 15

Occupational balance has been an important tenet underlying the practice of occupational therapy since the early 20th Century, when physicians prescribed "a balanced regimen of work" as part of a daily routine of activities "supervised by a new breed of health workers called occupational therapists" (Bryden & McColl, 2003, p. 29). In the present day, there is considerable interest in the concept of balance across occupational roles and occupational performance areas, and the concept of work-life balance is frequently addressed in the literature in many different fields.

Mine the Gold

In the literature on work-life balance, the ability of individuals to manage the demands of employment and family life predominantly address how perceived imbalance leads to distress. There is a temporal aspect to both work-life balance and occupational balance, suggesting that observing how people allocate their time is a worthwhile approach to measuring at least one aspect of balance. However, counting hours alone is overly simplistic because occupational balance is a perceived state, influenced by personal goals, values, and perspective, interacting with time and the sociocultural environment (Backman, 2004). There is emerging evidence that a satisfactory state of occupational balance is beneficial to health and well-being (Backman, 2004; Christiansen, 1996; Yerxa, 1998).

Become Systematic

Additional data are required, however, to verify a causal relationship between satisfactory occupational balance and well-being (Christiansen, 1996). Occupational therapists can contribute to this process by employing systematic approaches to assessment and interventions related to occupational balance. Sometimes clients may feel unable to effectively manage competing demands, as if their lives are "out of control." By creating a structure for analyzing time use systematically, we provide the opportunity to reframe this thinking and take action to regain a sense of efficacy over both daily routines and performance of occupations. By exploring individual perceptions regarding the meaning attributed to roles, occupations, and tasks that serve to organize one's day, we help clients to make more informed choices and achieve a sense of balance.

Use Evidence in Practice

Time use studies indicate that a person's well-being is associated with the activity patterns across days or weeks. By using time use measures, occupational therapists can collaborate with clients to gain insights about the supports and barriers to satisfactory engagement in daily occupations. A greater sense of occupational balance has been positively and significantly correlated with measures of health status and self-efficacy in a cross-sectional study of 237 adults with rheumatoid arthritis (RA). Participants who indicated their RA limited their ability to be productive also reported lower ratings of occupational balance than those who did not report work limitations (Backman, Kennedy, Chalmers & Singer, 2004). These types of studies provide the evidence necessary to inform clinical decision-making.

Make Occupational Therapy Contribution Explicit

Occupational therapists are concerned with maintaining or restoring performance of the occupations pertinent to the daily lives of individuals (and communities). Unlike the assessment of specific occupational performance areas or performance components, occupational balance considers performance across many areas, skills, and environments. Assessments of occupational balance make use of both quantitative and qualitative data to explain individual perspectives on time use and balance. They indicate our interest in uncovering aspects of occupational engagement that are satisfying or troublesome. Occupational therapists can then make recommendations for improving occupational balance and restoring a sense of well-being.

Engage in Occupation-Based, Client-Centered Practice

Taking time to measure how clients spend the day and understand how they derive pleasure from their unique constellation of occupations is part of a client-centered approach. This focus may empower clients and illustrates the occupational therapist's expertise in resolving problematic aspects of how they spend their days.

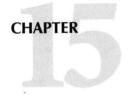

Occupational Balance
Measuring Time Use and Satisfaction Across Occupational Performance Areas

Catherine Backman, PhD, OT(C)

Measuring occupational balance is an interesting and thought-provoking endeavor. Scholars in fields such as social ecology, sociology, education, vocational counseling and psychology have examined time use and the meaning attributed to many aspects of everyday activity (Amundsen, 2001; Caproni, 1997; Kerka, 2001; Little, 2000; Perrons, 2003). Virtually all people work toward achieving a satisfactory balance of everyday activities, but it is difficult to identify precisely what a reasonable balance of occupations looks like. Thus, the traditional standardized test with normative data is unlikely to be developed for this concept. Achieving or working toward a balance among work, play, rest, and other activities is a familiar goal for many people, regardless of ability. Occupational balance is subjectively defined by individuals in terms of how they choose to spend time on valued, obligatory, and discretionary activities. Therefore, measurement of such a construct must be client-centered and take into account individual variation regarding what constitutes a "balanced" life. There are an infinite number of satisfying lifestyles, and the purpose of measuring occupational balance is to help people discover a balance that is right for them. Occupational balance is indicated by feelings of satisfaction, contentment or pleasure, while imbalance is characterized by feelings of distress or boredom as a result of being under or over-occupied (Townsend & Wilcock, 2004).

Measuring occupational balance is not as straightforward as the measurement of impairment (such as joint motion or muscle strength), nor is it as observable as discrete aspects of occupational performance (such as capac-ity to prepare a meal). It is not possible to place someone's daily occupations on a scale and observe whether or not balance has been achieved. However, it is possible to use various data collection procedures to obtain information about engagement in occupation and use this as a basis for problem identification and resolution with clients.

Ways of Measuring Occupational Balance

In an essay on balance in occupation, Christiansen (1996) offers three perspectives to thinking about balance, each of which suggests different approaches to measurement. The first relates to time use or how we structure our days and weeks. Questionnaires and diaries are measurement tools compatible with this approach. Measures of time use are briefly introduced in the following paragraphs. The second perspective considers chronobiology, or the naturally occurring rhythms of day and night, and their associated physiological responses. Although this perspective poses a theoretically interesting approach to understanding more about balance, no promising measurement tools were found to illustrate this perspective. The third perspective is a social ecology approach, which considers the environmental, social, and personal restraints and facilitators to how we engage in various activities. The writings of Csikszentmihalyi (1997), addressing "flow" and "optimal experience" appear to fall within the scope of this social ecological approach. Personal projects analysis (Little, 1983) and experience sampling method (Larson & Csikszentmihalyi, 1983) are two examples of assessing occupational balance that consider the context or environmental influences under which people act. The following provides an overview of time use and social ecological approaches to assessing occupational balance.

Time use refers to how people structure their days and may be assessed using questionnaires or diaries. The comment that "I have no time" to complete activities or pursue selected occupations seems to be a symptom of "I lack balance" in my life. Thus, time use approaches may provide data that more precisely identify the problem and potential solutions. One such approach is the Time Structure Questionnaire (TSQ) (Bond & Feather, 1988), a 26-item, self-administered questionnaire intended to assess "the degree to which individuals perceive their use of time to be structured and purposive" (p. 321). Individuals rate each item on a 1 to 7 scale, indicating the extent to which the item reflects their time use. Sample items include "Do you ever find that time just seems to slip away?" and "Do you plan your activities so that they fall into a particular pattern during the day?" Preliminary factor analysis suggested five aspects of time use measured by the TSQ: sense of purpose, structured routine, present orientation, effective organization, and persistence. If time use, and in particular these attributes of time use, appear to be important to a client's definition of occupational balance, the TSQ may be one way of evaluating the time-related aspect of occupational balance.

A more typical way to assess time use is with diaries or daily logs, such as the Occupational Questionnaire (OQ) (Smith, Kielhofner, & Watts, 1986) and the National Institutes of Health Activity Record (ACTRE) (Gerber & Furst, 1992). For both the OQ and the ACTRE, the client completes a diary by indicating the primary activity pursued in each half-hour increment of the day. The diary is kept for 2 days. Attributes of the activities and, in the case of the ACTRE, symptoms associated with each activity are assessed with specific questions following each entry on the diary sheet. Both of these tools provide an inventory of the types of activities the client pursues and may provide additional insight regarding how much time is spent on discretionary vs obligatory activities, possible sources of client dissatisfaction with time allocated to various activities, and ways to modify time use.

Harvey and Pentland (2004) summarize data from time use studies to describe what people do, for how long, and with whom. Most diaries are designed in half-hour increments and kept for periods of 2 to 7 days, and structured diaries are generally considered reliable. Depending on the issues one wishes to explore, diaries are also flexible, allowing for additional questions about the nature of the activities recorded, such as whether or not other people were involved in the activity. There is a great deal of data from population studies about time use, and many nations collect these data through regular national health and social surveys. Comparisons regarding time use and categories of occupations can then be made across sub-populations, such as age groups, genders, or regional communities. It is important to note that time use studies tend to focus on the primary activity or occupation in which the person was engaged at a particular moment in time, although some diary formats will also ask about secondary activities. The nature of occupation is such that multiple tasks may be occurring simultaneously, even tasks related to different occupations. For example, a mother may be simultaneously assisting her children with homework while preparing dinner and sorting through the mail to pay bills. Studies of mothers in particular have noted how occupations may be embedded in one another (Larson, 2000).

Another time use measure is the Structured Observation and Report Technique (SORT) (Rintala et al., 1984). The SORT is a subscale of the Longitudinal Functional Assessment System, which measures health status and functional performance of people with disabilities. The SORT is a cued recall record of the activities engaged in during a day and can be administered using either an interview or a diary format. Information about what the individual did, where, with whom, and for how long is recorded using the tool. Children's time use can be measured by interviewing the parents and validating the activities with the child. The SORT provides rich and specific data about activity patterns in individuals. Time use is only one part of the "balance equation" and each of the methods cited here recognize the limitations of time use alone, because they supplement this approach by attaining at least a little bit of descriptive data to further explain or elucidate aspects of occupation that may contribute to evaluating the concept occupational balance.

The social ecological perspective to studying occupation includes methods that examine engagement in goal-directed tasks, including the environmental, social, and personal restraints and resources that influence occupation. In this way, the relationship among daily occupations can be studied. Personal Projects Analysis (PPA) (Little, 1983) is an example of such an approach. PPA is not designed to account for the time people spend on activities, but instead focuses on the characteristics and interrelationships of the projects (occupations) in which the person is engaged. Briefly, PPA consists of three steps: project elicitation, rating the projects on various dimensions, and a cross-impact matrix. The project elicitation step asks the client to identify all goal-directed activities he or she is currently pursuing or about to begin working on. Projects may be in any area of life and range in scope from finding a job to getting a manicure. In step two, the client selects the 10 most relevant projects and rates them on a number of dimensions, such as the importance, enjoyment, and difficulty associated with each project. The approach is flexible enough to allow the addition or deletion of project characteristics in this step so that the characteristics of greatest interest to client and therapist are rated. The third step, the cross-impact matrix, asks the client to consider the relative impact of each project on each of the other projects. A project can have a positive, negative, or neutral effect on the client's pursuit of other projects.

The PPA requires a fair amount of introspection and has the potential to identify problematic occupations, desirable occupations, and conflict within a personal project system. It may therefore provide useful information for working with clients toward achieving a more satisfactory balance in daily occupations.

The use of the Experience Sampling Method (ESM) (Csikszentmihalyi & Larson, 1987; Larson & Csikszentmihalyi, 1983) was developed as a way to study people's experiences interacting in their natural environment and has been proposed as an approach to understanding engagement in daily activities. The objective is to obtain a sample of self-reports that are representative of moments in people's lives to identify and analyze how patterns in people's subjective experience relate to the wider conditions of their lives (Csikszentmihalyi & Larson, 1987; Larson & Csikszentmihalyi, 1983). The ESM is a research tool for studying what people do, feel, and think during their daily lives. Individuals carry electronic pagers and are signaled at random intervals. The signal is a cue to complete a form as soon as is feasible to describe the objective and subjective characteristics of the activity they were involved in at the time they were paged. The form asks several questions, such as level of involvement in the activity, mood, other people present, and the perceived challenge and value of the activity. An individual completes a series of forms during a pre-determined period of time, creating a set of various experiences with descriptions of their psychological state during each sampled activity.

Csikszentmihalyi & Csikszentmihalyi (1988) describe the ebb and flow of various activities of daily living in a way that parallels discussion of occupational balance in occupational therapy. Flow is defined as an intrinsically rewarding state of full involvement in an occupation, which in turn is considered a requirement of optimal experience or balance. If characteristics related to flow and optimal experience can be identified, then it may be possible to use this information to help clients achieve a better state of balance. Larson & Csikszentmihalyi (1983) provide an idiographic study using the ESM to document a woman's week, showing the ebb and flow of mood and involvement in the activities sampled. Such studies show how the individual spends time, provide a sample of thoughts and emotions associated with the activities, and illustrate the pattern of solitude and social activities throughout the week. This kind of archive may help identify patterns that reflect balance (or lack of balance) in occupation. The concept of flow and how it relates to the structure of everyday activities, work, leisure, and quality of life is discussed extensively elsewhere (Csikszentmihalyi, 1997).

SELECTED MEASURES OF OCCUPATIONAL BALANCE

In this section, the following tools are reviewed in Tables 14-1 through 14-5: the PPA, OQ, ACTRE, ESM, and SORT. These tools can be helpful to clients in examining how they spend time and the characteristics of the activities in which they engage so that they might change their time use, activity choices, or activity patterns in order to achieve greater satisfaction. None of these tools will result in a score that can be interpreted as "occupationally well-balanced" or "imbalanced."

Occupational therapists can use tools like those listed to document activity patterns or clarify issues related to their client's typical occupations. That is, these tools may be useful during the assessment phase of the occupational therapy process in order to clarify occupational performance issues that require intervention. For example, if symptoms seem to interfere with a client's ability to satisfactorily perform needed or desired activities, the OQ or ACTRE may help to clarify the extent of the problem and suggest possible modifications to time use, such as planning ahead. Or, if a client indicates dissatisfaction with his or her perceived imbalance of work and play, completing the PPA might yield very useful information about current goal-directed activities that enable the occupational therapist to coach the client toward a more satisfying balance of activities. Subsequent administration of these measures will help document changes as a result of intervention or other factors. As research tools, all of the instruments appear to provide information regarding how individuals engage in occupation and, therefore, are likely to enhance our understanding about activity patterns associated with health and illness.

FUTURE DIRECTIONS

Achieving balance among work, play, self-care, and rest is a goal with moving goal posts. As we move through life stages, our perception of what is important, meaningful, and deserving of our time and energy changes. The measurement of occupational balance is inexact, and the interpretation of the data generated by all of the methods discussed in this chapter requires careful consultation with the client in order to be useful in documenting current status and changes over time. Because culture, motivation, and life stage are all likely to influence one's perception of balance, the role of society, personality, and age might all be interesting lines of inquiry in future studies of occupational balance. It has also been suggested that the issue of balance is an issue of concern to a privileged segment of society (Kerka, 2001), because occupational choice and

Table 15-1

PERSONAL PROJECTS ANALYSIS (PPA)

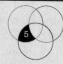

Source	Little, B. R. (1983). Personal projects: A rationale and a method for investigation. *Environment and Behavior,* 15, 273-309.
Important References	Christiansen, C., Backman, C., Little, B. R., & Ngyuen, A. (1999). Occupational and well-being: A study of personal projects. *American Journal of Occupational Therapy, 53,* 91-100.
	Christiansen, C. H., Little, B. R., & Backman, C. (1998). Personal projects: A useful approach to the study of occupation. *American Journal of Occupational Therapy, 52,* 439-446.
	Little, B. R., Lecci, L., & Watkinson, B. (1992). Personality and personal projects: Linking big five and PAC units of analysis. *Journal of Personality, 60,* 501-525.
	Palys, T. S., & Little, B. R. (1983). Perceived life satisfaction and the organization of personal project systems. *Journal of Personality and Social Psychology, 44,* 1221-1230.
Purpose	• Descriptive. PPA was developed for studying the stages of project inception, planning, action, and termination, as well as interproject impact and linkages with values and actions.
Type of Client	• Adolescents and adults of all ages.
Clinical Utility	
Format	• Self-report, paper, and pencil questionnaire administered following verbal or written instructions.
Procedures	• Respondent completes a 3-part questionnaire. Part 1 is a list of all goal-directed projects in which the client is currently engage or about to begin. In Part 2, the 10 most pertinent projects are rated on a 0 to 10 scale for various dimensions such as importance, enjoyment, and time adequacy. (There is some flexibility here as to how many dimensions are rated; a core set of 17 have been reported.) Part 3 is a cross-impact matrix in which each project is assessed regarding is impact on every other project.
	• Scoring consists of categorizing the listed projects from part 1, calculating means for each project dimension in part 2, and summing the cross-impact matrix ratings from part 3.
	• The cross-impact score indicates relative concordance or conflict within a project system, and is therefore a possible indicator of "occupational balance."
Completion Time	• 30 to 45 minutes for clients.
	• 10 to 15 minutes for scoring.
Standardization	• Instructions are available from the author, Dr. Brian Little, Social Ecology Department, Carleton University, Ottawa, ON. Formats for parts 1 and 2 are reprinted in Little, 1983; the format for the cross-impact matrix is in Christiansen et al., 1998. Little (1983) maintains a bank of comparative data.
Reliability	
Internal Consistency	• Adequate for project dimensions, averaging 0.70 (coefficient alpha), ranging from 0.53 for project stress to 0.77 for value congruency (Little et al., 1992).
Inter-Rater	• Not applicable, given nature of the tool.
Intra-Rater	• Not reported.
Test-Retest	• Adequate.
	• 24-hour interval Pearson's r ranged from 0.51 to 0.83 and 2 week interval ranged from 0.28 to 0.80.

continued

Table 15-1 (continued)

PERSONAL PROJECTS ANALYSIS (PPA)

Validity

Content
- Clients are able to report any and all projects, therefore, it is highly client-centered.
- 17 core dimensions appear to cover a broad range of characteristics of goal-directed activities.
- The method is sufficiently flexible that other dimensions may be added.
- Factor analysis suggests that project dimensions load on 5 factors: meaning, structure, efficacy, community, and stress, each of which appear to be relevant content

Convergent
- Not reported.

Construct
- PPA factor structure correlates moderately well with the NEO Personality Inventory and the Sense of Coherence Scale. Specific correlations are too numerous to list; see all Little references for details.
- It has been hypothesized that PPA scores would be associated with life satisfaction and depression; this has been established in several studies, see Christiansen et al., 1998 for a summary.

Strengths
- Easy to obtain and administer (to those with adequate reading and comprehension ability).
- Comprehensive description of occupations relevant to the individual client—increasing number of studies in the literature, from a range of investigators, are adding to the rigor of this tool.

Weaknesses
- Requires good literacy and cognitive skills on the part of the client, not suitable for those with cognitive impairment.
- Time to complete may be burdensome in some situations, depending on client priorities.

Final Word
- Great potential as a research tool for further exploring the concept of occupational balance.

---

allocation of time is a luxury that is not affordable to individuals living in poverty, for example.

The continued use and development of measures such as the PPA and ESM, especially with diverse populations, will no doubt provide a greater understanding of how occupation contributes to a sense of balance and general well-being. It would also be of interest to explore the concept of balance outside of industrialized nations. If occupation is a determinant of health, then a greater understanding of how people configure occupation in their daily lives would assist occupational therapists to enhance the health of their clients.

REFERENCES

Amundson, N. E. (2001). Three-dimensional living. *Journal of Employment Counseling, 38,* 114-127.

Backman, C. L. (2004). Occupational balance: Exploring the relationships among daily occupations and their influence on well-being. *Canadian Journal of Occupational Therapy, 71.*

Backman, C. L., Kennedy, S. M., Chalmers, A. & Singer, J. (2004). Participation in paid and unpaid work by adults with rheumatoid arthritis. *Journal of Rheumatology, 31,* 47-56.

Bond, M. J., & Feather, N. T. (1988). Some correlates of structure and purpose in the use of time. *Journal of Personality and Society Psychology, 55,* 321-329.

Bryden, P. & McColl, M. A. (2003). The concept of occupation: 1900 to 1974. In M. A. McColl, M. Law, D. Stewart, L. Doubt, N. Pollock, & T. Krupa (Eds.), *Theoretical basis of occupational therapy,* (2nd ed., pp. 27-37). Thorofare, NJ: SLACK Incorporated.

Caproni, P. (1997). Work/life balance: You can't get there from here. *Journal of Applied Behavioral Science, 33,* 46-56.

Christiansen, C. H. (1996). Three perspectives on balance in occupation. In R. Zemke & F. Clark (Eds.), *Occupational Science: The Evolving Discipline* (pp. 431-451). Philadelphia: F. A. Davis.

Christiansen, C., Backman, C., Little, B. R., & Ngyuen, A. (1999). Occupation and well-being: A study of personal projects. *American Journal of Occupational Therapy, 53.*

Table 15-2

OCCUPATIONAL QUESTIONNAIRE (OQ)

Source	Smith, N. R., Kielhofner, G., & Watts, J. H. (1986). The relationships between volition, activity pattern and life satisfaction in the elderly. *American Journal of Occupational Therapy, 40,* 278-283.
	May be downloaded from the Human Occupation Clearinghouse http://www.moho.uic.edu (select "other instruments based on MOHO" and then "download Occupational Questionnaire."
Important Reference	Kielhofner, G. (Ed.) (2002). *A model of human occupation. Therapy and application* (3rd ed.). Philadelphia: Lippincott Williams & Wilkins.
Purpose	• Descriptive.
	• Documents participation in occupations by half-hour intervals and describes clients' perceptions of type of occupation (work, play or leisure) and their sense of competence, value, and enjoyment attributed to each occupation.
Type of Client	• Adolescents and adults of all ages.
Clinical Utility	
Format	• A self-report, paper/pencil questionnaire.
Procedures	• The client completes a structured diary listing the primary occupation for each 30-minute time slot, then answers four additional questions on a 4 or 5 point nominal or ordinal scale (depending on the question).
	• Scoring consists of calculating proportion of time spent on occupations (grouped according to the four questions) and mean scores of the occupational characteristics assessed by the four questions.
Completion Time	• Approximately 20 minutes, in this author's experience with adults.
Standardization	• A brief manual would be useful to ensure consistent application and summarize findings from studies using the OQ subsequent to the original article. No published norms.
Reliability	
Internal Consistency	• Not reported.
Inter-Rater	• Not applicable, given the nature of the tool.
Intra-Rater	• Akin to test-retest.
Test-Retest	• Adequate in a pilot study of 20 elderly adults. Percent agreement for type of occupation was 87%, personal causation/competence 77%, value/importance 81%, and interest/enjoyment 77% (Smith et al., 1986).
Validity	
Content	• By nature a diary may include all occupations relevant to the individual, if he or she chooses to report them.
	• The classification, importance, competence, and enjoyment dimensions do not address all aspects of daily occupation, but represent an important first cut.
Convergent	• Not reported.
Construct	• Preliminary concurrent validity established in a pilot study of 18 college students who also completed the Household Work Study Diary. Percent agreement for values was 86%, interests 84%, and personal causation 92% (Smith et al., 1986).
	• An hypothesized association with life satisfaction was supported in a study of 60 adults aged 65 to 99 years with small but statistically significant correlations (Smith et al., 1986)

continued

Table 15-2 (continued)

OCCUPATIONAL QUESTIONNAIRE (OQ)

Strengths	• Easy to access, use and score- one of the earliest time use diaries designed from an occupational therapy perspective- compatible with theoretical approaches based on the Model of Human Occupation- additional references and access to fre quently asked questions is available through the MOHO clearinghouse.
Weaknesses	• Requires basic literacy, comprehension and cognitive skills, so may not be suitable for all clients.
	• Requires additional research to substantiate its fit with the MOHO, and utility as a tool for assessing occupational balance.
Final Word	• Probably best used in conjunction with an interview to fully understand the activity patterns and meaning associated with the responses on the OQ.

Christiansen, C. H., Little, B. R., & Backman, C. (1998). Personal projects: A useful approach to the study of occupation. *American Journal of Occupational Therapy, 52,* 439-446.

Csikszentmihalyi, M. (1997). *Finding flow.* New York: Basic Books.

Csikszentmihalyi, M., & Csikszentmihalyi, I. S. (Eds.). (1988). *Optimal experience: Psychological studies of flow in consciousness.* Boston: Cambridge University Press.

Csikszentmihalyi, M., & Larson, R. (1987). Validity and reliability of the Experience-Sampling Method. *Journal of Nervous and Mental Disease, 175,* 526-536.

Furst, G. P., Gerber, L. H., Smith, C., Fisher, S., & Shulman, B. (1987). A program for improving energy conservation behaviors in adults with rheumatoid arthritis. *American Journal of Occupational Therapy, 41,* 102-111.

Gerber, L. H., & Furst, G. P. (1992). Validation of the NIH Activity Record: A quantitative measure of life activities. *Arthritis Care & Research, 5,* 81-86.

Gerber, L., Furst, G., Shulman, B., et al. (1987). Patient education program to teach energy conservation behaviors to patients with rheumatoid arthritis: A pilot study. *Archives of Physical Medicine & Rehabilitation, 68,* 442-445.

Harvey, A. S., & Pentland, W. (2004). What do people do? In C. H. Christiansen & E. A. Townsend (Eds.), *Introduction to occupation: The art and science of living* (pp. 63-90). Upper Saddle River, NJ: Prentice Hall.

Kerka, S. (2001). The balancing act of adult life. ERIC Digest No. 229, Article EDO-CE-01-229. Retrieved June 1, 2004 from http://www.ericfacility.net/ericdigests/ ed459323.html

Kielhofner, G. (Ed.). (2002). *A model of human occupation. Therapy and application* (3rd ed.). Philadelphia: Lippincott Williams & Wilkins.

Larson, E. A. (2000). The orchestration of occupation: The dance of mothers. *American Journal of Occupational Therapy, 54,* 269-280.

Larson, R., & Csikszentmihalyi, M. (1983). The experience sampling method. In H.T. Reis (Ed.), *Naturalistic approaches to studying social interaction.* San Francisco: Jossey-Bass.

Little, B. R. (1983). Personal Projects: A rationale and method for investigation. *Environment and Behavior, 15,* 273-309.

Little, B. R. (1987). Personal Projects Analysis: A new methodology for counselling psychology. *Natcon, 13,* 591-614.

Little, B.R. (2000). Persons, contexts and personal projects. In S. Wapner, J. Demick, T. Yamamoto, & H. Minami (Eds.), *Theoretical perspectives in environment-behavior research.* New York: Kluwer Academic.

Little, B. R., Lecci, L., & Watkinson, B. (1992). Personality and personal projects: Linking big five and PAC units of analysis. *Journal of Personality, 60,* 501-525.

Palys, T. S., & Little, B. R. (1983). Perceived life satisfaction and the organization of personal project systems. *Journal of Personality and Social Psychology, 44,* 1221-1230.

Perrons, D. (2003). The new economy and the work-life balance: Conceptual explorations and a case study of new media. *Gender, Work and Organization, 10,* 65-93.

Rintala, D. H., Uttermohlen, D. M., Buck, E. L., Hanover, D., Alexander, J. L., Norris-Baker, C., Stephens, M. A. P., Willems, E. P., & Halstead, L. S. (1984). In A. S. Halpern & M. J. Fuhrer (Eds.), *Functional Assessment in Rehabilitation* (pp. 205-221). Baltimore: Paul H. Brookes.

Smith, N. R., Kielhofner, G., & Watts, J. H. (1986). The relationship between volition, activity pattern, and life satisfaction in the elderly. *American Journal of Occupational Therapy, 40,* 278-283.

Townsend, E., & Wilcock, A. (2004). Occupational justice. In C.H. Christiansen and E.A. Townsend, (Eds.), *Introduction to occupation. The art and science of living* (pp.243-273). Upper Saddle River, NJ: Prentice Hall.

Yerxa, E. J. (1998). Health and the human spirit for occupation. *American Journal of Occupational Therapy, 52,* 412-418.

Table 15-3

NATIONAL INSTITUTES OF HEALTH ACTIVITY RECORD (ACTRE)

Source	Gloria Furst, MPH, OTR, (e-mail) gfurst@cc.nih.gov (A request form may be downloaded from the Human Occupation Clearinghouse http://www.moho.uic.edu).
Important References	Furst, G. P., Gerber, L. H., Smith, C., Fisher, S., & Shulman, B. (1987). A program for improving energy conservation behaviors in adults with rheumatoid arthritis. *American Journal of Occupational Therapy, 41*, 102-111.
	Gerber, L. H., & Furst, G. P. (1992). Validation of the NIH Activity Record: A quantitative measure of life activities. *Arthritis Care & Research, 5*, 81-86.
	Gerber, L., Furst, G., Shulman, B., et al. (1987). Patient education program to teach energy conservation behaviors to patients with rheumatoid arthritis: A pilot study. *Archives of Physical Medicine and Rehabilitation, 68*, 442-445.
	Kielhofner, G. (Ed.) (2002). *A model of human occupation. Therapy and application* (3rd ed.). Philadelphia: Lippincott Williams & Wilkins.
Purpose	• Descriptive and evaluative.
	• An expansion of the OQ designed to describe the impact of pain and fatigue on performance of activities, and to be used as an outcome measure.
Type of Client	• Adolescents and adults of all ages.
Clinical Utility	
Format	• A self-report paper and pencil questionnaire, including a diary of occupations for each 30-minute time period over 2 days, together with several questions about perceptions and symptoms experienced while engaged in the occupation.
Procedures	• Verbal instructions and practice with a sample form are generally provided (and highly recommended) prior to clients taking the ACTRE home for completion. Written instructions are on the recording form.
	• A computer-based scoring method is available, using Excel for Windows or MacIntosh, available from NIH (see source).
Completion Time	• 40 to 60 minutes over 2 days. It is recommended that clients take 5 to 10 minutes at the mid-day meal, evening meal, and bed-time to complete the diary for the period of the day up to that point in time.
Standardization	• Complete instructions available from NIH. No published norms.
Reliability	
Internal Consistency	• Not reported.
Inter-Rater	• Not reported.
Intra-Rater	• Not reported
Test-Retest	• Not reported.
Validity	
Content	• By nature, a diary may include all occupations of relevance to the individual client, if he or she chooses to report them.
	• Questions address two major symptoms that may influence occupational performance.
	• Pain and fatigue, as well as aspects of importance, competence, and enjoyment, thereby providing a great deal of information to assist in planning occupational therapy intervention.
Convergent	• Not reported.

continued

Table 15-3 (continued)

NATIONAL INSTITUTES OF HEALTH ACTIVITY RECORD (ACTRE)

Construct	• Concurrent validity established in a pilot study of 21 adults with rheumatoid arthritis with three different "gold standard" measures: The Health Assessment Questionnaire's Activities and Lifestyle Index was used to validate pain, satisfaction, and difficulty/competence; the Feeling Tone Checklist was used to validate fatigue ratings; and the Pain Disability Index was used to validate pain ratings. • Spearman correlation coefficients were calculated, but just the significance levels and not the actual correlations were reported. All expected correlations were statistically significant except for ACTRE fatigue and the Feeling Tone Checklist during specific times of day.
Strengths	• A comprehensive diary based on a theoretical foundation specific to occupational therapy practice. • Readily available from NIH.
Weaknesses	• May seem complicated to some clients, so clear instruction and practice is necessary for many; not suitable for those with cognitive problems. • Limited work has been published to document the rigor of this tool. • In particular, if it is to be used as an outcome measure, test-retest reliability should be established.
Final Word	• The balance of time spent in rest and activity, as well as activities that are more or less meaningful to the client, is an important aspect of planning interventions for clients who need to manage symptoms like pain and fatigue in addition to planning their day's activities. The ACTRE has potential to help occupational therapists be systematic in their approach to working with clients on self-management strategies for living with chronic illness.

Table 15-4

EXPERIENCE SAMPLING METHOD (ESM)

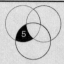

Source	Csikszentmihalyi, M., & Larson, R. (1987). Validity and reliability of the Experience Sampling Method. *Journal of Nervous and Mental Disease, 175*, 526-536.
Important References	Larson, R., & Csikszentmihalyi, M. (1983). The Experience Sampling Method. In H. T. Reis (Ed.), *Naturalistic approaches to studying social interaction*. San Francisco: Jossey-Bass.
	Csikszentmihalyi, M. (1997). Finding flow. *The psychology of engagement in every day life*. New York: Basic Books.
	Csikszentmihalyi, M., & Csikszentmihalyi, I. S. (Eds.). (1988). *Optimal experience: Psychological studies of flow in consciousness*. Boston: Cambridge University Press.
Purpose	• Descriptive.
	• ESM describes behavioral and intrapsychic aspects of daily activities, to obtain self-reports about people's experience as it occurs, minimizing reliance on memory.
	• Also describes the proportion of time devoted to various categories of occupation.
	• The objective is to identify and analyze how pattern's in people's subjective experience relate to the wider experience of their lives (Csikszentmihalyi & Larson, 1987).
Type of Client	• Adolescents and adults of all ages.
Clinical Utility	
Format	• A series of self-report forms that are completed over a pre-determined period of time (e.g., 1 week) every time a cue is received by beeper or pager. Signals are sent at random. The report forms then comprise a representative sample of various occupational experiences throughout the week.
Procedures	• The respondent is given a set of report forms and pager.
	• Each time a signal is received, the respondent completes a form describing the primary activity, environment, others present, and responds to a range of questions about mood, challenge, importance, and enjoyment associated with the occupation.
Completion Time	• A single form takes 2 minutes to complete. Typically, researchers issue 7 to 10 signals per day for 1 week, for a total self-report time commitment of about 2 hours. Time to code and score the data is not reported.
Standardization	• No published norms.
Reliability	
Internal Consistency	• Reported as impractical to assess.
Inter-Rater	• Percent agreement between coders of activities ranged from 88% to 96% (Csikszentmihalyi & Larson, 1987).
Intra-Rater	• Not reported.
Test-Retest	• For various affective dimensions, ranged from r=0.38 to 0.77.
Validity	
Content	• By virtue of randomly sampling experiences, ESM should include a representative description of activities or occupations.
	• Additional questions predominantly address affective aspects of experience.
Convergent	• Not reported.
Construct	• ESM discriminates between people with affective disorders and those without, for example, women with bulimia score lower than women without. Workers who are satisfied with their work score higher on the ESM questions related to level of involvement with rated activities than do workers who are less satisfied (Csikszentmihalyi & Larson, 1987).

continued

Table 15-4 (continued)

EXPERIENCE SAMPLING METHOD (ESM)

Strengths	• A systematic approach to sampling occupations over time, and selected affective attributes. • As a research tool, has potential to enhance our understanding of how people organize their time and choose their occupations.
Weaknesses	• Impractical for clinical use—The nature of random and frequent signaling to elicit responses may not appeal to some people; therefore, a selection bias may exist in those who participate in studies, and under-represent those who consider this approach awkward or invasive, and those with disabilities or impairment making form completion difficult.
Final Word	• Research evidence from studies using ESM has the potential to provide important information to advance occupational therapy theory and practice regarding occupational engagement and occupational balance (and imbalance).

Table 15-5

STRUCTURED OBSERVATION AND REPORT TECHNIQUE (SORT)

Source	Rintala, D. H., Uttermohlen, D. M., Buck, E. L., et al. (1984). In A. S. Halpern & M. J. Fuhrer (Eds.), *Functional assessment in rehabilitation* (pp. 205-221). Baltimore: Paul H. Brookes.
Important Reference	Quittner, A. L., & Opopari, L. C. (1994). Differential treatment of siblings: Interview and diary analyses comparing two family contexts. *Child Development, 65,* 800-814.
Purpose	• Descriptive.
	• SORT describes the unique constellation of a child's daily activities, including what they did, where, with whom, and how.
Type of Client	• Children and adolescents.
Clinical Utility	
Format	• Self-report questionnaire administered using an interview.
Procedures	• Respondents are asked to report on the activities they have completed over a specific period of time, usually the past 24 hours, and asked about other people present and the location of the activity.
Completion Time	• The interview takes 15 to 45 minutes. Time to code and score is not reported.
Standardization	• Instructions for administration are in the source article. No published norms.
Reliability	
Internal Consistency	• Reported as impractical to assess.
Inter-Rater	• Percent agreement between coders of activities ranged from 77% to 86% (Rintala et al., 1984).
Intra-Rater	• Not reported.
Test-Retest	• Not reported.
Validity	
Content	• By virtue of data collection method, content validity should be present.
Convergent	• Not reported.
Construct	• Self-report of activity agreed with independent observers from 77% to 83% of the time.
	• The SORT discriminates between different life experiences such as living at home or being in hospital.
	• The SORT has predicted activity levels post-discharge from a rehabilitation hospital, with a high correlation between in-hospital measures of independent activity and post-discharge measures. The SORT differentiates the time spent by mothers with a child with a chronic illness in comparison to healthy siblings.
Strengths	• One of the few tools designed specifically for children and youth.
	• As a research tool, has potential to describe how children and youth spend their time.
Weaknesses	• The SORT is a promising tool but requires further published information to assist with administration and interpretation.
Final Word	• The SORT presents the beginnings of a systematic approach to describing activity patterns in children.

Editors' Notes for Chapter 16

Mine the Gold

Both community integration and social support are multidimensional, theoretically complex constructs. The literature offers considerable discussion of both, from the 1960's to the present.

Become Systematic

These measures offer ways to systematically operationalize the social environment in occupational therapy practice.

Use Evidence in Practice

The evidence shows that these two constructs are highly influential for health, and presumably also for occupation.

Make Occupational Therapy Contribution Explicit

The social environment is critical for occupational performance. These measures offer ways to think about the social environment and act therapeutically to enhance its ability to support occupation.

Engage in Occupation-Based, Client-Centered Practice

These are all self-report measures that support client-centered practice and a focus on the environ-

16

MEASURING COMMUNITY INTEGRATION AND SOCIAL SUPPORT

Mary Ann McColl, PhD, OT Reg. (Ont.)

INTRODUCTION

Evidence accumulated over the past 40 years has shown incontrovertibly the importance of the social environment for health (Lomas, 1998). A number of theoretical constructs have been advanced that attempt to capture the essence of the social environment and its impact on health, all of which fall generally under the category of social capital (Putnam, 1995). The two that are discussed here are community integration and social support. Other aspects of the social environment that are not included in this chapter include social networks, social structures, social cohesion, and social outcomes (Djikers, 2000).

Community integration is arguably the ultimate goal of all occupational therapists—a situation where clients are happily and productively settled in a community that feels like a good fit (Kruzich, 1985). However, a clear definition of community integration is difficult to come by. Most of the definitions offered in the literature are multidimensional, and include three ideas: relationships with other people, independence in one's living situation, and activities to fill one's time (Bruininks, Chen, & Lakin, 1992; Carling, 1990; Halpern, 1985; Ittenbach, Bruininks, Thurlow, & McGrew, 1993; Jacobs, 1992; Johnston & Lewis, 1991; Rapp, Gowdy, Sullivan, & Wintersteen, 1988). In other words, community integration means having "something to do, somewhere to live, and someone to love." Although colloquial use has obscured the origins of this definition, its ability to communicate the essence of the construct is unmatched (McColl, Carlson, Johnston, Minnes, Shue, Davies, & Karlovits, 1998).

Social support is also a multidimensional construct, for which many definitions may be found in the literature. For our purposes, social support is defined as the experience of being "cared for and loved, valued, and esteemed, and able to count on others should the need arise" (Cobb, 1974; Friedland & McColl, 1987; McColl & Skinner, 1989). In particular, it should be distinguished from the more quantitative, structural concept of social networks, meaning the number and type of actual social contacts. There has been considerable research exploring the mechanism of social support, or the way it exerts an effect on health outcomes. Some researchers say support acts directly on health, prompting people to engage in positive health and help-seeking behaviors. Others say social support buffers the deleterious effects of stress on health, reducing the net effect of life events (Cohen & Wills, 1985). Still others provide evidence to suggest that the relationship between support and health is spurious, and that in fact, temperament and personal resiliency affect both support and health (Kendler, 1997; Kitamura, Kijima, Watanabe, Takezaki, & Tanaka, 1999).

To place these concepts within the framework of the World Health Organization's International Classification of Functioning, Disability and Handicap (ICF) (WHO, 2001), both represent dimensions of participation, or involvement in life situations. As defined here, the concept of integration encompasses learning and social problem-solving, undertaking multiple tasks and handling stress, communicating in a variety of styles and venues, getting around in the community, relating to others, and participating in community life. The concept of social support

Table 16-1

REINTEGRATION TO NORMAL LIVING INDEX

Source	Wood-Dauphinee, S., Opzoomer, A., Williams, J. I., Marchand, B., & Spitzer, W. O. (1988). Assessment of global function: The Reintegration to Normal Living Index. *Archives of Physical Medicine and Rehabilitation, 69*, 583-90.
Purpose	• To assess change in individuals or groups in terms of resumption of normal living patterns after onset of disability.
Type of Client	• Rehabilitation clients with sudden-onset disability.
Clinical Utility	
Format	• 11 statements with 10 cm. visual analogue response formats (fully describes my situation, does not describe my situation).
	• Total score of 110, converted to percents for ease of interpretation.
	• Can be self-administered or interviewed.
Completion Time	• Estimated at 5 to 10 minutes.
Reliability	
Internal Consistency	• Cronbach's alpha=0.90 to 0.95; principal components factor analysis supports one factor solution explaining 49% of variance.
Observer	• Significant agreement between patient and significant other.
Test-Retest	• Not reported.
Validity	
Content	• Developed on basis of three-stage empirical process involving consumers, professionals, and family members.
Criterion	• Scores related to work status and disease status, but not to living situation.
Construct	• Significant correlations with Quality of Life Index (Spitzer et al., 1981) and Affect Balance Scale (Bradburn, 1969).
Weaknesses	• Not standardized.
Strengths	• Scores easily interpreted and used in research and clinical practice; easy and quick to administer; well recognized in research and practice.

involves communication, interpersonal relationships and interactions, and community and social life.

The definitions above also place both constructs, community integration and social support, in the realm of experience. Thus, by definition, all of the measures reviewed here are self-report measures. Because we are interested in the experience of clients regarding support received and barriers and opportunities encountered in the community, we must rely on clients to tell us about their experience. Objective observation cannot provide a complete picture of either of these constructs.

Besides conforming with the definitions of integration and social support, four other criteria were applied in choosing the seven measures reviewed for the chapter. All measures had to:

1. Be currently used in practice, education, and/or research.

2. Have had recent research conducted on them or using them.

3. Have reasonable psychometric properties.

4. Be self-report format.

COMMUNITY INTEGRATION

This chapter reviews four measures for community integration. This is by no means an exhaustive list of available methods for measuring a topic as broad and all-encompassing as community integration; however, these four measures have been chosen because they meet the criteria outlined. They are presented here in the order in which they first appeared in the literature.

Reintegration to Normal Living Index

The Reintegration to Normal Living Index (RNL) (Table 16-1) (Wood-Dauphinee et al., 1988) is made up of 11 statements, such as "I participate in social activities as I feel necessary or important to me," and "I move around my community as I feel necessary." These items were devel-

	Table 16-2
	CRAIG HANDICAP ASSESSMENT AND REPORTING TECHNIQUE (CHART)
Source	Whiteneck, G., Charlifue, S., Gerhart, K., Overholser, D., & Richardson, G. (1992) Quantifying handicap: A new measure of long-term rehabilitation outcomes. *Archives of Physical Medicine and Rehabilitation, 73,* 519-26.
Purpose	• To measure the level of handicap experienced by an individual in a community setting.
Type of Client	• Designed for spinal cord injury; revised to include cognitive functioning and apply to other rehabilitation populations.
Clinical Utility	
Format	• Original: 27 questions with various response formats.
	• Revised: 34 items, including cognitive subscale.
	• Short form: 17 items.
Procedures	• Best when interview administered.
Completion Time	• Estimated at 30 minutes for long form, 15 for short form.
Reliability	
Internal Consistency	• Not reported.
Observer	• 0.69 to 0.84 correlations between patient and family member ratings.
Test-Retest	• 0.80 to 0.95 coefficient for subscales and total scale scores for 1 week interval; subject-proxy correlation=0.81.
Validity	
Content	• Based on WHO concept of handicap (WHO, 1981); not yet revised to reflect participation (WHO 2001).
Criterion	• Concordance with therapist ratings of high vs low handicap; concordance with CIQ.
Construct	• Rasch analysis supported underlying structure and linearity of CHART.
Strengths	• Very widely used and recognized.
	• Along with CIQ, considered an industry standard.
	• Used in Model Systems Database.
Weaknesses	• Scoring somewhat cumbersome.
	• Not consistent with recent ICF concept of participation.

oped with the input of health care consumers, family members, and professionals, all of whom contributed to the definition of the domain of the construct. Each of the items is scored on a 10-point visual analogue scale, anchored with the statements: "fully describes my situation" to "does not describe my situation." The RNL is quick and easy to administer and widely used in rehabilitation research and practice. Recent applications include typical rehabilitation populations, such as people with spinal cord injuries and acquired brain injuries (Harker, Dawson, Boschen, & Stuss, 2002), stroke, (Saladin, 2000), and geriatrics (Patrick, Perugini, & Leclerc, 2002). Recent research shows that patient reports of integration on the RNL are usually higher than those of significant others, and that agreement is relatively low (interclass correlation coeffi-

cient=0.36) (Tooth, McKenna, Smith, & O'Rourke, 2003). This suggests that the RNL may not be reliable for use as a proxy measure.

Craig Handicap Assessment and Reporting Technique

The Craig Handicap Assessment and Reporting Technique (CHART) (Table 16-2) (Whiteneck, Charlifue, Gerhart, Overholser, & Richardson, 1992) is a 27-item scale designed to correspond to the International Classification of Impairments, Disability, and Handicaps (ICIDH) (WHO, 1980) definition of handicap. Handicap is conceptualized as a disadvantage originating from a disability or impairment. This concept has been updated in

Table 16-3

COMMUNITY INTEGRATION QUESTIONNAIRE

Source	Willer, B., Rosenthal, M., Kreutzer, J. S., Gordon, W. A. & Rempel, R. (1993). Assessment of community integration following rehabilitation for traumatic brain injury. *Journal of Head Trauma Rehabilitation, 8*, 75-87.
Purpose	• The CIQ was developed to measure handicap as a function of community integration following brain injury.
Type of Client	• Developed for use in brain injury rehabilitation, but has been used more broadly in rehabilitation.
Clinical Utility	
Format	• 15 items in 3 scales—home integration, social integration and productive activities; three-point response options, different for each scale.
Procedures	• Not reported.
Completion Time	• Estimated at 10 minutes.
Reliability	
Internal Consistency	• 0.76 for total score; home subscale 0.84; social subscale 0.73; productivity subscale 0.35 (Willer, Linn, & Allen, 1994).
Observer	• Not reported.
Test-Retest	• 0.91 to 0.97 for clients and family members (retest period unspecified).
Validity	
Content	• Based on definition derived from literature; panel of 14 consumers, professionals, and researchers developed items in three sections.
Convergent	• Significant relationships with CHART subscales and total score (0.62 to 0.70).
Construct	• Discriminates between disabled and able-bodied samples on all three subscales.
Strengths	• Part of Model Systems Database; well known and recognized in research and practice; lots of evidence of psychometric values.
Weaknesses	• Concern about assumptions upon which it is based.

the recent ICF (WHO 2001), and to date, the CHART does not appear to have been similarly updated. The original CHART contained five subscales: physical independence, mobility, social integration, occupation, and economic self-sufficiency. In 1992, the Revised CHART was issued, to include a cognitive functioning scale, adding 7 new items. In 1998, the Short Form of the CHART was released, reducing the total number of items to 17, with only a 10% loss of predictive power. Items on the CHART tend to have yes/no, forced choice, or other quantitative response formats, such as "How many hours per week do you spend in home maintenance activities?" or "Can you use your transportation independently?" The CHART has been widely adopted and is now part of the Model Systems Database in the United States—a huge database involving major American rehabilitation facilities.

Community Integration Questionnaire

The Community Integration Questionnaire (CIQ) (Table 16-3) (Willer, Linn, & Allen, 1992) is a 15-item

measure that was designed for people with acquired brain injuries. It too was designed to conform to the WHO's 1981 concept of handicap, and is often used in combination with the CHART, with which it shares this theoretical base. Items on the CIQ include everyday functions such as, "Who prepares meals in your household?", "How many times a month do you participate in leisure activities?", and "Are you employed?". Items are divided into three subscales for home integration, social integration, and productivity. Most items have three possible response options, for a total score of 29. The CIQ is widely used and is valued for its quantitative properties and its ease of administration. Potential users however should be aware of some of the underlying assumptions of the CIQ scoring system. The score awards more points for doing activities alone than with others, for doing activities with friends than with family, and for interacting with able-bodied rather than disabled peers. If these assumptions are not applicable to the population of interest, therapists may wish to choose another measure.

Table 16-4

COMMUNITY INTEGRATION MEASURE

Source	McColl, M. A., & Davies, D. (1997). Psychometric properties of the Community Integration Measure. *Archives of Physical Medicine and Rehabilitation,* submitted.
Purpose	• A brief, client-centred measure of community integration, based on an empirically derived definition of integration.
Type of Client	• Developed for people with brain injury, but used successfully with other rehabilitation populations.
Clinical Utility	
Format	• 10 items each with 5 response options for a total score of 50 (eg, always agree, always disagree).
Procedure	• Self-administered or interview (phone or face to face).
Completion Time	• Average of 5 minutes.
Reliability	
Internal Consistency	• Cronbach's alpha=0.87; principal components factor analysis confirms one-factor solution explaining 44% variance.
Observer	• Not reported.
Test-Retest	• Not reported.
Validity	
Content	• Based on empirically derived model; uses client-centered language for items on community integration.
Criterion	• Correlates significantly with CIQ (Willer et al., 1992) r=0.32 (p<0.05).
Construct	• Discriminates between disabled and able-bodied samples (t=5.5; p<0.006). • Correlates significantly with ISEL (Cohen et al., 1985) r=0.42 (p<0.05).
Strengths	• Wording of questions taken from qualitative research makes language and ideas very accessible.
Weaknesses	• Not as well known as the CIQ, and potentially confused with it due to similarities in names.

Community Integration Measure

The Community Integration Measure (CIM) (Table 16-4) (McColl, Davies, Carlson, Johnston, & Minnes, 2001) is made up of 10 items, each with five response options from "always disagree" to "always agree." Items were derived from interviews with brain-injury survivors and their significant others about the experiences that led them to feel that they fit in with the community (McColl et al., 1998; Karlovits & McColl, 1999; McColl et al., 1999). These qualitative data furnished statements upon which items were based, such as, "I know my way around this community," "I can be independent in this community," and "There are people who I feel close to in this community." Administration and scoring of the CIM is quick and easy, and the measure has enjoyed a positive response in a number of rehabilitation populations. Minnes and colleagues (2003) explored the meaning of the concept of community integration by comparing findings on the CIM, CIQ and Assimilation, Integration, Marginalization, Segregation (AIMS) (Buell & Minnes, 1994). They found that the scores for the three measures, although purportedly measuring the same thing, did not correlate highly, and thus underlining the multidimensionality of the construct of community integration.

COMPARISONS OF THE FOUR MEASURES

The four measures have a number of notable similarities and some differences that make them more or less applicable in certain situations. An examination of the domains covered, the methods of administration, scoring, and psychometric properties highlight the commonalities and differences.

Domain

The domain of two of the measures (CHART and CIQ) is the WHO's 1981 notion of handicap. While this was initially a very useful idea for understanding the relationship between disabled individuals and communities, it has subsequently become obsolete with the publication of the ICF (WHO, 2001). Furthermore, the concept of handicap has been criticized, as it places too much emphasis on the individual and not enough on the community and environment as the locus of problems of community integration (McColl & Bickenbach, 1998). To date, neither instrument appears to have been updated to reflect participation explicitly, however, both clearly continue to serve the field well, primarily because they are well-known and extensively integrated into practice.

The domain of the other two instruments, the CIM and RNL, are empirically derived. Both used multi-stage processes to identify domains and language for the concept. Pilot testing in both cases ensured that the resulting instrument was conceptually and psychometrically sound.

Administration

Three of the measures, the CIM, CIQ, and RNL, are very short (5 to 10 minutes) and easy to administer. The CHART is a little longer but not prohibitively so (30 minutes), and a short form is now available which brings it into line with the other two.

Scoring

Scoring for the same three measures (CIQ, CIM, and RNL) is straightforward. Scores for the CIM and RNL are easily interpreted—one is out of 50 and the other out of 100. Scores for the CIQ, however, must be interpreted in light of the assumptions outlined above. Scoring of the CHART is considerably more complex than the other three.

Psychometric Properties

Psychometric properties and utility of all four measures have been satisfactorily addressed to the extent that therapists should be able to use any of the measures with a reasonable level of certainty.

SOCIAL SUPPORT

The chapter reviews three measures of social support, which conform to the definition stated earlier and to the criteria for inclusion. In addition, two of the measures have explicitly been developed or adapted for use with people with disabilities, and the third has been successfully used with typical rehabilitation populations. Therefore these three measures were chosen because they appear most applicable to occupational therapy.

Measures of social support have proliferated in the literature since the construct first achieved popularity in the early 1980s. Despite exhortations from leaders in the field that researchers should strive for consistency in measurement, it seems that each new research project necessitated a new measure of social support, often with a particular population in mind. The three measures presented here each focus on a different dimension of support: types of support, sources of support and evaluation of support.

Interpersonal Support Evaluation List

The Interpersonal Support Evaluation List (ISEL) (Table 16-5) (Cohen, Mermelstein, Kamarck & Hoberman, 1985) is a 40-item measure of social support that asks respondents about the types of support they have at their disposal: esteem support, tangible support, advice or guidance, and a sense of belonging. Items are all true/false response formats and ask participants to address situations such as, "There is someone I can trust for advice about household responsibilities," "There are several different people with whom I enjoy spending time," "If I were sick and needed someone to drive me to the doctor, I would have trouble finding someone," and "In general, people don't have much confidence in me." Items are worded in both positive and negative perspectives to avoid response biases. The ISEL has been adapted for use with people with disabilities, including the addition of several items that address disability-specific issues such as transportation, assistance with activities of daily living (ADL), and installation of household adaptations (McColl & Skinner, 1995). The adapted version offers three subscales: instrumental, informational, and emotional support.

Social Support Inventory for People With Disabilities

The Social Support Inventory for People with Disabilities (SSIPD) (Table 16-6) (McColl & Friedland, 1989) is a 35-item measure that focuses on five sources of support: intimate, family/friends, community associates, groups, and professionals. It was originally designed for use with people who had suffered a stroke (Social Support Inventory for Stroke Survivors [SSISS]; McColl & Friedland, 1989), but has subsequently been adapted for broader use. The measure asks seven questions about each sources of support: frequency, intensity, closeness, dependability, reciprocity, satisfaction with quality, and satisfaction with quantity. The SSIPD results in a score for each of the five sources, as well as summary scores for overall quantity and satisfaction. Further, it acknowledges that the presence of a disability requires different types of support and raises particular support issues. Recent research has confirmed the applicability of the SSIPD for a variety of applications with people with disabilities

Table 16-5

INTERPERSONAL SUPPORT EVALUATION LIST

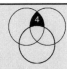

Source	Cohen, S., Mermelstein, R., Kamarck, T., & Hoberman, H. M. (1985). Measuring the functional components of social support. In I. G. Sarason & B. R. Sarason, (Eds.) *Social support: Theory, research & applications.* Boston: Martinus-Nijhoff.
Purpose	• To assess the perceived availability of social support to serve four functions.
Type of Client	• General population; adapted for people with spinal cord injuries.
Clinical Utility	
Format	• 40 items, with true/false response format.
	• 4 subscales corresponding to four types of support: tangible, esteem, appraisal, and belonging.
Completion Time	• Self- or interview-administered.
	• Estimated at 20 minutes.
Reliability	
Internal consistency	• Cronbach's alpha 0.77 to 0.86 for all subscales. Factor analysis supports four factor model corresponding to subscales.
Observer	• Not reported.
Test-retest	• 0.71 to 0.87 for 4-week interval; 0.67 to 0.87 for 2-day interval.
Validity	
Content	• Based on explicit theoretical framework for social support functions.
Criterion	• Correlates with Inventory of Socially Supportive Behaviors (r=0.46) (Barrera, Smadler & Ramsay, 1981); Family Environment Scale (r=0.30) (Moos & Moos, 1981), Partner Adjustment Scale (r=0.31) (Mermelstein, Lichtenstein, & McIntyre, 1983).
Construct	• Correlates with Rosenberg Self-Esteem Scale (r=0.74); Centre for Epidemiological Studies Depression Scale (r=0.37 to 0.47); Beck Depression Inventory (r=0.38 to 0.51).
	• Further research supports buffering theory of social support using ISEL (Cohen & Wills, 1985).
Strengths	• Widely used in research and practice, excellent psychometric properties, evidence from longitudinal studies.
Weaknesses	• Some confusion about scoring, multiple scoring systems available.

(Kim, Warren, Madill, & Hadley, 1999; Friedland, Renwick, & McColl, 1997; McColl & Skinner, 1989, 1995).

Interview Schedule for Social Interaction

The Interview Schedule for Social Interaction (ISSI) (Table 16-7) (Henderson, Duncan-Jones, Byrne, & Scott, 1980) is a 52-item measure based on the belief that individuals are likely to be more reflective and accurate in their responses in an interview situation than a self-administered one. The ISSI asks a series of questions about individuals with whom one has casual, close, and intimate associa-

tions, such as, "Would you prefer more or fewer friends like this?" and "Would you like to go out more or less often with friends from work?" The ISSI results in four scores, which have been shown to be very robust and meaningful: availability of attachments or close relationships (AVAT), adequacy of attachments (ADAT), availability of social interaction or more distant, diffuse relationships (AVSI), and adequacy of social interaction (ADSI). The ISSI has been used with a number of typical occupational therapy client groups, such as people with schizophrenia (Sorgaard Hansson, Heikkila, Vinding, Bjarnason, Bengtsson-Tops, et al., 2001), bipolar disorder (Johnson, Lundstrum, Aberg-Wistedt, & Mathe, 2003) and severe mental illness (Bengtsson-Tops & Hansson, 2003).

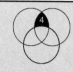

Table 16-6

SOCIAL SUPPORT INVENTORY FOR PEOPLE WITH DISABILITIES (SSIDP)

Source	McColl, M. A., & Friedland, J. (1989) Development of a multidimensional index for assessing social support in rehabilitation. *Occupational Therapy Journal of Research, 9(4)*, 218-34.
Purpose	• To assess amount and satisfaction for five sources of social support following stroke or other disability.
Type of Client	• Developed originally for use with stroke population (Social Support Inventory for Stroke Survivors (SSISS), but revised for use with all rehabilitation clients (SSIDP).
Clinical Utility	
Format	• 35 items—Same seven items for each of five sources of support.
	• Can be interview or self-administered.
Completion Time	• 20 minutes.
Reliability	
Internal Consistency	• Cronbach's alpha=0.85; multidimensional scaling explains 79% of variance.
Observer	• Not reported.
Test-Retest	• 0.91 on a 1-week interval.
Validity	
Content	• Based on theoretical model underlying and pilot-testing and consultation.
Criterion	• Correlates with ISSI ($r=0.48$; $p<0.01$).
Construct	• Negative correlations with depression (0.25 to 0.30; $p<0.05$).
Strengths	• Only measure found with detailed assessment of sources; items pertinent to people with disabilities.
Weaknesses	• Not well known; minimal research available.

COMPARISONS OF THE THREE MEASURES

The three measures of social support discussed above are also examined for similarities and differences that make them more or less applicable in certain situations. An analysis follows of the domains covered, the methods of administration, scoring, and psychometric properties.

Domain

The three measures chosen address different conceptualizations of social support in important ways. A great deal has been written about the necessity for clear operational definitions of social support, and these three measures address some of the issues raised in the literature (Alloway & Bebbington, 1987; Cohen & Wills, 1985; McColl, 1997; McColl & Skinner, 1989). Both the ISSI and the SSIPD address sources of support—the ISSI looks at two sources (attachments and integration) and the SSIPD looks at five sources (intimate, family, community, groups, and professionals). Both also look at qualitative and quantitative

dimensions: the ISSI considers availability and adequacy; the SSIPD considers amount and satisfaction. The ISEL, on the other hand, measures another important dimension of social support: types of support. The ISEL looks at the availability of supports, regardless of who they are, to fulfill specific support functions. Scoring systems are available for the three (instrumental, emotional, informational; McColl & Skinner, 1995) or four (plus appraisal; Cohen et al., 1985) type conceptualizations of support.

To achieve the kind of multidimensional measurement of social support recommended in the literature, it appears that more than one measure is necessary. Thus, these three offer some interesting possibilities. Adequate coverage of the concept should be able to be achieved by pairing the measures or by using all three.

Administration

The ISSI is designed to be administered by interview only, while the other two measures, the ISEL and the SSIPD, can both be self-administered or interview-administered. Administration of the ISSI is therefore somewhat more demanding and potentially costly, especially since it

Table 16-7

INTERVIEW SCHEDULE FOR SOCIAL INTERACTION

Source	Henderson, S., Duncan-Jones, P., Byrne, D. G., & Scott, R. (1980). Measuring social relationships: The Interview Schedule for Social Interaction. *Psychological Medicine, 10,* 723-34.
Purpose	• To assess availability and adequacy of social relationships.
Type of Client	• Developed for use in general population, but used extensively in medical and psychiatric research.
Clinical Utility	
Format	• 52 items with varying response formats; interviewer-administered.
	• Scoring results in four subscales: availability and adequacy of attachment and social integration (AVAT, ADAT, AVSI, ADSI).
Completion Time	• Average of 45 minutes.
Standardization	• Not standardized.
Reliability	
Internal Consistency	• Cronbach's alpha=0.67 to 0.81 for subscales; confirmatory factor analysis supports four-factor solution, with single second-order factor.
Observer	• Not reported.
Test-Retest	• 0.75 to 0.79 for four subscales.
Validity	
Content	• Based on Weiss' six provisions of social relationships (attachment, integration, nurturing, reassurance, dependability, guidance).
Criterion	• Subscale cores related in predictable ways to marital status and age.
Construct	• Significantly correlated in predictable ways with neuroticism and extraversion (Eysenck Personality Inventory); not significantly related to Crowne-Marlowe Social Desirability Inventory.
Strengths	• Well accepted by clinicians and patients; helped them to identify and analyze the primary group; scoring reflects multidimensional nature of construct.
Weaknesses	• Restricts consideration to two types of relationships—very close and diffuse.

takes an average of 45 minutes, compared to about 20 minutes for the other two.

Scoring

The ISEL results in either three or four scores, depending on the version chosen (McColl or Cohen, respectively). Each summarizes the availability of types of support. The ISSI results in four scores, describing the availability and adequacy of two sources of support. The SSIPD results in seven scores—five for sources of support and two for satisfaction with support. In all cases, scores are simply computed, readily interpretable, and easily understood.

Psychometric Properties

Again, the psychometric properties of all three measures are such that they could be used with confidence by therapists in practice, by researchers, or by administrators.

ISSUES IN MEASURING THE SOCIAL ENVIRONMENT

There are a number of issues associated with each of the constructs of social support and community integration that the therapist should consider in choosing to measure them. First, therapists will only be interested in either of these two constructs if they consider the social environment an appropriate target for occupational therapy intervention. In other words, unless therapists believe that occupational performance can be enhanced by better understanding the social environment within which it exists, they are unlikely to be interested in measuring social support or community integration. Instead, they will probably be more interested in measuring more focal or specific outcomes, such as particular occupational performance areas or performance components.

Furthermore, these two concepts only take on real meaning at the point where community living becomes a reality. Thus for inpatients in rehabilitation or acute care, these issues may seem remote and unwieldy. It is only at the point where discharge to the community can be conceived in a realistic way that assessment of the social environment makes sense. Thus, the use of community integration as an outcome for occupational therapists requires the long view of one's role with clients, beyond their transition to the community, and into a life that includes "someplace to live, something to do, and someone to love."

Having said that, the community can vary considerably in the scope and breadth. For most clients, it means their neighborhood, workplace, and home. It is defined geographically in terms of where they conduct most of their social interactions. However, for some clients, the community is smaller, while for others it is bigger. For clients living in a residential care facility, such as a group home or transitional center, the social environment may exist within the four walls of the facility. At the other extreme, for clients who work at a distance from their home, who travel extensively, or who are involved in advocacy and policy issues, whose important social ties are at a distance; the social environment may be much broader. It is important to recognize that environments can be defined in terms of geographical boundaries, but they can also be defined in relational terms, as communities of affiliation. Before measuring the social environment, and particularly community integration, it is important to understand what community means to a particular client and what reference points he or she is using.

In measuring social support, therapists may also wish to take account of the fact that they are often a part of the support system, and are not simply disinterested observers. Support is made up of both informal and formal sources. Informal sources are those with which the client has a personal relationship, usually made up of family, friends, neighbors, colleagues, and so on. These relationships would not be available to anyone else in the same way, because they are based on who the client is and who other people are in relation to him or her. Formal sources are those with which the client has a professional relationship, where it is the job of the support provider to offer a specific type of support. Obviously, occupational therapists are a part of the formal support systems of virtually all their clients. However, social support is usually dominated by informal sources, therefore therapists quickly become aware of the small part they play in the total support system.

Summary

In conclusion, this chapter offers seven instruments to assist therapists in assessing the social environment, particularly community integration and social support. These are constructs not routinely measured in occupational therapy, and yet they are arguably more important to the quality of life and overall functioning of clients than some that are more commonly assessed. Both constructs are conceptually complex and theoretically demanding. Both have had considerable development in the literature, often from other disciplines, especially psychology. Both constructs have been demonstrated to have a profound impact on the overall health and life satisfaction of people with disabilities. Future research in occupational therapy would be useful to elucidate the relationships between specific aspects of occupation and both community integration and social support.

References

Alloway, R., & Bebbington, R. (1987). The buffer theory of social support: A review of the literature. *Psychological Medicine, 17*, 91-108.

Bengtsson-Tops, A. & Hansson, L. (2003). Clinical and Social Changes in Severely Mentally ill Individuals admitted to an Outpatient Psychosis Team: an 18 month follow-up Study. *Scandinavian Journal of Caring Sciences, 17(1)*, 3-11.

Bradburn. (1969).

Bruininks, R. H., Chen, T. H., & Lakin, K. C. (1992). Components of personal competence and community integration for persons with mental retardation in small residential programs. *Research in Developmental Disabilities, 13*, 463-479.

Buell, M. K. & Minnes, P. (1994). An acculturation perspective on deinstutionalization, normalization and service delivery. *Journal on Developmental Disabilities, 3*, 94-107.

Carling, P. J. (1990). Major mental illness, housing and supports: The promise of community integration. *American Psychologist, 45(8)*, 969-975.

Cobb, S. (1974). A model for life events and their consequences. In B. S. Dohrenwend & B. P. Dohrenwend (Eds.), *Stressful life events: Their nature and consequences.* New York: John Wiley & Sons.

Cohen, S., Mermelstein, R., Kamarck, T., & Hoberman, H. M. (1985). Measuring the functional components of social support. In I. G. Sarason & B. R. Sarason (Eds.), *Social support: Theory, research & applications.* Boston: Martinus-Nijhoff.

Cohen, S., & Wills, T. A. (1985). Stress, social support and the buffering hypothesis. *Psychological Bulletin, 98*, 310-357.

Dijkers, M., Whiteneck, G., & El-Jaroudi, R. (2000). Measures of social outcomes in disability research. *Archives of Physical Medicine and Rehabilitation, 81*, S63-S80.

Friedland, J., & McColl, M. A. (1987). Social support and psychosocial dysfunction following stroke: Buffering effects in a community sample. *Archives of Physical Medicine and Rehabilitation, 68*, 475-480.

Friedland, J., Renwick, R., & McColl, M. A. (1996). Coping and social support as determinants of quality of life in HIV/AIDS. *AIDS Care, 8*, 15-31.

Halpern, A. S. (1985). Transition: A look at the foundations. *Exceptional Children, 51(6)*, 479-486.

Harker, W., Dawson, D., Boschen, K. A., & Stuss, D. (2002). A comparison of independent living outcomes following traumatic brain injury and spinal cord injury. *International Journal of Rehabilitation Research, 25,* 93-102.

Henderson, S., Duncan-Jones, P., Byrne, D. G., & Scott, R. (1980). Measuring social relationships: The Interview Schedule for Social Interaction. *Psychological Medicine, 10,* 723-734.

Ittenbach, R. F., Bruininks, R. H., Thurlow, M. L., & McGrew, K. S. (1993). Community integration of young adults with mental retardation: A multivariate analysis of adjustment. *Research in Developmental Disabilities, 14,* 275-290.

Jacobs, H. (1992). *Community integration and brain injury.* New Beginnings Conference, Ottawa, Ontario.

Johnson, L., Lundstrom, O., Aberg-Wistedt, A., & Mathe, A. A. (2003). Social Support in Bipolar Disorder: Its Relevance to remission and relapse. *Bipolar Disorders, 5(2),* 129-37.

Johnston, M. V., & Lewis F. D. (1991). Outcomes of community re-entry programmes for brain injury survivors. Part 1: Independent living and productive outcomes. *Brain Injury, 5,* 141-154.

Karlovits T. & McColl, M.A. (1999). Coping with community reintegration after severe ABI: A description of stressors and coping strategies. *Brain Injury, 14,* 212-8.

Kendler, K. (1997). Social support: A genetic-epidemiologic analysis. *American Journal of Psychiatry, 154(10),* 1398-1404.

Kim, P., Warren, S., Madill, H. & Hadley, M. (1999). Quality of life of stroke survivors. *Quality of Life Research, 8(4),* 293-301.

Kitamura, T., Kijima, N., Watanabe, K., Takezaki, Y & Tanaka, E. (1999). Precedents of perceived social support: Personality and early life experiences. *Psychiatry and Clinical Neurosciences, 53(6),* 649-54.

Kruzich, J. M. (1985). Community integration of the mentally ill in residential facilities. *American Journal of Community Psychology, 13(5),* 553-564.

Lomas, J. (1998). Social capital and health: Implications for public health and epidemiology. *Social Science Medicine, 47(9),* 1181-1188.

McColl, M. A. (1997). Social support and occupational therapy. In C. Christianson & C. Baum (Eds.), *Occupational therapy: Overcoming human performance deficits.* Thorofare, NJ: SLACK Incorporated.

McColl, M. A., & Bickenbach, J. (1998). *Introduction to disability.* London: W. B. Saunders.

McColl, M.A., Carlson, P., Johnston, J., Minnes, K., Shue, K., Davies, D., & Karlovits, T. (1998). The definition of community integration: Perspectives of people with brain injuries. *Brain Injury, 12,* 15-30.

McColl, M. A., & Davies, D. (1997) Psychometric properties of the Community Integration Measure. *Archives of Physical Medicine and Rehabilitation,* submitted.

McColl, M., Davies, D., Carlson, P., Johnston, J., Minnes, P. (2001). The community integration measure: Development and preliminary validation. *Archives of Physical Medicine and Rehabilitation, 82,* 429-434.

McColl, M.A., Davies, D., Carlson, P., Harrick, L., Johnston, J., Minnes, K., & Shue, K. (1999). Transitions to independent living after ABI. *Brain Injury, 13,* 311-30.

McColl, M. A., & Friedland, J. (1989). Development of a multidimensional index for assessing social support in rehabilitation. *Occupational Therapy Journal of Research, 9(4),* 218-234.

McColl, M. A., & Skinner, H. A. (1989). Concepts and measurement of social support in rehabilitation. *Canadian Journal of Rehabilitation, 2,* 93-107.

McColl, M. A., & Skinner, H. A. (1995). Assessing inter- and intra-personal resources for community living. *Disability and Rehabilitation, 17,* 24-34.

Minnes, P., Carlson, P., McColl, M., Nolte, M. L., Johnston, J., & Buell, K. (2003). Community Integration: A Useful construct, but what does it really mean? *Brain Injury, 17(2),* 149-159.

Paniak, C., Phillips, K., Toller-Lobe, G., Durand, A., & Nagy, J. (1999). Sensitivity of three recent questionnaires to mild traumatic brain injury: Related effects. *Journal of Head Trauma Rehabilitation, 14(3),* 211-219.

Patrick, L., Perugini, M., & Leclerc, C. (2002). Neuropsychological assessment and competency for independent living among geriatric patients. *Topics in Geriatric Rehabilitation, 17(4),* 65-77.

Putnam, R. D. (1995). Bowling Alone: America's Declining social capital. *Journal of Democracy, 6,* 65-78.

Rapp, C. A., Gowdy, E., Sullivan, W. P., & Wintersteen, R. (1988). Clint outcome reporting: The status method. *Community Mental Health Journal, 24(2),* 118-133.

Saladin, L. K. (2000). Measuring quality of life post-stroke. *Neurology Report, 24(4),* 133-9.

Sorgaard, K. W., Hansson, L, Heikkila, J., Vinding, H. R., Bjarnason, O., Bengtsson-Tops, A., et al. (2001). Predictors of social relations in persons with schizophrenia living in the community: A Nordic multicentre study. *Social Psychiatry and Psychiatric Epidemiology, 36(1),* 13-9.

Spitzer, S. L. (2003). Using participant observation to study the meaning of occupations of young children with autism and other developmental disabilities. *American Journal of Occupational Therapy, 57,* 66-76.

Tooth, L., McKenna, K. T., Smith, M.& O'Rourke, P. K. (2003). Reliability of Scores between stroke patients and significant others on the Reintegration to Normal (RNL) Index. *Disability and Rehabilitation, 25(9),* 433-440.

Whiteneck, G., Charlifue, S., Gerhart, K., Overholser, D., & Richardson, G. (1992). Quantifying handicap: A new measure of long-term rehabilitation outcomes. *Archives of Physical Medicine and Rehabilitation, 73,* 519-526.

Willer, B., Linn, R., & Allen, K. (1992). Community integration and barriers to integration for individuals with brain injury. In M. A. J. Finlayson & S. Garner (Eds.), *Brain injury rehabilitation: Clinical Considerations.* Baltimore: Williams & Wilkins.

Willer, B., Rosenthal, M., Kreutzer, J. S., Gordon, W. A., & Rempel, R. (1993). Assessment of community integration following rehabilitation for traumatic brain injury. *Journal of Head Trauma Rehabilitation, 8(2)*, 75-87.

Wood-Dauphinee, S., Opzoomer, A., Williams, J. I., Marchand, B. B., & Spitzer, W. O. (1988). Assessment of global function: The reintegration to normal living index. *Archives of Physical Medicine and Rehabilitation, 69*, 583-590.

WHO. (1980). *International classification of impairments, disability, and handicaps.* Geneva, Switzerland: Author.

WHO. (2001). *International classification of functioning, disability and health.* Geneva, Switzerland: Author.

Zhang, L., Abreu, B., Gonzales, V., et al. (2002). Comparison of the Community Integration Questionnaire, the Craig Handicap Assessment and Reporting Technique, and the Disability Rating Scale in traumatic brain injury. *Journal of Head Trauma Rehabilitation, 17(6)*, 497-509.

Editors' Notes for Chapter 17

Mine the Gold

Colleagues from other disciplines have provided information, research, and assessments to measure the influences of social, cultural, institutional, and physical environments. Occupational therapists combine this knowledge with our focus on persons doing occupations to assess environmental influences on performance.

Become Systematic

These measures enable occupational therapists to gather specific information about the environmental conditions that support or limit occupational performance.

Use Evidence in Practice

Use of environmental assessments aids therapists in understanding the complex relationship between person-environment and occupation-environment.

Make Occupational Therapy Contribution Explicit

Occupational therapists focus on environmental factors that support performance and make changes in the environment to improve performance.

Engage in Occupation-Based, Client-Centered Practice

The successful performance of day-to-day occupations is dependent on a supportive environment. Assessment and consideration of environmental factors facilitates clients in achieving their goals related to occupational performance.

MEASURING ENVIRONMENTAL FACTORS

Patricia Rigby, MHSc, OT Reg. (Ont.); Barbara Cooper, PhD;
Lori Letts, MA, OT Reg. (Ont.); Debra Stewart, MSc, OT Reg. (Ont.);
and Susan Strong, MSc, OT Reg. (Ont.)

The environment is integral to occupational therapy practice models and the International Classification of Functioning, Disability and Health (ICF) (World Health Organization [WHO], 2001). In occupational therapy, the environment influences human behavior and provides a context for occupational performance. Environment is broadly defined to include physical, social, cultural, economic, and organizational components. All activities and occupations undertaken by people occur within multiple environments. They are influenced by, and in turn have an impact upon environmental components. This reciprocal relationship of the person, his or her environment, and occupation is considered to be transactional, that is, to be so interwoven and interdependent that it cannot be teased apart. In occupational therapy, the outcome of the person-environment-occupation (PEO) relationship is known as occupational performance (Law, Cooper, Strong, Stewart, Rigby, & Letts, 1996). Occupational therapy interventions are primarily focused on facilitating and improving the occupational performance of people with disabilities or who are at risk for disabilities.

Similarly, the ICF classifies environmental factors as assistive products and technology; the natural and human-made environments; supports and relationships; attitudes; and services, systems and policies (WHO, 2001). These factors are included in the ICF to encourage the identification (through assessment) of environmental barriers and facilitators to the performance of daily occupations. The WHO hopes that new instruments will be created to assess both barriers and facilitators in the environment, which will be useful for various populations and age groups (WHO, 2001). The ICF also recognizes the importance of the environment in distinguishing between capacity and performance. The WHO proposes that a "standardized environment" can be used during assessment to measure a person's capacity for function (with the environment controlled). Capacity is different from performance, which is what a person does in his or her current environment (e.g., a familiar environment such as the person's home or community). The gap between performance and capacity is examined to identify the aspects of the environment that facilitate or create barriers to performance. Occupational therapists have employed a similar approach by comparing occupational performance across environments (e.g., comparing bath transfers in the hospital with bath transfers in a client's home) to identify the environmental resources or modifications that can be made to optimize performance (e.g., the installation of grab bars and the help of a trained attendant to assist with the bath transfer).

Occupational therapists are concerned with the goodness of PEO fit for their clients. In an environment where there is congruence, or a good fit between the P, E, and O components, the individual can carry out an occupation to the best of his or her ability and achieve optimal occupational performance. Conversely, environmental barriers can reduce the PEO fit and, thereby, affect occupational performance in a negative manner. A positive change in the congruence of any of the three components will result in a better fit of the respective interfaces, P-E, P-O, and O-E, and in improved occupational performance. A major goal of occupational therapy interventions is to improve PEO fit or the enabling factors that influence the individual's ability to carry out his or her chosen daily occupations. Often, environmental resources are more easily accessed and environmental barriers respond more readily to change, than using interventions to try and change the performance components of the person. However, adjustments in this area are often overlooked or limited to the physical environment (Law et al., 1996). See Section II for more in-depth information on this subject.

Historically, occupational therapy has viewed the person, the environment, and occupation as discrete elements, each contributing independently to the measurable outcomes of occupational performance. The qualities and attributes of the person have traditionally been assessed using a variety of tools, primarily standardized measures; the environment has been judged mostly from the perspective of physical accessibility, applying local or national standards for barrier-free design; and occupation has usually been evaluated employing observational methods within an occupational or task analysis. The profession is now moving toward using measures that assess the various interfaces of the PEO relationship in order to provide information on and improve our understanding of the complex phenomenon of occupational performance. To this end, both quantitative and qualitative data are required.

MEASUREMENT INSTRUMENTS

A variety of measurement tools are used in occupational therapy to provide information for 1) making clinical decisions (i.e., discriminating among factors), 2) evaluating (e.g., the PEO components and occupational performance), and 3) predicting outcomes. When choosing an instrument of measure, the occupational therapist must first consider the focus and purpose of the assessment, and then choose the most appropriate measure with the best psychometric and clinical utility properties available.

Problems with Measuring the Environment

It is difficult for any one instrument to measure something as multifaceted and complex as the environment and its dynamic influence on behavior. In addition, human limitations restrict us to gathering data at one point in time. We can improve upon this by comparing similar information gathered at multiple points in time and establishing patterns of relationships, by being accurate and comprehensive, and by ensuring that all important contributing factors are included in our evaluation. Most importantly, we can improve on our ability to assess the influence of the environment on occupational performance by having the environment rather than the person with disabilities be the focus or unit of measurement and by concentrating our examination on what is occurring at the person/environment and occupation/environment interfaces rather than on the PEO factors themselves.

The influence of time and the complexity of these issues mean that simple, short assessments are not likely to provide the depth and accuracy of information necessary for occupational therapists to evaluate accurately environmental effects on occupational performance. Specific, well-designed instruments may not always be available and choices may need to be made from among less than optimal measures. Under these circumstances, it is particularly important to be informed about the strengths and limitations of the instruments at your disposal.

Useful Instruments for Measuring the Environment

The 14 assessments presented in this chapter (Tables 17-1 to 17-14) have been selected as the best currently available for measuring the influence of the environment on occupational performance, especially at the PEO interfaces, and as possessing adequate to excellent psychometric properties and clinical utility. The Outcome Measures Rating Form (see Appendix B) was used to gather information for each instrument on: 1) the focus of the measurement, as indicated by the International Classification of Functioning, Disability and Health (ICF) framework (WHO, 2001); 2) clinical utility; 3) standardization; 4) reliability; 5) validity; and 6) strengths and weaknesses.

Most of the instruments that we have included are used by occupational therapists for clinical and/or research purposes. The measures are usually specific to a setting, and more than half address issues related to the home environment; the balance pertain to work, school, or health care environments. The measures have usually been developed for specific age groups, focusing mainly on children and seniors. They all address outcomes (occupational performance) as a function of the person living and operating within an environment.

We also identified a number of instruments, which are under development, and appear to have the potential to measure the person-environment relationship in a clinically useful manner, but for which insufficient psychometric information is currently available. These are discussed briefly in the next section. We have only included a few pertinent measures of social support as this topic is more fully addressed by McColl in Chapter 16 of this text.

INSTRUMENTS UNDER DEVELOPMENT

Health care providers are showing greater awareness of the influence of the environment on the daily performance of occupations. Consequently, several promising new assessments of the person and environment are under development. These include measures of the enabling or disabling qualities of the environment, measures to assess children's care and play environments, and tools to evaluate children's pleasure.

Table 17-1

HOME ENVIRONMENT

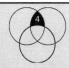

Sources	The Enabler Web site available at http://www.enabler.nu/index.html.
	Iwarsson, S., & Isacsson, A. (1996). Development of a novel instrument for occupational therapy assessment of the physical environment in the home methodologic study on The Enabler. *Occupational Therapy Journal of Research, 16(4)*, 227-244.
	Iwarsson, S., & Isacsson, A. (1995). *The enabler: Manual and assessment form.* The Swedish revised occupational therapy version. Available in English from Dr. S. Iwarsson, Lund University, Sweden, (Fax) 011-46 46 222 1959.
Important References	Cooper, B., Cohen, U., & Hasselkus, B. (1991). Barrier-free design: A review and critique of the occupational therapy perspective. *American Journal of Occupational Therapy, 45*, 344-350.
	Faange, A. & Iwarsson, S. (1999). Physical housing environment—development of a self-assessment instrument. *Canadian Journal of Occupational Therapy, 66(5)*, 250-260.
	Iwarsson, S., & Isacsson, A. (1998). Housing standards, environmental barriers in the home, subjective general apprehension of housing situation among the rural elderly. *Scandinavian Journal of Occupational Therapy, 3(2)*, 52-61.
	Iwarsson, S., Isacsson, A., & Lanke, J. (1998). ADL dependence in the elderly: The influence of functional limitations and physical environmental demand. *Occupational Therapy International, 5(3),* 1173-193.
	Iwarsson, S., Jensen, G., & Stahl, A. (2000). Travel Chain Enabler: Development of a pilot instrument for assessment of urban public bus transportation accessibility. *Technology and Disability, 12*, 3-12.
	Steinfeld, E., Shroeder, S., Duncan, J. et al. (1979). *Access to the built environment: A review of the literature.* Washington, DC: U.S. Government Printing Office.
Purpose	• To describe, evaluate, and predict the congruence or fit between an individual using mobility devices and his or her home environment. Measures multiple attributes.
	• Suitable for individual testing or surveys of populations.
Type of Client	• Designed for but not limited to use with older clients.
	• Suitable for any diagnostic category.
	• Additional clients: caregivers and other professionals, including architects and planners.
Clinical Utility	
Format	• Objective, norm-based assessment.
	• Interview, observation, performance, and size measurement techniques.
	• Noninvasive: Active client participation recommended with test.
	• Epidemiological data required when used with populations.
	• Phase 1 determines individual limitations in function and dependency on mobility devices.
	• Phase 2 identifies barriers in the physical environment.
	• Phases 1 and 2: Use dichotomous ratings (nominal).
	• Phase 3 juxtaposes the results of Phase 1 upon those of Phase 2 to develop a predictive functional accessibility score (ordinal: 4-point Likert scale) that can be validated through additional performance testing.
Procedures	• Rater should be trained.
	• Phase 1 and 3 easy to administer, score, and interpret.
	• Phase 2 is more difficult to score.

continued

Table 17-1 (continued)

HOME ENVIRONMENT

Completion Time	• Up to 2 hours depending on functional limitations and physical environment. In particular, Phase 2 can be time consuming to administer.
Standardization	• Manual available in English through author at the University of Lund, Sweden. • Outlines specific procedures for administration, scoring, and interpretation; provides evidence of reliability and validity.
Reliability	• Excellent.
Internal Consistency	• No evidence available.
Inter-Rater	• Three studies reported: Pilot 1 (n=416 occupational therapists and one building) 100% agreement for 46% environmental items and 81% to 94% agreement for 27% items. Pilot 2 (n=440 occupational therapists and 26 cases) overall mean Kappa=0.76 for person and 0.55 for environment. Pilot 3 (n=430 occupational therapists and 30 cases) mean Kappa 0.82 for person, 0.68 for environment (188 items), and 0.87 for accessibility problems; ICC range= 0.92 to 0.98 (Iwarsson & Isacsson, 1996).
Intra-Rater	• No evidence available.
Test-Retest	• ICC=0.92 to 0.98 (Iwarsson & Isacsson, 1996).
Validity	• Excellent.
Content	• Item selection based on literature review and expert opinion, and adjusted after pilot studies. • Includes: personal (15 items), functional ability (13), and dependence on mobility aids (2); 4 environmental subscales (188 items): outdoor conditions (33), entrances (49), and indoor conditions (100); and communication (6). • Phase 1 and 2 subscores can be used independently.
Convergent	• Swedish accessible housing standards provide the gold standard against which the environmental assessments are measured. No evidence available on how these were originally developed.
Construct	• Theoretical agreement for person-environment relationship (Lawton, 1986) and for construct of housing accessibility (Iwarsson & Isacsson, 1997; Iwarsson, Isacsson, & Lanke, 1998).
Strengths	• Meticulous development and testing. • Up-to-date Web site. • Widely used in Europe. • Phase 3 (interactive score) provides a predictive score (items weighted) of accessibility problems and measure of handicap resulting from the lack of congruence between the client and physical environment. • Useful for both clinical and research purposes. • Flexible (e.g., being adjusted for use as an assessment of accessibility for public travel) (Iwarsson, Jensen, & Stahl, 2000); development of a simplified self-administered assessment for clients that is conceptually compatible with the Enabler (Faange & Iwarsson, 1999).
Weaknesses	• Rater training more difficult to arrange outside Europe. • Phase 2 can be time consuming to administer.
Final Word	• North Americans might find this to be a very useful home environment assessment.

Table 17-2

HOME FALLS AND ACCIDENTS SCREENING TOOL (HOME FAST)

Source	Mackenzie, L., Byles, J., & Higginbotham, N. (2000). Designing the Home Falls and Accidents Screening Tool (HOME FAST): Selecting the items. *British Journal of Occupational Therapy, 63*, 260-269. (The appendix of the article includes all items of the HOME FAST along with definitions.)
Important References	Mackenzie, L., Byles, J., & Higginbotham, N. (2000). Designing the Home Falls and Accidents Screening Tool (HOME FAST): Selecting the items. *British Journal of Occupational Therapy, 63*, 260-269.
	Mackenzie, L., Byles, J., & Higginbotham, N. (2002a). Professional perceptions about home safety: Cross-national validation of the Home Falls and Accidents Screening Tool (HOME FAST). *Journal of Allied Health, 31(1)*, 22-28.
	Mackenzie, L., Byles, J., & Higginbotham, N. (2002b). Reliability of the Home Falls and Accidents Screening Tool (HOME FAST) for identifying older people at increased risk of falls. *Disability and Rehabilitation, 24*, 266-274.
Focus	• Modified ICF format.
Activity	• Many items relate to the abilities of the client (e.g., is the person able to get on an off the toilet easily and safely?), but focus on whether the environment is supportive of that task (e.g., toilet is of adequate height, rail exists beside toilet if needed).
Participation	• Not addressed.
Environmental Factors	• Home environment: floors, furniture, lighting, bathroom, storage, stairways/steps, and mobility.
Purpose	• Screening instrument designed to identify home hazards that may contribute to falls and therefore falls prevention interventions.
Type of Client	• Developed for use with a community-based population of older people.
Context	• Home refers to both inside and outside a person's residence.
Clinical Utility	
Format	• 25 items: Each item is scored as a hazard, not a hazard, or not applicable. Definitions are provided for each item to assist in scoring.
Procedures	• Clinicians use judgment and observation to identify home hazards.
Completion Time	• 20 to 30 minutes (Mackenzie et al., 2002b).
Cost	• Free.
Standardization	
Manual	• No manual available.
Norms	• No norms exist.
Reliability	• Adequate.
Internal Consistency	• Cronbach's alpha for the overall scale was 0.95 (Mackenzie et al., 2002b).
Observer	• Inter-rater reliability evaluated (n=40) using kappa for individual items and weighted kappa for the total number of hazards. The overall weighted kappa was 0.56 (considered fair to good agreement); kappas for individual items indicated that 4 items had excellent reliability; 20 had fair to good reliability; and one item (hazardous outside paths) had poor reliability (Mackenzie et al., 2002b).
Test-Retest	• Not yet tested.

continued

Table 17-2 (continued)

HOME FALLS AND ACCIDENTS SCREENING TOOL (HOME FAST)

Validity	• Adequate.
Content	• Based on compilation of items from the literature; field testing with 83 older adults; and review of content and field testing data by an expert panel to reduce the number of items (Mackenzie et al., 2000). Content was further examined through a cross-national validation (Australia, Canada and United Kingdom) that asked occupational therapists, physiotherapists and nurses to respond to a survey regarding the content and weighting of HOME FAST items (Mackenzie et al., 2002a).
Convergent	• Not yet tested. No gold standard exists.
Construct	• Initial evidence suggests that the HOME FAST may be useful in identifying relative risk for falls associated with exposure to home hazards, based on 99% confidence intervals (Mackenzie et al, 2000). However, further research in this area is required with larger sample sizes and with longitudinal information rather than cross-sectional data.
Strengths	• Can be quickly administered as a screening assessment.
	• Research has been conducted in various countries.
	• Initial psychometric research is positive.
Weaknesses	• Further examination of construct and predictive validity would strengthen our understanding of the measure.
Final Word	• The HOME FAST is a well-designed home hazards screening instrument that can be used in clinical practice and research. Its initial testing indicates good psychometric properties. To date most of the research has been conducted by the developers. As it becomes more widely known and used, it is anticipated that further data will be available from other researchers to confirm the findings to date.

The Environment-Independence Interaction Scale (EIIS) (Teel, Dunn, Jackson, & Duncan, 1997) is being developed to measure features of the rehabilitation environment that affect human performance. It is appropriate for adults receiving rehabilitation services in either home or institutional settings (Teel, 1999). The scale consists of 89 items organized into four environmental domains: physical (21 items), temporal (16 items), social (31 items), and cultural (21 items). There are four parallel versions of the EIIS: home-family, home-professional care provider, institutional-family, and institutional-professional care provider. Except for four dichotomous items, the remaining items are scored using a 5-point response scale with higher scores reflecting a rehabilitation environment that is more supportive of an individual's independence. Time to complete is 15 to 20 minutes.

Researchers are developing reliability estimates for the EIIS in both home and institutional settings. For validation, the Ecology of Human Performance framework (Dunn, Brown, & McGuigan, 1994) was used as a guide for conceptualization of the four environmental domains: physical, temporal, social, and cultural. Critical features of each domain were identified through interdisciplinary meetings and focus groups with rehabilitation professionals. Items were generated for each critical feature and then assessed for duplication or omission across the domains. The criteria used for determining inclusion were that an item was related to both home and institutional rehabilitation settings and that the content was within the knowledge base of the family and professional care providers who complete the scale. Information on the EIIS can be obtained from the University of Kansas School of Nursing.

The Environmental Utility Measure (EUM) (Danforth & Steinfeld, 2001) shows promise for assessing person-environment fit within the physical environment. It was developed to assess an individual's perception of his or her ease or difficulty in doing activities in various environmental settings. In addition the individual rates the acceptability of doing activities within those environments. For example, an individual might rate an environment difficult, but still acceptable given his or her impairments and expectations. Information on the EUM can be obtained from the Center for Inclusive Design and Environmental Access, School of Architecture and Planning.

The Home Occupational-Environment Assessment (HOEA) (Baum & Edwards, 1998) was designed to be used with individuals with cognitive or visual impairments in

Table 17-3

HOME ENVIRONMENT: HOME OBSERVATION FOR MEASUREMENT OF THE ENVIRONMENT (HOME) (REVISED EDITION)

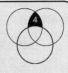

There are four versions: infant, early childhood, middle childhood, and early adolescent.

Source	Caldwell, B. M., & Bradley, R. H. (1984). Center for Child Development and Education. University of Arkansas at Little Rock, 33rd and University Avenue, Little Rock, AR, 72204, (Web) www.ualr.edu/~crtldept/home4.htm.
Important References	Bradley, R. H., & Caldwell, B. M. (1988). Using the HOME inventory to assess family environment. *Pediatric Nursing, 14,* 97-102.
	Bradley, R. H., Rock, S. L., Caldwell, B. M., & Brisby, J. A. (1989). Uses of the HOME Inventory for families with handicapped children. *American Journal on Mental Retardation, 94(3),* 315-330.
	Bradley, R. H., Corwyn, R. F., & Whiteside-Mansell, L. (1996). Life at home: same time, different places—An examination of the HOME Inventory in different cultures. *Early Development and Parenting, 6,* 1-19.
	Bradley, R. H., Corwyn, R. F., Caldwell, B. M., Whiteside-Mansell, L., Wasserman, G. A., Walker, T. B. & Mink, I. T. (2000). Measuring the home environments of children in early adolescence. *Journal of Research on Adolescence, 10,* 247-289.
	Elardo, R., & Bradley, R. H. (1981). The Home Observation for Measurement of the Environment (HOME) scale: A review of research. *Developmental Review, 1,* 113-145.
	Totsika, V., & Sylva, K. (2004). The Home Observation for Measurement of the Environment Revisited. *Child and Adolescent Mental Health, 9,* 25-40.

Focus
- Modified ICF format.

Activities
- Social behaviors and socialization.

Environmental Factors
- Physical: lighting, safety, size, location, equipment/technology/appliances/tools/toys.
- Social: stimulation, social support, communication, family organization.

Participation/Life Habits
- Interpersonal relations: family, relatives/friends, community life, use of services.

Purpose
- To describe and discriminate "the quality and quantity of stimulation and support for cognitive, social, and emotional development available to a child in the home environment" (Bradley et al., 1989, p. 314). Measures multiple attributes.

Type of Client
- Children and adolescents ages 0 to 15 with all diagnoses; respondents may include caregivers, service providers, and other professionals.

Context
- Home.

Clinical Utility

Format
- Interview and naturalistic observation; noninvasive, but requires active participation of client and caregiver.

Procedure
- Easy to administer and score; more complex to interpret. Training tapes are available and recommended.
- There are different subscales for each measure:

  Infant/toddler: responsivity, acceptance, organization, learning materials, involvement, and variety.

  Early childhood: learning materials, language stimulation, physical environment, responsivity, learning stimulation, modeling of social maturity, variety in experience, and acceptance.

  Middle childhood: responsivity, encouraging maturity, learning materials, active stimulation, emotional climate, physical environment, parental involvement, and family participation.

continued

Table 17-3 (continued)

HOME ENVIRONMENT: HOME OBSERVATION FOR MEASUREMENT OF THE ENVIRONMENT (HOME) (REVISED EDITION)

	Early adolescence: physical environment, learning materials, modeling, instructional activities, regulatory activities, variety of experience, acceptance, and responsivity.
Completion Time	• 90 to 120 minutes.
Standardization	• Both an administrative manual and a monograph (summary of research) are available.
	• Norms: 0 to 15 years. Norms available for typical children (Caldwell & Bradley, 1984) and for children with multiple handicaps (Bradley et al., 1989, p. 3).
Reliability	• Excellent.
Internal Consistency	• Cronbach's alpha for Infant/toddler version=0.89 total score and 0.44 to 0.89 for subscores; early childhood version=0.93 total score and 0.53 to 0.88 for subscores; middle childhood version=0.90 total score and 0.53 to 0.90 for subscores; early adolescent version=above 0.90 for total score.
Inter-Rater	• Average of 0.90% agreement in three studies and 0.9% to 0.96% in another (Bradley et al., 1989).
Test-Retest	• Not examined due to nature of the test (Bradley & Caldwell, 1988). Long-term stability between 6 to 24 months on total score was moderate (r=0.64).
Validity	• Excellent.
Content	• Statistical methods (content analysis, factor analysis, and item analysis) used (Elardo & Bradley, 1981).
Construct	• More than two studies that demonstrated confirmation of theoretical formulations.
Convergent	• Demonstrated adequate agreement with a gold standard measure.
Strengths	• Well-established measure, strong psychometrics with supporting research.
	• Applicable to broad range of ages and diagnoses.
Weaknesses	• Focuses on home environment, doesn't consider broader neighborhood or community.
Final Word	• Adequate to excellent clinical utility, excellent reliability and validity, easily available.

their homes. The authors developed this as a clinical checklist, and are currently integrating it with another instrument (C. Baum, personal communication, April 22, 2004).

The Home Assessment Profile (HAP) (Chandler, Duncan, Weiner & Studenski, 2001) is a new performance-based home assessment, which identifies and assesses the risk of hazards throughout the home, which may cause the older adult to fall. Interrater and test-retest reliability and predictive validity have been demonstrated (Studenski, Duncan, & Chandler, 1994; Sattin, Rodriguez, DeVito, & Wingo, 1998).

Bundy has developed The Test of Environmental Supportiveness (Bundy, 1999) to be used together with her Test of Playfulness (Bundy, 2002b;1996) to provide occupational therapists with a more complete picture of the play experience of any child whether or not the child has

a disability This tool examines both the human and non-human factors that help or hinder a child's play, and is described in more detail in Chapter 9. In a study of children with cerebral palsy playing in three different environments, the playfulness of each child was found to vary by environment (Rigby & Gaik, 2004). These findings reflect the dynamic nature of occupational performance and illustrate how the relationship among the child's abilities, what the child is doing, and the environmental factors are constantly changing.

The Assessment of Ludic Behavior involves an interview with a child's parent to discover what gives pleasure to a child with a physical disability (Ferland, 1997). There is a large focus on environmental factors (e.g., play partners, play setting, and materials) and play experiences. Reliability and validity testing has shown good results. The test is published in English and French.

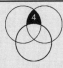

Table 17-4

LIFEASE SOFTWARE: EASE 3.2 BASIC AND EASE 3.2 DELUXE

Source	Lifease Web site: http://www.lifease.com/lifease-home.html. Author: Margaret Christenson, (e-mail) mchristenson@lifease.com.
Purpose	• Reviews personal needs and abilities and identifies potential home environment problems. Based on these data, develops best possible solutions.
Type of Client	• Aging population or adults with activity limitations.
Clinical Utility	
Format	• A computer-based tool (CD-format) using windows-based format. Can be conducted through an on-site home assessment with or without the client; or through an interview with the client, family or friend reviewing home information. Consumer version of Ease, LivAbility, available for purchase on the Web site: www.lifease.com.
Procedures	• Easy to administer using pop-up windows with checklists for selection of specific items in each room. Uses database of more then 4000 ideas and product solutions; offers instant reporting and information where products can be obtained. Searches the database by product, product description, or supplier.
Completion Time	• Varies depending on extent of activity limitations and number of rooms in the home.
Standardization	• Manual must be purchased. No gold standard exists.
Reliability	
Internal Consistency	• No evidence available.
Inter-Rater	• No evidence available.
Intra-Rater	• No evidence available.
Test-Retest	• No evidence available.
Validity	
Content	• Excellent item selection including comprehensive assessment of physical characteristics of home, functional actions needed for doing ADL at home, and provides a wide range of design and AT products and solutions. Constantly under review.
Convergent	• No evidence available.
Construct	• No evidence available.
Strengths	• Practical, comprehensive, popular. Electronic slides for occupational therapists available through company and AOTA.
Weaknesses	• Lacks psychometric testing.

MEASURES WORTHY OF CONSIDERATION BY OTs

There are measures of the environment that are used in different fields of practice in which OTs may work. An OT may want to become familiar with the measure even when they may not be the person administering it. For example, the Readily Achievable Checklist: A Survey for Accessibility (www.adaptenv.org) was developed for owners and managers of public buildings and businesses to identify barriers in their facilities. This survey tool is based on the Americans with Disabilities Act Accessibility Guidelines (ADAAG) and provides easy to use measurement guides to identify accessibility barriers, and suggestions for "readily achievable" access solutions. The occupational therapist can assist businesses to use this tool and set priorities for achieving accessibility.

In the fields of child health and children development there are a group of environmental rating scales published by the Frank Porter Graham (FGP) Child Development Institute, University of North Carolina at Chapel Hill that focus on the assessment of group programs for children of different ages. The four measures are: Infant-Toddler

Table 17-5

SAFETY ASSESSMENT OF FUNCTION AND THE ENVIRONMENT FOR REHABILITATION (SAFER TOOL) AND SAFETY ASSESSMENT OF FUNCTION AND THE ENVIRONMENT FOR REHABILITATION — HEALTH OUTCOME MEASUREMENT AND EVALUATION (SAFER-HOME)

Source
COTA Comprehensive Rehabilitation and Mental Health Services, 700 Lawrence Ave. West, Suite 362, Toronto, Ontario, M6A 3B4, (phone) 416-785-9230, (e-mail) info@cotarehab.ca.

Important References
Chui, T., Oliver, R., Marshall, L., & Letts, L. (2001). *Safety assessment of function and the environment for rehabilitation tool manual*. Toronto, ON: COTA Comprehensive Rehabilitation and Mental Health Services.

Chui, T., & Oliver, R. (2004). *Factor analysis and construct validity of the SAFER-HOME*. Manuscript submitted for publication.

Letts, L., & Marshall, L. (1995). Evaluating the validity and consistency of the SAFER Tool. *Physical and Occupational Therapy in Geriatrics, 13*, 49-66.

Letts, L., Scott, S., Burtney, J., Marshall, L., & McKean, M. (1998). The reliability and validity of the Safety Assessment of Function and the Environment for Rehabilitation (SAFER) Tool. *British Journal of Occupational Therapy, 61*, 127-132.

Focus
• Modified ICF format.

Activity/Participation
• Mobility, self-care, and instrumental activities of daily living within the home environment a focus.

Environmental Factors
• Focus on physical environment (safety, architecture, design) and social environment (supports from caregivers).

Purpose
• The SAFER Tool is designed to identify and describe safety concerns of individuals in their own homes and collect information to plan interventions and recommendations to improve safety (Chui et al., 2001). The SAFER-HOME is designed to measure change in safety over time (to evaluate the effectiveness of interventions to improve home safety).

Type of Client
• Originally developed for psychogeriatric population; later expanded to meet needs of adult clients with physical disabilities as well. Frequently used for clients with many diagnoses and complex needs.

Context
• Intended to be administered in the client's home.

Clinical Utility

Format
• Interview with client and/or caregivers, observation of task performance, naturalistic observation are used. The instrument is not standardized in administration format. SAFER Tool consists of 97 items. SAFER-HOME consists of 93 items. On the SAFER Tool each applicable item is scored as a problem or not a problem; the SAFER-HOME uses a four point rating scale for each item: no problem, mild problem, moderate problem, severe problem. There are 14 sections on the SAFER Tool: living situation, mobility, kitchen, fire hazards, eating, household, dressing, grooming, bathroom, medication, communication, wandering, memory aids, and general. Through factor analysis, the SAFER-HOME has been organized into 10 domains: meal preparation, awareness of safety hazards, mobility and toileting, cognitive impairment, homemaking support, emergency communication, functional communication, personal care, family assistance, and medication.

Procedures
• Home visit conducted with interview and observation.

Completion Time
• 45 to 90 minutes.

continued

Table 17-5 (continued)

SAFETY ASSESSMENT OF FUNCTION AND THE ENVIRONMENT FOR REHABILITATION (SAFER TOOL) AND SAFETY ASSESSMENT OF FUNCTION AND THE ENVIRONMENT FOR REHABILITATION— HEALTH OUTCOME MEASUREMENT AND EVALUATION (SAFER-HOME)

Cost	• SAFER: $100 for one manual and 10 forms; $20 for a package of 100 forms. (order form downloadable from www.cotarehab.ca). SAFER-HOME is not yet available for purchase.
Standardization	
Manual	• A manual for the SAFER Tool was published in 2001. It includes background information, administration instructions, guidelines for considering each item, potential recommendations for each item if identified as a problem, and four case studies to demonstrate how it can be used. As well, it describes future directions, including the development of the SAFER-HOME.
Norms	• There are no norms for the SAFER Tool. There is however information about a reference group of COTA clients. A table in the manual summarizes the SAFER tool results from 563 COTA clients, with a mean age of 78. The reference table provides 95th and 99th percentile totals for each section of the SAFER Tool and the Total Score.
Reliability	
Internal Consistency	• SAFER: Kuder-Richardson 20 estimate=0.83 (Letts & Marshall, 1995) SAFER-HOME: Coefficient alpha for total scores=0.8593; subscales ranged from 0.539 to 0.789 (Chui & Oliver, 2004)
Observer	• SAFER—Inter-rater reliability—Kappa or % agreement: acceptable to excellent for 92 items.
Test-Retest	• SAFER—Kappa or % agreement—acceptable to excellent for 90 items.
Validity	
Content	• For both the SAFER and the SAFER-HOME content validity has been established through review by experts and clinicians as well as statistical analysis of completed measures.
Criterion	• No evidence available (no gold standard exists).
Construct	• SAFER: Total scores have been associated with cognitive status and independent living in houses, but not directly to ADL or IADL. SAFER HOME: Total scores were compared to functional status scores using the SMAF. The correlation was weak, which confirmed that the SAFER HOME is measuring more than functional abilities.
Responsiveness	• Neither the SAFER nor the SAFER-HOME has yet undergone statistical testing of its responsiveness to change. It is hypothesized that the SAFER-HOME will be more sensitive to change with its 4-point rating for each item.
Strengths	• Comprehensive coverage of home safety. • Both the SAFER and SAFER-HOME developed and tested rigorously.
Weaknesses	• Length of administration a barrier in some practices. • Most of the research on the psychometrics are based out of the originating agency. • Further research on responsiveness to change needed.
Overall Utility	• Both instruments are unique in that they focus on all areas of safe function, with emphasis on the interaction between the skills and abilities of the person, and the home environment (including the physical characteristics and social support offered). Although the SAFER-HOME requires further research to examine its reliability and validity in more detail, it shows promise as an evaluative measure.

Table 17-6

Westmead Home Safety Assessment

Source	Co-ordinates Publications, a division of Co-ordinates Therapy Services Pty Ltd, P.O. Box 59, West Brunswick, Victoria, 3055, (phone) 011 61 3 93801127, (fax) 011 61 3 93874829, (Web) www.therapybookshop.com/coordinates.html.
Important References	Clemson, L. (1997). Home fall hazards: A guide to identifying fall hazards in the homes of elderly people and an accompaniment to the assessment tool. *The Westmead Home Safety Assessment*. West Brunswick, Victoria, Australia: Co-ordinates Publication.
	Clemson, L., Fitzgerald, M. H., & Heard, R. (1999). Content validity of an assessment tool to identify home fall hazards: The Westmead home safety assessment. *British Journal of Occupational Therapy, 62*, 171-179.
	Clemson, L., Fitzgerald, M. H., Heard, R., & Cumming, R. G. (1999). Inter-rater reliability of a home fall hazards assessment tool. *Occupational Therapy Journal of Research, 19*, 83-100.
Focus	• Modified ICF format.
Activity	• Activities included in the assessment but in terms of the physical environment as a hazard; client function is considered in terms of whether the activity is relevant to the client but functional abilities are not assessed.
Participation	• Not addressed.
Environmental Factors	• Physical environmental factors that may impact on the risk of falling (e.g., external and internal trafficways, general/indoors, living area, seating, bedroom, footwear, bathroom, kitchen, laundry, medication management).
Purpose	• To identify fall hazards in the home environments of older adults.
Type of Client	• Older adults, 65 years and older; all diagnoses. Respondents include clients, caregivers, service providers.
Context	• Home.
Clinical Utility	
Format	• Not a standardized assessment; 72 items are scored by the clinician based on interview, observation of task performance and naturalistic observation.
Procedures	• Complete during or immediately after a home visit; scoring is dichotomized; each item is rated as relevant or not; each relevant item is rated as a hazard or not; hazards are presented by type.
Completion Time	• One home visit required.
Cost	• $118.00 Australian.
Scale Construction	
Item Selection	• Items based on comprehensive literature review and expert opinion (Clemson, Fitzgerald, & Heard, 1999).
Weighting	• No.
Level of Measurement	• Nominal for each item; no summary score.
Subscales	• None, although the instrument is organized into different sections.
Standardization	
Manual	• The instrument is not standardized. The manual states that "the tool is an observational aid to assist therapists in systematically identifying hazards" (Clemson, 1997, p. 48). The manual provides operational definitions for a number of hazards.
Norms	• None.

continued

Table 17-6 (continued)

WESTMEAD HOME SAFETY ASSESSMENT

Reliability

Internal Consistency
- No evidence available.

Observer
- Inter-rater reliability tested in a sample of 21 clients' homes; kappa values of >0.75 for 34 items; and between 0.4 and 0.75 for 31 items; kappa could not be calculated for some items (Clemson et al., 1999).

Test-Retest
- No evidence available.

Validity

Content
- Established through content analysis of the literature and a rigorous expert review process (Clemson et al., 1999).

Criterion
- No evidence available (no gold standard exists).

Construct
- No evidence available.

Strengths
- Comprehensive assessment of home hazards specific to falls in older adults.

Weaknesses
- Does not address home hazards besides falls-further evaluation of reliability, construct validity and responsiveness to change would be helpful.

Overall Utility
- This instrument is one of the few instruments designed to exclusively focus on fall hazards in the home environment, and so is useful if fall hazards is a focus of intervention. It has been well developed and inter-rater reliability is good when training was provided. The manual supports its use in practice.

Environment Rating Scale, Revised Edition (Harms & Cryer, 2003) for children from birth to 2.5 years; Early Childhood Environment Rating Scale, Revised Edition (Harms, Clifford, & Cryer, 1998) for children ages 2.5 to 5 years; the Family Day Care Rating Scale (Harms & Clifford, 1989); and the School-Age Care Environment Rating Scale (Harms, Jacobs, & White, 1996) for ages 5 to 12 years. Another measure related to child health is The Playability Audit (Ontario Parks Association, 2001), which assesses the accessibility playgrounds for children of varying abilities. Although there is no report of its psychometric properties, it was developed by a group of experts and is administered in a standardized manner.

In occupational therapy practice with older adults there are a number of measures available that provide assessments of sheltered care or nursing home environments. Although these can be administered by occupational therapists, there is little evidence from the literature that occupational therapists are using them with any consistency. However, as practice shifts to focus more on environmental interventions to optimize occupational performance with older adults living in long term care (Cooper & Day, 2003), these may become more important to occupational therapy practice. The Multiphasic Environmental Assessment Procedure (MEAP) (Moos & Lemke, 1996) is a very comprehensive measure of sheltered care settings that has instruments that focus on the physical and architectur-

al features of the setting, the policy and programs offered, and includes five different instruments based on resident and staff reports, direct observations, and record reviews. The instrument is standardized, with norms from 262 community and 81 veteran facilities; with excellent reliability and validity. More recently, the Therapeutic Environment Screening Survey for Nursing Homes (TESS-NH) has been described in the literature (Sloane et al., 2002), as a descriptive instrument to assess physical environments for persons with dementia. It is available for download (http://www.unc.edu/depts/tessnh/index.html). The TESS-NH shows promise as an observational screening tool, which could be used by occupational therapists and others wanting to ensure physical environments are designed optimally. The psychometric research conducted to date is very encouraging (Sloane et al., 2002).

ADDITIONAL MEASUREMENT ISSUES

Some questions and issues about person-environment relations cannot be easily answered using standardized instruments of measure. For example, to describe the meaning of particular environments for people with disabilities, to determine the factors that provide environmental satisfaction for specific groups, or to explore how clients make choices are issues that may require a qualitative approach. However a few new tools address how

Table 17-7

POST-OCCUPANCY EVALUATION (POE)

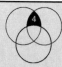

Source	Preiser, W. F. E., Rabinowitz, H. Z., & White, E. T. (1988). Social science. In *Post-occupancy evaluation*. New York: Van Nostrand Reinhold.
Important References	Cooper, B., Ahrentzen, S., & Hasselkus, S. (1991). Post-occupancy evaluation: An environment-behavior technique for assessing the built environment. *Canadian Journal of Occupational Therapy, 58(4)*, 181-188.
	Kennon, P. A., Bauer, J., & Parshall, S. (1988). Evaluating health care facilities. *Journal of Health Administration Education, 6(4 Pt 1)*, 819-831.
	Sundstrom, E., Bell, P. A., Busby, P. L. & Asmus, C. (1996). Environmental psychology 1989-1994. *Annual Review of Psychology, 47*, 485-512.
Purpose	• Evaluative/transactive: Examines the relationship and closeness of fit between people and their physical environments.
Type of Client	• All ages; all conditions.
Clinical Utility	
Format	• Survey, observation, and measurement.
	• Choice of methods and measures: appropriate for gathering information on user views and performance and on the building or context of user behavior.
	• Methods and measures targeted to meet agreed upon objectives for the POE.
Procedures	• Extent of procedures will vary according to scope of POE (indicative, investigative and diagnostic (Cooper et al., 1991). Specific model for approach described by Kennon, Bauer, & Parshall, 1988. This includes: 1) Establish purpose/objectives/scope of POE, 2) Collect and analyze relevant quantitative information, 3) Identify and examine relevant qualitative information, 4) Make an assessment, and 5) summarize recommendations.
Completion Time	• Variable: Dependent on depth and scope of POE.
Standardization	• Manual and norms dependent on measures chosen, building codes, etc.
Reliability	• Varies with instruments selected for use.
Internal Consistency	• See above.
Observer	• See above.
Test-retest	• See above.
Validity	• Varies with instruments selected for use.
Content	• See above.
Convergence	• See above.
Construct	• See above.
Strengths	• Used broadly and extensively in Environment-Behavior studies (e.g., hospital evaluations (Sundstrom et al., 1996).
	• Primarily used for home assessments by occupational therapists (Cooper et al., 1991).
	• Process provides critical information on person/environment fit crucial for maximizing the occupational performance of people with disabilities
	• Flexible in scope, depth, and focus of assessment.
	• Can be used for both evaluative and research purposes.
Weaknesses	• Process rather than an assessment per se, therefore only as good as the assessments used.

Table 17-8

CRAIG HOSPITAL INVENTORY OF ENVIRONMENTAL FACTORS (CHIEF) AND CHIEF SHORT FORM

Source	The Centre for Outcome Measurement in Brain Injury at Craig Hospital. Available at http://www.craighospital.org/Research/Disability/CHIEF%20Manual.pdf; http://www.craighospital.org/Research/Disability/DISCHIEF.asp; and http://www.tbims.org/ combi/chief/CHIEF.pdf
Important References	Whiteneck, G., Harrison-Felix, C. L., Mellick, D., Brookes, C. A., Charlifue, S., & Gerhart, K. A. (2004). Quantifying environmental factors: A measure of physical, attitudinal, service, productivity and policy barriers. *Archives of Physical Medicine and Rehabilitation, 85(8)*, 1324-35.
	Dijkers, M. P. J. M., Yavuzer, G., Ergin, S., Weitzenkamp, D., & Whiteneck, G. (2002). A tale of two countries: Environmental impact on social participation after spinal cord injury. *Spinal Cord, 40*, 351-362.
	Fougeyrollas, P. (1995). Documenting environmental factors for preventing the handicap creation process: Quebec contributions relating to ICIDH and social participation of people with functional differences. *Disability and Rehabilitation, 17*, 145-153.
	Whiteneck, G. G., Fougeyrolles, P., & Gerhart, K. A. (1997). Elaborating the Model of Disablement. In: M. Fuhrer (ed.), *Assessing medical rehabilitation practices: The promise of outcome research*. Baltimore, MD: Paul H. Brooks Publishing.
Focus	• Modified ICF format.
Activity	• Evaluation of environmental influences on accomplishment of daily activities and social roles.
Participation	• As defined within the ICIDH-2 (WHO, 1999, 2000).
Environmental Factors	• Five characteristics: accessibility, accommodation, resource availability, social support, and equality.
Purpose	• Evaluative: environmental characteristics which act to impede accomplishment of daily activities and social roles; to measure how individuals with a disability characterize the severity of perceived barriers (in the environment) to social participation.
Type of Client	• Individuals with physical and/or sensory impairments.
Clinical Utility	
Format	• Self-administered or administered by interview, either in person or by telephone; Can be administered through a proxy with primary respondent present and participating. Should not be administered to proxy alone.
	• CHIEF: 25 items; CHIEF Short-Form: 12 items.
Procedures	• No training required to administer, but advance review of material is recommended; easy to administer, score and interpret.
Completion Time	• CHIEF when self-administered is about 10 minutes, and interview is about 15 minutes. CHIEF Short Form when self-administered is about 5 minutes, and interview is about 10 minutes.
Cost	• Available from the Craig Hospital Web site at no cost.
Standardization	• Published as one inclusive manual, including psychometric properties.
Reliability	• Adequate.
Internal Consistency	• Cronbach's alpha values with the disability sample was 0.93 for the total score and ranged from 0.76 to 0.81 for the subscales.

continued

Table 17-8 (continued)

CRAIG HOSPITAL INVENTORY OF ENVIRONMENTAL FACTORS (CHIEF) AND CHIEF SHORT FORM

Inter-Rater	• Subject-proxy agreement was analyzed with resultant recommendation that proxies not be asked to complete CHIEF when subjects are unavailable to do so; ICCs for proxy-participant agreement ranged from 0.406 to 0.699 (total score ICC of 0.618).
Intra-Rater	• No evidence available.
Test-Retest	• One study completed; ICC of 0.926 for total score; individual item scores for frequency and magnitude scales range from 0.332 to 0.882.
Validity	• Adequate.
Content	• Based on review of the literature and consultation with experts. Four separate advisory panels (total of 32 participants) were convened, each focusing on a different area of disability issue (mobility, self-care, communication, and learning). Experts included academics, researchers, representatives from advocacy and policy implementation groups, and consumers.
Convergent	• No gold standard available for comparison.
Construct	• Addressed during study in which the subscales were established; was able to show differences in reported frequency and magnitude of environmental barriers between groups with a variety of impairments and activity limitations.
Strengths	• Very useful for assessing the frequency and magnitude of a broad range of environmental barriers.
	• Based on ICF and is a rare tool which addresses participation.
	• Comprehensive inventory of environmental factors.
	• Quick and easy to administer and score.
	• Appropriate for both population-based or individual-focused assessment and research.
	• Excellent preliminary evidence of psychometric properties.
	• Consistent with a client-centered perspective.
Weaknesses	• Had originally intended to measure both environmental facilitators and barriers, but focuses only on the environmental factors as barriers.
	• Scale for assessing magnitude of barriers has only 2-points (little vs big problem).
	• Further evaluation of psychometric properties needed.
Final Word	• The CHIEF is a very useful new tool which seeks a client's perspective whether the environment impedes participation in daily life. It is quick and easy to use and uses a client-centered perspective. It is readily available to the clinician from Craig Hospital Web site.

clients perceive the environment. These include, The Multidimensional Scale of Perceived Social Support (MSPSS), which assesses an individual's perceptions of the adequacy of their social supports; and the Craig Hospital Inventory of Environmental Factors (CHIEF) which assesses, from the clients perspective, how well the environment facilitates or hinders participation. See Chapter 5 for a discussion of qualitative methods that can be used to address a client's perspective. The results of qualitative studies augment our understanding and, in conjunction with standardized measures, greatly enrich our knowledge of the topic.

FUTURE RESEARCH

The gaps in knowledge on environmental measures identified by the review relate primarily to conceptual issues, instrument development, and methods of dissemination of information to the community.

Conceptual Issues

Environmental assessments take place at both the micro- and macro-level. The intimate, or micro-level, lies within the realm of professional service and requires prac-

Table 17-9

HOME AND COMMUNITY ENVIRONMENTS: MEASURE OF PROCESSES OF CARE (MPOC)

Source	King, S., Rosenbaum, P., & King, G. CanChild Centre for Childhood Disability Research, IAHS Building, McMaster University, 1400 Main Street West, Hamilton, ON, Canada, L8S 1C7, (Web) www.fhs.mcmaster.ca/canchild.
Important References	King, S., Rosenbaum, P., & King, G. (1995). Parents' perceptions of caregiving: Development and validation of a measure of processes of care. *Developmental Medicine & Child Neurology, 38,* 757-772.
	King, S., Rosenbaum, P., & King, G. (1996). *The Measure of Process of Care (MPOC): A means to assess family-centered behaviours of health care providers.* Hamilton, ON: McMaster University.
	King, S., King. G., & Rosenbaum, P. (2004). Evaluating health service delivery to children with chronic conditions and their families: Development of a refined measure of processes of care (MPOC-20). *Children's Health Care, 33,* 35-57.
Focus	• Modified ICF format.
Abilities/Disabilities; Activities	• Social skills and behaviors: social skills.
Environmental Factors	• Physical: lighting, safety, size, location, equipment/technology/appliances/tools/toys.
	• Social: Stimulation, social support, communication, family organization.
Participation/Life Habits	• Interpersonal relations: family, relatives/friends, community life, use of services.
Purpose	• To describe/discriminate among the components of care that have been shown to be important to caregivers. Can discern variations in parental experiences and perceptions of care and services and the extent to which certain behaviors of health care providers occur.
Type of Client	• Parent caregivers of children with long-term health or developmental problems; respondents are parent caregivers.
Context	• Home, community agency, rehabilitation center/health care setting, mail surveys.
Clinical Utility	
Format	• Questionnaire completed by caregiver, noninvasive. Active participation of client required.
Procedure	• Easy to administer, score, and interpret.
Completion Time	• 15 to 20 minutes for full MPOC; less time for MPOC-20.
Cost	• Manual and master for duplicating questionnaire $100.00 (Canadian).
Standardization	
Manual	• Excellent: Published manual outlines specific procedures for administration, scoring, interpretation, and evidence of reliability and validity.
Reliability	• Excellent.
Internal Consistency	• Excellent: Cronbach's coefficient alphas for full MPOC on the five scales range from 0.63 to 0.96 and 0.81 to 0.96 in two studies, and from 0.63 to 0.94 on the third (adequate to excellent). For MPOC-20: range is 0.77 to 0.87.
Inter-Rater	• N/A.
Intra-Rater	• No evidence.
Test-Retest	• Adequate to excellent: intra-class coefficients across the five subscales range from 0.78 to 0.88 after a 3-week interval for full MPOC; 0.81 to 0.86 for MPOC-20.

continued

Table 17-9 (continued)

HOME AND COMMUNITY ENVIRONMENTS:
MEASURE OF PROCESSES OF CARE (MPOC)

Validity	• Excellent.
Content	• Judgmental method used, including literature review, parental survey, and consultation with health care providers.
Convergent	• No evidence available.
Construct	• More than two well-designed studies have shown that the instrument conforms to prior theoretical relationships among characteristics or individuals.
	• Strength of Association for MPOC and stress=fair (r=-0.23 to 0.55 for full MPOC and -0.18 to 0.50 for MPOC-20); MPOC and satisfaction=poor to adequate (r=0.24 to 0.69 for full MPOC and 0.13 to 0.62 for MPOC-20); MPOC and social desirability (positive correlation)=significant difference on all scales between responses measuring reality and experience.
Strengths	• A psychometrically sound instrument to measure service provision.
	• Short version is easy and quick to administer.
Weaknesses	• Designed for use in pediatric services only.
Final Word	• Adequate to excellent clinical utility; excellent reliability and validity; easily available. Can be used in a variety of settings for research, program evaluation, and total quality management purposes. A companion tool is available for service providers to measure their implementation of family-centered services (MPOC-SP).

titioners to evaluate and adjust environments that promote occupational performance for individual clients. At the macro-level, environmental assessments are used to gather data from a population perspective and to predict the occupational performance of large groups. The theoretical bases used to develop measurement instruments must therefore reflect both levels of concern. In addition, they need to reflect the complex, dynamic aspects of the PEO relationship.

Measures

Instruments of measure can always be improved. The necessary process of establishing good psychometric data can be tedious, but is important, particularly for determining the clinical utility of these tools. Future measures need to be either more diverse or more flexible to allow them to be used with a variety of populations in a variety of settings. They must be more sensitive to detect change over time. Finally, measures are required that directly reflect the underlying theoretical bases and allow us to evaluate not only the relationships at the interfaces, but occupational performance itself. Meeting these goals is likely to be a long and multi-faceted process.

Dissemination

A clear theoretical base and good instruments of measure are useless if they are neither known nor used by the

clinical community. One strategy is to ensure that new practitioners are aware of these issues; another is to summarize the data using pragmatic, easily understood formats, much as we have done in the chapter. However, the task is complex and requires ongoing multifaceted solutions. The issue of how to improve the dissemination and integration of new measurement knowledge to the clinical community remains a challenge.

REFERENCES

Avallone, I., & Gibbon, B. (1998). Nurses' perceptions of their work environment in a nursing development unit. *Journal of Advanced Nursing, 27(6),* 1193-2-1.

Baker, GA., Carlisle, C., Riley, M., Tapper, J., & Dewey, M. (1992). The Work Environment Scale: A comparison of British and North American nurses. *Journal of Advanced Nursing, 17(6),* 692-8.

Baum, C. M. (2004). Personal communication.

Baum, C. M., & Edwards, D. F. (1998). *Guide for the Home Occupational-Environmental Assessment.* St. Louis, MO: Washington University Program in Occupational Therapy.

Boschen, K., Noreau, L., & Fougeyrollas, P. (1998). A new instrument to measure the quality of the environment for persons with physical disabilities. *Archives of Physical Medicine and Rehabilitation, 79,* 1331.

Bradley, R. H., & Caldwell, B. M. (1988). Using the HOME inventory to assess family environment. *Pediatric Nursing, 14,* 97-102.

Table 17-10

MEASURE OF QUALITY OF THE ENVIRONMENT (MQE)

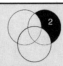

Source	Available via email from Kathy Boschen at boschen.kathy@torontorehab.on.ca or Luc Noreau at Luc.Noreau@rea.ulaval.ca
Important References	Fougeyrollas, P., Noreau, L., St Michel, G., & Boschen, K. (1999). *Measure of the Quality of the Environment, Version 2*. Author.
	Fougeyrollas, P., Noreau, L., & Boschen, K. (2002). Interaction of environment with individual characteristics and social participation: Theoretical perspectives and applications in persons with spinal cord injury. *Topics in SCI Rehabilitation, 7*, 1-16.
	Noreau, L., Fougeyrollas, P., & Boschen, K. (2002). Perceived influence of the environment on social participation among individuals with spinal cord injury. *Topics in SCI Rehabilitation, 7*, 56-72.
	Boschen, K., Noreau, L., & Fougeyrollas, P. (1998). A new instrument to measure the quality of the environment for persons with physical disabilities. *Archives of Physical Medicine and Rehabilitation, 79*, 1331.
Focus	• Modified ICF format.
Activity	• Evaluation of environmental influences on accomplishment of daily activities and social roles.
Participation	• Results of this evaluation expose obstacles contributing to participation restrictions.
Environmental Factors	• Defined broadly to include social, attitudinal, institutional, technical and physical factors in the environment.
Purpose	• To evaluate the environment's influence on the accomplishment of a person's daily activities and social roles in relation to his/her abilities and limitations.
Type of Client	• Developed for persons with physical disability, but has potential for broader applications.
Clinical Utility	
Format	• Interview with client within context of home, community, or workplace.
Procedures	• Client rates how much each environmental factor facilitates or is an obstacle to the accomplishment of daily activities and social roles. Major, moderate or minor facilitators and obstacles are identified.
Completion Time	• <30 minutes.
Standardization	• Manual includes basic scoring instructions; limited psychometric data provided.
Reliability	• Adequate.
Internal Consistency	• One study demonstrated moderate concordance scores across items.
Observer (Inter-Rater)	• N/A.
Observer (Intra-Rater)	• No evidence.
Test-Retest	• One study demonstrated moderate to good agreement.
Validity	Excellent.
Content	• Based conceptually on the Disability Creation Process model, followed by a thematic analysis by Whiteneck & Fougeyrollas and input from individuals with SCI and clinicians (Noreau, Fougeyrollas, & Boschen, 2002).
Convergent	• No evidence.
Construct	• Demonstrated ability to distinguish facilitators to social participation from environmental obstacles.

continued

Table 17-10 (continued)

MEASURE OF QUALITY OF THE ENVIRONMENT (MQE)

Strengths	• First tool to measure environmental facilitators and obstacles to social participation and accomplishment of daily activities. • Environment is defined broadly to include social, attitudinal, institutional, technical, and physical factors in the environment. • Tool is easy to administer. • Research evidence of validity and reliability. • Consistent with client-centered perspective.
Weaknesses	• Not published and only available from authors. • No method for summarizing scores. • No guidelines for interpreting scores. • Further examination of psychometric properties is recommended.
Final Word	• This is a promising new tool to assist therapists, together with their clients, to identify facilitators and obstacles to the client's participation in daily activities.

Bradley, R. H., Rock, S. L., Caldwell, B. M., & Brisby, J. A. (1989). Uses of the HOME inventory for families with handicapped children. *American Journal on Mental Retardation, 94(3),* 315-330.

Bradley, R. H., Corwyn, R. F., & Whiteside-Mansell, L. (1996). Life at home: same time, different places—An examination of the HOME Inventory in different cultures. *Early Development and Parenting, 6,* 1–19.

Bradley, R. H., Corwyn, R. F., Caldwell, B. M., Whiteside-Mansell, L., Wasserman, G. A., Walker, T. B., & Mink, I. T. (2000). Measuring the home environments of children in early adolescence. *Journal of Research on Adolescence, 10,* 247-289.

Brown, G. T., & Pranger, T. (1992). Predictors of burnout of psychiatric occupational therapy personnel. *Canadian Journal of Occupational Therapy, 59(5),* 258-67.

Bundy, A. C. (1999). *Test of environmental supportiveness.* Ft. Collins, CO: Colorado State University.

Bundy, A. C. (2002a). *Test of Environmental Performance.* Ft Collins, CO: Colorado State University.

Bundy, A. C. (2002b). *Test of Playfulness. Version 4.0.* Ft Collins, CO: Colorado State University.

Bundy, A. C. (1996). Play and playfulness. What to look for. In: L. D. Parnham & L. S. Fazio (Eds.), *Play in Occupational Therapy for Children.* St Louis: Mosby.

Byrne, M., Murphy, A. W., Plunkett, P. K., McGee, H. M., & Bury, G. (2003). Frequent attenders to an emergency department: a study of primary health care use, medical profile, and psychosocial characteristics. *Annals of Emergency Medicine, 41(3),* 309-18.

Caldwell, B. M., & Bradley, R. H. (1984). *Administration manual Home Observation for Measurement of the Environment* (Rev. ed.). Little Rock, AR: University of Arkansas.

Carlisle, C., Baker, G. A., Riley, M, & Dewey, M. (1994). Stress in midwifery: a comparison of midwives and nurses using the Work Environment Scale. *International Journal of Nursing Studies, 31(1),* 13-22.

Cecil, H., Stanley, M. A., Carrion, P. G., & Swan, A. (1995). Psychometric properties of the MSPSS and NOS in psychiatric outpatients. *Journal of Clinical Psychology, 51,* 593-602.

Chan, A. O., & Huak, C. Y. (2004). Influence of work environment on emotional health in a health care setting. *Occupational Medicine, 54(3),* 207-12.

Chandler, J. M., Duncan, P. W., Weiner, D. K., & Studenski, S. A. (2001). Special feature: The Home Assessment Profile—a reliable and valid assessment tool. *Topics in Geriatrics, 16,* 77-88.

Christenson, M. (2004). EASE3.2. Retrieved April 28, 2004 from http://www.lifease.com/lifease-home.html.

Chou, K. L. (2000) Assessing Chinese adolescents' social support: The Multidimensional Scale of Perceived Social Support. *Personality and Individual Differences, 28,* 299-307.

Chui, T., Oliver, R., Marshall, L., & Letts, L. (2001). *Safety assessment of function and the environment for rehabilitation tool manual.* Toronto, ON: COTA Comprehensive Rehabilitation and Mental Health Services.

Chui, T., & Oliver, R. (2004). *Factor Analysis and Construct Validity of the SAFER-HOME.* Manuscript submitted for publication.

Clara, I. P., Cox, B. J., Enns, M. W., Murray, L. T., & Torgrude, L. J. (2003). Confirmatory factor analysis of the multidimensional scale of perceived social support in clinically distressed and student samples. *Journal of Personality Assessment, 81(3),* 265-70.

Table 17-11

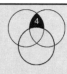

MULTIDIMENSIONAL SCALE OF PERCEIVED SOCIAL SUPPORT (MSPSS)

Source	Zimet, G. D., Dahlem, N.W., Zimet, S. G., & Farley, G. K. (1988). The Multidimensional Scale of Perceived Social Support. *Journal of Personality Assessment, 52(1)*, 30-41
Important References	Stanley, M. A., Beck, J. G., & Zebb, B. J. (1998). Psychometric properties of the MSPSS in older adults. *Aging & Mental Health, 2(3)*, 186-193.
	Zimet, G. D., Powell, S. S., Farley, G. K., Werkman, S., & Berkoff, K. A. (1990). Psychometric characteristics of the Multidimensional Scale of Perceived Social Support. *Journal of Personality Assessment, 55(3 & 4)*, 610-617.
Purpose	• Assess perceptions of social support adequacy from three sources: family, friends, significant other.
	• Developed after research indicated perceived social support has a stronger relationship to coping than objective ratings of contact.
	• Used in research to distinguish between groups, clinically to identify needs and recently as an outcome measure to evaluate treatment interventions.
Type of Client	• Adolescents, adults and older adults (55 to 82 years).
	• Individuals who have coping and life satisfaction issues (e.g., ABI caregivers, individuals with end stage renal disease).
	• Used with psychiatric conditions (generalized anxiety, depression, schizophrenia), post-surgical treatment (cardiac, cancer), marginalized groups (incarcerated women).
	• United States, Turkey, Italy, China, and Hong Kong.
Clinical Utility	
Format	• List/inventory of 12 statements of relationships with family, friends, significant other. Each item is rated on a 7-point Likert-type scale ranging from "very strongly disagree" (1) to "very strongly agree" (7).
	• MSPSS used in cultures other than Western have adjusted the instructions to contain culturally relevant meanings for "family" and "significant other" and translated item list into native language.
Procedures	• Responses are averaged to create total and subscale scores. Higher scores indicate higher perceived social support.
	• No training required.
Completion Time	• 2 to 5 minutes.
Standardization	• Self-explanatory, no published manual.
	• Published norms for the general adult Western population (Dahlem, Zimet, & Walker, 1991), general adult Italian (Prezza & Constantini, 1998; Prezza & Pacilli, 2002); Chinese students (Zhang & Norvilitis, 2002); psychiatry, surgical, and general population in Turkey (Eker, Arkar, & Yaldiz, 2000); adolescents in Hong Kong (Chou 2000) and Europe (Zimet et al., 1990); United States young and older adults with and without generalized anxiety (Stanley, Beck, & Zebb, 1998); young adults with and without significant psychopathology living in the community (Cecil, Stanley, Carrion, & Swan (1995); United States surgical patients with and without depression (Hann, Oxman, Ahles, Furstenberg, & Stukel, 1995; Oxman & Hull, 1997; Oxman, Freeman, Manheimer, & Stukel, 1994).
Reliability	
Internal Consistency	• Good; Cronbach's co-efficient alpha in above studies ranged consistently from 0.81 to 0.91.

continued

Table 17-11 (continued)

MULTIDIMENSIONAL SCALE OF PERCEIVED SOCIAL SUPPORT (MSPSS)

Inter-Rater	• Not reported.
Test-Retest	• Good; after 2 to 3months with 69 undergraduate psychology students: subscales (0.72, 0.85, 0.75), total score (0.85) (Zimet et al., 1988).
	• With 94 older adults with no diagnosable psychiatric disorder, subscales (friends 0.73, family 0.74) and total scale (0.70) were adequate, except significant other subscale was low (0.54) (Stanley, Beck, & Zebb, 1998).
Validity	
Content	• Principal component factor analysis confirmed subscale groupings with different groups and cultures (Zimet et al., 1988; Stanley, Beck, & Zebb, 1998; Zimet, et al., 1990; Cecil et al., 1995; Eker, Arkar, & Yaldiz, 2000; Zhang & Norvilitis, 2002; Clara, Cox, Enns, Murray, & Torgrude, 2003).
Convergent	• No evidence available.
Construct	• Negative relationships with Hopkins Symptom Checklist's levels of generalized anxiety (Zimet et al., 1988), poorer health amongst adolescent in-patients (Kazarian & McCabe, 1991), suicidal behavior (Soykan, Arapaslan, & Kumbaser, 2003) high use of emergency departments (Byrne, Murphy, Plunkett, McGee, & Bury, 2003) Positive relationships with health; compared to generalized anxiety in older adults (Stanley et al., 1998), or to significant psychopathology in young adults (Cecil et al., 1995), or to depression in surgical patients (Hann et al., 1995; Oxman & Hull, 1997; Oxman et al., 1994).
	• Positive relationships between marriage and significant other subscale with no differences on family or friend subscales for pediatric residents; positive relationships with family subscale and frequency among adolescents sharing concerns with mother (Zimet et al., 1990).
	• Marginalized groups have lower perceived social support (psychiatry: Eker, Arker,& Yaldiz, 2000; incarcerated women: Kane & DiBartolo, 2002).
	• Total scores correlate with self-esteem and life satisfaction (Prezza & Sgarro, 1992); spirituality and religiosity (Patel, Shah, Peterson, & Kimmel, 2002).
	• Related to age, marital status, sex, but not education amongst Italian general population (Prezza & Pacilli, 2002). Higher perceived social support in neighborhood population was significantly correlated with decreased incidence of childhood maltreatment (Coulton, Korbin, & Su, 1999) and Italians' sense of community (Prezza & Costantini, 1998). No correlation was found between size of Italian community (small town, small, large city) and perceived social support (Prezza & Costantini, 1998).
Strengths	• Simple to use and score in a short time.
	• Accumulating normative data and evidence for being transcultural.
	• Consistent with family-centered practice.
Weaknesses	• Need to be wary of socially desirable responses.
	• Requires evaluation of sensitivity to change.
Final Word	• Psychometrically sufficiently developed to begin to use clinically for needs assessment and outcome measurement in addition to research.
	• Dogan, Dogan, Tel, Coker, Polatoz and Dogan (2004) used the MSPSS in a battery of outcome measures to document changes in social interactions and family relationships after six home visits with individuals with schizophrenia living in Turkey.
	• Kane and DiBartolo (2002) used the MSPSS to accompany interviews of incarcerated women in the United States for a needs assessment and program planning.

Clemson, L. (1997). *Home fall hazards: A guide to identifying fall hazards in the homes of elderly people and an accompaniment to the assessment tool, the Westmead Home Safety Assessment.* West Brunswick, Victoria, Australia: Coordinates Publication.

Clemson, L., Fitzgerald, M. H., & Heard, R. (1999). Content validity of an assessment tool to identify home fall hazards: The Westmead home safety assessment. *British Journal of Occupational Therapy, 62,* 171-179.

Clemson, L., Fitzgerald, M. H., Heard, R., & Cumming, R. G. (1999). Inter-rater reliability of a home fall hazards assessment tool. *Occupational Therapy Journal of Research, 19,* 83-100.

Coulton, C., Korbin, J., & Su, M. (1999). Neighborhoods and child maltreatment: A multi-level study. *Child Abuse & Neglect, 23(11),* 1019-1040.

Cooper, B., Ahrentzen, S., & Hasselkus, B. (1991). Post-occupancy evaluation: An environment-behavior technique for assessing the built environment. *Canadian Journal of Occupational Therapy, 58(4),* 181-188.

Cooper, B., Cohen, U., & Hasselkus, B. (1991). Barrier-free design: A review and critique of the occupational therapy perspective. *American Journal of Occupational Therapy, 45,* 344-350.

Cooper, B. A., & Day, K. (2003). Therapeutic design of environments for people with dementia. In L. Letts, P. Rigby, & D. Stewart (Eds.), *Using environments to enable occupational performance* (pp. 253-268). Thorofare, NJ: SLACK Incorporated.

Corner, R., Kielhofner, G., & Lin, F. L. (1997). Construct validity of a work environment impact scale. *Work, 9,* 21-34.

Craig Hospital Research Department. (2001). *Craig Hospital Inventory of Environmental Factors (CHIEF) Manual Version 3.0.* Englewood, CO: Craig Hospital

Dahlem, N. W., Zimet, G. D., & Walker, R. R. (1991). The Mutlidimensional Scale of Perceived Social Support: A confirmatory study. *Journal of Clinical Psychology, 47,* 756-761.

Danford, G. S., & Steinfeld, E. (2001). *Environmental Utility Measure (EUMTM).* Buffalo, NY: Center for Inclusive Design and Environmental Access, SUNY.

Dijkers, M. P. J. M., Yavuzer, G., Ergin, S., Weitzenkamp, D., & Whiteneck, G. (2002). A tale of two countries: Environmental impact on social participation after spinal cord injury. *Spinal Cord, 40,* 351-362.

Dogan,, S., Dogan, O., Tel, H., Coker, F., Polatoz, O., & Dogan, F.B. (2004). Psychosocial approaches in outpatients with schizophrenia. *Psychiatric Rehabilitation Journal, 27(3),* 279-282.

Dunn, W., Brown, C., & McGuigan, A. (1994). The ecology of human performance: A framework for considering the effect of context. *American Journal of Occupational Therapy, 48,* 595-607.

Eker, D., Arkar, H., & Yaldiz, H. (2000), Generality of support sources and psychometric properties of a scale of perceived social support in Turkey. *Social Psychiatry & Psychiatric Epidemiology, 35,* 228-233.

Elardo, R., & Bradley, R. H. (1981). The Home Observation for Measurement of the Environment (HOME) Scale: A review of research. *Developmental Review, 1,* 113-145.

Faange, A., & Iwarsson, S. (1999). Physical housing environment—development of a self-assessment instrument. *Canadian Journal of Occupational Therapy, 66(5),* 250-260.

Ferland, F. (1997). *Play, children with disabilities and occupational therapy: The Ludic Model.* Ottawa, Ontario: University of Ottawa Press.

Fielding, J., & Weaver, S. M. (1994). A comparison of hospital- and community-based mental health nurses: Perceptions of their work environment and psychological health. *Journal of Advanced Nursing, 19(6),* 1196-204.

Fougeyrollas, P. (1995). Documenting environmental factors for preventing the handicap creation process: Quebec contributions relating to ICIDH and social participation of people with functional differences. *Disability and Rehabilitation, 17,* 145-153.

Fougeyrollas, P., Noreau, L., St Michel, G., & Boschen, K. (1999). *Measure of the Quality of the Environment, Version 2.* Author.

Fougeyrollas, P., Noreau, L & Boschen, K. (2002). Interaction of environment with individual characteristics and social participation: Theoretical perspectives and applications in persons with spinal cord injury. *Topics in SCI Rehabilitation, 7,* 1-16.

Hann, D. M., Oxman, T. E., Ahles, T. A., Furstenberg, C. T., & Stukel, T. A. (1995). Social support adequacy and depression in older patients with metastatic cancer. *Psycho-oncology, 4,* 213-221.

Harms, T., & Clifford, R. M. (1989). Family Day Care Rating Scale manual. Available from: www.fpg.unc.edu/~ecers.

Harms, T., Clifford, R. M., & Cryer, B. (1998). *Early Childhood Environment Rating Scale—Revised (ECERS—R) manual.* New York: Teachers College Press.

Harms, T., & Cryer, B. (2003). *Infant/Toddler Environment Rating Scale—Revised Edition (ITERS-R) manual.* New York: Teachers College Press.

Harms, T., Jacobs, E. V., & White, D. R. (1996). *School Age Care Environment Rating Scale manual.* New York: Teachers College Press.

Holahan, C. J., Moos, R. H., Holahan, C. K., & Brennan, P. L. (1997). Social context, coping strategies, and depressive symptoms: An expanded model with cardiac patients. *Journal of Personality and Social Psychology, 72,* 918-928.

Humphreys, K., Finney, J., & Moos, R. (1994). Applying a stress and coping framework to research on mutual help organizations. *Journal of Community Psychology, 22,* 312-327.

Iwarsson, S., & Isacson, A. (1995). *The enabler: Manual and assessment form.* The Swedish revised occupational therapy version. Available in English from Dr. S. Iwarsson, Lund University, Sweden, (Fax) 011-46 46 222 1959.

Iwarsson, S., & Isacson, A. (1996). Development of a novel instrument for occupational therapy assessment of the physical environment in the home methodologic study on The Enabler. *Occupational Therapy Journal of Research, 16(4),* 227-244.

Table 17-12

LIFE STRESSORS AND SOCIAL RESOURCES INVENTORY —ADULT FORM (LISRES-A)

Source	Psychological Assessment Resources, 16204 N. Florida Ave., Lutz, FL, 33549, (phone) 800-331-8378 or (813) 968-3003 (Web) www.parinc.com, .
Important References	Moos, R. H. (2000). *Life stressors and social resources inventory, and coping responses inventory: An annotated bibliography.* Retrieved April 13, 2005 at www.parinc.com.
	Holahan, C. J., Moos, R. H., Holahan, C. K. & Brennan, P. L. (1997). Social context, coping strategies and depressive symptoms: An expanded model with cardiac patients. *Journal of Personality & Social Psychology, 72,* 918-928.
	Humphreys, K., Finney, J & Moos, R. (1994). Applying a stress and coping framework to research on mutual help organizations. *Journal of Community Psychology, 22,* 312-327.
	Moos, R., Fenn, C., Billings, A., & Moos, B. (1989). Assessing life stressors and social resources: Applications to alcoholic patients. *Journal of Substance Abuse, 1,* 135-152.
Purpose	• To provide an inventory or profile of an individual's life context, specifically life stressors and social resources. Used to identify issues, and to monitor and evaluate social resource/stress reduction interventions.
Type of Client	• Adults 18 years and older.
	• Healthy adults; or psychiatric, substance abuse, or medical patients.
Clinical Utility	
Format	• Self-report of stable and new life stressors and social resources in nine domains: physical health, home/neighborhood, financial, work, spouse/partner, children, extended family, friends, and social activities.
	• 200 items in 8-page item booklet are responded to using dichotomous and likert-type scales, marked in 2-part answer/profile form.
	• Manual=$34 (USD); item booklets=$32/10 pkg; hand-scorable answer/profile Forms=$48/25 pkg + 7% sales tax and shipping.
Procedures	• Can be administered in groups or individually as a structured interview with individuals below sixth grade reading or comprehension.
	• No formal training in clinical or counseling psychology required.
	• There are 16 subscales: 9 life stressors (measure 8 domains and provides an index of negative life events) and 7 social resources (measures 6 of the 8 domains and provides an index of positive life events). Subscales can be used independently. No summary score or total score.
Completion Time	• 30 minutes to administer, 15 minutes to score.
Standardization	• Normed on 1884 adults (1181 men and 703 women).
	• Clear, comprehensive instructions with manual for administration, scoring, and interpretation.
Reliability	• Adequate.
Internal Consistency	• Stressor Scales: 0.77 to 0.93.
	• Social Resources Scales: 0.50 work item; 0.82 to 0.92 for the rest.
Inter-Rater	• N/A.
Intra-Rater	• N/A.
Test-Retest	• Stability at 4- and 7-year follow-ups: moderate to high for all scales except work, negative, and positive events.

continued

Table 17-12 (continued)

LIFE STRESSORS AND SOCIAL RESOURCES INVENTORY —ADULT FORM (LISRES-A)

Validity	• Excellent.
Content	• Original items from literature search and research with two pilot studies (18 months apart) involving depressed patients, alcoholic patients, arthritic patients, and healthy adults from which indices were developed.
Convergent	• No evidence available.
Construct	• Sociodemographic variables correlate with stressors and resources consistent with prior studies.
	• Discriminative between diagnosis, treatment outcomes and health seeking in adults with substance-abuse, depression, cardiac, and arthritic conditions.
	• Research using measure supports theoretical constructs concerning interrelationships amongst stress, resources and coping.
	• Evaluation of AA self-help groups confirmed friendly networks and coping style mediates effects of group (Humphreys et al., 1994); increased peer support associated with less distress and police involvement for alcoholics (Moos, Finney, & Moos, 2000)
Strengths	• Examines both stressors and social supports in one tool- Modified ICIDH format.
	• Well standardized.
	• Internally consistent, relatively stable tool.
Weaknesses	• Further research needed with broader populations.
	• No spirituality items.
Final Word	• Helpful to examine the process of stress and coping; has been used successfully to evaluate social support groups.

Iwarsson, S., & Isacsson, A. (1998). Housing standards, environmental barriers in the home, subjective general apprehension of housing situation among the rural elderly. *Scandinavian Journal of Occupational Therapy, 3*(2), 52-61.

Iwarsson, S., Isacsson, A., & Lanke, J. (1998). ADL dependence in the elderly: The influence of functional limitations and physical environmental demand. *Occupational Therapy International, 5(3),* 1173-193 .

Iwarsson S., Jensen A., & Stahl G. (2000). Travel Chain Enabler: Development of a pilot instrument for assessment of urban public bus transportation accessibility. *Technology and Disability, 12,* 3-12.

Kane, M., & DiBartolo, M. (2002). Complex physical and mental health needs of rural incarcerated women. *Issues in Mental Health Nursing, 23,* 209-229.

Kazarian, S. S., & McCabe, S. B. (1991). Dimensions of social support in the MSPSS: factor structure, reliability and theoretical implications. *Journal of Community Psychology, 19,* 150-160.

Kennon, P. A., Bauer, J., & Parshall, S. (1988). Evaluating health care facilities. *Journal of Health Administration Education, 6(4 Pt 1),* 819-831.

King, S., King. G., & Rosenbaum, P. (2004). Evaluating health service delivery to children with chronic conditions and their families: Development of a refined measure of processes of care (MPOC-20). *Children's Health Care, 33,* 35-57.

King, S., Rosenbaum, P., & King, G. (1995). Parents' perceptions of care giving: Development and validation of a measure of process. *Developmental Medicine & Child Neurology, 38,* 757-772.

King, S., Rosenbaum, P., & King, G. (1996). *The Measure of Process of Care (MPOC): A means to assess family-centered behaviors of health care providers.* Hamilton, Ontario, Canada: Neurodevelopmental Clinical Research Unit, McMaster University and Chedoke-McMaster Divisions of the Hamilton Health Sciences Corporation.

Koran, L. M., Moos, R. H., & Zasslow, M. (1983). Changing hospital work environments: an example of a burn unit. *General Hospital Psychiatry, 5(1),* 7-13.

Law, M., Cooper, B., Strong, S., Stewart, D., Rigby, P., & Letts, L. (1996). The Person-Environment-Occupation Model: A transactive approach to occupational performance. *Canadian Journal of Occupational Therapy, 63(1),* 9-23.

Table 17-13

WORKPLACE ENVIRONMENT: WORK ENVIRONMENT IMPACT SCALE

Source	Moore-Corner, R. A., Kielhofner, G., & Olsen, L. (1998). *Model of Human Occupation.* Clearinghouse: University of Illinois at Chicago.
Important References	Corner, R., Kielhofner, G., & Lin, F. L. (1997). Construct validity of a work environment impact scale. *Work, 9,* 21-34.
	Olsen, L. (1998). *The Work Environment Impact Scale: Construct validity with a psychiatric population.* Unpublished master's thesis. University of Illinois at Chicago.
Focus	• Modified ICIDH format.
Environmental Factors	• Physical: transportation, safety, lighting, time, equipment/technology/appliances/tools, sound, architecture /accessibility/design.
	• Social: attitudes, social climate, social support, communication, integration, expectations.
	• Economic: income security.
	• Institutional: institutional climate, program structure/policies.
Participation/Life Habits	• Work: paid occupation, search for employment.
Purpose	• To describe how individuals with disabilities experience and perceive their work environment. Measures multiple attributes.
Type of Client	• Adults over age 18 whose work has been interrupted by an injury or illness or who are experiencing difficulty on the job.
Context	• Workplace.
Clinical Utility	
Clarity of Instructions	• Excellent: clear, comprehensive, concise, and available.
Format	• Noninvasive, requires active participation of client but no equipment.
	• Semi-structured interview and standardized rating scale used.
Procedure	• Complex to administer, score, and interpret. Examiner qualifications not addressed but would require good interviewing skills and professional training for formulation needed for summary of results.
Completion Time	• Requires 30 minutes to conduct interview, and 10 to 15 minutes to complete summary.
Cost	• $30.00 (USD) + 5% sales tax and shipping.
Scale Construction	
Item Selection	• Adequate: the 17 items include most of the relevant characteristics of attributes.
Subscales	• Items are categorized as environmental qualities facilitating return to work, environmental qualities inhibiting return to work, recommended reasonable accommodations, worker's goals, and request for occupational therapy involvement.
Weighting	• No.
Level of Measurement	• Ordinal: 4-point Likert scales that are collapsed to produce a dichotomous summary.
Standardization	
Manual	• Excellent: published and outlines specific procedures for administration, scoring, interpretation; evidence of reliability and validity.
Norms	• N/A.

continued

Table 17-13 (continued)

WORKPLACE ENVIRONMENT: WORK ENVIRONMENT IMPACT SCALE

Reliability

Rigor	• Adequate: one published study on reliability.
Internal Consistency	• Adequate: 100% fit with expected response pattern of Rasch model.
Inter-Rater	• No evidence available.
Test-Retest	• No evidence available.

Validity

Rigor	• Adequate: One to two studies supporting validity.
Content	• Adequate: Has content validity, but no specific method was used.
Construct	• Adequate: One to two studies confirm theoretical formulations. Valid for workers with psychiatric disabilities: those with greater satisfaction, performance, and health had a higher degree of match with their occupational environment.
Criterion	• No evidence available.
Responsiveness	• No evidence available.
Overall Utility	• Adequate: anecdotal evidence only on clinical utility for planning work-related interviews.

Lawton, M. P. (1986). *Environment and aging.* Albany, NY: Centre for the Study of Aging.

Letts, L., & Marshall, L. (1995). Evaluating the validity and consistency of the SAFER tool. *Physical and Occupational Therapy in Geriatrics, 13,* 49-66.

Letts, L., Scott, S., Burtney, J., Marshall, L., & McKean, M. (1998). The reliability and validity of the Safety Assessment of Function and the Environment for Rehabilitation (SAFER) tool. *British Journal of Occupational Therapy, 61,* 127-132.

Mackenzie, L., Byles, J., & Higginbotham, N. (2000). Designing the Home Falls and Accidents Screening Tool (HOME FAST): Selecting the items. *British Journal of Occupational Therapy, 63,* 260-269.

Mackenzie, L., Byles, J., & Higginbotham, N. (2002a). Professional perceptions about home safety: Cross-national validation of the Home Falls and Accidents Screening Tool (HOME FAST). *Journal of Allied Health, 31(1),* 22-28.

Mackenzie, L., Byles, J., & Higginbotham, N. (2002b). Reliability of the Home Falls and Accidents Screening Tool (HOME FAST) for identifying older people at increased risk of falls. *Disability and Rehabilitation, 24,* 266-274.

Maloney, J. P., Anderson, F. D., Gladd, D. L., Brown, D. L., & Hardy, M. A. (1996). Evaluation and comparison of health care Work Environment Scale in military settings. *Military Medicine, 161(5),* 284-9.

Maloney, J. P., Anderson, F. D., Gladd, D. L., Brown, D. L., & Hardy, M. A. (1996). Evaluation and comparison of healthcare Work Environment Scale in military settings. *Military Medicine, 161(5),* 284-9.

Maloney, J. P., Bartz, C., & Allanach, B. C. (1991). Staff perceptions of their work environment before and six months after an organizational change. *Military Medicine, 156(2),* 86-92.

Moos, R. H. (2000). Life Stressors and Social Resources Inventory, and Coping Responses Inventory. Annotated Bibliography. Retrieved March 15, 2005 from www.par-inc.com

Moos, R. (1994a). *Work Environment Scale manual* (3rd ed.). Palo Alto, CA: Consulting Psychologists Press.

Moos, R. (1994b). *The Social Climate Scales. A user's guide* (2nd ed.). Palo Alto, CA: Consulting Psychologists Press.

Moos, R. (1986). Work as a human context. In M. S. Pallack & R. O. Perloff (Eds.), *Psychology and Work: Productivity, Change and Employment. Master lecture series.* (Vol. 5, pp. 9-52). Washington, DC: American Psychological Association

Moos, R., Fenn, C., Billings A., & Moos, B. (1989). Assessing life stressors and social resources: Applications to alcoholic patients. *Journal of Substance Abuse, 1,* 135-152

Moos, R., Finney, J., & Moos, B. (2000). Inpatient substance abuse care and the outcome of subsequent community residential and outpatient care. *Addiction, 95,* 833-846.

Moos, R. H., & Lemke, S. (1996). *Evaluating residential facilities: The Multiphasic Environmental Assessment Procedure.* Thousand Oaks, CA: Sage.

Noreau, L., Fougeyrollas, P., & Boschen, K. (2002). Perceived influence of the environment on social participation among individuals with spinal cord injury. *Topics in SCI Rehabilitation, 7,* 56-72.

Olsen, L. (1998). *The Work Environment Impact Scale: Construct validity with a psychiatric population.* Unpublished master's thesis. University of Illinois at Chicago.

Ontario Parks Association. (2001). *The playability tool kit.* Hamilton, ON: Ontario Parks Association.

Table 17-14

WORK ENVIRONMENT SCALE (WES)

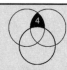

Source	Career/Lifeskills Resources Inc., 116 Viceroy Rd., Unit B1, Concord, ON, L4K 2M2, (Web) www.career-lifeskills.com/products_services/atpr/corpcultdev/cpp-59000. html, (phone) 905-760-0111 or 877-680-0200 (Toll-free in Canada).
Important References	Moos, R. (1986). Work as a human context. In M.S. Pallack & R.O. Perloff (Eds.), *Psychology and work: Productivity, change and employment. Master lecture series*. (Vol 5, pp. 9-52). Washington, DC: American Psychological Association.
	Moos, R. (1994a). *Work Environment Scale manual* (3rd ed.). Palo Alto, CA: Consulting Psychologists Press.
	Moos, R. (1994b). *The Social Climate Scales. A user's guide* (2nd ed.). Palo Alto, CA: Consulting Psychologists Press.
Purpose	• Measure workers' perceptions of a workplace's social environment.
Type of Client	• Adults, all diagnosis working in competitive employment or vocational rehabilitation settings. Employers and service providers can also complete scales.
	• Individuals, groups, or organizations with social-ecological interventions.

Clinical Utility

Format
- Self-report Format: Booklet of 90 statements about the work environment with items related to 10 subscales (9 items each): worker involvement, coworker cohesion, supervisor support, autonomy, task orientation, work pressure, clarity, managerial control, innovation, physical comfort.
- On an answer sheet, the items have a 2-point answer format—true-false. There are three versions or forms that can be used together or individually. Using the Real Form (Form R) people indicate how they view the current workplace environment.
- On the Ideal Form (Form I) people rate the ideal workplace and on the Expected Form (Form E) people endorse what they imagine a new, unfamiliar workplace to be.
- Manual, 3rd edition=$80.95 (Canadian); answer sheets=$31.75 pkg/25; reusable booklets=$56.90 pkg/25; Scoring Key=$28.70

Procedures
- Hand scored using a plastic overlay template/key, the same key for all versions; scores are summed within each subscale and often graphed by subscale.
- For interpretation, subscales are grouped by theoretical dimensions (Moos, 1986): Relationship dimension (involvement, coworker cohesion, supervisor support), personal growth dimension (autonomy, task orientation, work pressure), system maintenance and change dimension (clarity, managerial control, innovation, physical comfort). Interpretation by a professional with clinical training (e.g., OT) recommended.
- Patterns and trends are discussed with respondents, including perceptions and their stability over time, contrasts of worker and employer/service provider perceptions or between worker's real, ideal or expected scores, and comparisons of different work settings.

Completion Time
- 15 to 20 minutes to complete and 5 to 10 minutes to score; discussion unlimited.

Standardization
- Published manual (Moos, 1994a) and kits with directions for administration, scoring, interpretation.
- Norms available for comparison based on >8,300 employees in 116 work groups, including health care, general offices, light manufacturing services.

continued

Table 17-14 (continued)

WORK ENVIRONMENT SCALE (WES)

Reliability	• Excellent: More than two well-designed studies completed with adequate to excellent reliability values.
Internal Consistency	• Adequate: Pearson >0.60.
Inter-Rater	• Not applicable.
Intra-Rater	• Not applicable.
Test-Retest	• Adequate: Intra-class coefficient >0.70.
Validity	• Excellent.
Content	• Items were originally selected from a large group of Social Climate Scales (Moos, 1994b) and under went multiple revisions and factor analysis; face of items is recognizably meaningful to readers and relate to the tool's purpose.
Convergent	
Construct	• Able to measure changes in workplaces over time during organizational change in several independent studies (e.g., Tommasini, 1992; Maloney, Bartz, & Allanach, 1991; Koran, Moos, & Zasslow, 1983). Discriminates between workplace environments (nursing units: Avallone & Gibbon, 1998; military hospitals: Maloney, Anderson, Gladd, Brown, & Hardy, 1996; hospital & community environments: Fielding & Weaver, 1994) and work practice models (Thomas, 1992).
	• Identifies significant differences in views between worker groups (astronauts & ground crews: Salnitskiy et al., 2001; head, staff & agency nurses: Maloney et al., 1996; midwives & nurses: Carlisle, Baker, Riley, & Dewey, 1994) Subscales are predictive of work satisfaction, quality of life, staff burnout and emotional health in several independent studies (e.g., Trief, Aquilino, Paradies, & Weinstock, 1999; Brown & Pranger, 1992; Chan & Huak, 2004).
	• Confirms theoretical formulations of peer and supervisory support moderating anxiety about burnout (Turnipseed, 1998); of cultural differences in perceptions of rules and pressures (Staten, Mangalindan, Saylor, & Stuenkel, 2003).
Strengths	• Standardized with impressive psychometric properties and readily available, portable.
	• Promotes discussion and identifies clients' views.
	• Useful on an individual basis, groups or with organizations.
Weaknesses	• Intervention plans are not directly clear from scores alone, requiring discussion with respondents to relate trends/patterns to daily workplace events/issues requiring intervention.
	• Further research needed to identify interactional effects between demographic variables and subscales (Baker et al., 1992).
Final Word	• A well-standardized, reliable tool that can be useful for obtaining workers' perceptions of the social work environment for individual worker's rehabilitation, matching individuals and work environments; organizational development; and evaluating program change.

Oxman, T. E., Freeman, D. H., Manheimer, E. D., & Stukel, T. (1994). Social support and depression after cardiac surgery in elderly patients. *American Journal of Geriatric Psychiatry, 4,* 309-323.

Oxman, T. E., & Hull, J. G. (1997;). Social support, depression and activities of daily living in older heart surgery patients. *Journal of Gerontology, 52B,* 1-114.

Patel, S. S., Shah, V. S., Peterson, R. A., & Kimmel, P. L. (2002). Psychosocial variables, quality of life, and religious beliefs in ESRD patients treated with hemodialysis. *American Journal of Kidney Disease, 40(5),* 1013-22.

Preiser, W. F. E., Rabinowitz, H. Z., & White, E. T. (1988). *Post-occupancy evaluation.* New York: Van Nostrand Reinhold.

Prezza, M., & Costantini, S. (1998). Sense of community and life satisfaction: Investigation in three different territorial contexts. *Journal of Community and Applied Social Psychology, 8,* 181-194.

Prezza, M., & Pacilli, M. G. (2002). Perceived social support from significant others, family and friends and several socio-demographic characteristics. *Journal of Community & Applied Social Psychology, 12,* 422-429.

Rigby, P., & Gaik, S. (2004). *The stability of playfulness across environmental settings: A pilot study.* Manuscript submitted for publication.

Kanas, N., Salnitskiy, V., Weiss, D. S., et al. (2001). Crew member and ground personnel interactions over time during Shuttle/Mir space missions. *Aviation, Space and Environmental Medicine, 72:*453-461.

Sattin R. W., Rodriguez, J. G., deVito, C. A., Wingo, P. A. (1998). Home environmental hazards and the risk of fall injury events among community-dwelling older persons. *Journal of the American Geriatric Society, 46,* 669-676

Sloane, P. D., Mitchell, C. M., Weisman, G., et al. (2002). The Therapeutic Environment Screening Survey for Nursing Homes (TESS-NH): An observational instrument for assessing the physical environment of institutional settings for persons with dementia. *Journal of Gerontology, Social Sciences, 57B,* S69-S78.

Soykan, A., Arapaslan, B., & Kumbasar, H. (2003). Suicidal behavior, satisfaction with life, and perceived social support in end-stage renal disease. *Transplant Procedures, 35(4),* 1290-1291.

Stanley, M. A., Beck, J. G., & Zebb, B. J. (1998). Psychometric properties of the MSPSS in older adults. *Aging & Mental Health, 2(3),* 186-193.

Staten, D. R., Mangalindan, M. A., Saylor, C., & Stuenkel, D. L. (2003). Staff nurse perceptions of the work environment: a comparison among ethnic backgrounds. *Journal of Nursing Care Quality, 18(3),* 202-8.

Steinfeld, E., Shroeder, S., Duncan, J. et al. (1979). *Access to the built environment: A review of the literature.* Washington, DC: U.S. Government Printing Office.

Strong, S., Rigby, P., Law, M., Cooper, B., Letts, L., & Stewart, D. (1999) Clinical applications of the Person-Environment-Occupation Model. *Canadian Journal of Occupational Therapy, 66,* 122-130

Studenski, S., Duncan, P. W., Chandler, J, et al. (1994). Predicting falls: the role of mobility and nonphysical factors. *Journal of the American Geriatric Society, 42(3),* 297-302.

Sundstrom, E., Bell, P. A., Busby, P. L. & Asmus, C. (1996). Environmental Psychology 1989-1994. *Annual Review of Psychology, 47,* 485-512.

Teel, C. (1999). Challenges in the measurement of the rehabilitation environment. *Rehabilitation Outlook, 4(2),* 3, 5.

Teel, C., Dunn, W., Jackson, S., & Duncan, P. W. (1997). The role of the environment in fostering independence: Conceptual and methodological issues in developing an instrument. *Topics in Stroke Rehabilitation, 4(1),* 28-40.

Thomas, L. H. (1992). Qualified nurse and nursing auxiliary perceptions of their work environment in primary, team and functional nursing wards. *Journal of Advanced Nursing, 17(3),* 373-82.

Tommasini, N. R. (1992). The impact of a staff support group on the work environment of a specialty unit. *Archives of Psychiatric Nursing, 6(1),* 40-7.

Totsika, V., & Sylva, K. (2004). The Home Observation for Measurement of the Environment Revisited. *Child and Adolescent Mental Health, 9,* 25–40.

Trief, P. M., Aquilino, C., Paradies, K., & Weinstock, R. S. (1999). Impact of the work environment on glycemic control and adaptation to diabetes. *Diabetes Care, 22(4),* 569-74.

Turnipseed, D. L., (1998). Anxiety and burnout in the healthcare work environment. *Psychological Report, 82(2),* 627-42.

Whiteneck, G. G., Harrison-Felix, C. L., Mellick, D. S., Brooks, C. A., Charlifue, S. B., & Gerhart, K. A. (in press). Quantifying environmental factors: A measure of physical, attitudinal, service, productivity and policy barriers. *Archives of Physical Medicine and Rehabilitation.*

Whiteneck, G. G., Fougeyrolles, P., & Gerhart, K. A. (1997). Elaborating the Model of Disablement. In M. Fuhrer (Ed.) *Assessing medical rehabilitation practices: The promise of outcome research.* Baltimore, MD: Paul H. Brooks Publishing Co.

WHO. (2001). *International classification of functioning, disability and health.* Geneva: author. Retrieved April 20, 2004 from http://www.who.int/classification/icf

Zhang, J., & Norvilitis, J. M. (2002). Measuring Chinese psychological well-being with Western developed instruments. *Journal of Personality Assessment, 79(3),* 492-511.

Zimet, G. D., Dahlem, N. W., Zimet, S. G., & Farley, G. K. (1988). The Multidimensional Scale of Perceived Social Support. *Journal of Personality Assessment, 52(1),* 30-41

Zimet, G. D., Powell, S. S., Farley, G. K., Werkman, S., & Berkoff, K. A. (1990). Psychometric characteristics of the Multidimensional Scale of Perceived Social Support. *Journal of Personality Assessment, 55(3 & 4),* 610-617.

SECTION III

USING MEASUREMENT IN PRACTICE

Section II provided a comprehensive review of the many occupational performance and environmental assessments and measures available to occupational therapists. This section will discuss ways in which therapists might construct viable plans for measuring occupational performance of individuals within various service settings and structures. Examples of using measurement in different practice arenas will be described. As well, the importance of educating policy makers about occupational therapy and ways in which measurement can be used by occupational therapists to influence policy decisions are explored. Section III ends with a review of the importance of using measurement in occupational therapy practice and a discussion of some challenges in ensuring that measurement is integrated into practice.

Editors' Notes for Chapter 18

Mine the Gold

Occupational scientists have begun to conduct research that examines the practices of occupational therapists that consider themselves to practice from an occupation-based perspective within traditional service systems, as well as innovative community-based settings. Occupational therapists use this research to reflect on their own practices as they are influenced by socio-cultural practice contexts.

Become Systematic

Within systems, therapists practice from a client-centered, occupation-based perspective by consistently incorporating ethnographic interviewing, occupational history profiling and ecological assessment/observation of occupational performance in natural contexts.

Use Evidence in Practice

By consistently incorporating evidence that illustrates ethnographic interviewing, occupational history profiling, and ecological assessment/observation, therapists focus their interventions to increase engagement in occupation in context and social participation, outcomes that are increasingly valued in health and social policy-making.

Make Occupational Therapy Contribution Explicit

Within traditional and innovative communities of practice, occupational therapists frame assessment, treatment and outcomes to highlight occupational therapy's unique biopsychosocial training and perspective that bridges traditional institutional systems and individuals' social worlds.

Engage in Occupation-Based, Client-Centered Practice

Occupational therapists select ethnographic and ecological assessments that examine the individual's ability to perform occupations and participate in daily life and the social world, as well as barriers to desired performance and satisfaction.

18

MEASURING OCCUPATIONAL PERFORMANCE WITHIN A SOCIOCULTURAL CONTEXT

Pollie Price, PhD, OTR/L

SERVICE SYSTEMS INFLUENCE SOCIOCULTURAL CONTEXTS AND COMMUNITIES OF PRACTICE

Institutional service settings are socio-cultural contexts that are largely organized and driven by socio-cultural and historico-political factors. For example, perspectives about health and disability, the political nature of medical insurance and the definition of "education" in a particular national society are socio-cultural and historic-political factors that influence service systems. Occupational therapists contend with many parameters as they attempt to provide best practice occupational therapy services within particular socio-cultural contexts that are organized around these larger forces. Some of these parameters include the mission of the institution, payment systems' criteria for admission and outcomes, policies for providing services for under- and uninsured, and productivity standards. Institutions are also communities of practice in which practitioners from various disciplines, backgrounds and perspectives negotiate the "joint enterprise" (Wenger, 1998), including underlying assumptions, language, and routines of the social practice. Some of these parameters include the focus and standards of service, how services are scheduled and provided, and what counts as acceptable outcomes.

Each of these parameters influence practice uniquely in each service setting. For example, payment systems and service delivery models are quite different in school, acute rehabilitation, community mental health, and innovative community-based settings. In this chapter, we will discuss the influences of these service parameters on measurement approaches in early intervention/public education, rehabilitation settings, community-mental health and innovative community-based contexts, demonstrating how to address socio-cultural challenges in a way that takes the best advantage of occupational therapy expertise and equips therapists to take up and sustain client-centered, occupation-based practices.

INSTITUTIONAL PARAMETERS INFLUENCE MEASUREMENT OPTIONS WITHIN COMMUNITIES OF PRACTICE

Disciplines and systems function with theoretical and operational assumptions respectively. Within systems, there are two operational assumptions that affect the measurement process: 1) systems change regularly with socio-cultural and historico-political changes, and 2) professionals derive their own assumptions from actions emerging from their community of practice (Wenger, 1998).

The first operational assumption that affects measurement is that service settings change regularly. These changes are typically the result of internal (e.g., organizational) or external (e.g., legislation, billing/funding) forces that influence the particular service setting's operations. It is critical that professionals remain apprised of the setting's internal and external parameters so that decision-making and planning are consistent with the setting. For example, in 1997, Medicare funding in the United States changed for skilled nursing facilities (Boerkoel, 1998). Before the

Balanced Budget Act of 1997 was passed, occupational, physical, and speech therapy services were reimbursed on a fee-for-service basis after they were delivered (retrospective payment). Because of this reimbursement pattern, skilled nursing facilities encouraged all disciplines to provide skilled therapy for all residents in order to increase revenue. Under the new system of prospective payment, therapists are required to complete their assessments within the first 48 hours of admission, determine the intensity of care, and determine the rehabilitative needs of the resident. Under these circumstances, occupational therapists have had to adjust measurement strategies in order to determine the type, frequency, and duration of services and likely outcomes very quickly.

PROFESSIONAL ASSUMPTIONS INFLUENCE MEASUREMENT OPTIONS WITHIN COMMUNITIES OF PRACTICE

Most professionals, including occupational therapists, do not practice alone; professional practices are social and socially constructed. Recent studies of communities of practice (Lave & Wenger, 1999; Wenger, 1998) have focused in depth upon how ideologies, roles and routines of a community of practice are formed and maintained, and how newcomers are initiated and brought in to those communities. Social practices are created and sustained by individuals who share a vision of "what they are up to"—a joint enterprise (Wenger, 1998). The joint enterprise involves the enactment of a shared repertoire that supports the rules, standards and goals of the enterprise. New members are mentored into the repertoires, routines and discourses of the community; however, they also bring their own knowledge, experiences and personal agendas that, in turn, shape the enterprise. Wenger (1998) concluded that shared repertoires are always in flux and continuously negotiated by participants with different perspectives and personal agendas. Studies in occupational therapy have concluded that the socio-cultural context of a practice has a significant impact on the reasoning and actions of practitioners (Barris, 1984; Schell, 1998, 1999).

Occupational therapists have historically cared about the contexts in which their service recipients undergo intervention and recovery; however they have not been particularly reflective about how the practice context influences how they envision their roles and carry out their work. Practices both shape and are shaped by physical, temporal-historical, socio-cultural, and political conditions, and these conditions encourage some practices and constrain others. Some settings may be more conducive to and supportive of client-centered, occupation-based practices than others; professionals may have to be more reflexive, creative and socially savvy in some settings in order to effect client-centered, occupation-based practices.

Practitioners enter a community of practice, bringing their own theoretical perspectives, practical experiences, and personal agendas. After some time of negotiating possibilities in changing routines and discourses, there is a blending of perspectives that lead, to a greater or lesser degree, to changes in the routines and discourses of the community of practice. Practitioners settle into routines and patterns that become largely tacit and based on assumptions. If the negotiated joint enterprise does not honor a client-centered, occupation based perspective, occupational therapists may feel constrained in the types of measurements they might use to frame their intervention plans and outcomes; they may feel pressured to use assessments that focus more on circumscribed functional performances, and underlying body structures and functions. In medical setting, the push toward evidence-based practice tends to focus service toward more component-driven assessment and intervention. To date, little evidence has been produced in occupational therapy that would support outcomes concerned with quality of life, improved ability to engage in occupation or participate in social life (Pierce, 2003), although Goldstein-Lohman, Kratz, and Pierce (2003) provided a cogent example of integrating specific evidence-based intervention into an occupation-based program.

Professionals plan their measurement strategies based on their interpretations of the setting's beliefs, values, and policies. These interpretations, if not questioned, may be based on assumptions. For example, if a school district creates a complex process for submitting referrals for comprehensive assessment, professionals might interpret this action as an indication that the district wishes to restrict the identification of children who have special needs. Based on this interpretation, occupational therapists might stop participating in pre-assessment teams and using screening checklists with teachers.

The assumptions that professionals make within practice contexts can restrict or misguide them from providing best practice measurement of occupational performance. For example, if you believe that "they won't let you" conduct a home visit as part of discharge assessment, or "won't pay for" a community assessment, or "don't want you in the classroom" to conduct skilled observations of a student's participation in context, a therapist may not pursue best practice options for measurement.

INTERSECTION OF SOCIO-CULTURAL CONTEXT AND BEST PRACTICE ASSESSMENT

As previously stated, institutional settings are largely organized and driven by socio-cultural and historico-political systems, such as perspectives about health and disability, the political nature of medical insurance and the definition of "education" in a particular national society. Institutions are also communities of practice in which practitioners from various disciplines, backgrounds, and perspectives negotiate the "joint enterprise" (Wenger, 1998), including underlying assumptions, language and routines of the social practice. Each practice context has both kinds of influences that guide general parameters for practice in that setting. We have selected educational, medical/rehabilitative, and community contexts to illustrate the broad range of factors that affect measurement practices. We will describe some potential issues that might influence occupational performance measurement selection and implementation in these socio-cultural contexts and provide an illustration of occupational performance measurement in these settings that honors both the setting parameters and the implementation of best practice occupational therapy measurement.

Educational Systems: Early Intervention and Public Education Settings

In the United States, the purpose of the educational system is to provide a free, appropriate, public education (FAPE) for all children and youth in the least restrictive environment (LRE). This purpose emanates from federal laws that outline children's rights to services regardless of their disability; the laws extend services from birth to age 21 and include early intervention, preschool, grade school, high school, and vocational programs. States, community cooperatives, and local education agencies operate these programs with money from local, state and federal sources. The agencies receive apportionments based on total numbers of children in the school district (or other service, e.g., early intervention program), children with disabilities, specially trained personnel and aides/other support services. The local agency then has the responsibility to "purchase" the services needed for all the children for that year (Dunn, 2000).

The focus of educational systems is education. Although this seems obvious, the meaning of this statement is critical to the success of occupational therapy in this system. The occupational therapy profession grew out of medical model services, so it has been challenged to change the focus to be relevant to educational systems.

Educational systems call upon practitioners to be educationally relevant, that is, to apply expertise in service to the children's educational needs and goals. With this focus, there may be areas of occupational therapy expertise that are not appropriate for the educational environment; it is our responsibility to be vigilant in identifying relevant (and therefore irrelevant) service options.

The educational system requires its professionals to focus on the children's educational experiences, so occupational therapists have to come to understand the particular team's perspective on "relevant educational experiences and goals" for the child. This information provides a filter for selecting measurement strategies that are consistent with the team's perspective and the Occupational Therapy Practice Framework (American Occupational Therapy Association [AOTA], 2002). Therefore, best practice measurement in educational systems must include interviews with the child, teacher, and parent, and an ecological assessment (i.e., skilled observation in natural contexts for that performance) of the child's ability to participate in relevant learning contexts, including but not limited to classroom, playground, lunchroom, library, bathroom, music, art, and gym. Measurement would include observation of the activities a student might have to perform in order to participate successfully (use the restroom independently, carry a tray in the lunchroom, find and play with a friend on the playground, interact quietly in the library). One such measure that a therapist could use is the School Function Assessment, which was designed to "measure a student's performance of functional tasks that support his or her performance in the academic and social aspects of an elementary school program" (Edwards & Baum, 2001, p. 80). An ecological approach encourages the therapist to keenly observe "the child and the context and consider the impact of each part on the other" (Dunn, 2000, p. 2). Measurement also includes comparisons of behavioral and educational performance expectations to other children's performance, and the child's strengths and barriers for participation within relevant contexts. Therapists only measure performance skills and patterns (i.e., motor, process, communication/interaction, habits, routines, and roles) and underlying body functions and structures (AOTA, 2002) when they are suspected be barriers to participation in context and performances of interest.

In some cases, the occupational therapist would have participated on a pre-assessment team (i.e., a team that meets with the classroom teachers to solve problems in learning strategies and participation prior to comprehensive assessment for special education services) and may have a good understanding of the child's performance problems. Within these initial data gathering strategies, the therapist could determine possible adaptations to the tasks or environments that would support the child's

Table 18-1

SUMMARY OF CONTEXT DATA

	Code*
Cultural	
They come from African-American heritage.	?
They live in a middle-class neighborhood near urban core.	s
Physical	
Tanisha lives with her parents.	s
Aunt drives her to and from school.	s
Social	
Both parents work outside the home and express stress with managing home while caring for Tanisha and her younger brother.	b
Parents are very anxious about Tanisha's "learning disabilities" and are unsure about Tanisha's transition to a full day of school.	?
Parents have limited experience with the IEP process.	?
They have a child who is younger than Tanisha.	?
They have a lot of family in the area.	?
Aunt picks up both children daily, takes Tanisha to school.	s
Personal	
Tanisha is a 4-year old girl who lives with her middle class parents.	s
Tanisha has just entered preschool.	s
Spiritual	
Tanisha's parents are Jehovah's Witnesses and the family attends church regularly.	?
Temporal	
Tanisha is 4 years old.	?
Virtual	
Tanisha watches television but does not play on the computer.	?

*Code: s=supporting factor, b=barrier to performance, ?=requires further assessment.

engagement and participation in learning and social contexts and identify the performance skills and patterns that might be interfering with successful performance at school. Based on these hypotheses, the therapist might review other test data, observe the student in another setting, such as home (McDermott, 1996), conduct follow-up interviews, or test the child with a perceptual, memory, socialization, cognitive or motor test. The therapist would then interpret these data in light of the initial educational participation and performance concern so the team could make an appropriate overall educational plan.

Case Example

Tanisha is a child who seemed to be developing normally until she began talking. It became apparent that her language expression was limited, and by the time she entered preschool, she had not yet learned basic concepts, such as shapes and colors. The preschool team referred Tanisha for evaluation by the school district resource team due to concerns with her ability to interact with peers.

The occupational therapist on the team decided to assess Tanisha's occupational performance by observing her participate in a game of Barnyard Bingo with her teacher and a few of her classmates. Within this naturally occurring activity, the therapist was able to observe how Tanisha's skills supported or interfered with her ability to participate with her peers.

To summarize, the therapist observed that Tanisha did not initiate engagement, did not verbally or socially interact or participate in the game, and was largely ignored by her peers, with the exception of her friend Lisa. Based on these insights, the therapist generated a range of possible intervention strategies. Tables 18-1, 18-2, and 18-3 summarize measurement data on Tanisha to illustrate how to combine skilled observations, interview data, and history information within the educational setting.

Table 18-2

SUMMARY OF COMMENTS FROM INTERVIEWS, OBSERVATIONS, AND ASSESSMENT

Performance Skills/ Patterns	*Basic & Instrumental ADL*	*Education/Work/ Productive Activity*	*Play/Leisure/Social Participation*
Motor	Tanisha eats and drinks typically; she dresses when her mom picks out clothes; she needs help to bathe thoroughly; she helps to feed their dog and set the table.	Tanisha colors, cuts, uses glue typically; holds and scribbles with pencil and crayon; makes eye contact with teacher and/or therapists when her name is called.	Tanisha swings, climbs, and runs like a typical 4-year-old.
Process	According to mom, Tanisha needs a lot of help to start and finish her daily routine; Tanisha indicates to her teacher when she needs to use the restroom; eats snacks like a typical child.	Tanisha has difficulty following 3-step directions to complete an art project; requires step-by-step verbal cues and a visual model; functional communication is poor; does not interact with books.	Tanisha often requires repetition to learn the rules for structured games; knows and attempts to sing a few childhood songs; looks at picture books.
Communication/ Interaction	Tanisha accepts affection from her family and church members, makes eye contact when spoken to, follows her parents' directives, touches her brother and gives him toys, attempts to say words to express wants and needs.	Tanisha does not initiate interaction with teacher outside of restroom needs; shows withdrawing from from tasks.	Tanisha does not initiate interaction with peers; she will play a structured game with others but does not interact verbally or socially; she does not interact on the playground; she will play alongside her friend Lisa.
Habits/Routines/ Roles	Tanisha does not have established routines, but will participate in self-care and household routines with help. Tanisha participates in family and church activities.	Tanisha seems to like being in the classroom; does seem to be aware of and follow class rhythm and routine.	Tanisha routinely stands on the periphery of her peers can participate in structured games with support.

Best practice occupational therapy assessment in school settings must consider all factors that may interfere with a student's ability to participate in learning and social opportunities at school. As noted in Table 18-1, the therapist noted several aspects of Tanisha's profile that needed further assessment. First, because both parents worked full time outside the home, had a second child younger than Tanisha and had expressed stress in managing at home, the therapist felt it important to observe the family's routines and interactions to identify if there were any interventions or modifications that would reduce the parents' stress, improve their feeling of successfully managing the home, and increase opportunities for family "play" time. The ther-

apist observed that, with the exception of the time the family spent at church, the parents were consumed by other aspects of managing the home and seemed to have little time or energy to play with Tanisha and her younger brother. Tanisha spent time watching TV, and with the exception of handing toys to her brother, had little opportunity to explore or develop competence with toys, and almost no opportunity to play and socialize with other children her age.

Secondly, the therapist had observed that Tanisha was largely disinterested in the play and social environment at school, and did not initiate exploration of her environment. Based on these observations, the therapist decided

Table 18-3

SUMMARY OF OCCUPATIONAL PERFORMANCE ANALYSIS

Task Performance Being Measured: Red Rover Game During Outside Play

Individual's Performance	Typical Performance
Tanisha stands on the periphery, does not join in, does not show enthusiasm.	Teacher divides the children into two teams by having having them count off by twos. Children are showing varying levels of excitement for the game.
She cannot identify her number, relying on the teacher to assign her to a team.	Each child waits for his or her turn and calls out the number, sometimes the teacher has to remind someone to pay attention.
Tanisha joins her team reluctantly, standing by her friend Lisa.	The teacher instructs them to stand in two rows about 10 feet apart.
Tanisha is reluctant to hold hands, but when teacher encourages her, she does so. She does not chant the rhyme with the others and does not call out names. Her name is never called.	Children hold hands tightly, chant the rhyme, and call the name of a child on the other team to break through their line. If the child breaks through the line, then he or she picks someone to take back to his or her team.
No one tries to break through between her and her partners.	If the child fails to break through, he or she joins that team.

to "play" with Tanisha (observe Tanisha in her context) in her home to see what kinds of activities and interactions most engaged Tanisha. This approach is consistent with the participant observation approach Spitzer (2003) used to understand the occupations of young children with autism. By playing with Tanisha, following her lead, sometimes introducing her to new toys and props and watching her responses, the therapist found that Tanisha particularly enjoyed listening, dancing, and humming to childhood music tapes and playing with the hats, scarves, and gloves that the therapist had brought with her. These observations helped the therapist to make questions to the teacher and her parents about ways they might enrich Tanisha's experiences in order to increase her engagement and participation with her peers in the classroom and on the playground.

Medical/Rehabilitation Systems

Medical/rehabilitative systems is a broad term that encompasses many types of institutions, programs, and services, including in- and outpatient services provided in hospitals, skilled-nursing facilities, free-standing rehabilitation centers, other community locations, and consumer homes. A comprehensive team (e.g., psychiatrist, neuropsychologist, psychologist, medical social worker, nurse, occupational therapist, speech/language pathologist, physical therapist, and art/music/recreation/horticultural therapist) or a smaller team of professionals provides

services in these systems. Professional services are funded differently for different disciplines; some services are not funded by reimbursement systems, but when the services are valued and deemed necessary by the team and facility, they may provided as part of a per diem rate.

Programs are funded differently depending upon the setting and population, and as intimated earlier in this chapter, reimbursement patterns are continuously changing. For example, in the United States, medical services for persons over 65 and individuals with chronic disabilities are supported by Medicare funds at a fixed rate for diagnosis, acuity of problems and rehabilitation needs, or for individual services. If the individual is funded by private insurance, generally, services are reimbursed at a per diem rate, or contracted rate that has been negotiated between the facility and the insurance company. Although worker's compensation may still reimburse on a fee for service basis, after services have been delivered, the number of private insurance companies using fee for service reimbursement is dwindling.

Each of these reimbursement structures calls upon professionals to conduct their measurement strategies a little differently. For example, when a funding source is paying based on individual services rendered (i.e., fee for service), there is an incentive to conduct discipline- specific assessments because each one will be paid for. If there is a flat rate based either on diagnosis, as in the case of Medicare, or at a per diem rate, as is the case for most private insurance, the teams are more likely to construct an overall assessment strategy that yields the most information with the least amount of time spent.

When considering best practice measurement in medical/rehabilitative systems, occupational therapists have to understand the mission, service orientation and reimbursement structures for the particular setting. This information provides a filter for selecting measurement strategies that will determine the skilled contribution of occupational therapy for the individual in that setting. Best practice measurement must include an interview with the patient or family/significant others to gain a sense of the person's life, adaptive strategies, priorities for this stage of recovery and for moving to the next level of recovery and care, as well as outcome expectations. Best practice measurement must also include an ecological assessment of the individual's performance for negotiating the immediate environment. In each stage of recovery and transition, occupational therapists keep their focus on what the person wants or needs to do in order to determine the best intervention to increase satisfying performance. One factor that is paramount to consider in rehabilitation systems is the service recipient's diagnosis and stage of recovery. Medical status corresponds with level of care and type of facility. For example, a person who has just had a cerebrovascular accident, hip replacement, or psychotic episode will require intensive medical management of his or her illness or disability in an intensive care or medical/surgical unit of a hospital. Therefore, individuals in these settings are more limited due to instability of body regulation, medical precautions, lower tolerance for activities and reduced capacities in general. Measurement issues in acute care situations are related to maintaining the person's physiological stability and, therefore, must be brief. When persons are more stable and further along in their recovery, they can tolerate more intensive evaluation and intervention. It is important to emphasize that although therapists must address immediate, acute needs of individuals, the special and unique contribution that occupational therapists make is their consideration of long-range planning to reconnect individuals to their lives.

Best practice measurement would still include formal and informal interviews about the person's occupational history, preferences and priorities. Best practice contextualizes acute therapy procedures within a narrative understanding of who the person is and what they care about in their daily lives (Mattingly, 1991; 1992; 1993). Therapists using a client-centered, occupation-based perspective acknowledge the person as an occupational being and help the person understand the relationship of the therapy procedures to the person's life and priorities.

As a person stabilizes medically, he or she will move to a less restrictive environment, such as a rehabilitation unit or home. The occupational therapist would assess per-

formance of other activities that the client wants or needs to do within the typical temporal and physical contexts in which the person typically performs them. When measurement in the individual's natural context is not feasible, the therapist must try to approximate or simulate the natural conditions as much as possible (Pierce, 2003), including cultural, physical, social, personal, spiritual, temporal, and virtual aspects (AOTA, 2002). The assessment would include a sampling of meaningful activities that the person identifies as priorities and might include washing, dressing, clothing care, meal preparation, accessing a favorite chair to watch television, surfing the Internet, gardening, engaging in a hobby, or visiting with others. The occupational performance assessment at this point of the person's recovery focuses on identifying barriers to satisfying engagement in living. This is done through formal interviewing (Law, Baptiste, McColl, Polatjko, & Pollack, 1990; Spencer, Krefting, & Mattingly, 1993) and informal narrative interactions (Clark, 1993; Crepeau, 1991; Mattingly, 1991, 1994; Jackson, 1998) as well as observations of performance and participation. Ultimately, the occupational therapist would assess performances and identify interventions that would remove barriers and create adaptive strategies and systems (Frank, 1996; Spencer, Davidson, & White, 1996) for participation and performance of desired in all natural settings of home and community.

Influences that Affect Decision-Making in Rehabilitation Systems

There are many issues that affect professionals' decision making in rehabilitation systems. Because health care systems are changing rapidly, occupational therapy professionals serving in rehabilitation systems are often more vulnerable to inaccurate assumptions that influence decisions. The Functional Independence Measure (FIM), developed for inpatient acute rehabilitation service programs, was adopted by Medicare as tool that would guide assessment, goal setting, and measurement of outcome effectiveness in inpatient rehabilitation settings. Medicare reimbursement in acute rehabilitation programs is now based on diagnosis and general guidelines for likely course of outcome and length of stay. These changes in Medicare policy have been rapidly adopted by many medical insurance programs and substantially influenced reimbursement patterns, and therefore, service delivery in all inpatient rehabilitation settings. As service outcomes have been driven to be more measurable, service recipients began to be moved through levels of care at a faster pace and lengths of stay shortened. For example, when a person reaches a minimum level of assistance with activities of daily living (ADL) on the FIM scale, he or she is no longer eligible for inpatient rehabilitation, irrespective of social resources to provide that assistance (McKesson Health Solutions, 2003).

These changes in health care policy and practice are often incongruent with a client-centered, occupation-based occupational therapy practice. One of the theoretical assumptions in occupational therapy is that engagement in meaningful, relevant, and age-appropriate activity provides a therapeutic medium for adapting, learning or resuming occupations and life roles. The FIM scale does not provide much opportunity for individualizing goals or therapeutic activities based on the service recipient's preferences or priorities. Therapists may feel constrained and conflicted in measurement and intervention planning by a service setting's outcome measure that does not address or respect an individual's goals or priorities.

In many medical and rehabilitation systems, with the increasing emphasis on using evidence-based research, and because of the nature of much of evidence-based research, the overall emphasis of assessment and intervention is geared toward reducing pathology and impairments that result from pathology. Occupational therapists are concerned with helping persons successfully and adaptively resume life roles and occupations. Occupational therapists have a unique biopsychosocial perspective that bridges the medical and social arenas. Occupational therapists need to recognize this broader perspective in order to articulate the significant contribution they bring to the long-term outcomes and to negotiate more client-centered, occupation-based outcomes. This means that even during acute phases of recovery, occupational therapists will be discussing issues of living a satisfying life. Therapists must feel comfortable offering these types of data to the measurement processes throughout the phases of recovery and rehabilitation. Many other team members use highly technical, specialized equipment that measures changes in body functions, including computerized temperature, pulse, and blood pressure monitors, as well as computerized measures of balance and strength. In this biomedical world, occupational therapists face the seduction of taking up high-tech standardized measurement rather than assessing the individual's ability to perform occupations and participate in daily life. It is important to remember that no one else will be addressing daily life, an area that is important to the service recipient and family.

With the rapid adoption and wide use of the FIM scale as an outcomes measure, coupled with shorter lengths of stay, occupational therapists may be conflicted about what their intervention should focus on, the performance areas on the FIM scale or the occupations, priorities and preferences of the person. In this author's facility, assessment forms, conference notes, and progress notes have evolved such that they compel therapists to write goals and progress that address items on the FIM scale. This is a dilemma in many acute rehabilitation settings, as goals and outcomes provide a lens for interventions. Although it is likely that the FIM will continue to be the "gold standard"

for medical reimbursement, documentation forms and procedures must include the individual's goals and priorities, and must acknowledge the individual as a person with an occupational history. The occupational therapists in this author's setting have considered ways to modify existing forms and documentation systems in ways that would support t ethnographic interviewing. They document and report patient's social roles, occupational history, adaptive strategies, and goals, which helped the therapists to narratively link a person's therapy assessments and interventions to his or her life and priorities. These changes in documentation and reporting have helped to shape their perspectives to a more client-centered, occupation-based lens, and enabled them to more creatively use meaningful activities and occupations and natural contexts for intervention (Jackson, 1998; McLaughlin-Gray, 1998). With a client-centered, occupation-based perspective, occupational therapists will be able to make explicit the unique and complex perspective and contribution to service recipients, families, and team members.

Case Example

John recognized that he was having difficulty driving and walking during a typical day at work as a graphics consultant. Until this time, John enjoyed his life as a single, self-espoused student of the Buddhist religion and Asian languages. He was active in a local Buddhist temple, which he considered his community. John expected to quickly return to his previous lifestyle and level of independence. Occupational therapy evaluation and treatment was ordered as part of a comprehensive rehabilitation program. Best practice assessment included gathering information about the context, tasks, his strengths and barriers as they interacted to create performance. The following tables illustrate a way to summarize the data gleaned from John's assessment (Tables 18-4 through 18-6).

Occupational therapy assessment focused on identifying supports and barriers for relevant occupational performances, including his ability to safely perform his self-care, and remember safety information. As his ability to safely perform his bathing, dressing and toileting improved, simple instrumental activities of daily living (IADL) such as the ability get simple meals, perform laundry, access and sustain his attention in computer tasks and organize and follow through with a daily schedule were assessed.

Best practice occupational therapy assessment in rehabilitation settings should include, as much as is possible, assessment of occupational performance in the individual's natural contexts to identify potential barriers and possible adaptive strategies. In addition to assessing John's ability to negotiate his home environment (see Table 18-6), the therapist also took John to a local grocery store to assess his ability to negotiate the store in his wheelchair, secure

Table 18-4

SUMMARY OF CONTEXT DATA

	Code*
Cultural	
John is a Caucasian man who was born on the East coast and relocated to the West coast as an adult.	?
John has immersed himself in a Buddhist community temple and studies Asian languages.	s
Physical	
John lives in an efficiency apartment with a half flight of stairs.	b
The apartment is small and cluttered, with low light.	b
He sleeps on a mattress on the floor that he props up against the wall during the day.	b
His laundry facility is down the half flight of stairs, several steps down the walkway, through a locked door.	b
Garbage bin and carport are also down the stairs and 100 feet.	b
Social	
John is divorced, with no children, no local family.	?
He is interested in resuming dating.	s
He socializes with co-workers and friends he has made at the Temple.	s
He has a language tutor.	?
Personal	
John is 56, college graduate, and works as a computer consultant.	s
He is a lifelong learner.	s
Spiritual	
John considers himself a Buddhist; uses herbs and mediates daily.	?
Temporal	
John is late middle-aged, young at heart.	?
Virtual	
John is fluent on the internet for research, communication.	s
He is fluent on the computer for designing graphics.	s

*Code: s=supporting factor, b=barrier to performance, ?=requires further assessment.

and carry desired items and interact with store personnel and the public when making requests or purchase, and identify or create adaptive strategies. The therapist was able to see subtle lapses in problem solving, and therefore, assisted John in figuring out how he might secure groceries when he returned home. Through ethnographic interviewing (Jackson, 1998; Law, et al, 1990; Spencer et al., 1993) and ongoing narrative storytelling and storymaking (Clark, 1993; Mattingly, 1991, 1994), therapists will come to understand the individual's occupational history and their social roles and relationships that the individual wishes to resume. Through these kinds of narrative interactions, John's therapist came to understand that he was eager to return to driving, work and his Buddhist community. He spoke frequently about wishing to resume dating relations with women. Best practice occupational therapy assessment would also consider outpatient options or community resources that will enable the individual to continue to adapt and improve occupational performances toward their desired occupations, social roles, and relationships. In John's case, the therapist provided driving assessment information and alternative transportation resources, and referred John to the community re-entry program to continue to address his priorities to return to driving, work, and community life.

Table 18-5

SUMMARY OF COMMENTS FROM INTERVIEWS, OBSERVATIONS, AND ASSESSMENT

Performance Skills/ Patterns	Basic & Instrumental ADL	Education/Work/ Productive Activity	Play/Leisure/Social Participation
Motor	John is able to stand for short periods to complete bathing, dressing, toileting with contact guard for balance and safety; he needs reminders to plan his daily schedule, including recording his therapy schedule, getting his medications, and identifying time for computer work and studying language.	John is able to type words slowly with his non-dominant left hand. He is able to carry his flash card box, manipulate cards, and copy characters.	John got to groups and participated in them from his wheelchair.
Communication/ Interaction	John is able to ask for medications and interact with nurses, therapists, and doctors about his medical and therapy needs and goals.	John independently interacted with his employer and co-workers on the telephone.	John was quite outgoing and friendly. He enjoyed talking and sometimes dominated conversations.
Habits/Routines/ Role	After a couple of days of cuing, John managed his daily routine: showering, dressing and grooming, getting his therapy schedule, and and asking for his medications.	John scheduled in time to study his languages, keyboard on the computer, and do research.	John saw himself as a leader and encourager of others, taking a prominent role in support and activity groups.

Community Systems: Independent Living, Community Mental Health, Employment Settings

The purpose of community service agencies is to support individuals in their pursuit of productive and satisfying lives. Individual agencies might have a more focused perspective, but they share this overall enterprise. For example, employment settings emphasize work activities, but support might include finding ways to use transportation options to get to work, encouraging socialization as part of the workday, or development of specific work-related skills and patterns to enhance job performance. Community mental health and independent living programs focus on removing social barriers and enhancing skills and patterns so that individuals can achieve optimum participation in relevant and meaningful life activities, including managing homes, securing employment, negotiating communities, and finding a place in the social world (Rebiero, Day, Semeniuk, O'Brien & Wilson, 2001).

Community agencies are generally non-profit, generally have altruistic missions, and receive their financial support from public and private sources (e.g., through grants, service contracts and donations). They typically have professional and community members serving on either advisory or policy-making boards in support of their work. Occupational therapists working within such settings are paid a salary from the public and private sources just mentioned. Although there are a small amount of Medicaid funds (in the United States) available for medically relevant services, most occupational therapy services are provided as a part of the facility's services. In other countries such as Canada, funding for community agencies is often provided through a universal health and social service system. This is because of the community-based, client-centered focus as opposed to a biomedical focus, which predominates the health care systems in the United States.

Community settings (e.g., supervised or independent-living programs, transitional placement agencies, and employment settings) are well suited to the core values, philosophy, and expertise of the occupational therapist. When individuals wish to live or work within the community, they can profit from the functional and adaptive approach of the occupational therapist. Therapists de-emphasize remediation of body structures and functions while focusing on designing interventions that will help

---

Table 18-6

SUMMARY OF OCCUPATIONAL PERFORMANCE ANALYSIS

Task Performance Being Measured: Therapeutic Outing to Home

Individual's Performance	Typical Performance
John could walk with is walker from the carport to the stairs leading to his apartment.	Middle-aged adult would open the car door, get out of the car, walk to the stairs, climb the stairs with
With some difficulty, he was able to climb 6 steps, using the handrail. John was able to unlock his door, open the sliding door, and enter his apartment. Once in, John had some difficulty walking through the apartment with his walker due to clutter on the floor. He made comments about how he could rearrange things. Using his walker, with difficulty, John was able to carry trash down the stairs and 50 feet along the walkway, open the back gate, and open the lid to the dumpster. He was able to unlock and open the door to the laundry room. He identified that he would use detergent discs, and carry laundry in a bag that would hang from his walker.	or without the rail, unlock the sliding door, and enter He would be able to walk around or over the clutter. He would carry the trash down the stairs, along the walkway, open the gate, open the lid to the dumpster, and put the trash in. He would carry the laundry basket and soap down the stairs, put the basket on the on the ground to unlock and open the door, carry the basket into the laundry room, and put the laundry in the wash.
John had difficulty thinking about how he might manage his daily life once home, thinking he would be walking, driving, and working within 2 weeks. He would need to develop some new routines and relationships with his friends and co-workers. With encouragement, he identified and contacted friends who could help him secure groceries and other needed items once home. John secured hospital transportation in order to attend the outpatient community re-entry program upon discharge.	He would manage his life in his usual and customary manner, driving or getting a ride into the community to secure needed items, and to interact with friends and co-workers.

---

individuals develop competent occupational performances and effective adaptive strategies in order to manage their own resources and daily lives and improve social participation. As with other systems, this emphasis guides the measurement process toward a more contextual and directed problem-solving approach to address specific life challenges.

When providing best practice measurement, occupational therapists must investigate barriers to independent occupational performance (e.g., inability to carry out meal planning) and, considering alternatives that tap individual adaptive strengths, provide adequate environmental cues or modify the task for easier performance. Occupational therapists must conduct assessments in a way that enables them to make recommendations that support engagement in occupation to support participation in the person's social context.

For example, in a mental health community re-entry program, occupational therapists are likely to begin the

assessment process by interviewing the case manager and consumer about the life situation of concern. It would be very important for the occupational therapy assessment to include skilled observation of the life activity in the individual's natural context (e.g., home, work, grocery store). In some cases, the therapist would also include measures such as those discussed in other sections of this text (e.g., ecological assessment, criterion-referenced occupational performance measures). Based on assessment information, occupational therapy outcome goals and intervention plans must focus on reducing contextual and social barriers and enhancing individuals' abilities to participate in, perform and manage relevant daily life activities and roles, and access future occupational opportunities.

Case Example

Maggie wanted to live on her own and work in her community. Occupational therapy was requested to assist with this transition. Occupational therapy assessment

Table 18-7

SUMMARY OF CONTEXT DATA

*Code**

Cultural

Maggie lives in the middle-class, Irish-American neighborhood in which she grew up.   s

She knows many people in her apartment and in her community (e.g., grocery, bank, craft shop).   s

Physical

Maggie lives in a community apartment with a roommate.   s

Apartment is ground level with level entrance.   s

Laundry facility 100 feet from front door.   s

Bus stop is at the corner in front of the apartment building.   ?

Library is two buildings down on the same side of the street.   s

Social

Maggie's roommate does shopping with Maggie.   ?

They share cooking, cleaning, and laundry.   s

Maggie works at the local library in circulation.   ?

She wants to attend a singles' group at church and a pottery group at a local craft shop.   ?

She and her mother attend church mass and then dine out each Saturday evening.   b

Mother comes by the apartment daily.   b

Personal

Maggie is a 24-year-old library circulation clerk who graduated from high school at 19.   ?

Spiritual

Although Maggie attends mass weekly, her spiritual beliefs are not clear.   ?

Temporal

As a young adult, Maggie wants to live on her own.   ?

She wants to date and expand her involvement in leisure activities.   s

She wants to get an associate's degree as a library technician.   ?

Virtual

Maggie engages in Internet dating chat rooms a couple of times per week.   ?

*Code: s=supporting factor, b=barrier to performance, ?=requires further assessment.

focused on identifying supports and barriers for participation in relevant occupational performances (e.g., grocery shopping, money management, accessing transportation, work, and social relationships). Best practice assessment included gathering information about the context, activities and occupations, and Maggie's strengths and limitations as they interacted to create performance. The following tables illustrate a way to summarize the data gleaned from Maggie's assessment (Tables 18-7, 18-8, 18-9).

Best practice occupational therapy assessment in community systems often involves numerous visits in order to uncover the primary barriers and possible intervention options. As noted in Table 18-8, the occupational thera-

pist identified tasks that require further assessment. Based on the information Maggie gave the therapist in the initial interview, the therapist had some hunches about possible barriers to Maggie living, working and socializing independently in her community. First, the therapist felt that Maggie's life opportunities would be enhanced if she had increased access to places in her community, including church and the grocery store. Maggie revealed in the initial interview that she often felt awkward when communicating with people that she did not know, but emphasized wanting to begin dating again and attend pottery classes at a local pottery shop. Finally, the therapist was unsure about the nature of the relationships between Maggie and

Table 18-8

Summary of Comments From Interviews, Observations, and Assessment

Performance Skills/ Patterns	Basic & Instrumental ADL Grocery shopping.	Education/Work/ Productive Activity Job at library, wants to attend school.	Play/Leisure/Social Participation Attending church, wants to take up pottery.
Motor	Roommate drives. Looks for oncoming traffic. Moves cart effectively, but slowly, in store; roommate loads groceries into and out of car, and carries them to the apartment.	Walks to library. Moves through library effectively, but slowly, to put books on shelves. Can lift up to three books at a time.	Mother drives. Moves effectively, but slowly, out of church with mother. Holds hymnal, prayer book, and program.
Process	Tries many strategies for communication. Recognizes safety issues.	Once supervisor sorts books to be restacked by section, she is able to find the correct section and place the book correctly.	Sings hymns, reads, and recites prayers.
Communication/ Interaction	Uncomfortable/awkward when talking with new people.	Communication is awkward when people ask for help.	Interacts easily with friends and acquaintances; this is the church in which she grew up.
Habits/Roles/ Routines	Maggie and her roommate develop a weekly menu and grocery list each Sunday evening and shop Monday evenings.	Maggie showers each morning, dresses neatly for work, and arrives for work on time. Although she performs, she follows the library's routines, takes breaks and lunch with another coworker.	Maggie and her mother have attended church most every Sunday since Maggie was a young girl. She knows and follows the sequence of the mass.

her mother, and Maggie and her roommate. Although Maggie mentioned wanting to learn to become a library assistant, the therapist decided to wait on further assessment in that area since Maggie is satisfied with her current position at the library. In addition, because Maggie and her roommate both stated their satisfaction with their apartment management, the therapist deferred further assessment on laundry, cooking, and cleaning.

The therapist subsequently contacted the case manager and social worker to ask them to explore financial and community resources (e.g., Medicaid funding for special transportation services, securing funding, and setting up a referral for a driving assessment with a certified driving instructor). The therapist then asked Maggie if she might consider the city bus system as one option for getting places in the community. When Maggie indicated that she might consider that option, the therapist suggested that they take a bus trip to the grocery store where Maggie could purchase food to make dinner for a couple of friends

she knew from church. Maggie became excited about this idea, called her friends to set a date, and then called the therapist to arrange the trip to the grocery store. The therapist understood that by assessing Maggie's performance within the natural context, she would be able to test out her hunches about Maggie's occupational performance barriers, discover Maggie's adaptive strategies, and begin to identify intervention options.

Innovative Community-Based Practice

Several scholars (Hocking, 2001; Pierce, 2001, 2003; Toth-Fejel, Toth-Fejel, & Hedricks, 1998) have argued that occupational therapy assessment and intervention is most powerful when implemented in an individual's natural context and when engaged in the individual's occupations. Fidler (2000) suggested that therapists should remove their practices altogether from hospitals and prac-

Table 18-9

SUMMARY OF OCCUPATIONAL PERFORMANCE ANALYSIS

Task Performance Being Measured: Therapeutic Outing to Home

Individual's Performance	Typical Performance
Maggie depends on roommate for transportation to the grocery store.	Caucasian young adult would drive self, ride with another, or walk.
Roommate verbally cues Maggie to look at the item on the list and compare to the category on the aisle marker.	Task requires selected attention, ability to walk through the store with cart, topographical memory, categorization.
Maggie finds and selects the most cost-effective item.	Task requires the ability to find and select the needed item; some might select the most cost-effective item.
Maggie depends on roommate to ask for items they can't find.	Task requires problem-solving, generalization, and self-expression.
Maggie pushes cart slowly but effectively through the store, retrieves items from shelf, roommate moves grocery sacks from cart to car and into apartment.	Person would have the motor skills to retrieve items off the shelves, place items on the grocery belt, and move sacks from cart into car and into apartment.

tice in environments in which they can engage in more potent therapy. Pierce (2003) asserted that "the most effective occupational therapy is provided in settings on which occupational therapists can operate from their true culture that values the subjective experience and perspective of the client over their own as experts" (p. 207). Clark (1993) provided a powerful example of an innovative course of intervention with Penny Richardson that was unfettered by the constraints, requirements and service guidelines of the medical reimbursement system.

A word of caution is required here, lest we oversimplify our emerging understanding of "occupation" and its use in practice. Therapists choose therapeutic activities and contexts based on complex tacit reasoning (Fleming, 1994a). Researchers (Jackson, 1998; Jackson, Carlson, Mandel, Zemke, & Clark, 1998; McLaughlin-Gray, 1996; Rebiero et al., 2001) have shown that the use of a variety of activities, occupations and contexts lead to successful occupational outcomes. To say that assessment and intervention is most powerful when done in the individual's natural context as the individual engages in his or her occupations does not reflect the complexity of the therapeutic process, oversimplifies therapists' reasoning and simply does not hold up in all cases.

The following case example comes from the author's own dissertation research (Price, 2003) in which I examined the occupation-centered practice of Nancy, an experienced occupational therapist who fashioned her own pri-

vate practice as an "after school club". While she accepted many forms of traditional reimbursement, she also accepted private pay, often on a flexible schedule, as with the following child, Hannah and her mother, Susan.

Case Example

One day as Hannah and her mother Susan drove by an elementary school playground, Hannah told her mother she wanted to go to school. This would be any mother's dream and expectation, except that since the time Hannah was a tiny baby, she was terrified of and would scream, cry and hide her face around anyone but her mother. When Hannah was around two and a half years old, Susan took her to a psychologist who referred her to Nancy for assessment. Occupational therapy assessment included an interview with Susan, Hannah's mother, and observation of Hannah in a small group of peers her age to identify strengths and barriers for participation in childhood activities with others. Tables 18-10 to 18-12 illustrate a way to summarize the data gleaned from Hannah's assessment.

As is true with all of occupational therapy practice, assessment and intervention is iterative, that is to say, it is not linear. Even when therapists can obtain a good occupational history from which to launch intervention, therapists' first attempts at creating meaningful therapeutic interventions are often trail and error and require multiple revision and adjustments. Such was the situation with Hannah and Nancy. Nancy started by having Hannah participate in a small group with a very few children her age.

Table 18-10

SUMMARY OF CONTEXT DATA

	Code*
Cultural	
Hannah's parents were both educated, middle and upper-middle class professionals.	?
Physical	
Her family lived in a second-story apartment in an affluent suburb of Los Angeles.	?
The apartment was cluttered with art and percussion instruments.	s
Hannah's room was Victorian, with lace curtains and bed spread, a small white wooden table and chairs, and wall art that she had made with her father.	s
Social	
Hannah had a close relationship with her mother, and with her Nanny.	s
At the time of the study, Hannah and Nancy had a trusting, reciprocal relationship.	s
Hannah did not initiate interactions with other children, but was beginning to tolerate their presence and mutually engage in parallel play with support.	b
Personal	
Hannah was 4 years old, attending a small group with one other boy, waiting to start preschool.	s
Spiritual	
Unknown whether Hannah's family had a spiritual practice.	?
Temporal	
Hannah was 4 years old, developing normally with exception of socially.	b
Virtual	
Hannah watched Disney and other childhood videos on a small TV in her room.	?

*Code: s=supporting factor, b=barrier to performance, ?=requires further assessment.

Hannah screamed. Nancy changed the therapeutic conditions, seeing Hannah individually with Susan present. Hannah screamed. With Hannah on her lap, Nancy helped her turn the pages of a book, and when Hannah became distraught, they would retreat to the safe room next door, away from the demands of the intervention, and there Nancy taught Hannah to breathe. Little by little, Hannah developed trust in Nancy and began to play more spontaneously and joyously with her. At this point, Nancy again changed the therapeutic conditions, moving their therapy sessions to Hannah's park, where she could learn to be around other children. At first, Hannah would stay on the baby swings, where she knew no one her age would approach her, then gradually moved to the slide and the big girl swings. By the end of the summer, she was tolerating other children playing next to her, although, according to Nancy, she still did not initiate interaction.

At this point, Nancy again changed the therapeutic conditions, having Hannah participate in a small group with one other child, Evan, who did not have much language, and who Hannah could sort of take care of. With

Nancy's support, Hannah was able to engage in and sustain short periods of reciprocal play with Evan. When Hannah started school, Nancy again changed the therapeutic conditions and had her start participating in a larger group with a "mix of real calm kids, and there's the kids with more jazzy behaviors, ...a little cross section of what you'd probably find in a school, out on the playground..." I observed as Nancy and Hannah engaged in a therapeutic process in which Hannah would retreat, get stuck, get engaged, sustain engagement, while Nancy used several narrative micro-processes to keep Hannah moving forward (see Table 18-11 for an example of one session). Ultimately, Hannah told Nancy she did not want to go to the group, which might have been seen as a clinical failure. Simultaneously, Nancy observed Hannah participating in her preschool classroom (Table 18-12). Hannah's mother, Susan, talked about many areas of progress that she had seen in Hannah that she attributed to Nancy's intervention, such as feeling safe, having the tools to break into social groups, talking to neighbors, hugging friends, making two new friends in the summer school program, and

Table 18-11

Summary of Comments From Interviews, Observations, and Assessment

Performance Skills/ Patterns	Basic & Instrumental ADL	Education/Work/ Productive Activity	Play/Leisure/Social Participation
Motor	Hannah asked when she needed to use the restroom. She needed some help with hygiene. Hannah had a good appetite and could eat and drink on her own.	Hannah moved stiffly through the little kid's group room. At times, she needed Nancy's help with hand-over-hand support or motoring to start engaging.	Hannah's play repertoire was limited; she did not like to pretend that Play-Doh could be food; she usually completed activities without physical help.
Process		Hannah could often complete painting activities once she had started them.	Although Hannah usually knew what to do, she often needed Nancy's support to initiate and sustain engagement with the others.
Communication		Hannah would accept and pass glitter paint.	Hannah would accept and pass Mr. Potato Head; she occasionally made eye contact with others as they initiated interaction with her, and would verbally respond with modeling, but would not initiate verbal interaction or eye contact on her own, except with Nancy.
Habits/Routines/ Roles		Hannah trusted and respected Nancy and wanted to show Nancy what she had worked on in between sessions.	Hannah had a compulsive need for order, which, according to Nancy, might make her a little rigid and bossy. When Hannah became overwhelmed with social situations, she would pull at her fingers and bury her head in her mother's lap.
			Hannah wanted to participate with the others and became sad when she couldn't.

running off to play on the swings with her best buddy, Franco.

In summary, a more complex understanding of best practice occupational therapy assessment is that assessment is iterative with interventions. In Nancy and Hannah's case, although careful with Susan's private pay arrangement, Nancy had no constraint of medical or educational reimbursement or service parameters. Nancy had

the freedom to see Hannah and create therapeutic conditions that she hoped would keep Hannah moving toward her goal of going to preschool. Nancy tried one context, graded expectations and did with Hannah, building a rapport and relationship with her. When Hannah became comfortable with one situation, Nancy changed the context, activity and social demands to expand her play repertoire and social participation with peers. Although

Table 18-12

SUMMARY OF OCCUPATIONAL PERFORMANCE ANALYSIS

Task Performance Being Measured: Participating in the Classroom: Snack, Free Play, and Circle Time

Individual's Performance	**Typical Performance**
"She's having a snack and giggling with another girl."	Preschooler would either sit with a friend or be directed to a seat; she would spontaneously show her snack and silliness would likely ensue.
"It looks to me like she's basically going up, making the initial contact, the kids seem to like her, they approach her a lot of the time, but it looks like she's having some difficulty carrying through."	Preschoolers "explore a lot, they want to do everything and then they'll settle down on a favorite thing... kids... scope out other kids... they'll go play with some."
Hannah approached girls building with large cardboard bricks, joined in, but never said anything.	Preschoolers sometimes talk about what they are up to or creating.
"When she went to circle time, the girls were inviting her to sit with them, and they were joking saying, "Don't sit here, sit here"..., she was confusesd and she sat down next to the quiet little boy, and she looked kind of frozen. The boys were kind of jabbing each other, and the girls were looking around making side comments. She looked a little stressed and her eyes got big, and she opened her mouth like to take in some air... then after the activity started... she participated fully, and laughed and had a good time... Hannah only looked at the teacher."	Preschooler often spontaneously sits in the circle, sometimes next to a friend, sometimes directed to a spot. Preschooler may need redirection to pay attention and participate.

Hannah removed herself from participating in the group with the boys, she could experience the progress she had made with Nancy:

Hannah: After my birthday I get, I'll be four and a half, 'cause Christmas comes at my birthday, huh momma? Four and a half.

Susan: You'll be 4 at Christmas (gestured 4).

Hannah: I'm gonna have a blankie party. And everyone's gonna bring their girl blankies.

Pollie: That sounds like fun. Like a slumber party?

Hannah: Yes.

Pollie: With girlfriends?

Hannah: And then uh, everyone's gonna bring their purses and blankies.

Susan: Oh, yeah!

Pollie: That sounds like a fun party. The best kind.

Hannah's plans for her birthday party revealed that Hannah herself knew how far she had come. Even she thought of herself as the kind of friend that would have blankie parties with girlfriends.

SUMMARY

This chapter has highlighted some of the parameters that influence best practice in education, medical/rehabilitation, community-based service systems, and innovative community practices. The missions, scope of services and outcomes, billing and reimbursement, and operational structures and functions that support or constrain best practice measurement were described, as they are configured differently in different settings.

Occupational therapists operate out of a theoretical assumption that when individuals engage in meaningful and goal-directed activity, they learn or resume relevant occupations and life roles. This perspective is either supported or constrained by the operational assumptions and processes of socio-cultural systems or communities of practice. Many service systems, especially those funded by federal and state governments, HMOs, or private insurance companies, change regularly, thus influencing the role and scope of occupational therapy services. Many times, interpretations of policies or procedures are outdated, inaccurate or are transmitted though informal channels, many times as assumptions, influencing best practice decisions.

Some potential issues that might arise within particular socio-cultural settings have been described. The author has attempted to provide a template to guide occupational performance measurement in these particular settings in ways that honor both the setting parameters and the implementation of best practice occupational therapy.

The author has emphasized that occupational therapists must take several actions in order to provide relevant, valuable and expert occupational therapy measurement. First, therapists must have an understanding of the mission, service orientation and reimbursement structures for the setting. Second, therapists must frame their assessment services in a way that meets the facility's needs, making sure to addresses the occupational performance and life roles, needs and desires of individuals. Therapists must resist the urge to reduce their perspectives to biomedical restoration of underlying body structures and functions and learn to articulate and set outcomes, goals, and interventions at the level of skills and patterns that will support occupational and life role performance to support social participation. Third, therapists must keep abreast of changes in order to accurately interpret them and reconfigure occupational therapy assessment to meet the needs of the facility while maintaining their commitments to service recipients and best practice. Occupational therapists may draw supports from the *Occupational Therapy Practice Framework* (AOTA, 2002), World Health Organization, (2001); *AOTA Code of Ethics, Standards of Practice,* (1998) and the numerous official documents that are intended to shape best occupational therapy practice (AJOT, November/ December 2003).

This information provides a filter for selecting measurement strategies that will determine the skilled contribution of occupational therapy for the individual in a particular socio-cultural service context. Best practice measurement across all settings must include an interview with the service recipient, family, and other service providers in order to gain a sense of the person's life, adaptive strategies, priorities and outcome expectations. Best practice measurement must also include an ecological assessment of the individual's performance within the natural contexts in which they normally occur whenever possible, or make their best effort to creatively simulate the natural social conditions and activity demands (Pierce, 2003). Therapists measure performance skills and patterns (i.e., motor, process, communication/interaction, habits, roles, and routines) (AOTA, 2002) when therapists suspect that they are possible barriers to occupational performance and social participation. Ultimately, it is the unique and skilled ability of the occupational therapist to select measurement strategies that will enable him or her to identify any barriers and possible interventions to enhance individuals' satisfaction and participation in relevant occupations and life roles. It is imperative for occupational therapists to strengthen client-centered, occupation-based approaches and make explicit the unique and important contribution that occupational therapists make to help individuals bridge institutional settings and their own social worlds.

This author's own research (Price, 2003) concluded that occupational therapists, because of their education that combines biopsychosocial theories, activity analysis and a focus on enabling participation in occupation with others in social worlds, are particularly and uniquely suited to bridge biomedical, educational and other institutional systems with an individual's social and occupational world, a role Fleming (1994b) noted as "transporter." While some pioneer occupational therapists create and expand innovative, community-based practices that are unfettered by the constraints of traditional institutional funding and outcome measures, it is equally important to strengthen client-centered, occupation-based approaches and make explicit the unique and important contribution that occupational therapists make to help individuals transcend institutional settings and participate most fully in their own social worlds.

REFERENCES

AOTA. (1998). *Reference manual of the official documents of the American Occupational Therapy Association, Inc.* (7th ed.). Bethesda, MD: Author.

AOTA. (2002). Occupational therapy practice framework: Domain and process. *American Journal of Occupational Therapy, 56,* 609-639.

Barris, R. (1984) Toward an image of one's own: Sources of variation in the role of occupational therapists in psychosocial practice. *American Journal of Occupational Therapy Research, 4,* 3-23.

Boerkoel, D. (1998). A clinician's survival guide to the prospective payment system. *Gerontology Special Interest Section Quarterly, 21,* 1-4.

Clark, F. (1993). Occupation embedded within a real life: Interweaving occupational science and occupational therapy. 1993 Eleanor Clark Slagle Lecture. *American Journal of Occupational Therapy, 47,* 1067-1078.

Crepeau, E. B. (1991). Achieving intersubjective understanding: An example from an occupational therapy treatment session. *American Journal of Occupational Therapy, 44,* 1016-1024.

Dunn, W. (2000). *Best practice occupational therapy: in community service with children and families.* Thorofare, NJ: SLACK Incorporated.

Edwards, D. & Baum, C. (2001). Occupational performance: Measuring the perspectives of others. In: M. Law, C. Baum, and W. Dunn (Eds.). *Measuring occupational performance: Supporting best practice in occupational therapy.* Thorofare, NJ: SLACK Incorporated.

Fidler, G. (2000). Beyond the therapy model: Building our future. *American Journal of Occupational Therapy, 54,* 99-101.

Fleming, M. H. (1994a). Conditional reasoning: Creating meaningful experiences. In C. Mattingly & M.H. Fleming (Eds.), Clinical reasoning: Forms of Inquiry in a therapeutic practice, (pp. 197-235). Philadelphia: F. A. Davis.

Fleming, M., H., (1994b). A commonsense practice in an uncommon world. In C. Mattingly & M. H. Fleming (Eds.). Clinical reasoning Forms of inquiry in a therapeutic practice (pp. 94-115). Philadelphia: F. A. Davis.

Frank, G. (1996). The concept of adaptation as a foundation for occupational science research. In R. Zemke & F. Clark (Eds.), *Occupational science: The evolving discipline* (pp. 47-55). Philadelphia: F. A. Davis.

Goldstein-Lohman, H., Kratz, A., & Pierce, D. (2003). A study of occupation-based practice. In D. Pierce (Ed.). *Occupation by design: Building therapeutic power.* Philadelphia: F. A. Davis.

Hocking, C. (2001). The issue is—Implementing occupation-based assessment. *American Journal of Occupational Therapy, 55,* 463-469.

Jackson, J. (1998). The value of occupation as the core of treatment: Sandy's experience. *American Journal of Occupational Therapy, 52,* 466-473.

Jackson, J., Carlson, M., Mandel, D., Zemke, R., & Clark, F. (1998). Occupation in lifestyle redesign: The well-elderly study occupational therapy program. *American Journal of Occupational Therapy, 52,* 326-336.

Lave, J. & Wenger, E. (1999). *Situated learning: Legitimate peripheral participation.* Cambridge: Cambridge University Press.

Law, M., Baptiste, S., McColl, M.A., Polatjko, H.& Pollack, N. (1990). The Canadian occupational performance measure: An outcome measure for occupational therapy. *Canadian Journal of Occupational Therapy, 57,* 82-87.

Mattingly, C. (1991). The narrative nature of clinical reasoning. *American Journal of Occupational Therapy, 45,* 998-1005.

Mattingly, C. (1994). The narrative nature of clinical reasoning. In C. Mattingly & M. H. Fleming (Eds.), *Clinical reasoning: Forms of inquiry in a therapeutic practice.* Philadelphia: F. A. Davis Company.

Mattingly, C. (1998). *Healing dramas and clinical plots: The narrative structure of experience.* Cambridge: Cambridge University Press.

McDermott, J. P. (1996). The acquisition of a child by a learning disability. In S. Chaiklin & J. Lave (Eds.), *Understanding practice* (pp. 269-305). New York: Cambridge University Press.

McKesson Health Solutions. (2003). *InterQual level of care: Rehabilitation criteria adult and pediatric.* Newton, MA: McKesson Corporation.

McLaughlin-Gray, J. (1998). Putting occupation into practice: Occupation as ends, occupation as means. *American Journal of Occupational Therapy, 52,* 354-364.

Pierce, D. (2003) *Occupation by design: Building therapeutic power.* Philadelphia: F. A. Davis.

Pierce, D. (2001). Occupations by design: Dimensions, therapeutic power, and creative process. *American Journal of Occupational Therapy, 55,* 249-259.

Price, P. (2003). Occupation-centered practice: Providing opportunities for becoming and belonging. Unpublished doctoral dissertation, University of Southern California, Los Angeles.

Rebeiro, K. L., Day, D. G., Semeniuk, B., O'Brien, M. K., & Wilson, B. (2001). Northern Initiative for social action: An occupation-based mental health program. *American Journal of Occupational Therapy, 55,* 493-500.

Schell, B. (1999). *The effects of practice context on occupational therapists' clinical reasoning.* Unpublished manuscript.

Schell, B. (1998). Clinical reasoning: The basic of practice. In: M. E. Neistadt & E. B. Crepeau (Eds.), *Willard And Spackman's Occupational Therapy* (9th Ed.). Philadelphia: Lippincott.

Spencer, J. C., Davidson, H., & White, V. (1996). Continuity and change: Past experience as adaptive repertoire in occupational adaptation. *American Journal of Occupational Therapy, 50,* 526-534.

Spencer, J. C., Krefting, L., & Mattingly, C. (1993). Incorporation of ethnographic methods in occupational therapy assessment. *American Journal of Occupational Therapy, 7,* 303-309.

Spitzer, S. L. (2003). Using participant observation to study the meaning of occupations of young children with autism and other developmental disabilities. *American Journal of Occupational Therapy, 57,* 66-76.

Toth-Fejel, G. E., Toth-Fejel, G. F., & Hedricks, C. A. (1998)). Case report—Occupation-centered practice in hand rehabilitation using the experience sampling method. *American Journal of Occupational Therapy, 52,* 381-385.

Wenger, E. (1998). *Communities of practice: Learning, meaning & identity.* Cambridge: Cambridge University Press.

WHO. (2001). International classification of functioning, disability, and health. Retrieved March 21, 2005 from http://www3.who.int/icf/icftemplate.cfm.

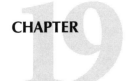

USING INFORMATION TO INFLUENCE POLICY

Carolyn Baum, PhD, OTR/C, FAOTA; Sue Baptiste, MHSc, OT Reg. (Ont.), FCAOT; and Mary Law, PhD, OT Reg. (Ont.), FCAOT

"In order for a profession to maintain its relevancy it must be aware of the times, interpreting its contribution to mankind in accordance with the needs of the times."

Geraldine L. Finn, OTR
Eleanor Clarke Slagle Lecture (1972)

A recent article on the cover of *USA Today* (July 16-18, 2004 edition) reported a decision by Medicare to redefine obesity as a medical condition. This change could allow coverage of treatment for obesity. What the decision means is that coverage of treatment is possible *"but only if scientific research proves them effective and a national Medicare panel agrees."* This was a welcome decision for those who will benefit. The relevance of this decision to occupational therapy is that the decision was tied to coverage for those services that document effectiveness. The demonstration of effectiveness will be central to the determination of coverage for treatments from now on. *Occupational therapists must use measures to document the effectiveness of their interventions.*

This chapter is intended to help the reader understand the importance of the use of occupational performance measures to educate policymakers about occupational therapy and its contribution to health care and explore methods and strategies for influencing policy decisions that will ensure that occupational therapy is a viable service in the future. This chapter provides a background for the use of occupational therapy measurement information in the policy arena and highlights key discussion issues for future consideration by the profession. We hope that it

will foster the discussion of issues that require the attention of occupational therapists.

Occupational therapists can influence the health of their communities by taking knowledge of occupational performance into new arenas of health care. It is the occupational therapist's responsibility to help policy-makers understand how occupational therapy's unique contribution to occupational performance reduces health care costs, as it directs its services to help individuals with or at risk for disabilities to live independently. These functions can be achieved in many ways, from challenging insurance denials, encouraging professional direction, and stimulating laws and regulations, to becoming involved in consumer groups and advocacy-oriented organizations that share the same concerns for persons with disabilities.

All public policy initiatives require the practitioner to become involved in the communities in which they live and work and educate people about the benefits of occupational therapy as they interact with people whose job or interest it is to improve the health and lives of the people in that community. This is possible when data regarding the performance needs of persons with disabilities have been collected and summarized at a level that policy-makers can understand.

A PROFESSION'S RESPONSIBILITY

Occupational therapy (as reflected in us as professionals) has the professional responsibility to address the needs of our societies as it struggles with issues of chronic disease, disability, and handicapping situations. To societies, these issues mean lost productivity and costly services; to individuals, they mean poorer health and compromised well-being. A brief review of the health issues of Canada and the United States will set a context to examine what occupational therapists can do to highlight our contribution to helping both society and the individuals who can benefit from our interventions.

About 45 million Americans, or one in 6, and one of seven Canadians over the age of 15 years, about 3.4 million people (Statistics Canada, 2002) have a physical or mental impairment that interferes with their daily activities, yet only 25% are so severe that they cannot work or participate in their communities. Disability is now a public health problem, affecting not only individuals with disabling conditions and their immediate families, but also society (Pope & Tarloff, 1991).

The problems associated with chronic disease and disability are so prevalent that in 2000 the American government published the *Healthy People 2010 Objectives* with priorities to challenge communities and health professionals to promote prevention strategies for their citizens. A number of the objectives should be of interest to occupational therapists, including:

1. Improving functional independence of its citizens.
2. Preventing the ill from becoming disabled.
3. Encouraging physical activity.
4. Reducing the number of persons 65 and over who have difficulty performing two or more personal care activities.
5. Reducing deaths caused by motor vehicle crashes.
6. Reducing fall related injuries.
7. Increasing the proportion of providers of primary care who routinely evaluate people aged 65 and over for impairments of vision, hearing, cognition, and functional status.

In Canada, the federal government has worked to improve the health and participation of Canadians through health promotion strategies (Health and Welfare Canada, 1986, 1987). Health is viewed as much more than the absence of disease, and many provinces in the country have set health goals for their populations. One example is the province of Ontario, where the health goals include an emphasis on health promotion and disease prevention; building healthy, supportive communities; reducing illness, disability, and death; improving the physical environment; and ensuring accessible and affordable health services for all (Premier's Council on Health, Well-Being and Social Justice, 1993).

Two specific initiatives have become milestones in the further development of health care systems in Canada over the past 5 years. *The Health of Canadians—The Federal Role* was a report that came out of the Standing Senate Committee on Social Affairs, Science and Technology,

chaired by Michael Kirby within which there were clear and commanding recommendations made regarding several key areas requiring attention (Health Canada, 2002a). These recommendations encompassed: the restructuring of the current hospital and doctor system to enhance efficiency and effectiveness through the provision of timely care of a high quality; an aim to reduce wait times for major procedures and hospitalizations, or the available resources to enable patients to obtain such services elsewhere; the expansion of public insurance plans to include coverage of palliative needs as well as those services required following catastrophic events; more federal investment and support of the total health care endeavors from services to research and development; suggestions for increasing federal revenue to allow such investment to take place; and, clear warning of the outcomes if such recommendations should not be heeded. Close on the heels of the Kirby Report, came the Romanow Report (Health Canada, 2002b) within which were articulated detailed, costed recommendations with time frames for implementation that aimed to preserve the long-term sustainability of Canada's universally accessible, publicly funded health care system. These recommendations were framed within three high level themes: that strong leadership and enhanced governance structures and processes are imperative to maintain the Canadian Medicare model and realize its essential nature as a national asset; that the system itself must become more accountable to the Canadians to whom it provides service through being more efficient and responsive to their needs; and that some investments of a strategic nature need to be made at the onset of any change in order to reap the benefits over time, and to ensure sustainability. Early the following year, Canada's Provincial Prime Ministers agreed to a new health plan to improve access to quality care for all Canadians. The Government of Canada will provide $34.8 billion over five years to relieve immediate pressures on the health care system, to enhance drug plan coverage for primary care, home care and catastrophic needs and for the purchase of diagnostic and medical equipment, and investment in information technology. Provincial governments will report to citizens on how health care dollars are being spent to improve health care in Canada (Health Canada, 2003).

RAISING ISSUES IN PUBLIC FORUMS

As society builds strategies to manage its needs, occupational therapists must be able to answer some important questions that will place occupational therapy in a key position in the new health system. Most importantly, we need to be able to address key issues in public forums to educate the policy-makers that make decisions about the allocations of resources that pay for occupational therapy services. The following are offered as examples, each question is related to an area where occupational therapists currently work and must have the data to retain our positions.

- What occupational performance measures document the activity participation, instrumental activity levels and effectiveness of environmental modifications that will allow older adults to retain their independence in their communities?

- Do people who receive occupational therapy services demonstrate productive work behaviors, are they able to problem solve, manage multiple tasks and can they sustain productivity with environmental or job modifications?

- Do those who receive occupational therapy service, and engage in community life, experience fewer secondary health conditions?

- What impact does assistive technology have on community participation?

- Does occupational therapy improve the child's participation in the classroom, in the family, and in community activities?

It is through public policy that support is garnered for community living, that children with disabilities gain access to services, that the mentally ill have access to programs that give them the skills for living, and that individuals with disabilities gain access to the services that will help them learn to live and work as productive individuals. Governments provide funding for all of these programs.

Because occupational therapy is so closely linked to the legislative process, it is important for therapists to be informed and involved. The therapists' responsibilities go beyond their relationship with their clients and beyond their role as health care professionals. As citizens in a democracy, they also have a responsibility to propose policy and raise the issues that affect necessary legislation. To become vitally involved in the political system, each therapist must take the responsibility of gaining the skills necessary to influence policy. Such skills are acquired by mobilizing resources and learning the workings of the system in which the policy will be changed.

A Changing Definition of Health and a Changing Mechanism for Delivery of Health Services

Geraldine Finn, in her 1972 Slagle lecture, stated that a profession is measured by how it addresses the needs of the time. This time in history is complicated by issues such as violence and abuse, mental illness, joblessness, increased numbers of welfare recipients, chronic disease, inadequate day care and parenting skills, and an aging population—all in addition to the problems of access to health care services. Many of the problems are such that they also involve problems in occupational performance, thereby creating opportunities and responsibilities for occupational therapists.

Health has been redefined as physical, mental, and social well-being and the individual's ability to function optimally in his or her environment (Health and Welfare Canada, 1986). "Health depends not only on health care but also on other factors including individual behavior, genetic makeup, exposure to health threats, and social and economic conditions" (Durch, Bailey, & Stoto, 1997, p. 24). It is through the process of engagement in occupation that people develop and maintain health (Law, Steinwender, & LeClair, 1998). Conversely, lack of occupation causes a breakdown in habits that leads to physiological deterioration and lessens the ability to perform competently in daily life (Kielhofner, 1992). As occupational therapists, we seek to understand the mechanisms supporting the performance of persons' actions in everyday life. To understand occupational performance, the individual's characteristics; the environment; the nature of the meaning of the activities, task, and roles that the individual wants or needs to perform; and the impact these factors have on health must be understood. As we assume our roles in communities, we need to employ our knowledge of the factors that contribute to successful occupational performance: such knowledge comes from the use of measures that documents successful occupational performance.

The changes in the health system require occupational therapists to focus our concerns on the long-term health needs of the people we serve and to help them develop healthy behaviors to improve their health and to minimize the health care costs associated with disabling conditions. We must initiate efforts to work with others in the community to integrate a range of services that promote, protect, and improve the health of the public. These efforts will require occupational therapists to work collaboratively with individuals in the client's environment (family, teachers, independent living specialists, employers, neighbors, friends) to assist them in obtaining the skills and make the modifications to remove barriers that create social disadvantage. This requires occupational therapy personnel to reframe how we think about occupational therapy, from a biomedical to a sociomedical context, and take an active role in building healthy communities (Baum & Law, 1997).

Health care is in a turbulent period, which some equate to a revolution. Health care systems have developed within an environment and culture that are constantly adapting to new situations and being modified by new economics. Over the past two decades we have seen new payment structures and a greater emphasis on promoting health, basically because healthier people use fewer health services.

The transition to a community health paradigm is in progress, but it is occurring slowly because of the great symbolic power of the biomedical system in Western society. Currently, the system is organized around concepts of impairment. In the impairment model, people look to the medical system to "fix the problem." With chronic disease and disability, the focus must shift to one that will enable individuals to do what is necessary to support their daily life in spite of their disease or disability. This is occupational therapy's focus on daily life, and it creates a leadership opportunity.

It is important to recognize that the orientation of the evolving system fits well within the values of occupational therapy. If occupational therapy could design a health system, it would focus on wellness and have its outcomes organized around well-being, function, and life satisfaction. It would focus on capabilities, allowing patients or clients to exercise personal responsibility and participate in their own care. An occupational therapy-friendly system would be community-centered and involve collaboration and coordinated services. Occupational therapists can contribute to the design of the new health system by working with our institutions to build programs that support the health care system's mission. Such an approach will significantly expand whom we will describe as the consumer.

The health community is becoming more receptive to occupational therapy's concepts and interventions, but it still requires a political effort on the part of all occupational therapists to influence the development of the new health system and to secure their places in that system. Although great strides have been made in developing new therapies to help the disabled person function independently, they will have been made in vain if therapists are denied access to the clients who need occupational therapy services.

EXPANSION OF THE TRADITIONAL MEDICAL MODEL

As health institutions become responsible for the health of the population they serve, they are investigating means of implementing health education and health promotion programs. Occupational therapists must make our contribution to health known to those who have needs. The following section identifies potential users of occupational service. It is presented in the hope that occupational therapists will explore how they can participate in the development of an expanding health system either as an employee of large health systems or as a private entrepreneur. Each of the following requires the expertise of an occupational therapist practicing or consulting from an occupational performance perspective. Following each description are questions to help you reflect on the occu-

pational performance issues that you could address with the potential consumer—the questions also ask you to reflect on the occupational performance measures that would provide you with the data to have those discussions.

Industry

Industry needs productive workers; this means workers without injuries and workers who attend work regularly. Occupational therapists can identify jobs that pose a risk for for injury, recommend environmental changes, and accommodations that support productive workers. In addition, occupational therapists can work with employees to plan for retirement and especially help employees learn skills to manage their aging parents.

Discussion Issues

What are the occupational performance issues that occupational therapists can address that will meet industries' need to have productive workers? Think about the aging population, individuals with disability who want to work, and the need for workers to work in teams. What are key occupational performance measures that will document occupational therapy's contribution?

Social Security Administration

Social Security disability determinations, and the access to other social programs and funding, have historically been based on physical capacity as determined by physicians, often without the person receiving rehabilitation, to help him or her overcome disabilities that limit his or her potential for work. In the next decade we will see disability determinations redesigned to be functionally based. This change in approach will require occupational therapists to have the skills to implement a functional assessment paradigm.

Discussion Issues

What are the occupational performance issues that occupational therapists can address that will meet the needs of governments, in particular, social service agencies? Think about the need to develop expertise in functional assessment and build assessment centers that can address this need, and perhaps help people who want to work understand their options for work within their capabilities. What occupational performance measures will document the person's capacity for work?

Hospital/Community Health System

For years, hospitals functioned under a fee-for-service approach, where all services were delivered with a specific fee attached. Occupational therapists charged for services and, for the most part, hospitals collected; actually, occupational therapy, together with physical therapy, was a profit center for hospitals. There were no financial incentives to help people gain the skills to function outside the medical community, as every time patients came back for services, the fees for services generated new income. Strategies in health financing have changed. The new systems must operate with heavily discounted fees or through a prospective fee paid to the facility. Now the hospital must retain monies to achieve a profitable or sustainable business. This approach creates a financial incentive to practice prevention. Occupational therapists can help prevent secondary conditions that limit health and quality of life and, at the same time, help facilities decrease the cost of care.

Discussion Issues

What are the occupational performance issues that will limit the development of secondary conditions? How could you introduce prevention into existing treatment programs? How could you increase the participation of the family in planning the care and acquiring the skills to manage their loved ones in order to avoid secondary conditions? What occupational performance measures and issues would document the self management strategies that would show evidence of a reduction in secondary conditions?

Schools

Occupational therapists have traditionally been in the schools. Federal laws in the United States have made occupational therapy a related service to ensure that children developed the capacity to participate in their educational experiences. The problems faced by our schools today require occupational therapists to expand their role. Teenage violence, abusive behavior, teen pregnancy, drug and alcohol abuse, and teen suicide are all symptoms of impaired occupational performance. The occupational therapist can serve as a consultant to school administration and teachers to enable children to engage in meaningful and productive tasks. Central to the occupational therapist's role in the school is to foster the development of vocational and instrumental life skill training that will support the child with a developmental disability as he or she enters the adult world.

Discussion Issues

What are the occupational performance issues that children and adolescents experience that you could address in service, educational, and/or consultative models? How would you include children, teachers, and parents in the development of programs? How could you increase the participation of the family in planning the care and acquiring the skills to foster the development and maturation of their children? What occupational performance measurements will document the importance of occupational therapy in models to enable children to acquire the skills to make the transition to adulthood?

City and County Government

Our cities and small towns are facing many problems, some of which relate directly to health. Communities are populated with older adults, many of whom are poor. How does a person continue to live independently when normal changes of aging alter sensory and cognitive systems? An occupational therapist can be a major resource for individuals, for families, and for communities to structure the environment that makes it possible for the person to live in the community. The difference between staying at home and going to a nursing home may be as simple as having the proper equipment and training so that they can take care of themselves at home. Traditionally, housing is an issue of county government and monies for older adult programs come from the federal agency Housing and Urban Development (HUD). Grants to HUD can support occupational therapists to perform assessments, modifications, and training functions. Most older adults want to continue to be productive. Where can they go if something they want to do is difficult (e.g., driving, golf, reading problems due to macular degeneration, fishing, etc.)? An occupational therapy approach to support independence could be a valuable resource for the older adult in the community. Another problem facing our communities relates to the increase in domestic crime and mental illness. Victims of abuse and those with mental illness make up a large percentage of the homeless population. Communities have established shelters as intermediate housing. Persons who want to move to independent status need skills— skills that occupational therapists can facilitate in self-management, home maintenance, job readiness, and approaches to parenting. Such programs are being supported by HUD, usually through county government. The addition of occupational therapists to community teams expands the fine work that social workers have performed to implement skill training and successful experiences that lead to productive living.

Discussion Issues

What are the occupational performance issues of adults at risk experience that you could address in a service, educational, and/or consultative model? How would you include participants, including county leaders, in the development of programs? What would you measure to demonstrate a need for occupational therapy in building healthier communities?

Penal Institutions

Society is struggling with a problem of incarceration. Our penal institutions are full and people are receiving limited sentences because there is no room. What skills do criminals need to leave the penal institution with skills to work, to participate in families, and engage in recreational pursuits? Occupational therapists have had some experience working with those who are or have been incarcerated. This is an area that is ripe for those who want to apply their knowledge of behavior and organize to address issues of vocation and life readiness.

Discussion Issues

What are the occupational performance issues that limit individuals who have committed crimes? Who would you contact to explore the potential of working with incarcerated individuals? What would be the occupational performance issues that would be measured to document occupational therapy's role with incarcerated individuals?

Architecture or Engineering Firms or Individuals

With over 50 million people with disabilities (Brandt & Pope, 1997) and the implementation of the Americans with Disabilities Act, architecture and engineering firms are being asked more and more to build environments that meet universal design concepts. Occupational therapists can play an important consulting role in building and interior design functions for these firms. Not only do architects and engineers need to meet physical accessibility standards, they need to consider sensory capacity of older adults and work specifically with persons with disabilities to maximize the fit with their environment. We will see major technology centers develop to help persons with disabilities explore the potential of technology to support the meaningful activities in their lives. Occupational therapists can partner with rehabilitation engineers to help individuals become independent in the use of effective technologies.

Discussion Issues

What are the occupational performance issues that you could address in service, educational, and/or consultative models with architects and/or engineers? Where could you interact with architects and engineers to learn more about what they do? What would be the occupational performance issues that should be measured in a consultative role?

Retirement Communities

In this new millennium, a very large cohort of adults will be aging. The baby boom of the late 1940s to mid 1960s will create the largest number of older adults in the history of the world. With these numbers comes opportunities. Where would you interact with individuals who operate retirement communities? Retirement communities have emerged to serve a current need; the new volume of older adults will support even greater growth. One problem with these retirement communities is that older persons enter the community as healthy, productive older adults and they continue to age. The problems of aging may limit independence. The occupational therapist can

be a resource to these communities to make adaptations, accommodations, and encourage older adults to remain active and fit for the activities that are meaningful and important to the residents.

Discussion Issues

What are the occupational performance issues that would help older adults stay independent and engaged in community activities? What occupational performance measures would document the independence and engagement of older adults?

Public Information

Consumers are becoming educated. Are occupational therapists educating consumers? Are we writing books, teaching courses at the junior colleges, teaching community education courses, appearing on talk shows? How about a talk show, *Remaining Active, Strategies for Independence in Later Years?* Do we have unique knowledge that will help people live meaningful and productive lives?

Discussion Issues

What are the occupational performance issues that limit an individual's abilities to live independent and meaningful lives? What knowledge could we share to help people with chronic diseases and disabilities retain or regain their social activities? Who would you look to in order to obtain the knowledge and skills to carry out these functions? Who would you contact to explore the potential to conduct community health education? What occupational performance measures would document social engagement?

Day Care Facilities (Child and Adult)

Enriched environments foster development and maintenance of health. Occupational therapists could be developing and operating enriched day care centers—even intergenerational centers. In the past, day care facilities have been primarily funded by public monies. For the first time, many families have four living generations; day care will be a strategy that supports the fulfillment of their commitments to family. Also, in the past decade we have seen the development of long-term care insurance. Monies will be available to fund day care. What would be different about an occupational therapy-developed day care environment for children or adults?

Discussion Issues

What are the occupational performance issues that could be addressed in day care programs? What would be unique about an occupational therapy-oriented day care model? What occupational performance measure would be central to a day care program?

Examples of Influencing Policy

The following examples illustrate the use of measurement to influence policy decisions related to continuous quality improvement and health service administration.

Use of Measurement for Continuous Quality Improvement and Program Evaluation

A large teaching hospital was undergoing massive reorganization and restructuring. The external consultants had completed a large part of their overall review, and it was becoming particularly obvious that there had to be some radical shifts in how work was approached to ensure that savings anywhere near the size required would be accomplished. Many strategies were discussed, one of the key options being to address any potential reductions in the length of stay of patients within the inpatient wards. While the idea of practice guidelines was not a new one, there were many within the health care teams who felt that this would lead to prescribing standardized care and remove the option for responding to the unique needs of each patient. Nevertheless, the concept of developing practice guidelines for some specific patient populations was deemed to be both sensible and possible within a relatively short time frame.

Historically, practice guidelines have been part of medical decision-making for a very long time. Their role was mainly to summarize information regarding accepted practice rather than attempt in any way to change these practices. By definition, such guidelines simply evolved (Eddy, 1990). In more recent years, there have been massive changes in both the development and application of practice guidelines. Most of these changes have been in response to the dramatic increase in knowledge and complexity with which health care practitioners are presented. There is also an increase in the importance of evidence in the determination of practice, and the evaluation of that evidence is becoming more demanding and rigorous. The interdisciplinary team of the inpatient orthopaedic floor began a process of developing a practice guideline for patients requiring hip replacement. The process was anything but simple, with many periods of extreme disagreement and dissatisfaction. However, after approximately 1 year, the team was ready to apply the hip replacement practice guideline. This particular guideline covered patient contact from the time of registration at a preoperative clinic through to discharge and home management. During the development of the guideline, there was a parallel initiative that sought to gain "buy-in" from all potential users of the orthopaedic inpatient service. This process was fraught with pitfalls and concerns; regardless, the practice guideline was launched 1 year after the inception

of the idea. Evaluation was built into the overall project design, and, after 6 months of follow-up, it was determined that the guidelines had accomplished much of their original purpose. Concerns still remain for some team members, mainly seated within the fear that individual patient needs will be subsumed in order to meet the guideline expectations.

It must be remembered, however, that practice guidelines need to be based on the methods of science and utilized in a fashion that ensures that patients' preferences are paramount in the choices among plausible treatment options (Wennberg, 1991).

Use of Measurement for Budgeting, Reimbursement, or Administrative Purposes

As part of creating a management system that would be readily responsive to continuous demands for profiles of practice and service, the director of a large occupational therapy department determined that all staff within the department should understand and be committed to a combined mission of service, education, research, and administration. In order to speed the journey toward this goal, the senior team developed a set of underlying principles, including baseline standards and criteria against which all staff would be measured. These standards were developed with consideration for:

- The main role the individual filled within the department (e.g., clinical, educational).
- The level of educational preparedness (e.g., diploma, baccalaureate, graduate, community college certificate).
- The position (e.g., senior, staff, specialist, manager).
- The client population being served (e.g., adult neurology, pediatric head injury, outpatient psychiatry).

Using the outcomes of this analysis, the senior team determined what the expectations would be for achievement during a year, as part of preparation for the annual performance appraisal and professional development plan. For example:

- Staff, prepared at a bachelor's level and who had mostly clinical responsibilities, were also expected to be involved with student learning, either as a clinical preceptor or in a more formal role such as tutor; similarly, their commitment to research would be small but would include being available to help with pilot-testing new instruments or data collection; administrative responsibilities would include completing their own workload measurement forms and fulfilling management needs on their clinical units.
- Other staff who had graduate preparation, with mostly administrative or educational responsibilities,

were expected to maintain a clinical caseload in more of a specialist or consultation capacity; they may be involved actively in furthering their own research interests but would be active participants in the research endeavors of others.

Once this system was in place and all staff were used to seeing their working world against this broad backdrop, then the basis for a strong staff development component of an overall quality assurance program was established. The expectations and scope of practice for all staff were converted into a set of broad-base common indicators against which the accomplishments of a work experience would be considered. At all times, a clear overview of staff accomplishments, commitments, and responsibilities was available in answer to requests from administrative colleagues. At budget times, this allowed for an ease in defining where staff time was being spent, which in turn could be related to the workload measurement system as a second level of detail. In many cases, these data were helpful in determining where additional resources should be deployed at times of contingency, where opportunities for enhanced professional opportunities should be given, and where merit increases should apply.

Across the spectrum, from recruitment to appraisal to retention and further development, this model served both the individual and the department (hence the organization) well.

SHAPING THE FUTURE

The profession of occupational therapy continues to grow, not only by generating knowledge of occupation and its effect on performance, but also by demonstrating how important it is for people with occupational performance dysfunction to have access to occupational therapy services. The process of sharing information about occupational therapy is called technology transfer. Occupational therapy is an applied science, and its application must be known to the individuals who can benefit from it. The results of our research will give credence to our profession's image as a necessary health service if the people who influence the evolving health care system have access to those results. It is every occupational therapist's responsibility to transfer information about occupational therapy's technology to consumers, to providers, and to the public policy-makers.

REFERENCES

Baum, C. M., & Law, M. (1997). Occupational therapy practice: Focusing on occupational performance. *American Journal of Occupational Therapy, 51,* 277-288.

Brandt, E. N. Jr., & Pope, A. M. (1997). *Enabling America: Assessing the role of rehabilitation science and engineering.* Washington, DC: National Academy Press.

Durch, J. S., Bailey, L. A., & Stoto, M. A. (Eds.). (1997). *Improving health in the community: A role for performance monitoring.* Washington, DC: National Academy Press.

Eddy, D. M. (1990). Clinical decision-making: from theory to practice. Practice policies: What are they? *Journal of the American Medical Association, 263*(6), 877-880.

Finn, G. (1972). The occupational therapist in prevention programs. *American Journal of Occupational Therapy, 26,* 59-66.

Health and Welfare Canada. (1986). *Achieving health for all: A framework for health promotion.* Ottawa, Ontario: Government of Canada.

Health and Welfare Canada. (1987). *Active health report.* Ottawa, Ontario: Government of Canada.

Health Canada. (2002a). *The Health of Canadian—The Federal Role.* Ottawa, On: Author.

Health Canada. (2002b) *Building on values: The future of health care in Canada.* Ottawa,On: Author.

Health Canada (2003). *Health care renewal accord.* Ottawa, On: Author.

Kielhofner, G. (1992). *Conceptual foundations of occupational therapy.* Philadelphia: F. A. Davis.

Law, M., Steinwender, S., & LeClair, L. (1998). Occupation, health and well-being. *Canadian Journal of Occupational Therapy, 65*(2), 81-91.

Pope, A. M., & Tarloff, A. R. (Eds.). (1991). *Disability in America: Toward a national agenda for prevention.* Washington, DC: National Academy Press.

Premier's Council on Health, Well-Being and Social Justice (1993). *Our environment, our health.* Toronto, Ontario: Province of Ontario.

Statistics Canada. (1992). *Canadian health and activity limitation survey.* Ottawa, Ontario: Statistic Canada.

Weise, E. (2004). Medicare redefines obesity as medical; Change could allow coverage of treatment. *USA Today.* July 16-18.

Wennberg, J. E. (1991). Unwanted variations in the rules of practice. *Journal of the American Medical Association, 265*(10), 1306-1307.

20

CHALLENGES AND STRATEGIES IN APPLYING AN OCCUPATIONAL PERFORMANCE MEASUREMENT APPROACH

Mary Law, PhD, OT Reg. (Ont.), FCAOT; Carolyn Baum, PhD, OTR/C, FAOTA; and Winnie Dunn, PhD, OTR, FAOTA

The purpose of this chapter is to discuss the importance of using an occupational performance measurement approach in occupational therapy practice and address some of the challenges in ensuring that measurement is integrally woven into our practice.

Incorporating outcome measurement into every occupational therapy practice is no longer a choice made by individual therapists. With increased pressure for fiscal accountability, changing accreditation and regulatory standards, increased responsibility to ensure competent practice, and increased expectations from consumers, occupational therapists must have reliable and valid methods to document the effects of their practice. Since participation is our desired outcome with the persons we serve, valid and reliable outcome measurement of participation is the way to provide this documentation.

It is our hope that this book will help student occupational therapists and occupational therapists in practice develop measurement strategies that are efficient and inform both their practice and their colleagues and consumers about the practice of occupational therapy. Let us conclude our dialogue by examining questions about measurement, its implementation, and the challenges inherent in the effective use of measurement that more clearly represents the core philosophy of occupational therapy.

WHY DO WE NEED TO ENSURE THAT MEASUREMENT IS INTEGRAL TO OUR PRACTICE?

Identity

From the earliest time in the history of occupational therapy, occupational therapists have placed value on enabling persons to engage in occupations that are important to them within their daily lives. The profession of occupational therapy began with recognition that there is an important and significant relationship between occupation, health, and well-being. Unfortunately, these early values were displaced during the middle of the 20th century when occupational therapists began to focus their treatment on changing impairments such as mood, range of motion, and strength, rather then enabling engagement in occupation. Because of this shift in focus, the outcomes that were measured during therapy emphasized changes in impairment or performance components, rather than measuring the impact of these component changes on participation outcomes. Beginning in the 1970s, occupational therapy had shifted back to its roots with a renewed emphasis on interventions designed to facilitate clients to perform chosen occupations in the environments in which they live, work, and play.

This shift back to our roots, however, has not been complete. Even today, in many practice locations, occupational therapy practice remains in conflict between the core values of the profession (i.e., a focus on enabling and providing opportunities for improved occupational performance and more satisfaction with living) and the demands of some settings which compel therapists to remain focused on addressing the impairments of individuals.

The entire health system is now focusing on function, well-being, and quality of life. The World Health Organization (WHO) International Classifications of Functioning, Disability and Health (ICF) (2001) emphasizes activity and participation as critical features of a comprehensive view of healthy living. This expansion of the traditional medical model view from "fixing impairments" or "cure" towards function, well being and quality of life requires occupational therapy to take a leadership role in identifying what a person needs and wants to do and the environmental supports that make that doing possible. Our unique contribution goes beyond impairment at the activity and participation level that provides and supports performance, and removes the barriers that limit an individual's participation in life activities. It is this uniqueness that gives us our identity. Charles Christiansen, in his 1999 Eleanor Clarke Slagle Lecture, reminds us that what we do shapes our identities of ourselves and what others perceive us to be (Christiansen, 1999). Our measurement approach has everything to do with that identity.

Furthermore, with a new focus on participation, more and more occupational therapists will have the opportunity to provide services in community settings not previously served by occupational therapy. Our ability to contribute to and provide leadership within these new systems will be possible by having a strong identity that is associated with performance and participation. Conducting measurement that addresses performance in context will make that expertise clear to everyone.

Uniqueness

A shift is occurring toward a focus on function as one of the primary indicators of intervention effectiveness (Ware, 1993; 2003). What, then, is the unique contribution of occupational therapy in service systems? A careful review of the Institute of Medicine report Enabling America (Brandt & Pope, 1997) identifies nursing, physical therapy, engineering, and occupational therapy as disciplines that focus on improving the function of the person with a disability. The goal of promoting function is shared by occupational therapy, physical therapy, nursing, social work, psychology, and medicine, among others (Fisher, 1992).

It is our perspective that makes our contribution unique. Occupational therapists understand and analyze the relationship between persons, the occupations they choose to do, and the environments in which persons carry out these occupations. Occupational therapists identify the supports and barriers to a person's chosen occupation and can collaborate with that person and his or her family to ensure successful participation in these occupations. Unlike other disciplines, we are making our best contribution when we stand at the intersection between the person and his or her desired participation. Occupational therapists are the only discipline whose focus is on activity as distinct from the environment. Other disciplines are more likely to focus on the person's ways of handling participation or on the environment's characteristics related to desired performance. Occupational therapy, through its focus on the interaction between persons and environment, enables the team to use the best aspects of the person and the environment to support performance.

Core Knowledge

At the core of what we do is what we know—our specialty is occupational performance. Our subspecialty may be in working with children, older adults, persons with mental illness, or individuals with hand injuries or spinal cord injuries. Our core knowledge is not who or what we treat—it is how our knowledge will empower our clients to achieve their objectives in performing occupations of their choice.

Therefore, it is impossible to address a person's engagement in daily occupations without a strong understanding of what the person wants and needs to do and knowledge of how performance components and environmental factors influence that person's performance. Occupational therapists often describe themselves as taking a holistic approach to care; This approach comes from having knowledge of the factors that contribute to the occupational performance of the individual or community that we are serving. We must use measurement tools to gather the information to support our unique contribution to the health and well-being of those we serve. Hopefully, this text has provided knowledge and strategies to enable the practitioner to employ the type of measurement in his or her daily practice with clients of different diagnoses, cultures, and social situations that reflect our interest and expertise in the person's ability to perform, the environment's capacity to support desired performance, and the task's characteristics to enable successful performance. It is only in creating congruence between what we say is our expertise and what others observe in our measurement and intervention strategies that we inform others about ourselves.

Evidence of Making a Difference

Occupational therapy clients come to receive intervention that will enable them to conduct their lives in a successful and satisfying way. They expect that our interventions are effective, appropriate to their needs, and cost-efficient. In addition to our clients' expectations, there is a need for increased accountability in all service systems and from regulatory bodies. Just as others expect it, occupational therapists must expect themselves to employ best practices. As described earlier in this book, best practice combines research evidence with clinical reasoning and client's values and preferences to provide effective occupational therapy intervention. In such an evidence-based practice, therapists use research knowledge while collaborating with clients to identify occupational performance needs, analyze the reasons for participation difficulties, and provide intervention to improve occupational performance.

Knowledge of the effectiveness of interventions is drawn from the research literature and from an active outcome measurement protocol within each occupational therapist's practice. It is important for every therapist to employ outcome measurement strategies that will enable him or her to acquire evidence of whether or not occupational therapy intervention is effective as it is happening. Every occupational therapist needs to know if their intervention has made a difference overall for their clients. Our more traditional strategies of measuring performance components will not provide this evidence, because the relationship between improved component skills and participation has not been demonstrated. Occupational therapists will serve themselves better to make the direct link between the measurement of performance in context and the intervention process.

Focus on Societal Needs: Quality of Life, Well-Being

About 50 million Americans, or one in five, and 3.4 million Canadians, or 14.6% (Statistics Canada, 2002), have a physical or mental impairment that interferes with their daily activities, with 41% of them are so severe that they cannot work or participate in their communities. Disability is a public health problem that affects not only individuals and their immediate families, but also society (Brandt & Pope, 1997; Pope & Tarloff, 1991).

There are a number of issues facing society that occupational therapists can address. Persons with chronic disease, illness, and neurological or mental health conditions need the resources and skills to lead productive lives and participate with family as they live and work in their communities. Children present another challenge. Those with chronic disease and disability need the support to grow into adulthood with the skills to achieve independence in

their lives. Technology has made independence possible for those who previously were not physically capable of independent living. Workers continue to have injuries, and more and more are suffering needless injuries from the movements required in their jobs. Providing workers with the skills to avoid injuries is becoming basic to employee education programs in many industries. Not only do people miss work because of injury, more and more are finding it difficult to manage aging parents on a day-to-day basis. This creates important opportunities for occupational therapists who focus on occupational performance and employ measurement strategies focused on what people need and want to do.

Hospitals have joined into health care networks and, as the funding systems approach payment based on covered lives, they are building programming to ensure that the communities they serve are healthy. Health costs less than illness. Occupational therapists can play key roles in supporting healthy communities by helping their clients attain the knowledge to prevent secondary conditions. This often means building community follow-up programs and linking clients to community resources and independent living centers to help them gain the confidence and skills to perform the activities and roles that are meaningful to them. Occupational therapists play a role in facilitating community independence and can provide important contributions to a population-based approach to health.

Occupational therapists have traditionally played a role in the school systems based on legal mandates, but with an occupational performance perspective, occupational therapy personnel can have an expanded role. Society is looking for ways to prepare children with the skills and behaviors for life. For example, occupational therapists can play a role with children who have behavior disorders by helping them achieve satisfaction in meaningful tasks that provide an outlet for their frustration and a forum to highlight their strengths, rather than continuing to expect them (and their teachers) to struggle within a context that amplifies limitations in performance. Within the context of schools, occupational therapists are also sources of knowledge to improve classroom organization, teaching modifications and building planning in service to all the students and teachers within the school. Expanding our roles beyond the traditional service to persons with specific disabilities   provides opportunities for occupational therapy knowledge to support a more successful and satisfying experience for everyone.

Our towns and cities are facing a crisis with the increase in older adults who need housing and supportive services to live independently. Occupational therapists are a natural resource to support the health, fitness, and social needs of older adults who are at risk for losing their independence. Occupational therapists are also important resources for families as they struggle to make good decisions about support mechanisms for their older family members. Occupational performance must be the focus of identifying problems that limit full participation in community life.

Society is progressively developing a universal environment that makes the disabilities we identify today transparent; this means that the barriers that prohibit successful participation are being removed for everyone. For example, although curb cuts have been installed to comply with the Americans with Disabilities Act (ADA), they are used by many more citizens without traditional "disabilities" (e.g., parents with strollers, or adults who wish to avoid joint trauma from stepping off the curb). Occupational therapists have the expertise to work with architects, engineers, and city planners to remove barriers that place unnecessary restraints on individuals. The measurement models we are recommending in this text provide an entry into community planning. Occupational therapists who employ an occupational performance approach will demonstrate immediate relevance for this societal evolution. At the center of all of these issues is occupation. Society's problems become exaggerated when its citizens cannot work, cannot care for themselves, and cannot care for others.

What Are the Major Challenges to Incorporating Measurement Into Occupational Therapy Practice?

Where to Start

What if you have not been exposed to the measures that answer the questions about how persons engage in occupations of their choice within many different environments in their community? Start by thinking about the type of outcome measure you need to evaluate occupational performance outcomes. What occupations do your clients want or need to perform? There is a need to move beyond impairment level measures and exert our uniqueness in helping people achieve their occupational objectives.

We suggest that you start by developing an understanding of the principles of measurement and how measurement is used in occupational therapy. Review Chapter 3 in this text and the decision-making process for measurement outlined in the chapter. Get together with colleagues and focus on one area of your practice to determine an outcome measure that you could use. Don't try to do everything at once. Choose an instrument that you think will strengthen your understanding of your client's issues and use it. Discuss with your colleagues how you

might implement a measurement model that will illustrate the unique contribution of occupational therapy to your institution's program. If you start identifying one measure to incorporate into your practice and then try others, outcome measurement will soon become an integral part of what you do everyday as an occupational therapist.

In these discussions, you will also want to identify measures or data collection procedures that you can stop using so that your assessment does not become unmanageable. For example, if you begin with a performance in context measure, this may inform you about a narrower focus for further assessment, thus reducing what you have to use as follow-up assessment. You might also have data from other sources (e.g., observation, referral, other discipline's tests) that give you what you need without duplicating effort.

What if I Don't Have Time?

Measurement tools must have clinical utility in order to be incorporated into occupational therapy assessment and to be useful for intervention planning. Review the measures identified in this book to determine which are most efficient for your practice. Many assessments included in this text are self-reports and can be completed and brought to the occupational therapy session for the therapist and clients to review together. The caregiver instruments provide a way to engage the caregiver in the planning process and help the therapist to ensure that intervention addresses true occupational performance issues. Remember this—although some measures take time to do, the information from occupational performance measures can save time during occupational therapy intervention. For example, use of the Canadian Occupational Performance Measure to identify a client's occupational performance issues leads to more focused assessment strategies and intervention and thus increases client motivation and saves time in the long run.

The Protocols Used in Our Facility Do Not Include Measurement

People establish protocols to find the most effective and efficient way to serve a particular group. The occupational therapist and other health care professionals must be vigilant in adapting protocols to include measurement strategies and data that facilitate life planning, such as discharge decisions, transitions from school to work, and other factors that address the client's participation. Since we have to generate data about the cost-effectiveness of our interventions, such as reduced health care usage overall, outcome measurement contributes to both positive intervention planning and documentation for effectiveness. Other health professionals want to add measures to answer their specific questions; occupational therapists can join with colleagues to be sure the right measures are being used to document the effectiveness of the interventions.

My Team Expects Certain Information From Me (e.g., Range of Motion Data)

Over time, team members come to expect certain roles from their colleagues. Changing these roles can be difficult; you can meet with the team to explicitly discuss the occupational therapist's role. Such a discussion is an opportunity for you to highlight the focus that occupational therapists place on occupational performance and how measurement of this concept can provide information to the team about clients' functioning. The occupational therapist also needs to highlight expectations for the other team members. Physical therapists contribute knowledge of movement, speech-language pathologists contribute knowledge of communication, and occupational therapists contribute knowledge of occupational performance.

Another strategy is to find ways to incorporate information from other disciplines into your reporting mechanisms. Sometimes more than one team member comes to the meeting with similar data; although this is validating, it can also be wasteful. Team members must have trust in each other's ability to gather information, and we demonstrate our trust by using data collected by others in our characterization of the person's status and our interpretation of the meaning of that data for performance needs.

Third, occupational therapists can use a transition strategy. We can report on performance in context with our "new" measures and include comments on the "expected" data from our observations. This strategy makes the link between component function and performance. For example, if you begin to incorporate the School Function Assessment into your measurement strategy, you can comment on the functional range of motion the child demonstrates in the same tasks from your observations of that task. With the new, and more expansive participation information along with the expected information, the team can learn about the broader possibilities for affecting change.

Most Outcome Measures Do Not Apply to My Clients

While it is true that there are some low-incidence populations that are not well-represented in assessment samples, this issue is not as critical for measures that focus on performance in context. Some of the measures in this book emphasize the characteristics of the environment, thus making them relevant to whatever environment the person exists within. Others focus on the performance itself; again, systematic ways of recording performance can be

helpful to any therapist serving any population. Some of the measures require significant others, including family and other service providers, to complete the information about the individual you are serving; in these cases, applicability is related to the informant's interest and ability to complete the forms with or without the therapist's assistance. Traditional standardized measures of the person's skills and abilities does limit applicability when your client doesn't match the sample in the measure. However, with performance in context, these same restrictions aren't relevant; contexts are what they are, regardless of the person's characteristics. Additionally, obtaining information about performance, making whatever the person does relevant for the assessment process. The measurement strategies we are recommending in this book set therapists free from former restraints.

One other comment is critical here. The central focus of occupational therapy practice is performance in daily life; everything we do must support this focus. Therefore, when we drift very far from this goal, we must ask ourselves whether we are still providing occupational therapy. There are many things an occupational therapist might know how to do from specialized training. It doesn't make it occupational therapy just because an occupational therapist performs the task. It is only occupational therapy when the focus is performance of occupations within daily life.

What Measure Do I Use?

The most appropriate outcome measure in each client's situation depends on what information you need to build a client-centered care plan. By reading through the book, we are sure that you have found a number of instruments that would help you help your clients. The reviews we have prepared will help you to have confidence in the measures that you choose. We have also reviewed several individualized measurement strategies that can be used in almost all intervention encounters. You will have to try some to find the ones that are congruent with your team's style; that is a great way to get others committed to this transition, because they will "own" the process with you.

What Happens to All My Other Knowledge (e.g., Testing of Performance Components)?

Some therapists worry that they will lose the skills that they have developed in testing specific performance components. In fact, you will still need these skills, but may use them at different points in the therapeutic process. As outlined in Chapter 3, the first step in the measurement process is to use an assessment to enable clients to identify occupational performance issues for intervention. After that has been completed, the therapist needs to gather information about performance components and environmental factors that are either helping or hindering the client's occupational performance. It is at this stage, therefore, that other knowledge, such as testing performance components and environmental assessment, is required. You may also find that you will have a more focused performance component assessment because you will see that only certain aspects will be relevant to particular performance. For example, the family might provide cues and supports during the personal hygiene rituals that make testing perceptual and memory skills irrelevant to getting teeth brushed and hands washed (e.g., including a game or song in the morning ritual, which the parents enjoy). Although occupational therapy knowledge is holistic, you do need to know how the person's impairment is limiting his or her occupational performance, and then you can focus energy appropriately.

We Have No Money to Buy Assessments

This is a common dilemma in occupational therapy practice today. One of the ways to address this issue is to ensure that you use the assessments that you purchase often. If this is the case, you can justify the purchase because it provides the outcome information you need. It is important to review the measurement carefully, as there may be assessments that are similar but less costly. Many of the assessments we have discussed are in the public domain and do not need to be purchased. Others can be purchased at quite a low price, under $100.

The Focus on Occupational Performance Outcomes in Occupational Therapy—Is This Just a Trend That Will Go Away Soon?

Occupational performance has been the focus of the profession since it began in 1918. The person-environment perspective is implicit in occupational therapy values and is reflected now in the way in which all outcomes of health are measured in well-being, satisfaction, and quality of life. This is an expertise for which we are recognized.

What Do I Write in My Reports and How Do I Ensure Reimbursement?

National health policies within the United States such as Medicare and most payment systems recognize individuals' progress to the level that they were achieving prior to their illness or injury. Documentation must focus on how the person is making progress and achieving function to overcome the impairments caused by the illness or injury.

One strategy involves measuring and documenting the occupations that the person can now perform in light of the impairments that were causing difficulty in performance. However, some systems are offering a lump sum for the person's care, such as HMOs and some Medicare systems. In these systems, there is currently less concern for specific outcomes by the reimbursement agent; the service agencies have the responsibility to decide what interventions will yield them the most efficient and effective way of releasing the person from care because less time in care means better use of the money available. Balancing between efficient use of resources on a person's behalf and providing quality care will be the challenge for these systems. Your documentation needs to reflect both a respectfulness for efficient use of resources and your concern for the person's performance. For example, in discussing cooking as a desired outcome, you can write about the home instructions for practice, include information about safety in the home to "reduce the chances for accidents," thereby reducing re-hospitalization, and discuss the changes in other status due to the person's increased participation. You must tailor your documentation to the particular system without losing track of the occupational therapy focus.

These situations make the need for evidence about our contributions to efficiency and effectiveness even more critical. Your documentation of each case can provide portions of the evidence that can develop into a convincing argument. In addition, these situations make it even more critical for occupational therapists to illustrate their unique contributions explicitly. It is no wonder that some rehabilitation endeavors are viewing occupational therapy and physical therapy as duplication of service when they both document measurement of the same person-variable data. We must be willing to take the risk to shine the light on our differences in perspective through documentation and to contribute to databases that can show reduction in use of health care dollars across time with increased independence. Emphasize the person's ability to care for him- or herself, which requires less home care follow-up and fewer re-admissions and re-occurrences.

When documenting for children and families, we must be better about projecting outcomes across time, even toward adulthood. Supporting the team to make these projections provides a yardstick for prioritizing how to spend the child's time at various stages in development. It is very easy to get caught up in reaching milestones without continuing to consider whether these skills are contributing to long-term planning.

Another pitfall to avoid when serving children and families is measuring only to determine the child's eligibility for services. We primarily use status measures of the child's skills to establish a discrepancy between capacity and performance. However, these measures do not guide practice.

The measures we have included in this text provide information for intervention planning, and many of them provide a means for including the family in the data collection process. When families have something explicit to contribute, they become full members of the team as the law intended.

Teaching the Next Generation of Occupational Therapists

One of the biggest challenges for our profession is to determine the best strategies for passing along best practices to our developing colleagues and, at the same time, provide information to our practicing colleagues. Educators must take a leadership role in making best practice information available to both groups. This book is a great resource for students and their teachers because it guides you through the rationale and application of best practices in measurement (i.e., to make sure that our measurement approaches clearly reflect the core concepts of occupational therapy). For faculty, we urge you to use this book as your resource for exploring occupation-centered practice. Students can complete many of the measures on their own families and friends and discuss what insights they gained from using them. You can work with the students on groups of measures that might become a packet for fieldwork placements. If you have meetings with your supervising therapists, you can make the measures available for them to review and discuss.

For new graduates, using this book to build your initial repertoire of measures will prepare you to implement these best practices on fieldwork and in your work. The student's biggest challenge after learning these best practices is how to handle fieldwork and initial job situations that are using more traditional performance component measurements. First and foremost, students and new graduates must feel empowered to effect change in these systems by having studied and practiced the appropriate measures and by preparing a rationale for why the alternatives you offer are worth a try. We recommend that students use this topic as one of their teaching/inservice opportunities for the staff; your supervisors take students because they want to keep current, so take advantage of this. We also recommend that you include some of these measures along with others traditionally used and prepare to point out the utility of the additional information to your supervisor and the team. These strategies both inform the therapist of new information and invite the systems to try a new way.

REFERENCES

Brandt, E. N. Jr., & Pope, A. M. (1997). *Enabling America: Assessing the role of rehabilitation science and engineering.* Washington, DC: National Academy Press.

Christiansen, C. (1999). *Defining lives: Occupation as identity — An essay on relationships, competence and the creation of meaning.* Eleanor Clarke Slagle Lectureship, American Occupational Therapy Association, Indianapolis, IN, April 1999.

Fisher, A. G. (1992). The Foundation—Functional measures, part 1: What is function, what should we measure, and how should we measure it? *American Journal of Occupational Therapy, 46(2),* 183-185.

Pope, A. M., & Tarloff, A. R. (Eds.). (1991). *Disability in America: Toward a national agenda for prevention.* Washington, DC: National Academy Press.

Statistics Canada. (2002). *A profile of disability in Canada, 2001.* Ottawa, ON: Statistics Canada.

Ware, J. E. (1993). Measures for a new era of health assessment. In: A. L. Stewart & J. E. Ware (Eds.), *Measuring functioning and well-being* (pp. 3-12). Durham, NC: Duke University Press.

Ware, J. E. Jr. (2003) Conceptualization and measurement of health-related quality of life: Comments on an evolving field. *Archives of Physical Medicine and Rehabilitation, 84(4 Suppl 2),* 43-51.

WHO. (2001). *International classification of functioning, disability, and health (ICF).* Geneva, Switzerland: Author.

LIST OF MEASURES
(ALPHABETICAL)

Activities Scale for Kids (ASK), 190-191

Activity Card Sort (ACS), 115-116, 258-259

ADL Situational Test, 238

Adolescent Role Assessment, 278

Arnadottir OT-ADL Neurobehavioral Evaluation (A-ONE), 192-193

Arthritis Impact Measurement Scales (AIMS), 194-196

Assessment of Ludic Behaviors (ALB), 134

Assessment of Motor and Process Skills (AMPS), 239

Assessment of Occupational Functioning—Collaborative Version, 280-281

Barthel Index (BI), 197-199

Canadian Occupational Performance Measure (COPM), 86, 173

Caregiver Assessment of Functional Dependence and Upset (CAFU), 240

Child Behaviors Inventory of Playfulness (CBIP), 138-139

Child Health Questionnaire (CHQ), 200-201

Child-Initiated Pretend Play Assessment (ChIPPA), 142-143

Children's Assessment of Participation and Enjoyment (CAPE), 110-111, 265-266

Children's Health Assessment Questionnaire (CHAQ), 206-208

Community Integration Measure, 305

Community Integration Questionnaire, 305

Coping Inventory for Children, 98

Craig Handicap Assessment and Reporting Technique (CHART), 121-122, 270-271, 304

Craig Hospital Inventory of Environmental Factors (CHIEF) and CHIEF Short Form, 329-330

Direct Assessment of Functional Abilities (DAFA), 242

Direct Assessment of Functional Status (DAFS), 241

Early Coping Inventory, 99

Experience Sampling Method (ESM), 296-297

Extended Activities of Daily Living Scale (EADLS), 243

Feasibility Evaluation Checklist, 177

Functional Autonomy Measurement System (SMAF), 202-203

Functional Behavior Profile (FBP), 102-103

Functional Independence Measure (FIM) & WeeFIM, 204-207

Health Assessment Questionnaire (HAQ), 208-210

Home and Community Environments: Measure of Processes of Care (MPOC), 331-332

Home Environment, 317-320

Home Environment: Home Observation for Measurement of the Environment, Revised Edition (HOME), 321-322

Home Falls and Accidents Screening Tools, 320-321

Home Observation for Measurement of the Environment (HOME), 148-149

Interest Checklist and Activity Checklist, 263-265

Interpersonal Support Evaluation List, 307

Interview Schedule for Social Interaction (ISSI), 309

Job Content Questionnaire (JCQ), 167-168

Juvenile Arthritis Functional Assessment Report (JAFAR). 211-212

Juvenile Arthritis Functional Assessment Scale (JAFAS), 211-212

Juvenile Arthritis Self-Report Index (JASI), 213-214

Katz Index of Activities of Daily Living, 215-216

Kitchen Task Assessment (KTA), 244

Leisure Activity Profile (LAP), 269

Leisure Boredom Scale, 253

Leisure Competence Measure (LCM), 254-255

Leisure Diagnostic Battery, 272-273

Leisure Diagnostic Battery (LDB), 274-275

Leisure Satisfaction Questionnaire/Leisure Satisfaction Scale (LSS), 256-257

Lifease Software: Ease 3.2 Basic and Ease 3.2 Deluxe, 323

Life Habits Assessment (LIFE-H), 119-120

Life Role Salience Scale, 282

Life Stressors and Social Resources Inventory—Adult Form (LISRES-A), 338-339

London Handicap Scale, 117-118

Measure of Quality of the Environment, 333-334

Melville Nelson Self-Care Assessment, 217-218

Memory and Behavior Problems Checklist: Revised, 101-102

Multidimensional Scale of Perceived Social Support (MSPSS), 335-336

National Institutes of Health Activity Record (ACTRE), 294-295

Occupational Circumstances Assessment-Interview and Rating Scale (OCAIRS), 87

Occupational Performance History Interview II, 84, 171-172

Occupational Questionnaire (OQ), 292-293

Occupational Role History, 279

Occupational Self-Assessment, 85

Parenting Stress Index (PSI), 95-96

Patient Specific Function Scale (PSFS), 219-220

Pediatric Activity Card Sort (PACS), 114, 135, 260-261

Pediatric Evaluation of Disability Inventory (PEDI), 221-223

Pediatric Interest Profiles: Survey of Play for Children and Adolescents, 133, 263

Perceived Efficacy and Goal Setting System (PEGS), 88

Performance Assessment of Self-Care Skills (PASS), 245

Person in Environment System, 283

Personal Care Participation Assessment and Resource Tool (PC-PART), 124-126

Personal Projects Analysis (PPA), 290-291

Physical Self-Maintenance Scale (PSMS), 220-222

Play History, 131-132

Post-Occupancy Evaluation (POE), 328

Preferences for Activities of Children (PAC), 267-269

Reintegration to Normal Living Index, 302

Revised Knox Preschool Play Scale (PPS-R), 140-141

Role Checklist, 284

Safety Assessment of Function and the Environment for Rehabilitation (SAFER), 324-325

Safety Assessment of Function and the Environment for Rehabilitation—Home Outcome Measurement and Evaluation (SAFER-HOME), 324-325

School Function Assessment (SFA), 96-97, 112-113

Social Problem Questionnaire, 281

Social Support Inventory for People with Disabilities (SSIDP), 308

Spinal Function Sort, 175-176

Structured Assessment of Independent Living Skills (SAILS), 246

Structured Observation and Report Technique (SORT), 298

Test of Environmental Supportiveness (TOES), 146-147

Test of Grocery Shopping Skills, 247

Test of Playfulness (ToP) Version 4, 136-137

Transdisciplinary Play-Based Assessment (TPBA) 2nd Ed., 144-145

Valpar Component Work Samples (VCWS), 174

Vineland Adaptive Behavior Scales (VABS), 100

Westmead Home Safety Assessment, 326-327

Work Environment Scale (WES), 342-344

Worker Role Interview, 169-170

Workplace Environment: Work Environment Impact Scale, 340-341

World Health Organization—Disability Schedule II (WHO-DAS II), 123

B

LIST OF MEASURES BY OCCUPATIONAL PERFORMANCE AREA

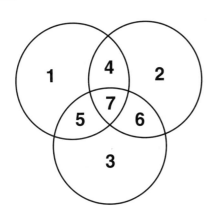

PEO DIAGRAMS LINKED TO OUTCOME MEASURES

Space 1 illustrates the person variables alone. Measures of performance components would fit here.

Space 2 illustrates the environmental variables alone. This would include measures of the features of the environment, such as are included in Chapter 17.

Space 3 illustrates the occupation variables alone. There are no measures of this type in this book.

Space 4 represents the intersection of person and environment. Measures in this category will inform you about how the person fits into or responds to environmental conditions. Various chapters include measures of this type.

Space 5 represents the intersection of person and occupation. Measures in this category will inform you about the person's interests and needs for occupational performance. Various chapters will introduce these measures to you.

Space 6 represents the intersection of occupation and the environment. Measures in this category address the capacity of environments to support particular tasks and the

match between tasks and environments. This classification is not used in the this book.

Space 7 represents the intersection of all three variables, occupational performance. Many of the measures in this section capture this relationship, and therefore are very useful tools for intervention planning in natural environments.

Space 1

Child Behaviors Inventory of Playfulness (CBIP), 138-139

Child Health Questionnaire (CHQ), 200-201

Leisure Boredom Scale, 253

Memory and Behavior Problems Checklist: Revised, 101-102

Space 2

Home Falls and Accidents Screening Tool (HOME FAST), 319-321

Home and Community Environments: Measure of Processes of Care (MPOC), 331-332

Life Stressors and Social Resources Inventory—Adult Form (LIS-RES-A), 338-339

Measure of Quality of the Environment (MQE), 333-334

Safety Assessment of Function and the Environment for Rehabilitation (SAFER), 324-325

Safety Assessment of Function and the Environment for Rehabilitation—Health Outcome Measurement and Evaluation (SAFER-HOME), 324-325

Westmead Home Safety Assessment, 326-327

Workplace Environment: Work Environment Impact Scale, 340-341

Space 4

Coping Inventory for Children, 98

Early Coping Inventory, 99

Home Environment, 317-321

Home Observation for Measurement of the Environment (HOME), 148-149

Interpersonal Support Evaluation List, 307

Interview Schedule for Social Interaction (ISSI), 309

Lifease Software: Ease 3.2 Basic and Ease 3.2 Deluxe, 323

Multidimensional Scale of Perceived Social Support (MSPSS), 335-336

Parenting Stress Index (PSI), 95-96

Post-Occupancy Evaluation (POE), 328

Social Support Inventory for People with Disabilities (SSIDP), 308

Test of Environmental Supportiveness (TOES), 146-147

Work Environment Scale (WES), 342-343

Space 5

Activities Scale for Kids (ASK), 190-191

Activity Card Sort (ACS), 115-116, 258-259

ADL Situational Test, 238

Adolescent Role Assessment, 278

Arnadottir OT-ADL Neurobehavioral Evaluation (A-ONE), 192-193

Arthritis Impact Measurement Scales (AIMS), 194-196

Barthel Index (BI), 197-199

Caregiver Assessment of Functional Dependence and Upset (CAFU), 240

Child-Initiated Pretend Play Assessment (ChIPPA), 142-143

Community Integration Measure, 305

Community Integration Questionnaire, 304

Craig Handicap Assessment and Reporting Technique (CHART), 121-122, 270-271, 303

Direct Assessment of Functional Status (DAFS), 241

Experience Sampling Method (ESM), 296-297

Extended Activities of Daily Living Scale (EADLS), 243

Functional Behavior Profile (FBP), 102-103

Interest Checklist and Activity Checklist, 263-264

Juvenile Arthritis Functional Assessment Report (JAFAR), 211-212

Juvenile Arthritis Functional Assessment Scale (JAFAS), 211-212

Juvenile Arthritis Self-Report Index (JASI), 213-214

Leisure Diagnostic Battery, 273

Leisure Satisfaction Questionnaire/Leisure Satisfaction Scale (LSS), 256-257

Life Role Salience Scale, 282

London Handicap Scale, 117-118

National Institutes of Health Activity Record (ACTRE), 294-295

Occupational Questionnaire (OQ), 292-293

Patient Specific Function Scale (PSFS), 219-220

Pediatric Activity Card Sort (PACS), 114, 135, 260-261

Pediatric Interest Profiles: Survey of Play for Children and Adolescents, 133, 262

Personal Projects Analysis (PPA), 245

Preferences for Activities of Children (PAC), 267-268

Reintegration to Normal Living Index, 302

Role Checklist, 284

Social Problem Questionnaire, 281

Spinal Function Sort, 175-176

Structured Assessment of Independent Living Skills (SAILS), 246

Test of Grocery Shopping Skills, 247

Test of Playfulness (ToP) Version 4, 136-137

Valpar Component Work Samples (VCWS), 174

Vineland Adaptive Behavior Scales (VABS), 100

Space 7

Assessment of Ludic Behaviors (ALB), 134

Assessment of Motor and Process Skills (AMPS), 239

Assessment of Occupational Functioning—Collaborative Version, 280-281

Canadian Occupational Performance Measure (COPM), 86, 173

Children's Health Assessment Questionnaire (CHAQ), 208-210

Children's Assessment of Participation and Enjoyment (CAPE), 110-11, 265-266

Craig Hospital Inventory of Environmental Factors (CHIEF) and CHIEF Short Form, 329-330

Direct Assessment of Functional Abilities (DAFA), 244

Feasibility Evaluation Checklist, 177

Functional Autonomy Measurement System (SMAF), 202-203

Functional Independence Measure (FIM) & WeeFIM, 204-207

Health Assessment Questionnaire (HAQ), 208-210

Job Content Questionnaire (JCQ), 167-168

Katz Index of Activities of Daily Living, 215-216

Kitchen Task Assessment (KTA), 244

Leisure Activity Profile (LAP), 269

Leisure Competence Measure (LCM), 254-255

Leisure Diagnostic Battery (LDB), 274-275

Life Habits Assessment (LIFE-H). 119-120

Melville Nelson Self-Care Assessment, 217-218

Occupational Circumstances Assessment-Interview and Rating Scale (OCAIRS), 87

Occupational Performance History Interview II, 84, 171-172

Occupational Role History, 279

Occupational Self-Assessment, 85

Pediatric Evaluation of Disability Inventory (PEDI), 221-223

Perceived Efficacy and Goal Setting System (PEGS), 88

Performance Assessment of Self-Care Skills (PASS), 245

Person in Environment System, 283

Personal Care Participation Assessment and Resource Tool (PC-PART), 124-126

Physical Self-Maintenance Scale (PSMS), 224-225

Play History, 131-132

Revised Knox Preschool Play Scale (PPS-R), 140-141

School Function Assessment (SFA), 96-97, 112-113

Structured Observation and Report Technique (SORT), 300

Transdisciplinary Play-Based Assessment (TPBA) 2nd Ed., 144-145

Worker Role Interview, 169-170

World Health Organization-Disability Schedule II (WHO-DAS II), 123

LIST OF MEASURES BY SOURCE/ AUTHOR

Amatea, E. S., Cross, E. G., Clark, J. E., & Bobby, C. L., Life Role Saliance Scale, 282

American Guidance Service Inc., Vineland Adaptive Behavior Scales (VABS), 100

Arnadottir, G., Arnadottir OT-ADL Neurobehavioral Evaluation (A-ONE), 192-193

Baron, K., Kielhofner, G., Ienger, A., Goldhammer, V. & Wolenski, J., Occupational Self-Assessment, 85

Baum, C., & Edwards, D. F., Kitchen Task Assessment (KTA), 244

Baum, C., Activity Card Sort (ACS), 115-116, 258-259

Baum, C., Functional Behavior Profile (FBP), 102-103

Behnke, C., & Fetkovich, M. M., Play History, 131-132

Black, M. M., Adolescent Role Assessment, 280

Bosche, K., Measure of Quality of the Environment (MQE), 333-334

Bradley, R., & Caldwell, B. M., Home Observation for Measurement of the Environment (HOME), 148-149

Bryze, K., Play History, 131-132

Bundy, A., Test of Environmental Supportiveness (TOES), 146-147 (9)

Bundy, A., Test of Playfulness (ToP) Version 4, 136-137

Caldwell, B. M., & Bradley, R. H., Home Environment: Home Observation for Measurement of the Environment (HOME) (Revised Edition), 321-322

Canadian Occupational Therapy Association, Pediatric Activity Card Sort (PACS), 114, 135, 260-261

Canadian Occupational Therapy Association Comprehensive Rehabilitation and Mental Health Services, Safety Assessment of Function and the Environment for Rehabilitation (SAFER Tool), 324-325

Canadian Occupational Therapy Association Comprehensive Rehabilitation and Mental Health Services, Safety Assessment of Function and the Environment for Rehabilitation—Health Outcome Measurement and Evaluation (SAFER-HOME), 324-325

Career/Lifeskills Resources Inc., Work Environment Scale (WES), 342-343

Centre for Outcome Measurement in Brain Injury at Craig Hospital, Craig Hospital Inventory of Environmental Factors (CHIEF), and CHIEF Short Form, 329-331

Center for Rehabilitation Effectiveness, Pediatric Evaluation of Disability Inventory (PEDI), 221-223

Centre d'expertise, Functional Autonomy Measurement System (SMAF), 202-203

Centre interdisciplinaire de recherche en réadaptation et intégration sociale, Life Habits Assessment (LIFE-H), 119-120

Cohen, S., Mermelstein, R., Kamarck, T., & Hoberman, H. M., Interpersonal Support Evaluation List, 307

Co-ordinates Publications, Westmead Home Safety Assessment, 326-327

Corney, R. H., & Clare, A. W., Social Problem Questionnaire, 281

Csikszentmihalyi, M., & Larson, R., Experience Sampling Method (ESM), 296-297

Data System (Marita Kloseck), Leisure Competence Measure (LCM), 254-255

Deshpande, S., Kielhofner, G., Henriksson, C., Haglund, L., Olson, L., Forsyth, K., & Kulkarni, S., Occupational Circumstances Assessment-Interview and Rating Scale (OCAIRS), 87

Dickerson, A. E., Role Checklist, 284

Employment Potential Improvement Corporation, Spinal Function Sort, 175-176

Ferland, F., Assessment of Ludic Behaviors (ALB), 134

Fisher, A. G., Assessment of Motor and Process Skills (AMPS), 239

Florey, L. L., & Michelman, S. M., Occupational Role History, 279

Fries, J. F., Health Assessment Questionnaire (HAQ), 208-210

Furst, G., National Institutes of Health Activity Record (ACTRE), 294-297

Gitlin, L. N., Roth, D. L., Burgio, L., et al., Caregiver Assessment of Functional Dependence and Upset (CAFU), 240

Hamera, E., & Brown, C., Test of Grocery Shopping Skills, 247

Health Act, Child Health Questionnaire (CHQ), 200-201

Henderson, S., Duncan-Jones, P., Byrne, D. G., & Scott, R., Interview Schedule for Social Interaction (ISSI), 309

Holm, M. B., & Rogers, J. C., Performance Assessment of Self-Care Skills (PASS), 245

Howe, S., Levinson, J., Shear, E., Hartner, S., McGirr, G., Schulte, M., & Lovell, D., Juvenile Arthritis Functional Assessment Report (JAFAR), 211-212

Idyll Arbor Inc., Leisure Satisfaction Questionnaire/Leisure Satisfaction Scale (LSS), 256-257

Idyll Arbor, Inc., Leisure Diagnostic Battery, 272-273

Iso-Ahola, S. E., & Weissinger, E., Leisure Boredom Scale, 253

Iwarsson, S., & Isacsson, A., Home Environment, 317-320

Karagiozis, H., Gray, S., Sacco, J., Shapiro, M., & Kawas, C., Direct Assessment of Functional Abilities (DAFA), 242

Karasek, R. A., Job Content Questionnaire (JCQ), 167-168

Katz, S., Ford, A. B., Moskowitz, R. W., Jackson, B. A., & Jaffe, M. W., Katz Index of Activities of Daily Living, 215-216

Kielhofner, G., Mallinson, T., Crawford, C., Nowak, M., Rigby, M., Henry, A., & Walens, D., Occupational Performance History Interview II, 84, 171-172

King, S., Rosenbaum, P., & King, G., Home and Community Environments: Measure of Processes of Care (MPOC), 331-332

Knox, S., Revised Knox Preschool Play Scale (PPS-R), 140-141

Law, M., Baptiste, S., Carswell, A., McColl, M. A., Polatajko, H. & Pollock, N., Canadian Occupational Performance Measure, 86, 173

Lawton, M. P., & Brody, E. M., Physical Self-Maintenance Scale (PSMS), 222-223

LDB Project, Leisure Diagnostic Battery (LDB), 274-275

Lifease Corporation, Lifease Software: Ease 3.2 Basic and 3.2 Deluxe, 323

Linder, T. W., Transdisciplinary Play-Based Assessment (TPBA) 2nd Ed., 144-145

Little, B. R., Personal Projects Analysis (PPA), 290-291

Loewenstein, D., Amigo, E., Duara, R., et al., Direct Assessment of Functional Status (DAFS), 241

Lovell, D. J., Howe, S., Shear, E., Hartner, S., McGirr, G., Schulte, M., & Levinson, J., Juvenile Arthritis Functional Assessment Scale (JAFAS), 211-212

Mackenzie, L., Byles, J., & Higginbotham, N., Home Falls and Accidents Screening Tools, 319-320

Mahoney, S. I., & Barthel, D. W., Barthel Index (BI), 197-199

Mahurin, R. K., DeBittignies, B. H., & Pirozzolo, F. J., Structured Assessment of Independent Living Skills (SAILS), 246

Mann, W. C. & Talty, P., Leisure Activity Profile (LAP), 269

McColl, M. A., & Davies, D., Community Integration Measure, 305

McColl, M. A., & Friedland, J., Social Support Inventory for People with Disabilities (SSIDP), 308

Medical Outcomes Trust, London Handicap Scale, 117-118

Meenan, R. F., Arthritis Impact Measurement Scales (AIMS2), 194-196

Mellnick, D., Craig Handicap Assessment and Reporting Technique (CHART), 121-122, 270-271, 303

Melville, D. L., & Nelson, L. L., Melville Nelson Self-Care Assessment, 217-218

Missiuna, C., Pollock, N., & Law, M., Perceived Efficacy and Goal Setting System (PEGS), 88

Moore-Corner, R. A., Keilhofner, G., & Olsen, L., Workplace Environment: Work Environment Impact Scale, 340-341

No author, Interest Checklist & Activity Checklist, 263-264

Nouri, F. M. & Lincoln, N. B., Extended Activities of Daily Living Scale (EADLS), 243

Oakley, F., Kielhofner, G., Barris, R., & Reichler, R., Role Checklist, 284

PART Group, Personal Care Participation Assessment and Resource Tool (PC-PART), 124-126

Preiser, W. F. E., Rabinowitz, H. Z., & White, E. T., Post-Occupancy Evaluation (POE), 328

Program in Occupational Therapy, Feasibility Evaluation Checklist, 177

Psychological Assessment Resources, Inc., Parenting Stress Index (PSI), 95-96

Psychological Assessment Resources, Life Stressors and Social Resources Inventory—Adult Form (LISRES-A), 338-339

Psychological Corporation, Children's Assessment of Participation and Enjoyment (CAPE), 110-111, 265-266

Psychological Corporation, Preferences for Activities of Children (PAC), 267-269

Psychological Corporation, School Function Assessment (SFA), 96-97, 112-113

Rintala, D. H., Uttermohlen, D. M., Buck, E. L., et al., Structured Observation and Report Technique (SORT), 298

Rogers, C. S., Impara, J. C., Frary, R. B., et al., Child Behaviors Inventory of Playfulness (CBIP), 138-139

Rogers, J. C., & Holm, M. B., Performance Assessment of Self-Care Skills (PASS), 245

Rogers, J. C., Holm, M., Goldstein, G., McCue, M., & Nussbaum, P., Performance Assessment of Self-Care Skills (PASS), 245

Scholastic Testing Service, Inc., Coping Inventory for Children, 98

Scholastic Testing Service, Inc., Early Coping Inventory, 99

Singh, G., Athreya, B. H., Fries, J. F., & Goldsmith, D. P., Children's Health Assessment Questionnaire (CHAQ), 206-208

Skurla, E., Rogers, J. C., & Sunderland, T., ADL Situational Test, 238

Smith, N. R., Kielhofner, G., & Watts, J. H., Occupational Questionnaire (OQ), 292-293

Stagnitti, K. Child-Initiated Pretend Play Assessment (ChIPPA), 142-143

Stratford, P., Gill, C., Westaway, M., & Binkley, J., Patient Specific Function Scale (PSFS), 217-219

Takata, N., Play History, 131-132

Teri, L., Truax, P., Logsdon, R., Uomoto, J., Zarit, S., Vitaliano, P. P., Memory and Behavior Problems Checklist: Revised, 101-102

Therapy Skill Builders, Pediatric Interest Profiles: Survey of Play for Children and Adolescents, 133, 263

Uniform Data System for Medical Rehabilitation, Functional Independence Measure (FIM) & WeeFIM, 202-204

Valpar International Corporation, Valpar Component Work Samples (VCWS), 174

Velozo, C. A., Kielhofner, G., & Fisher, G., Worker Role Interview, 169-170

Watts, J. H., & Madigan, J. M., Assessment of Occupational Functioning-Collaborative Version, 280-281

Whiteneck, G., Charlifue, S. Gerhart, K., Overholser, D., & Richardson, G., Craig Handicap Assessment and Reporting Technique (CHART), 121-122, 270-271, 303

Willer, B., Rosenthal, M., Kreutzer, J. S., Gordon, W. A. & Rempel, R., Community Integration Questionnaire, 304

Williams, J. B. W., Karls, J. M., & Wandrei, K., Person in Environment System, 283

Wood-Dauphinee, S., Opzoomer, A., Williams, J. I., Marchand, B., & Spitzer, W. O., Reintegration to Normal Living Index, 302

World Health Organization., World Health Organization—Disability Schedule II (WHO-DAS II), 123

Wright, F. V., Law, M., Crombie, V., Goldsmith, C., Dent, P., & Shore, A., Juvenile Arthritis Self-Report Index (JASI), 211-212

Young, N. L., Activities Scale for Kids (ASK), 190-191

Zimet, G. D., Dahlem, N.W., Zimet, S. G., & Farley, G. K., Multidimensional Scale of Perceived Social Support (MSPSS), 335-336

LIST OF MEASURES MAPPED TO THE INTERNATIONAL CLASSIFICATION OF FUNCTIONING

GENERAL TASKS AND DEMANDS

Activities Scale for Kids (ASK), 190-191

Activity Card Sort (ACS), 115-116, 258-259

Adolescent Role Assessment, 278

Arnadottir OT-ADL Neurobehavioral Evaluation (A-ONE), 192-193

Arthritis Impact Measurement Scales (AIMS), 194-196

Assessment of Ludic Behaviors (ALB), 239

Assessment of Motor and Process Skills (AMPS), 239

Assessment of Occupational Functioning—Collaborative Version, 280-281

Barthel Index (BI), 197-199

Canadian Occupational Performance Measure (COPM), 86, 173

Caregiver Assessment of Functional Dependence and Upset (CAFU), 240

Child Behaviors Inventory of Playfulness (CBIP), 138-139

Child Health Questionnaire (CHQ), 208-210

Child-Initiated Pretend Play Assessment (ChIPPA), 142-143

Children's Assessment of Participation and Enjoyment (CAPE), 110-111, 265-266

Children's Health Assessment Questionnaire (CHAQ), 208-210

Community Integration Measure, 305

Community Integration Questionnaire, 304

Coping Inventory for Children, 98

Craig Handicap Assessment and Reporting Technique (CHART), 121-122, 270-271, 303

Direct Assessment of Functional Abilities (DAFA), 242

Direct Assessment of Functional Status (DAFS), 241

Early Coping Inventory, 99

Experience Sampling Method (ESM), 296-297

Extended Activities of Daily Living Scale (EADLS), 243

Feasibility Evaluation Checklist, 177

Functional Autonomy Measurement System (SMAF), 202-203

Functional Behavior Profile (FBP), 102-103

Health Assessment Questionnaire (HAQ), 208-210

Home Observation for Measurement of the Environment (HOME), 148-149

Interest Checklist & Activity Checklist, 263-264

Interpersonal Support Evaluation List, 307

Interview Schedule for Social Interaction (ISSI), 309

Job Content Questionnaire (JCQ), 167-168

Juvenile Arthritis Functional Assessment Report (JAFAR), 211-212

Juvenile Arthritis Functional Assessment Scale (JAFAS), 211-212

Juvenile Arthritis Self-Report Index (JASI), 213-214

Katz Index of Activities of Daily Living, 215-216

Kitchen Task Assessment, 244

Leisure Activity Profile (LAP), 269

Leisure Boredom Scale, 253

Leisure Competence Measure (LCM), 254-255

Leisure Diagnostic Battery, 273-274

Leisure Diagnostic Battery (LDB), 274-275

Leisure Satisfaction Questionnaire/Leisure Satisfaction Scale (LSS), 256-257

Life Habits Assessment (LIFE-H), 119-120

London Handicap Scale, 117-118

Melville Nelson Self-Care Assessment, 217-218

Memory and Behavior Problems Checklist: Revised, 101-102

National Institutes of Health Activity Record (ACTRE), 294-295

Occupational Circumstances Assessment-Interview and Rating Scale (OCAIRS), 87

Occupational Performance History Interview II, 84, 171-172

Occupational Questionnaire (OQ), 292-293

Occupational Role History, 279

Occupational Self-Assessment, 85

Parenting Stress Index (PSI), 95-96

Patient Specific Function Scale (PSFS), 219-220

Pediatric Activity Card Sort (PACS), 114, 135, 260-261

Pediatric Evaluation of Disability Inventory (PEDI), 221-223

Pediatric Interest Profiles: Survey of Play for Children and Adolescents, 133, 262

Perceived Efficacy and Goal Setting System (PEGS), 88

Performance Assessment of Self Care Skills (PASS), 245

Person in Environment System, 283

Personal Projects Analysis (PPA), 290-291

Physical Self-Maintenance Scale (PSMS), 224-225

Play History, 131-132

Preferences for Activities of Children (PAC), 267

Reintegration to Normal Living Index, 302

Revised Knox Preschool Play Scale (PPS-R), 140-141

Role Checklist, 284

School Function Assessment (SFA), 96-97, 112-113

Social Problem Questionnaire, 281

Social Support Inventory for People with Disabilities (SSIDP), 308

Spinal Function Sort, 175-176

Structured Assessment of Independent Living Skills (SAILS), 246

Structured Observation and Report Technique (SORT), 298

Test of Grocery Shopping Skills, 247

Test of Playfulness (ToP) Version 4, 136-137

Transdisciplinary Play-Based Assessment (TPBA) 2nd Ed., 144-145

Valpar Component Work Samples (VCWS), 174

Vineland Adaptive Behavior Scales (VABS), 100

Worker Role Interview, 340-341

World Health Organization-Disability Schedule II (WHO-DAS II), 123

COMMUNICATION

ADL Situational Test, 238

Arnadottir OT-ADL Neurobehavioral Evaluation (A-ONE), 192-193

Assessment of Ludic Behaviors (ALB), 134

Assessment of Occupational Functioning—Collaborative Version, 280-281

Canadian Occupational Performance Measure (COPM), 86, 173

Caregiver Assessment of Functional Dependence and Upset (CAFU), 240

Child-Initiated Pretend Play Assessment (ChIPPA), 142-143

Children's Assessment of Participation and Enjoyment (CAPE), 110-111, 266-266

Coping Inventory for Children, 98

Direct Assessment of Functional Abilities (DAFA), 242

Direct Assessment of Functional Status (DAFS), 241

Experience Sampling Method (ESM), 296-297

Functional Autonomy Measurement System (SMAF), 202-203

Functional Independence Measure (FIM) & WeeFIM, 204-207

Home Observation for Measurement of the Environment (HOME), 321-322

Life Habits Assessment (LIFE-H), 119-120

National Institutes of Health Activity Record (ACTRE), 294-295

Occupational Questionnaire (OQ), 292-293

Patient Specific Function Scale (PSFS), 219-220

Pediatric Evaluation of Disability Inventory (PEDI), 221-223

Performance Assessment of Self Care Skills (PASS), 245

Personal Projects Analysis (PPA), 291-292

Preferences for Activities of Children (PAC), 267-268

Revised Knox Preschool Play Scale (PPS-R), 140-141

School Function Assessment (SFA), 96-97, 112-113

Structured Assessment of Independent Living Skills (SAILS), 246

Structured Observation and Report Technique (SORT), 298

Test of Playfulness (ToP) Version 4, 136-137

Transdisciplinary Play-Based Assessment (TPBA) 2nd Ed., 144-145

Valpar Component Work Samples (VCWS), 174

Vineland Adaptive Behavior Scales (VABS), 100

World Health Organization—Disability Schedule II (WHO-DAS II), 123

MOBILITY

Activities Scale for Kids (ASK), 190-191

Activity Card Sort (ACS), 115-116, 258-259

ADL Situational Test, 238

Arnadottir OT-ADL Neurobehavioral Evaluation (A-ONE), 192-193

Arthritis Impact Measurement Scales (AIMS), 194-196

Assessment of Ludic Behaviors (ALB), 134

Assessment of Motor and Process Skills (AMPS), 239

Assessment of Occupational Functioning—Collaborative Version, 280-281

Barthel Index (BI), 197-199

Canadian Occupational Performance Measure (COPM), 86, 173

Child Health Questionnaire (CHQ), 200-201

Children's Assessment of Participation and Enjoyment (CAPE), 110-111, 265-266

Children's Health Assessment Questionnaire (CHAQ), 208-210

Craig Handicap Assessment and Reporting Technique (CHART), 121-122, 270-271, 303

Early Coping Inventory, 99

Experience Sampling Method (ESM), 296-297

Extended Activities of Daily Living Scale (EADLS), 243

Functional Autonomy Measurement System (SMAF), 202-203

Health Assessment Questionnaire (HAQ), 208-210

Interest Checklist and Activity Checklist, 263-264

Job Content Questionnaire (JCQ), 167-168

Juvenile Arthritis Functional Assessment Report (JAFAR), 211-212

Juvenile Arthritis Functional Assessment Scale (JAFAS), 211-212

Juvenile Arthritis Self-Report Index (JASI), 213-214

Katz Index of Activities of Daily Living, 215-216

Leisure Activity Profile (LAP), 269

Leisure Competence Measure (LCM), 254-255

Leisure Diagnostic Battery, 272-273

Leisure Diagnostic Battery (LDB), 274-275

Life Habits Assessment (LIFE-H), 119-120

London Handicap Scale, 117-118

National Institutes of Health Activity Record (ACTRE), 294-295

Occupational Questionnaire (OQ), 292-293

Patient Specific Function Scale (PSFS), 219-220

Pediatric Activity Card Sort (PACS), 114, 135, 260-261

Pediatric Evaluation of Disability Inventory (PEDI), 221-223

Perceived Efficacy and Goal Setting System (PEGS), 88

Performance Assessment of Self Care Skills (PASS), 245

Personal Care Participation Assessment and Resource Tool (PC-PART), 124-126

Personal Projects Analysis (PPA), 290-291

Physical Self-Maintenance Scale (PSMS), 224-225

Preferences for Activities of Children (PAC), 267-268

Revised Knox Preschool Play Scale (PPS-R), 140-141

School Function Assessment (SFA), 96-97, 112-113

Spinal Function Sort, 175-176

Structured Assessment of Independent Living Skills (SAILS), 246

Structured Observation and Report Technique (SORT), 308

Transdisciplinary Play-Based Assessment (TPBA) 2nd Ed., 144-145

Valpar Component Work Samples (VCWS), 174

Vineland Adaptive Behavior Scales (VABS), 100

Worker Role Interview, 169-170

World Health Organization—Disability Schedule II (WHO-DAS II), 123

SELF-CARE

Activities Scale for Kids (ASK), 190-191

Activity Card Sort (ACS), 115-116, 258-259

ADL Situational Test, 238

Arnadottir OT-ADL Neurobehavioral Evaluation (A-ONE), 192-193

Arthritis Impact Measurement Scales (AIMS), 194-196

Assessment of Motor and Process Skills (AMPS), 239

Assessment of Occupational Functioning—Collaborative Version, 280-281

Barthel Index (BI), 197-199

Canadian Occupational Performance Measure (COPM), 86, 173

Caregiver Assessment of Functional Dependence and Upset (CAFU), 240

Child Health Questionnaire (CHQ), 200-201

Children's Health Assessment Questionnaire (CHAQ), 208-210

Craig Handicap Assessment and Reporting Technique (CHART), 121-122, 270-271, 303

Direct Assessment of Functional Abilities (DAFA), 242

Direct Assessment of Functional Status (DAFS), 241

Experience Sampling Method (ESM), 296-297

Extended Activities of Daily Living Scale (EADLS), 243

Functional Autonomy Measurement System (SMAF), 202-203

Functional Independence Measure (FIM) & WeeFIM, 204-207

Health Assessment Questionnaire (HAQ), 208-210

Interest Checklist and Activity Checklist, 263-264

Juvenile Arthritis Functional Assessment Report (JAFAR), 211-212

Juvenile Arthritis Functional Assessment Scale (JAFAS), 211-212

Juvenile Arthritis Self-Report Index (JASI), 213-214

Katz Index of Activities of Daily Living, 215-216

Kitchen Task Assessment, 244

Life Habits Assessment (LIFE-H), 119-120

London Handicap Scale, 117-118

Melville Nelson Self-Care Assessment, 217-218

Memory and Behavior Problems Checklist: Revised, 101-102

National Institutes of Health Activity Record (ACTRE), 296-297

Occupational Performance History Interview II, 84, 171-172

Occupational Questionnaire (OQ), 292-293

Occupational Self-Assessment, 85

Patient Specific Function Scale (PSFS), 219-220

Pediatric Activity Card Sort (PACS), 114, 135, 260-261

Pediatric Evaluation of Disability Inventory (PEDI), 221-223

Performance Assessment of Self Care Skills (PASS), 245

Personal Care Participation Assessment and Resource Tool (PC-PART), 124-126

Personal Projects Analysis (PPA), 292-293

Physical Self-Maintenance Scale (PSMS), 222-223

Reintegration to Normal Living Index, 302

School Function Assessment (SFA), 96-97, 112-113

Structured Assessment of Independent Living Skills (SAILS), 246

Structured Observation and Report Technique (SORT), 298

Vineland Adaptive Behavior Scales (VABS), 100

World Health Organization—Disability Schedule II (WHO-DAS II), 123

DOMESTIC LIFE

Activity Card Sort (ACS), 115-116, 258-259

Adolescent Role Assessment, 278

Arthritis Impact Measurement Scales (AIMS), 194-196

Assessment of Motor and Process Skills (AMPS), 239

Assessment of Occupational Functioning—Collaborative Version, 280-281

Canadian Occupational Performance Measure (COPM), 86, 173

Caregiver Assessment of Functional Dependence and Upset (CAFU), 240

Children's Assessment of Participation and Enjoyment (CAPE), 110-111, 265-267

Community Integration Questionnaire, 304

Direct Assessment of Functional Abilities (DAFA), 242

Direct Assessment of Functional Status (DAFS), 241

Experience Sampling Method (ESM), 296-297

Extended Activities of Daily Living Scale (EADLS), 243

Functional Autonomy Measurement System (SMAF), 202-203

Functional Independence Measure (FIM) & WeeFIM, 204-207

Interest Checklist & Activity Checklist, 177

Juvenile Arthritis Functional Assessment Report (JAFAR), 211-212

Juvenile Arthritis Functional Assessment Scale (JAFAS), 211-212

Juvenile Arthritis Self-Report Index (JASI), 213-214

Katz Index of Activities of Daily Living, 215-216

Life Habits Assessment (LIFE-H), 119-120

London Handicap Scale, 117-118

National Institutes of Health Activity Record (ACTRE), 294-295

Occupational Performance History Interview II, 84, 171-172

Occupational Questionnaire (OQ), 292-293

Occupational Self-Assessment, 279

Parenting Stress Index (PSI), 95-96

Patient Specific Function Scale (PSFS), 219-220

Personal Care Participation Assessment and Resource Tool (PC-PART), 124-126

Personal Projects Analysis (PPA), 290-291

Preferences for Activities of Children (PAC), 267-268

Role Checklist, 284

Structured Observation and Report Technique (SORT), 298

Test of Grocery Shopping Skills, 247

World Health Organization—Disability Schedule II (WHO-DAS II), 123

INTERPERSONAL INTERACTIONS AND RELATIONSHIPS

Activity Card Sort (ACS), 115-116, 258-259

Adolescent Role Assessment, 278

Assessment of Occupational Functioning—Collaborative Version, 280-281

Canadian Occupational Performance Measure (COPM), 86, 173

Child Behaviors Inventory of Playfulness (CBIP), 138-139

Child Health Questionnaire (CHQ), 200-201

Child-Initiated Pretend Play Assessment (ChIPPA), 142-143

Children's Assessment of Participation and Enjoyment (CAPE), 110-111, 265-266

Community Integration Questionnaire, 305

Coping Inventory for Children, 98

Craig Handicap Assessment and Reporting Technique (CHART), 121-122, 270-271, 303

Direct Assessment of Functional Abilities (DAFA), 242

Early Coping Inventory, 99

Experience Sampling Method (ESM), 296-297

Extended Activities of Daily Living Scale (EADLS), 243

Functional Behavior Profile (FBP), 102-103

Home Observation for Measurement of the Environment (HOME), 148-149

Interpersonal Support Evaluation List, 307

Interview Schedule for Social Interaction (ISSI), 309

Job Content Questionnaire (JCQ), 167-168

Leisure Activity Profile (LAP), 269

Leisure Competence Measure (LCM), 254-255

Leisure Diagnostic Battery, 272-273

Leisure Satisfaction Questionnaire/Leisure Satisfaction Scale (LSS), 274-275

Life Habits Assessment (LIFE-H), 119-120

London Handicap Scale, 117-118

Memory and Behavior Problems Checklist: Revised, 101-102

National Institutes of Health Activity Record (ACTRE), 294-295

Occupational Questionnaire (OQ), 292-293

Parenting Stress Index (PSI), 95-96

Patient Specific Function Scale (PSFS), 219-220

Pediatric Evaluation of Disability Inventory (PEDI), 221-223

Pediatric Interest Profiles: Survey of Play for Children and Adolescents, 133, 262

Perceived Efficacy and Goal Setting System (PEGS), 88

Person in Environment System, 283

Personal Projects Analysis (PPA), 291-292

Play History, 131-132

Preferences for Activities of Children (PAC), 114, 135, 260-261

Reintegration to Normal Living Index, 302

Revised Knox Preschool Play Scale (PPS-R), 140-141

Role Checklist, 284

School Function Assessment (SFA), 96-97, 112-113

Social Problem Questionnaire, 283

Social Support Inventory for People with Disabilities (SSIDP), 308

Structured Assessment of Independent Living Skills (SAILS), 246

Structured Observation and Report Technique (SORT), 298

Test of Grocery Shopping Skills, 247

Test of Playfulness (ToP) Version 4, 136-137

Transdisciplinary Play-Based Assessment (TPBA) 2nd Ed., 144-145

Valpar Component Work Samples (VCWS), 174

Vineland Adaptive Behavior Scales (VABS), 100

World Health Organization—Disability Schedule II (WHO-DAS II), 123

Learning and Applying Knowledge

Activity Card Sort (ACS), 115-116, 258-259

Adolescent Role Assessment, 278

Assessment of Ludic Behaviors (ALB) 134

Assessment of Motor and Process Skills (AMPS), 239

Assessment of Occupational Functioning—Collaborative Version, 280-281

Canadian Occupational Performance Measure (COPM), 86, 173

Child-Initiated Pretend Play Assessment (ChIPPA), 142-143

Children's Assessment of Participation and Enjoyment (CAPE), 110-111, 265-266

Coping Inventory for Children, 98

Direct Assessment of Functional Abilities (DAFA), 242

Early Coping Inventory, 99

Experience Sampling Method (ESM), 296-297

Functional Autonomy Measurement System (SMAF), 202-203

Functional Behavior Profile (FBP), 102-103

Interest Checklist and Activity Checklist, 263-264

Interpersonal Support Evaluation List, 307

Job Content Questionnaire (JCQ), 167-168

Kitchen Task Assessment, 244

Leisure Activity Profile (LAP), 269

Leisure Boredom Scale, 253

Leisure Competence Measure (LCM), 254-255

Leisure Diagnostic Battery, 272-273

Leisure Diagnostic Battery (LDB), 274-275

Leisure Satisfaction Questionnaire/Leisure Satisfaction Scale (LSS), 256-257

Life Habits Assessment (LIFE-H), 119-120

London Handicap Scale, 117-118

Memory and Behavior Problems Checklist: Revised, 101-102

National Institutes of Health Activity Record (ACTRE), 294-295

Occupational Questionnaire (OQ), 292-293

Occupational Role History, 279

Patient Specific Function Scale (PSFS), 219-220

Pediatric Activity Card Sort (PACS), 114, 135, 260-261

Perceived Efficacy and Goal Setting System (PEGS), 88

Performance Assessment of Self Care Skills (PASS), 245

Personal Projects Analysis (PPA), 290-291

Play History, 131-132

Preferences for Activities of Children (PAC), 267-268

Reintegration to Normal Living Index, 302

Revised Knox Preschool Play Scale (PPS-R), 140-141

School Function Assessment (SFA), 96-97, 112-113

Structured Assessment of Independent Living Skills (SAILS), 246

Structured Observation and Report Technique (SORT), 300

Test of Grocery Shopping Skills, 247

Transdisciplinary Play-Based Assessment (TPBA) 2nd Ed., 144-145

Valpar Component Work Samples (VCWS), 174

Vineland Adaptive Behavior Scales (VABS), 100

Worker Role Interview, 169-170

Major Life Areas

Activity Card Sort (ACS), 115-116, 258-259

Adolescent Role Assessment, 278

Arthritis Impact Measurement Scales (AIMS), 194-196

Assessment of Occupational Functioning—Collaborative Version, 280-281

Canadian Occupational Performance Measure (COPM), 86, 173

Caregiver Assessment of Functional Dependence and Upset (CAFU), 240

Children's Assessment of Participation and Enjoyment (CAPE), 110-111, 265-266

Community Integration Questionnaire, 304

Craig Handicap Assessment and Reporting Technique (CHART), 121-122, 270-271, 303

Direct Assessment of Functional Abilities (DAFA), 242

Direct Assessment of Functional Status (DAFS), 241

Early Coping Inventory, 99

Experience Sampling Method (ESM), 296-297

Feasibility Evaluation Checklist, 177

Interpersonal Support Evaluation List, 307

Job Content Questionnaire (JCQ), 167-168

Juvenile Arthritis Functional Assessment Report (JAFAR), 211-212

Juvenile Arthritis Functional Assessment Scale (JAFAS), 211-212

Juvenile Arthritis Self-Report Index (JASI), 213-214

Leisure Activity Profile (LAP), 269

Life Habits Assessment (LIFE-H), 119-120

Life Role Salience Scale, 282

Life Stressors and Social Resources Inventory—Adult Form (LISRES-A), 338-339

London Handicap Scale, 117-118

National Institutes of Health Activity Record (ACTRE), 294-295

Occupational Performance History Interview II, 84, 171-172

Occupational Questionnaire (OQ), 292-293

Occupational Role History, 279

Occupational Self-Assessment, 85

Patient Specific Function Scale (PSFS), 219-220

Pediatric Activity Card Sort (PACS), 114, 135, 260-261

Perceived Efficacy and Goal Setting System (PEGS), 88

Performance Assessment of Self Care Skills (PASS), 245

Personal Projects Analysis (PPA), 290-291

Preferences for Activities of Children (PAC), 267-268

Reintegration to Normal Living Index, 302

Role Checklist, 284

Social Problem Questionnaire, 281

Spinal Function Sort, 175-176

Structured Assessment of Independent Living Skills (SAILS), 246

Structured Observation and Report Technique (SORT), 298

Valpar Component Work Samples (VCWS), 174

Vineland Adaptive Behavior Scales (VABS), 100

Worker Role Interview, 169-170

COMMUNITY, SOCIAL, AND CIVIC LIFE

Activity Card Sort (ACS), 115-116, 258-259

ADL Situational Test, 240

Adolescent Role Assessment, 278

Arthritis Impact Measurement Scales (AIMS), 194-196

Assessment of Occupational Functioning—Collaborative Version, 280-281

Canadian Occupational Performance Measure (COPM), 86, 173

Caregiver Assessment of Functional Dependence and Upset (CAFU), 240

Children's Assessment of Participation and Enjoyment (CAPE), 110-111, 265-266

Community Integration Measure, 305

Community Integration Questionnaire, 304

Coping Inventory for Children, 98

Craig Handicap Assessment and Reporting Technique (CHART), 121-122, 270-271, 303

Direct Assessment of Functional Abilities (DAFA), 242

Direct Assessment of Functional Status (DAFS), 241

Early Coping Inventory, 99

Experience Sampling Method (ESM), 296-297

Functional Autonomy Measurement System (SMAF), 202-203

Functional Behavior Profile (FBP), 102-103

Home Observation for Measurement of the Environment (HOME), 148-149

Interest Checklist and Activity Checklist, 263-264

Interpersonal Support Evaluation List, 307

Interview Schedule for Social Interaction (ISSI), 309

Juvenile Arthritis Functional Assessment Report (JAFAR), 211-212

Juvenile Arthritis Functional Assessment Scale (JAFAS), 211-212

Juvenile Arthritis Self-Report Index (JASI), 213-214

Katz Index of Activities of Daily Living, 215-216

Leisure Activity Profile (LAP), 269

Leisure Competence Measure (LCM), 254-255

Leisure Diagnostic Battery, 272-273

Leisure Satisfaction Questionnaire/Leisure Satisfaction Scale (LSS), 256-257

Life Habits Assessment (LIFE-H), 119-120

Life Role Salience Scale, 282

Life Stressors and Social Resources Inventory—Adult Form (LISRES-A), 338-339

London Handicap Scale, 117-118

Memory and Behavior Problems Checklist: Revised, 101-102

Multidimensional Scale of Perceived Social Support (MSPSS), 335-336

National Institutes of Health Activity Record (ACTRE), 294-295

Occupational Questionnaire (OQ), 292-293

Patient Specific Function Scale (PSFS), 219-220

Pediatric Activity Card Sort (PACS), 114, 135, 260-261

Pediatric Evaluation of Disability Inventory (PEDI), 221-223

Perceived Efficacy and Goal Setting System (PEGS), 88

Person in Environment System, 283

Personal Projects Analysis (PPA), 290-291

Play History, 131-132

Preferences for Activities of Children (PAC), 267-268

Role Checklist, 284

Structured Observation and Report Technique (SORT), 298

Vineland Adaptive Behavior Scales (VABS), 100

World Health Organization—Disability Schedule II (WHO-DAS II), 123

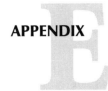

APPENDIX

OUTCOME MEASURES RATING FORMS AND GUIDELINES

OUTCOME MEASURES RATING FORM
CANCHILD CENTRE FOR DISABILITY RESEARCH
INSTITUTE OF APPLIED HEALTH SCIENCES, MCMASTER UNIVERSITY
1400 MAIN STREET WEST, ROOM 408
HAMILTON, ONTARIO, CANADA L8S 1C7
Fax (905) 522-6095
lawm@mcmaster.ca

To be used with: Outcome Measures Rating Form Guidelines (CanChild, 2004)

Name and initials of measure: _____

Author(s): _____
_____

Source and year published: _____
_____

Date of review: _____

Name of reviewer: _____

1. Focus

A. *Focus of measurement—Using the ICF framework*

❏ Body functions................. Are the physiological functions of body systems (includes psychological functions).

❏ Body structures................. Are anatomical parts of the body such as organs, limbs, and their components.

❏ Activities and participation....Activity is the execution of a task or action by an individual. Participation is involvement in a life situation.

❏ Environmental factors...........Make up the physical, social and attitudinal environment in which people live and conduct their lives.

B. *Attribute(s) being measured—Check as many as apply.*

This list is based on attributes cited in the ICF, 2001: WHO.

Body Functions

Global mental functions

❏ Consciousness   ❏ Intellectual   ❏ Temperament and personality

❑ Orientation   ❑ Global psychosocial   ❑ Energy and drive
❑ Sleep

Specific mental functions
❑ Attention   ❑ Thought   ❑ Mental functions of language
❑ Memory   ❑ Higher level cognitive   ❑ Experience of self and time
❑ Psychomotor   ❑ Calculation   ❑ Perceptual
❑ Mental function of sequencing complex measurements

Sensory functions and pain
❑ Seeing and related   ❑ Hearing and vestibular

Voice and speech functions
❑ Voice   ❑ Fluency and rhythm of speech
❑ Articulation   ❑ Alternative vocalization

Functions of the cardiovascular, hematological, immunological, and respiratory systems
❑ Cardiovascular   ❑ Respiratory system
❑ Hematological and   ❑ Additional functions and sensations of the
   immunological systems   cardiovascular and respiratory systems

Functions of the digestive, metabolic and endocrine systems
❑ Related to the digestive   ❑ Related to metabolism
   system   and the endocrine system

Genitourinary and reproductive functions
❑ Urinary   ❑ Genital and reproductive

Neuromuscular and movement-related functions
Joints and Bones   ❑ Mobility of joint   ❑ Mobility of bone
                       ❑ Stability of joint

Muscle   ❑ Muscle power   ❑ Muscle endurance
                       ❑ Muscle tone

Movement   ❑ Motor reflex   ❑ Involuntary movement
                       ❑ Involuntary movement   ❑ Sensations related to muscle
                          reaction   and movement
                       ❑ Control of voluntary   ❑ Gait patterns
                          movement

Functions of the skin and related structures
Skin   ❑ Protection   ❑ Other functions
                       ❑ Repair   ❑ Sensations
Hair   ❑ Function of the hair
Nails   ❑ Function of nails

Body Structures
Structures of the nervous system
❑ Brain   ❑ Spinal cord and related structures
❑ Meninges   ❑ Sympathetic nervous system
❑ Parasympathetic nervous system

Eye, ear, and related structures
❑ Eye socket   ❑ Around eye   ❑ Middle ear
❑ Eyeball   ❑ External ear   ❑ Inner ear

Structures involved in voice and speech

❑ Nose   ❑ Pharynx
❑ Mouth   ❑ Larynx

Structures of the cardiovascular, immunological, and respiratory systems

Cardiovascular system   ❑ Heart   ❑ Veins
                              ❑ Arteries   ❑ Capillaries

Immune system   ❑ Lymphatic vessels ❑ Lymphatic nodes
                              ❑ Thymus   ❑ Spleen
                              ❑ Bone marrow

Respiratory system   ❑ Trachea   ❑ Lungs
                              ❑ Thoracic cage   ❑ Muscles of respiration

Structures related to the digestive, metabolic, and endocrine systems

❑ Salivary glands   ❑ Pancreas   ❑ Intestines
❑ Oesophagus   ❑ Liver   ❑ Endocrine glands
❑ Stomach   ❑ Gall bladder

Structures related to the genitourinary and reproductive systems

❑ Urinary system   ❑ Pelvic floor   ❑ Reproductive system

Structures related to movement

❑ Head and neck   ❑ Shoulder region   ❑ Lower extremity
❑ Upper extremity   ❑ Trunk   ❑ Pelvic region
❑ Additional musculoskeletal structures related to movement

Skin and related structures

❑ Skin   ❑ Skin and glands
❑ Nails   ❑ Hair

Activities and Participation

Learning and applying knowledge

Purposeful sensory   ❑ Watching   ❑ Other purposeful sensing
                              ❑ Experiences   ❑ Listening

Basic learning   ❑ Copying   ❑ Rehearsing
                              ❑ Learning to read   ❑ Learning to write
                              ❑ Learning to calculate ❑ Acquiring skills

Applying knowledge   ❑ Focusing attention ❑ Calculating
                              ❑ Thinking   ❑ Solving problems
                              ❑ Reading   ❑ Making decisions
                              ❑ Writing

General tasks and demand

                              ❑ Undertaking a single task   ❑ Undertaking multiple tasks
                              ❑ Carrying out daily routine   ❑ Handling stress and other psychological demands

Communication

                              ❑ Receiving (verbal, nonverbal, written, formal sign language)
                              ❑ Producing (verbal, nonverbal, written, formal sign language)
                              ❑ Conversation and use of communication devices and techniques

Mobility

- ❏ Changing and maintaining body position
- ❏ Walking and moving
- ❏ Carrying, moving, and handling objects
- ❏ Moving around using transportation

Self-care

- ❏ Washing oneself
- ❏ Caring for body parts
- ❏ Toileting
- ❏ Dressing
- ❏ Eating
- ❏ Drinking

Looking after one's health

- ❏ Ensuring oneself physical comfort
- ❏ Maintaining one's health
- ❏ Managing diet and fitness

Domestic life

Acquisition of necessities

- ❏ Acquiring a place to live
- ❏ Acquisition of goods and services

Household tasks

- ❏ Preparing meals
- ❏ Doing housework
- ❏ Caring for household objects and assisting others

Interpersonal interactions and relationships

General

- ❏ General interpersonal interactions (basic and complex)

Particular interpersonal

- ❏ Informal social relationships
- ❏ Relating with strangers

Relationships

- ❏ Family relationships
- ❏ Intimate relationships
- ❏ Formal relationships

Major life areas

Education

- ❏ Informal
- ❏ Preschool
- ❏ School

Work and employment

- ❏ Apprenticeship
- ❏ Acquiring, keeping, and terminating a job
- ❏ Renumerative employment
- ❏ Non-renumerative employment

Economic life

- ❏ Basic economic transactions
- ❏ Complex economic transactions
- ❏ Economic self-sufficiency

Community, social and civic life

Community

- ❏ Community life

Recreation and leisure

- ❏ Play
- ❏ Sports
- ❏ Arts and culture
- ❏ Crafts
- ❏ Hobbies
- ❏ Socializing

Civic

- ❏ Religion and spirituality
- ❏ Human rights
- ❏ Political life and citizenship

Environmental Factors

Products and technology

- ❏ Communication
- ❏ Culture, recreation, and sport
- ❏ Design, construction, and buildings for public use
- ❏ Religion and spirituality
- ❏ Education
- ❏ Products or substances for personal consumption
- ❏ Design, construction, and buildings for private use
- ❏ Land development
- ❏ Employment
- ❏ Products and technology for personal use in daily living
- ❏ For personal indoor and outdoor mobility and transportation
- ❏ Assets

Natural environment and human-made changes to environment

☐ Physical geography   ☐ Sound   ☐ Human events

☐ Flora and fauna   ☐ Air quality   ☐ Time-related changes

☐ Natural events   ☐ Population   ☐ Vibration

☐ Light   ☐ Climate

Support and relationships

☐ Immediate family   ☐ Extended family   ☐ Friends

☐ Health professionals   ☐ Other professionals   ☐ Strangers

☐ People in positions of authority   ☐ People in subordinate positions   ☐ Personal care providers and personal assistants

☐ Acquaintances, peers, colleagues, neighbors, and community members   ☐ Domesticated animals

Attitudes

☐ Of immediate family   ☐ Of extended family   ☐ Of friends

☐ Of strangers   ☐ Of health professionals   ☐ Of health-related professionals

☐ Of people in positions of authority   ☐ Of people in subordinate positions   ☐ Of personal care providers and personal assistants

☐ Of acquaintances, peers, colleagues, neighbors, and community members   ☐ Societal attitudes   ☐ Social norms, practices, and ideologies

Services, systems, and policies

☐ Production of consumer goods   ☐ Architecture and construction   ☐ Associations and organizations

☐ Open space planning   ☐ Social security   ☐ Clvil protection

☐ Utilities   ☐ Health   ☐ Economic

☐ Transportation   ☐ Labor and employment   ☐ General social support

☐ Legal   ☐ Housing   ☐ Education and training

☐ Media   ☐ Communication   ☐ Political

C. Does this measure assess a single attribute or multiple attributes?

☐ Single

☐ Multiple

D. Check purposes that apply and indicate (*) primary purpose of the measure

☐ To describe or discriminate

☐ To predict

☐ To evaluative

Comments:_____

_____

E. Perspective—Indicate possible respondents

☐ Client   ☐ Other professional

☐ Caregiver/parent   ☐ Other

☐ Service provider

F. Population measure designed for:

Age: Please specify all applicable ages if stated in the manual

❐ Infant (birth to <1 year)   ❐ Adult (>18 years to <65 years)

❐ Child (1 year to <13 years)   ❐ Senior (>65 years)

❐ Adolescent (13 to <18 years) ❐ Age not specified

Diagnosis:

List the diagnostic group(s) for which this measure is designed to be used:_____

_____

_____

G. Evaluation context—Indicate suggested/possible environments for this assessment

❐ Home   ❐ Education setting   ❐ Community

❐ Workplace   ❐ Community agency   ❐ Rehabilitation center/health care setting

❐ Other_____

2. Clinical Utility

A. Clarity of Instructions (Check one of the ratings)

❐ Excellent: Clear, comprehensive, concise, and available

❐ Adequate: Clear, concise, but lacks some information

❐ Poor: Not clear and concise or not available

Comments:_____

_____

B. Format (check applicable items)

❐ Interview

❐ Naturalistic observation

❐ Task performance

❐ Questionnaire: ❐ Self completed

                            ❐ Interview administered

                            ❐ Caregiver completed

❐ Other_____

Physically invasive: ❐ Yes   ❐ No

Active participation of client: ❐ Yes   ❐ No

Special equipment required: ❐ Yes   ❐ No

C. Time to complete assessment: _____ *minutes*

Administration: ❐ Easy   ❐ More complex

Scoring: ❐ Easy   ❐ More complex

Interpretation: ❐ Easy   ❐ More complex

(Consider time, amount of training, and ease)

D. Examiner qualifications: Is formal training required for administering and/or interpreting?

❐ Required   ❐ Recommended   ❐ Not required

❐ Not addressed

E. Cost (Canadian Funds)

Manual: $_____

Score sheets: $_____ for _____ sheets

Indicate year of cost information:_____

Source of cost information:_____

F. Manual (check one of the ratings)

❏ Excellent: Published manual which outlines specific procedures for administration, scoring and interpretation, evidence of reliability and validity

❏ Adequate: Manual available and generally complete but some information is lacking or unclear regarding administration, scoring and interpretation, evidence of reliability and validity

❏ Poor: No manual available or manual with unclear administration, scoring and interpretation, no evidence of reliability and validity

G. Overall Clinical Utility

❏ Excellent: Excellent manual or published document, acceptable to client, feasible to purchase, administer, score, and interpret

❏ Adequate: Adequate to excellent manual or published document; some area of concern in terms of feasibility recost, time, complexity, acceptability

❏ Poor: Poor/no manual or not feasible due to major concerns of cost, time, complexity, or acceptability

3. Scale Construction

A. Which specific domain does this measure assess?

❏ Physical   ❏ Psychological   ❏ Social

❏ School functioning   ❏ Environmental   ❏ Personal care

❏ Other

B. Item Selection (check one of the ratings)

❏ Excellent: Included all relevant characteristics of attribute based on comprehensive literature review and survey of experts

❏ Adequate: Included most relevant characteristics of attribute

❏ Poor: Convenient sample of characteristics of attribute

Comments:_____

_____

C. Weighting

Are the items weighted in the calculation of total score?   ❏ Yes   ❏ No

If yes, are the items weighted?   ❏ Implicitly   ❏ Explicitly

D. Level of Measurement

❏ Nominal   ❏ Ordinal   ❏ Interval

❏ Ratio

Scaling method (Likert, Guttman, etc.):_____

Number of items:_____

Indicate if subscale scores are obtained: ❏ Yes   ❏ No

If yes, can the subscale scores be used alone?

Administered: ❏ Yes   ❏ No

Interpreted: ❏ Yes   ❏ No

List subscales: Number of items:

_____   _____

_____   _____

_____   _____

_____   _____

_____   _____

4. Standardization

A. Norms available (N/A for instrument whose purpose is only evaluative)

❏ Yes   ❏ No   ❏ N/A

Age: Please specify all applicable ages for which norms are available

❏ Infant (birth to <1 year)   ❏ Adult (>18 years to <65 years)

❏ Child (1 year to <13 years)   ❏ Senior (>65 years)

❏ Adolescent (13 to <18 years)

Populations for which it is normed:

_____

_____

Size of sample: n = _____

5. Reliability

A. Rigor of standardization studies for reliability (check one of the ratings)

❏ Excellent: More than 2 well-designed reliability studies completed with adequate to excellent reliability values

❏ Adequate: 1 to 2 well-designed reliability studies completed with adequate to excellent reliability values

❏ Poor: Reliability studies poorly completed, or reliability studies showing poor levels of reliability

❏ No evidence available

Comments:_____

_____

B. Reliability Information

Type of reliability	Statistic used	Value	Rating (excellent, adequate, poor)
_____	_____	_____	_____
_____	_____	_____	_____
_____	_____	_____	_____

*Guidelines for levels of reliability coefficient (see instructions)

Excellent: >0.80   Adequate: 0.60 to 0.79   Poor: <0.60

6. Validity

A. Rigor of standardization studies for validity (check one of the ratings)

❏ Excellent: More than 2 well-designed validity studies supporting the measure's validity

❏ Adequate: 1 to 2 well-designed validity studies supporting the measure's validity

❏ Poor: Validity studies poorly completed or did not support the measure's validity

❏ No evidence available

Comments:_____

_____

B. Content validity (Check one of the ratings)

❏ Excellent: Judgmental or statistical method (e.g., factor analysis) was used and the measure is comprehensive and includes items suited to the measurement purpose

Method: ❏ Judgmental   ❏ Statistical

❏ Adequate: Has content validity but no specific method was used

❏ Poor: Instrument is not comprehensive

❏ No evidence available

C. Construct validity (Check one of the ratings)

❏ Excellent: More than 2 well-designed studies have shown that the instrument conforms to prior theoretical relationships among characteristics or individuals

❏ Adequate: 1 to 2 studies demonstrate confirmation of theoretical formulations

❏ Poor: Construct validation poorly completed, or did not support measure's construct validity

❏ No evidence available

Strength of association:_____

_____

D. Criterion validity (Check ratings that apply)

❏ Concurrent   ❏ Predictive

❏ Excellent: More than 2 well-designed studies have shown adequate agreement with a criterion or gold standard

❏ Adequate: 1 to 2 studies demonstrate adequate agreement with a criterion or gold standard measure

❏ Poor: Criterion validation poorly completed or did not support measure's criterion validity

❏ No evidence available

Criterion measure(s) used: _____

_____

Strength of association:_____

_____

E. Responsiveness (Check one of the ratings)

❏ Excellent: More that 2 well-designed studies showing strong hypothesized relationships between changes on the measure and other measures of change on the same attribute.

❏ Adequate: 1 to 2 studies of responsiveness

❏ Poor: Studies of responsiveness poorly completed or did not support the measure's responsiveness

❏ N/A

❏ No evidence available

Comments:_____

_____

7. Overall Utility
(Based on an Overall Assessment of the Quality of This Measure)

❏ Excellent: Adequate to excellent clinical utility, easily available, excellent reliability, and validity

❏ Adequate: Adequate to excellent clinical utility, easily available, adequate to excellent reliability, and adequate to excellent validity

❏ Poor: Poor clinical utility, not easily available, poor reliability and validity

Comments/notes/explanations:_____
_____
_____
_____

Materials Used for Review/Rating

Please indicate the sources of information used for this review/rating:

❒ Manual
❒ Journal articles (attach or indicate location)
   ❒ By author of measure
   ❒ By other authors

List sources:_____
_____
_____
_____

❒ Books: Provide reference
❒ Correspondence with author (attach)
❒ Other sources:_____
_____
_____
_____

OUTCOME MEASURES RATING FORM GUIDELINES
CanChild Centre for Childhood Disability Research
Institute of Applied Health Sciences, McMaster University
1400 Main Street West. Room 408
Hamilton, Canada L8S 1C7
fax (905) 522-6095
lawm@mcmaster.ca
Prepared by: Mary Law, Ph.D. O.T.(C)

For further discussion of issues: Law, M. (1987). Measurement in occupational therapy: Scientific criteria for evaluation. *Canadian Journal of Occupational Therapy*, 54, 133-138.
General information: Name of Measure, Authors, Source and Year.

1. Focus

A. *Focus of measurement*. Use the ICF framework to indicate the focus of the measurement instrument that is being reviewed. The definitions are as follows:

- Body Functions: Are the physiological functions of body systems (including psychological functions).
- Body Structures: Are anatomical parts of the body such as organs, limbs and their components.
- Activities and Participation: Activity is the execution of a task or action by an individual. Participation is involvement in a life situation.
- Environmental Factors: Make up the physical, social and attitudinal environment in which people live and conduct their lives.

B. *Attributes being measured*. The rating form lists attributes organized using the ICF framework. Check as many attributes as apply to indicate what is being measured by this instrument.

C. *Single or multiple attribute*. Check the appropriate box to indicate whether this measure assesses a single attribute only or multiple attributes.

D. *List the primary purpose for which the scale has been designed*. Secondary purposes can also be listed but the instrument should be evaluated according to its primary purpose (i.e., discriminative, predictive, evaluative).

Discriminative. A discriminative index is used to distinguish between individuals or groups on an underlying dimension when no external criterion or gold standard is available for validating these measures.

Predictive. A predictive index is used to classify individuals into a set of predefined measurement categories... either concurrently or prospectively, to determine whether individuals have been classified correctly.

Evaluative. An evaluative index is used to measure the magnitude of longitudinal change in an individual or group on the dimension of interest. (Kirshner, B. & Guyatt G. (1985). A methodological framework for assessing health indices. *Journal of Chronic Diseases*, 38, 27-36.)

E. *Perspective*. Indicate the possible respondents.

F. *Population for which it is designed (AGE)*. If no age is stated, mark as age unspecified. List the diagnostic groups for which the measure is used.

G. *Evaluation context*. Refers to the environment in which the assessment is completed. Check all possible environments in which this assessment can be completed.

2. Clinical Utility

A. *Clarity of instructions*. Check one of the ratings. Excellent: clear, comprehensive, concise and available; Adequate: clear, concise but lacks some information; Poor: not clear and concise or not available.

B. *Format*. Check all applicable items to indicate the format of data collection for the instrument. Possible items include naturalistic observation, interview, a questionnaire (self-completed, interview administered or caregiver-completed) and task performance.

Physically invasive. Indicates whether administration of the measure requires procedures that may be perceived as invasive by the client. Examples of invasiveness include any procedure that requires insertion of needles or taping of electrodes, or procedures which require clients to take clothing on or off.

Active participation of client. Indicate whether completion of the measure requires the client to participate verbally or physically.

Special equipment required. Indicate whether the measurement process requires objects which are not part of the test kit and are not everyday objects. Examples of this include stopwatches, a balance board or other special equipment.

C. *Time to complete the assessment.* Record in minutes. For *Administration, Scoring,* and *Interpretation,* consider the time and the amount of training and the ease with which a test is administered, scored and interpreted, and indicate whether these issues are easy or more complex. For *Administration, Scoring,* and *Interpretation* to be rated as easy, each part of the task should be completed in under 1 hour with minimal amount of training and is easy for the average service provider to complete.

D. *Examiner qualifications.* Indicate if formal training is required for administering and interpreting this measure.

E. *Cost.* In Canadian funds, indicate the cost of the measurement manual and score sheets. For *score sheets,* indicate the number of sheets obtainable for that cost. List the *source* and the year of the cost information so readers will know if the information is up to date.

3. Scale Construction

A. *Item selection.* Check one of the ratings. Excellent: included all relevant characteristics of the attribute based on comprehensive literature review and survey of experts—a comprehensive review of the literature only is enough for an excellent rating, but a survey of experts alone is not enough; Adequate: included most relevant characteristics of the attribute; Poor: convenient sample of characteristics of the attribute.

B. *Weighting.* Indicate whether the items in the tool are weighted in the calculation of the total score. If items are weighted, indicate whether the authors have weighted these items implicitly or explicitly. Implicit weighting occurs when there are a number of scales and each have a different number of items and the score is obtained by simply adding the scores for each item together. Explicit weighting occurs when each item or score is multiplied by a factor to weight its importance.

C. *Level of measurement.* State whether the scale used is *nominal* (descriptive categories), *ordinal* (ordered categories), or *interval* or *ratio* (numerical) for single and for summary scores. Indicate the *scaling method* that was used and the *number of items* in the measure. Indicate if *subscale scores* are obtained. Indicate whether the subscales can be administered alone and the scores interpreted alone. In some cases, the scores can be interpreted alone, but the whole measure must be administered first. List the subscales with the number of items and indicate if there is evidence of reliability and validity for the subscales so that the scores can be used on their own. Standardization is the process of administering a test under uniform conditions.

4. Standardization

A. *Manual.* Check one of the ratings. Excellent: published manual which outlines specific procedures for administration; scoring and interpretation; evidence of reliability and validity. Adequate: manual available and generally complete but some information is lacking or unclear regarding administration; scoring and interpretation; evidence of reliability and validity. Poor: no manual available or manual with unclear administration; scoring and interpretation; no evidence of reliability and validity.

B. *Norms.* Indicate whether norms are available for the instrument. Please note that instruments which are only meant to be evaluative do not require norms. Indicate all ages for which norms are available, the *populations* for which the measure has been normed (e.g., children with cerebral palsy, people with spinal cord injuries), and indicate the *size of the sample* that was used in the normative studies.

5. Reliability

Reliability is the process of determining that the test or measure is measuring something in a reproducible and consistent fashion.

A. *Rigour of standardization studies for reliability.* Excellent: More than 2 well designed reliability studies completed with adequate to excellent reliability values; Adequate: 1 to 2 well-designed reliability studies completed with adequate to excellent reliability values; Poor: No reliability studies or poorly completed, or reliability studies showing poor levels of reliability.

B. Reliability information. Internal Consistency: the degree of homogeneity of test items to the attribute being measured. Measured at one point in time. Observer: 1) Intra-observer—Measures variation which occurs within an observer as a result of multiple exposures to the same stimulus, 2) Inter-observer—Measures variation between two or more observers. Test-Retest: Measures variation in the test over a period of time.

Complete the table and reliability information by filling in the *type of reliability* that was tested (internal consistency, observer, test-retest); the *statistic* that was used (e.g., Cronbach's coefficient alpha, kappa coefficient, Pearson correlation, intra-class correlation); the *value* of the statistic that was found in the study; and the *rating* of the reliability. Guidelines for levels of the reliability coefficient indicate that it will be rated excellent if the coefficient is greater than 0.80, adequate if it is from 0.60 to 0.79, and poor if the coefficient is less than 0.60.

6. Validity

A. Rigour of standardization studies for validity. Excellent: More than 2 well designed validity studies supporting the measure's validity; Adequate: 1 to 2 well designed validity studies supporting the measure's validity; Poor: No validity studies completed, studies were poorly completed or did not support the measure's validity.

B. Content validity. Check one of the ratings. *Content validity*: the instrument is comprehensive and fully represents the domain of the characteristics it claims to measure. (Nunnally, J.C. (1978). *Psychometric theory*. New York: McGraw-Hill.) Excellent: Judgmental or statistical method (e.g. factor analysis) was used and the measure is comprehensive and includes items suited to the measurement purpose; Adequate: Has content validity but no specific method was used; Poor: Instrument is not comprehensive. *Method*: Note whether a judgmental (e.g., consensus methods) or statistical method (e.g., factor analysis) of establishing content validity was used.

C. *Construct validity.* The measurements of the attribute conform to prior theoretical formulations or relationships among characteristics or individuals. (Nunnally, J.C. (1978). *Psychometric theory*. New York: McGraw-Hill.) Excellent: More than 2 well-designed studies have shown that the instrument conforms to prior theoretical relationships among characteristics or individuals; Adequate: 1 to 2 studies demonstrate confirmation of theoretical formulations; Poor: No construct validation completed. Indicate the *strength of association* of the findings for construct validity by listing the value of the correlation coefficients found.

D. *Criterion validity.* Check one of the ratings. *Criterion validity*: The measurements obtained by the instrument agree with another more accurate measure of the same characteristic, that is, a criterion or gold standard measure. (Nunnally, J. C. (1978). *Psychometric theory*. New York: McGraw-Hill.) Indicate whether the type of criterion validity which was investigated is concurrent, predictive, or both. Excellent: More than 2 well-designed studies have shown adequate agreement with a criterion or gold standard; Adequate: 1 to 2 studies demonstrate adequate agreement with a criterion or gold standard measure; Poor: No criterion validation completed. Indicate the *strength of association* of the evidence for criterion validity by listing the values of the correlation coefficients which were found in the criterion validity studies. Using the information from the assessment that has been completed on this measure, check the appropriate rating to give an overall assessment of the quality of the measure.

E. *Responsiveness.* Check one of the ratings (applicable only to evaluative measures). *Responsiveness*: The ability of the measure to detect minimal clinically important change over time. (Guyatt, G., Walter, S. D., & Norman, G. R. [1987]. Measuring change over time: Assessing the usefulness of evaluative instruments. *Journal of Chronic Diseases*, 40, 171-178.) Excellent: More that 2 well-designed studies showing strong hypothesized relationships between changes on the measure and other measures of change on the same attribute; Adequate: 1 to 2 studies of responsiveness; Poor: No studies of responsiveness; N/A: Check if the measure is not designed to evaluate change over time.

7. Overall Utility

Excellent: Adequate to excellent clinical utility, easily available, excellent reliability and validity. *Adequate:* Adequate to excellent clinical utility, easily available, adequate to excellent reliability and adequate to excellent validity. *Poor:* Poor clinical utility, not easily available, poor reliability, and validity.

8. Materials Used

Please indicate and list the sources of information that were used for this review. By listing sources of information and attaching appropriate journal articles or correspondence with authors, it will be easier to find further information about this measure if it is required.

INDEX

accuracy, sources of, 69

activities of daily living (ADL), 94, 109, 179–225, 353. *See also* Extended Activities of Daily Living (EADL) Scale; Instrumental Activities of Daily Living (IADL)

Activities Scale for Kids (ASK), 25, 190–191, 386, 390, 391, 392

Activity Card Sort (ACS), 115–116, 258–259, 386, 387, 390, 391, 392, 393, 394, 395

activity specific ADL instruments, 180–181

acuity issues, 50–51

ADL instruments, 180–183, 190–225

ADL Situational Test, 233, 234, 236, 238, 386, 388, 391, 392, 395

administrative policy, 373–374

Adolescent Leisure Interest Profile (ALIP), 133

Adolescent Role Assessment, 277–278, 386, 387, 390, 392, 393, 394, 395

adult day care, 372

Adult Sensory Profile, 57, 61–62

aging, impacting impairment, 50

agnosia, 51–52

Alzheimer's disease, 232–233

Amatea, E. S., 282, 387

American Guidance Service Inc., Vineland Adaptive Behavior, 100, 387

Americans with Disabilities Act (ADA), 372, 378

Accessibility Guidelines (ADAAG), 323

Amigo, E., 241, 388

anomia, testing of, 54

AOTA Code of Ethics, Standards of Practice, 364

aphasia, testing of, 54

Arnadottir, G., 192–193, 387

Arnadottir OT-ADL Neurobehavioral Evaluation (A-ONE), 192–193, 386, 387, 390, 391, 392

Arthritis Impact Measurement Scales (AIMS), 194–196, 386, 388, 390, 391, 392, 394, 395

assessment, 38

    client-centered, 83–87

    of outcome measurement, 41–42

    of performance components and environmental conditions, 35–36

Assessment of Ludic Behavior (ALB), 130, 132, 134, 137, 322, 386, 387, 390, 391, 394

Assessment of Motor and Process Skills (AMPS), 234, 237, 239, 386, 387, 390, 392, 394

Assessment of Occupational Functioning (AOF), 279, 282
    —Collaborative Version (AOF-CV), 279–281, 282, 386, 389, 390, 391, 392, 393, 394, 395

Athreya, B. H., 208–210, 388

audition testing, 54

Balanced Budget Act of 1997, 347–348

Baptiste, S., 86, 173, 388

Baron, K., 85, 387

Barris, R., 284, 388

Barthel, D. W., 197–199, 388

Barthel Index (BI), 180, 197–199, 386, 388, 390, 391, 392

Baum, Carolyn, 93, 102–103, 115–116, 244, 258–259, 387

Behnke, C., 387

best practices

    in community settings, 357–359

    defining, 9–10

five key actions for, 46–47

in medical/rehabilitation systems, 353

in rehabilitation setting, 354–355

sociocultural context in, 349–363

Bing, R. K., 5–6

Binkley, J., 219–220, 389

biopsychosocial theory, 364

Black, M. M., 277, 278, 387

Bobby, C. L., 282, 387

Boschen, Kathy, 333–334, 387

Boston Naming Test, Consortium to Establish a Registry for Alzheimer's Disease (CERAD) version of, 54, 55

Bradley, R. H., 321–322, 387

Brody, E. M., 224–225, 227, 388

Brown, C., 61–62, 247, 388

Bruininks-Oseretsky Test of Motor Proficiency (BOTMP), 24, 49

Bryze, K., 387

BTE Work Simulators, 161

Buck, E. L., 298, 388

budgeting decisions, 373–374

Bundy, Anita, 146–147, 322, 387

Burgio, L., 240, 388

Burke, Janice, 279–282

Buros Mental Measurement Yearbook, 56

Byles, J., 319–320, 388

Byrne, D. G., 309, 388

Caldwell, B. M., 321–322, 387

Canada, health promotion strategies in, 368

Canadian Association of Occupational Therapists (CAOT), 81

Canadian Model of Occupational Performance, 15

Canadian Occupational Performance Measure (COPM), 39, 84–85, 87, 109, 173, 182, 193, 233–239, 241, 378, 386, 388, 390, 391, 392, 393, 394, 395

Canadian Occupational Therapy Association, 114

Comprehensive Rehabilitation and Mental Health Services, Safety Assessment of Function and the Environment for Rehabilitation—Health Outcome Measurement and Evaluation (SAFER-HOME), 326–327, 387

Comprehensive Rehabilitation and Mental Health Services, Safety Assessment of Function and the Environment for Rehabilitation (SAFER Tool), 326–327, 387

Pediatric Activity Card Sort (PACS) of, 114, 135, 262–263, 387

Career/Lifeskills Resources Inc., 344–345, 387

Caregiver Assessment of Functional Dependence and Upset (CAFU), 229, 233, 235, 236, 240, 386, 388, 390, 391, 392, 393, 394, 395

caregivers, 82, 93, 94

Carswell, A., 86, 173, 388

case studies, 70

Center for Inclusive Design and Environmental Access, School of Architecture and Planning, 320

Center for Outcome Measurement in Brain Injury at Craig Hospital, 331–332, 387

Center for Rehabilitation Effectiveness, 221–223, 387

Centre d'expertise, Functional Autonomy Measurement System (SMAF), 202–203, 387

Centre interdisciplinaire de recherche en réadaptation et intégration social, Life Habits Assessment (LIFE-H), 119–120, 387

Charlifue, S., 270–271, 303–304, 389

Child Behaviors Inventory of Playfulness (CBIP), 130, 132–137, 138–139, 385, 388, 390, 393

Child Health Questionnaire (CHQ), 200–201, 385, 388, 390, 391, 392, 393

Child-Initiated Pretend Play Assessment (ChIPPA), 130, 137, 142–143, 386, 389, 390, 391, 393, 394

children

ADL instruments for, 181

client-centered approach with, 87–88

recognizing performance impairments in, 54–56

self-reported health status of, 94

Children's Assessment of Participation and Enjoyment (CAPE), 110–111, 265–266, 386, 388, 390, 391, 393, 394, 395

Children's Autism Rating Scale (CARS), 60

Children's Health Assessment Questionnaire (CHAQ), 208–210, 386, 388, 390, 391, 392

Christiansen, Charles, 5, 14, 376

chronobiology, 287

civic life measures, 395

Clare, A. W., 281, 387

Clark, J. E., 282, 387

classroom, occupational performance analysis in, 363

client

definition of, 89

identification of performance issues by, 33–35

insights of, 88–89

needs of, 12–13

Client and Clinician Assessment of Performance (CCAP), 76

client-centered approach, 8–9, 81–90, 86–87, 193, 232

advantages and disadvantages of, 82–83

assumptions of, 82

with children, 87–88

Occupational Circumstance Assessment Interview and Rating Scale in, 85–86

of occupational performance, 83–84, 154–156

client-identified ADL activities, 180

Client-Oriented Role Evaluation, 85

clinical reasoning, 70–71

Cochrane Collaboration databases, 30–31
cognitive impairment, 51–53, 236–237
cognitive status, 228
Cohen, S., 307, 387
communication measures, 31, 391
communities of practice, 347–348
community-based practice, innovative, 359–363
community environments, 331–332
  OT models for, 11–15
  performance assessment in, 356–359
community health system, 370–371
community integration, 301–306, 310
Community Integration Measure (CIM), 305, 306, 386, 388, 390, 395
Community Integration Questionnaire (CIQ), 304–305, 306, 386, 389, 390, 393, 394, 395
community life measures, 395
"compare to self" paradigm, 29
Consortium to Establish a Registry for Alzheimer's Disease (CERAD), 54
constraint negotiation strategies, 250–251
Contemporary Task-Oriented Approach Model, 14–15
continuous quality improvement, 373
controlled setting, 67–68
Cook, Dr. Joanne, 67
Co-ordinates Publications, Westmead Home Safety Assessment, 328–329, 387
Coping Inventory for Children, 98, 385, 388, 390, 391, 393, 394, 395
Corcoran, M. A., 76
core knowledge, 376
Corney, R. H., 281, 387
Craig Handicap Assessment and Reporting Technique (CHART), 121–122, 270–271, 303–304, 306, 386, 388, 389, 390, 391, 392, 393, 394, 395
Craig Hospital Inventory of Environmental Factors (CHIEF)/CHIEF Short Form, 329–330, 386, 387
Crawford, C., 84, 171–172, 388
credibility, 69
criterion measurement, 25
Crombie, V., 213–214, 389
Cross, E. G., 282, 387
Csikszentmihalyi, M., 109, 249, 287–288, 289, 296–297, 387

Dahlem, N. W., 335–336, 389
Daniels, D., 63
data
  analysis of, 65–66, 74–75
  further collection of, 18
  word vs numbers, 68
Data System (Marita Kloseck), Leisure Competence Measure (LCM), 256–257, 387
Davies, D., 305, 388

day care facilities, 372
DeBittignies, B. H., 246, 388
decision-making process, 39–43, 353–356
dementia, 51–52, 233
Dent, P., 213–214, 389
dependability, 69
depression, 52, 54
description, 74–75
Deshpande, S., 87, 387
Developmental Test of Visual Motor Integration, 56
Dickerson, A. E., 387
Direct Assessment of Functional Abilities (DAFA), 233, 234, 236, 242, 386, 388, 390, 391, 392, 393, 394, 395
Direct Assessment of Functional Status (DAFS), 234, 236, 241, 386, 388, 390, 391, 392, 393, 394, 395
disability, 3
  ADL instruments for, 181
  Nagi model of, 227
  proxy vs self-reports on, 94
  quality of life with, 377–378
  WHO classification of, 107
documentation
  to ensure reimbursement, 380–381
  of quantitative information, 74
domestic life measures, 392–393
Duara, R., 241
Duncan-Jones, P., 309, 388
Dunn, W., 58, 61–62, 63
Dura, R., 388

Early Childhood Environment Rating Scale, Revised Edition, 327
Early Coping Inventory, 99, 385, 388, 390, 391, 393, 394, 395
ecological validity, 25–28
Ecology of Human Performance Model, 13
Educational Resource Information Clearinghouse (ERIC), 43
educational systems, 349–352
Edwards, D. F., 244, 387
effort testing, 159–160
Employment Potential Improvement Corporation, Spinal Function Sort, 175–176, 387
employment settings, 356–359
Engelhardt, Tristam, 107
environment, 315
  assessment of, 35–36, 316–343
Environment-Independence Interaction Scale (EIIS), 320
environmental context, 25–28, 27, 89–90, 231
environmental factors, measuring, 315–343
Environmental Utility Measure (EUM), 320
ergonomic-based assessment, 154–155
ethnography, 66, 70–71
evaluation, 70–71

evidence, 31, 46
evidence-based health care, 2
evidence-based practice
    challenges of providing, 30–31
    in functional capacity assessment, 164
    measurement information for, 21, 22, 29–30
Experience Sampling Method (ESM), 287–288, 289, 291,
        296–297, 386, 387, 390, 391, 392, 393, 394, 395
experimental tradition, 67
Extended Activities of Daily Living (EADL) Scale, 234,
        237, 241, 243, 386, 388, 390, 391, 392, 393

family context, 93
Family Day Care Rating Scale, 327
Farley, G. K., 335–336, 389
Feasibility Evaluation Checklist, 177, 386, 388, 390, 394
Fetkovich, M. M., 387
Finn, Geraldine, 369–370
Fisher, A. G., 239, 387
Fisher, G., 169–170, 389
Fleming, M., 75–76
Florey, L. L., 278–279, 387
flow, 249, 287–288
Ford, A. B., 215–216, 388
Forsyth, K., 87, 387
Frary, R. B., 388
free appropriate, public education (FAPE), 349
Freland, F., 387
Frenchay Aphasia Screening Test (FAST), 54, 55
Friedland, J., 308, 388
Fries, J. F., 208–210, 387, 388
functional assessment, 162–163
Functional Assessment Network (FAN), 161
Functional Autonomy Measurement System (SMAF), 202–
        203, 386, 387, 390, 391, 392, 393, 394, 395
Functional Behavior Profile (FBP), 93, 95, 102–103, 386,
        387, 390, 393, 394, 395
functional capacity evaluation, 160–165
Functional Communication Profile, 54
Functional Impairment Battery (FIB), 53–54
Functional Independence Measure (FIM) and WeeFIM,
        93–94, 204–207, 353–354, 386, 389, 391, 392, 393
functional intervention, 251
functional levels, 152–154
functional literacy testing, 54
functional mobility reports, 94
Furst, Gloria, 294–295, 388

general task and demands measures, 390–391
Gerhart, K., 270–271, 303–304, 389
Geriatric Depression Scale, 55
Geriatric Depression Scale Short Form (GDS-SF), 54
Gill, C., 219–220, 389
Ginzburg, Eli, 277

Gitlin, L. N., 76, 240, 388
Goldhammer, V., 85, 387
Goldsmith, C., 213–214, 389
Goldsmith, D. P., 208–210, 388
Goldstein, G., 245, 388
Gordon, W. A., 389
government, occupational therapists in, 371
Graham, Frank Porter, 323–327
Gray, S., 242, 388
grounded theory, 66

Haglund, L., 87, 387
Hamera, E., 247, 388
Hamilton Rating Scale for Depression, 54
Hartner, S., 388
health
    changing definition of, 369–370
    participation and, 108
Health Act, Child Health Questionnaire (CHQ), 200–
        201, 388
Health Assessment Questionnaire (HAQ), 208–210, 386,
        387, 390, 391, 392
The Health of Canadians—The Federal Role, 368
health services delivery, 369–370
Healthy People 2010 Objectives, 368
hearing loss, 52–53
Henderson, S., 309, 388
Henriksson, C., 87, 387
Henry, A., 84, 171–172, 388
Higginbotham, N., 319–320, 388
Hoberman, H. M., 307, 387
Holm, M. B., 245, 388
Home and Community Environments: Measure of Proc-
        esses of Care (MPOC), 385, 388
Home Assessment Profile (HAP), 322
home care pilot study, 75–76
Home Environment: Home Observation for Measurement
        of the Environment (HOME) Revised Edition,
        321–322, 387
home environment measures, 317–318, 331–332, 386, 388
Home Falls and Accidents Screening Tool (HOME
        FAST), 319–320, 385, 388
Home Observation for Measurement of the Environment
        (HOME), 130, 139, 148–149, 386, 387, 390, 391,
        393, 395
Home Occupational-Environment Assessment (HOEA),
        320–322
hospital/community health system, 370–371
household context, 93
Housing and Urban Development (HUD) grants, 371
Howe, S., 388

Idyll Arbor Inc., Leisure Satisfaction Questionnaire/
        Leisure Satisfaction Scale (LSS), 258–259, 388

lenger, A., 85, 387
impairments
    ADL instruments for, 181
    identifying, 53–54
    impact of, 50–52, 53
    measuring at performance component level, 49–50
    in older adults, 55
Impara, J. C., 388
independence, 26, 51
independent living settings, 356–359
individualized outcomes, evaluating, 71
industry workers, 370
Infant-Toddler Environment Rating Scale, Revised Edition, 323–327
Infant Toddler Sensory Profile, 63–64
information, influencing policy, 367–374
Institute of Medicine, Enabling America report, 376
institutional barriers, 250–251
institutional parameters, 347–348
Instrumental Activities of Daily Living (IADL), 94, 228, 234, 237, 354
    vs activities of daily living, 109
    client-centered versus standard approaches to, 232
    considerations in measuring, 228–232
    definition of, 179, 227–228
    measuring performance in, 157, 232–247
    purpose of, 229–230
Integrated Disability and Safety Management system, 157
intelligence scales, 56
Interdisciplinary Assessment Data, 54–56
interdisciplinary systems models, 10
Interest Checklist and Activity Checklist, 386, 388, 390, 392, 393, 394, 395
International Classification of Functioning (ICF), 107, 108, 109
    environmental factor classification in, 315–316
    measures mapped to, 390–395
    for occupational therapy measurement, 12
International Classification of Functioning, Disability and Health, WHO (ICF), 1, 10–11, 301–302, 376
International Classification of Impairments, Disability and Handicaps, WHO, 303–304, 306
interpersonal interaction measures, 393
Interpersonal Support Evaluation List (ISEL), 306, 307, 308–309, 386, 387, 390, 393, 394, 395
interventions
    effectiveness of, 377
    implementing, 18
Interview Schedule for Social Interaction (ISSI), 307–309, 386, 388, 390, 393, 395
interviews, 73–74
    in community-based practice, 359, 362
    in medical/rehabilitation setting, 356
    in public education setting, 351

vs quantitative data, 68
    semi-structure, 278
intrinsic motivation, 251
investigator role, 69–70
Isacsson, A., 317–318, 388
Iso-Ahola, S. E., 253, 388
Iwarsson, S., 317–318, 388

Jackson, B. A., 215–216, 388
Jackson, E., 250–251
Jaffe, M. W., 215–216, 388
Job Content Questionnaire (JCQ), 157, 167–168, 386, 388, 390, 392, 393, 394
job demands analysis (JDA), 157
job descriptions, 156
Job Match System, 157
job requirement levels, 152–154
Juvenile Arthritis Functional Assessment Report (JAFAR), 211–212, 386, 388, 390, 392, 393, 394, 395
Juvenile Arthritis Functional Assessment Scale (JAFAS), 211–212, 386, 388, 390, 392, 393, 394, 395
Juvenile Arthritis Self-Report Index (JASI), 213–214, 386, 389, 390, 392, 393, 394, 395
    Part 2 of, 193

Kamarck, T., 307, 387
Karagiozis, H., 242, 388
Karasek, R. A., 167–168, 388
Karls, J. M., 283, 389
Karnofsky Performance Scale, 94
Katz, S., 215–216, 388
Katz Index of Activities of Daily Living, 180, 215–216, 386, 388, 390, 392, 393, 395
Kaufman Assessment Battery for Children (KABC), 56
Kawas, C., 242, 388
Kids Play Survey (KPS), 133
Kielhofner, G., 5, 13–14, 84, 85, 87, 169–170, 171–172, 279–282, 284, 292–293, 340–341, 387, 388, 389
King, G., 331–332, 388
King, S., 331–332, 388
Kirby Report, 368
Kitchen Task Assessment (KTA), 39, 233, 235, 236, 244, 386, 387, 390, 392, 394
Klein Bell ADL assessment, 180
knowledge, learning and applying, 394
knowledgeable informants, 72
Knox, S., 140–141, 388
Kreutzer, J. S., 389
Kulkarni, S., 87, 387

language assessment, 51, 54, 56
language naming deficits, 51–52
Lansky Play-Performance Scale, 94
Larson, R., 289, 296–297, 387

Law, M., 86, 88, 109, 173, 213–214, 388, 389

Lawton, M. P., 224–225, 227, 388

LDB Project, Leisure Diagnostic Battery (LDB), 274–275, 388

Learning & Applying Knowledge, 107

learning measures, 394

least restrictive environment (LRE), 349

leisure, 249

   barriers to, 250–251

   performance assessment in, 249–275

Leisure Ability Model, 251

Leisure Activity Profile (LAP), 269, 386, 388, 390, 392, 393, 394

Leisure Boredom Scale (LBS), 253, 385, 388, 390, 394

Leisure Competence Measure (LCM), 254–255, 386, 387, 390, 392, 393, 394, 395

Leisure Diagnostic Battery (LDB), 272–273, 274–275, 386, 388, 390, 392, 393, 394, 395

leisure education, 251

Leisure Satisfaction Questionnaire/Leisure Satisfaction Scale (LSS), 256–257, 386, 388, 390, 393, 394, 395

Levinson, J., 388

Life Habits Assessment (LIFE-H), 119–120, 386, 387, 390, 391, 392, 393, 394, 395

life history, 66

Life Role Salience Scale, 282, 386, 387, 394, 395

Life Stressors and Social Resources Inventory—Adult Form (LISRES-A), 338–339, 385, 388, 394, 395

Lifease Corporation, Lifease Software: Ease 3.2 Basic and 3.2 Deluxe, 286, 323, 325, 388

Lighthouse Near Acuity Card, 55

Lincoln, N. B., 243, 388

Linder, T. W., 144–145, 388

Link-Nelson Occupational Therapy Evaluation for Skilled Nursing Facilities

   Melville Nelson Self-Care Assessment (SCA) of, 217–218

literacy, 53

Little, B. R., 290–291, 388

Loewenstein, D., 241, 388

Logsdon, R., 101–102, 389

London Handicap Scale, 117–118, 386, 388, 390, 392, 393, 394, 395

Longitudinal Functional Assessment systems, Structured Observation and report Technique (SORT) subscale of, 288

Lovell, D. J., 388

Mackenzie, L., 319–320, 388

Madigan, J. M., 279–281, 389

Mahoney, S. I., 197–199, 388

Mahurin, R. K., 246, 388

major life areas measures, 394–395

Mallinson, T., 84, 171–172, 388

Mann, W. C., 269, 388

Marchand, B., 302–303, 389

Mattingly, C., 75–76

maximal effort measurement, 159–160

McColl, M. A., 86, 173, 305, 308, 316, 388

McCue, M., 245, 388

McGill, G., 388

McMaster Model, 164

meaningfulness, 28, 67, 68

measure analysis worksheets, 47

Measure of Processes of Care (MPOC), 331–332

Measure of Quality of the Environment (MQE), 333–334, 385, 387

measurement, 3–18

   central considerations in, 22–25

   client-centered approach to, 8–9

   costs of, 380

   criteria for, 28–31

   critical review of, 43

   environmental context and ecological validity in, 25–28

   goals in, 17–18

   guiding decisions about, 33–43

   interpreting results of, 38, 42–43

   issues and practice of, 21–31

   list of, 383–384

   mapped to International Classification of Functioning, 390–395

   need for in practice, 21–22

   by occupational performance area, 385–386

   in occupational therapy, 45–47

   principles of, 378

   setting framework for, 21–25

   by source/author, 387–389

   strategies for, 16–18

   validity and reliability of, 22–23

measurement information

   establishing integrity of, 49–57

   for evidence-based practice, 29–30

   medical model, expansion of, 370–372

Medical Outcomes Trust, London Handicap Scale, 117–118, 388

medical records, 230, 231–232

medical/rehabilitation systems, 352–353

Medicare

   Canadian model of, 368

   in rehabilitation systems, 353

   reimbursement for, 347–348, 352–353

Meenan, R. F., 388

Mellnick, Dave, 121–122, 388

Melville, D. L., 388

Melville Nelson Self-Care Assessment (SCA), 217–218, 386, 388, 390

Memory and Behavior Problems Checklist: Revised, 101–102, 385, 389, 390, 392, 394, 395 memory testing, 54

mental health community settings, 356–359

Mermelstein, R., 307, 387

Meyer, Adolph, 3, 4, 5, 6

Michelman, S. M., 278–279, 387

Missiuna, C., 88, 388

mobility measures, 391–392

Model of Human Occupation (MOHO), 13–14, 83, 84, 279, 282

Model Systems Database, U.S., CHART in, 304

Moore-Corner, R. A., 340–341, 388

Moorhead, Linda, 279

Moskowitz, R. W., 215–216, 388

Motor Free Test of Visual Perception, 56

motor impairments, 52

Multidimensional Scale of Perceived Social Support (MSPSS), 330, 335–336, 386, 389, 395

Multiphasic Environmental Assessment Procedure (MEAP), 327

Nagi model of disablement, 227

National Health Interview Survey on Disability, 94

National Institutes of Health Activity Record (ACTRE), 288, 289, 294–295, 386, 388, 390, 391, 392, 393, 394, 395

National Occupational Classification and Dictionary of Occupational Titles, 156–157

natural setting, 67–68, 74

naturalistic research, 66–70

needs and measurement approaches, 16

Nelson, L. L., 388

Nouri, F. M., 243, 388

Nowak, M., 84, 171–172, 388

Nussbaum, P., 245, 388

Oakley, Frances, 282–283, 284, 388

objective investigation, 69–70

observations

    community-based, 359, 362

    documenting, 74

    in medical/rehabilitation setting, 356

    in public education setting, 351

    in qualitative evaluation, 73

    strengths and limitations of information from, 231

occupation, 5–7

occupation-based, client-centered practice, 2, 47

occupational balance, 287

    future directions for, 289–291

    measures of, 289–298

    ways of measuring, 287–289

Occupational Circumstances Assessment-Interview and Rating Scale (OCAIRS), 85–86, 87, 386, 387, 390

Occupational History, 279

occupational performance

    definition of, 7–8

    identifying goals of, 40–41, 43

    identifying problems in, 49–50

    measures of

        challenges and strategies in, 375–381

        in classroom, 363

        client-centered perspective on, 81–90, 154–156

        listed by area, 385–386

        in public education setting, 352

        qualitative, 65–77

        in sociocultural context, 347–364

        in therapeutic outing to home, 357, 360

    participation and, 107–108

Occupational Performance History Interview II (OPHI), 83, 84, 87, 171–172, 386, 388, 391, 393, 394

Occupational Questionnaire (OQ), 288, 289, 292–293, 386, 388, 391, 392, 393, 394, 395

occupational role assessment, 277–284

Occupational Role History, 278–279, 386, 387, 391, 394

Occupational Self-Assessment (OSA), 83–84, 85, 86–87, 386, 387, 391, 392, 393, 394

occupational storytelling, 71

occupational therapists, 381

occupational therapy

    central concepts for, 6–10

    within community environments, 11–15

    core knowledge of, 376

    measures of, 1–2, 15–16, 45–47

    philosophical influences on, 4–6

    in public education setting, 349–352

    roots of, 375–376

Occupational Therapy Practice Framework, 349, 364

older adults

    ADL instruments for, 181

    impairment of, 52–55

Olsen, L., 87, 340–341, 397-388

optimal experience, 287–288

Opzoomer, A., 302–303, 389

outcome measurement, 24–25, 40–43, 379

    guiding decisions about, 33–43

    interpreting, 40

    selection of, 36–37, 39

Outcome Measures Rating Form, 316, 396–405

    guidelines for, 406–409

Outcomes Assessment Information Set (OASIS), 76

Overholser, D., 270–271, 303–304, 389

pain assessment, 158–159

parental reports, 94

Parenting Stress Index (PSI), 95–96, 386, 388, 391, 393

PART Group, Personal Care Participation Assessment and Resource Tool (PC-PART), 124–126, 388

participation, 107–108
  interdisciplinary systems models for, 10
  measurement of, 107–126
  supports and barriers to, 27–28
Patient Specific Function Scale (PSFS), 193, 219–220, 386, 389, 391, 392, 393, 394, 395
Peabody Individual Achievement Test-Revised, 54
Pediatric Activity Card Sort (PACS), 114, 130, 132, 135, 260–261, 386, 391, 392, 394, 395
Pediatric Evaluation of Disability Inventory (PEDI), 182, 221–223, 386, 387, 391, 392, 393, 395
Pediatric Interest Profiles, 130, 132
Survey of Play for Children and Adolescents, 133, 262–264, 386, 389, 391, 393
penal institutions, 371–372
Perceived Efficacy and Goal Setting System (PEGS), 87–88, 386, 388, 391, 392, 393, 394, 395
perceived freedom, 251
performance
  assessment by areas of, 35
  within community environments, 11–15
  comparisons to external standards, 28–29
  impaired
    in children, 54–56
    in older adults, 52–54
  sensory processing and, 56–57
Performance Assessment of Self-Care Skills (PASS), 39, 233, 235, 237, 245, 386, 388, 391, 392, 394
Performance Assessment of Self-Care Skills (PASS-Clinic or Home versions), 229
performance-based assessment, 35–36
  impairment issues impacting, 50–52
  strengths and limitations of, 230
performance-capacity gap, 315
performance measurement
  of activities of daily living, 179–225
  context for, 49–50
  of IADLs, 227–247
  testing of, 379–380
performance outcomes
  identified by other person or group, 35
  identified by person, 33–35
  measurement stages of, 34–38
person-environment integration, 26–28
person-environment-occupation framework, 45–46, 164
person-environment-occupation (PEO) diagrams linked to outcome measures, 385–386
person-environment-occupation (PEO) model, 14, 107, 151–154, 155, 315–316
Person in Environment System, 283, 386, 389, 391, 393, 395
person-occupation measurement, 160–165
person variables, evaluation of, 27

Personal Care Participation Assessment and Resource Tool (PC-PART), 124–126, 386, 388, 392, 393
personal causality, 251
Personal Projects Analysis (PPA), 287–291, 386, 388, 391, 392, 393, 394, 395
Physical Demands Analysis (PDA), 157
physical disability measures, 233–241
Physical Self-Maintenance Scale (PSMS), 224–225, 386, 388, 391, 392
Pirozzolo, F. J., 246, 388
play, 129–130
  activity assessment, 132
  measuring performance in, 129–149
  supportiveness of environment for, 137–139, 146–149
Play History, 130, 131–132, 386, 387, 389, 391, 393, 394, 395
Playability Audit, 327
player, approach of to play, 132–137
playfulness assessment, 132–137
Polatajko, H., 86, 173, 388
policy, information influencing, 367–374
Pollock, N., 86, 88, 173, 388
population-based time use surveys, 109
Post-Occupancy Evaluation (POE), 328, 386, 388
practice-based qualitative approaches, 70–71
practice measurements, 345
Pre-Teen Play Survey (PPS), 133
prediction, 67
Preferences for Activities of Children (PAC), 267–268, 386, 388, 391, 392, 393, 394, 395
Preiser, W. F. E., 328, 388
presbycusis, 52–53
process measurement, 24, 71
professional assumptions, 348
professional responsibility, 367–368
Program in Occupational Therapy, Feasibility Evaluation Checklist, 177, 388
programs, evaluating outcomes for, 40–43
protocols, measurement strategies in, 378–379
proxy reports, 93–94, 230, 231
psychiatric illness measures, 233–241
Psychological Assessment Resources
  Life Stressors and Social Resources Inventory—Adult Form (LISRES-A), 340–341, 388
  Parenting Stress Index (PSI), 95–96, 388
Psychological Corporation
  Children's Assessment of Participation and Enjoyment (CAPE), 110–111, 267–268, 388
  Preferences for Activities of Children (PAC), 269–270, 388
  School Functional Assessment (SFA), 96–97, 112–113, 388
psychosocial status, 52

public education setting, 349–352
public forums, raising issues in, 368–369
public information, 372

qualitative measurement, 66, 75–76
    for occupational performance, 65–77
    practice-based uses of, 70–71
    principles and purpose for, 72–75
qualitative research designs, 65–66
quality improvement, evaluating, 71
quality of life, 377–378
    interdisciplinary systems models for, 10
    participation and, 108
    reports on, 94
quantitative data, 68
questions, asking right, 72–73

Rabinowitz, H. Z., 328, 388
Rapid Estimate of Adult Literacy in Medicine (REALM), 54
Rasch analysis, 83, 84, 85, 182
Readily Achievable Checklist: A Survey for Accessibility, 323
reading ability, 53
REALM test, 55
reasoning, types of, 76
recreation participation, 251
reflective questions, 34–35
rehabilitation systems, decision-making in, 353–356
Reichler, R., 284, 388
Reilley's Model of Occupational Behavior, 13–14
Reilly, Mary, 5, 277
reimbursement, 352–353, 373–374, 380–381
Reintegration to Normal Living Index, 302–303, 306, 386, 389, 391, 392, 393, 394
relationship measures, 393
reliability, 69
Rempel, R., 389
responsiveness, 25
Resumption of Activities of Daily Living Scale (RADL), 160
retirement communities, 372
Revised Classification of Jobs, 156
Revised Knox Preschool Play Scale (PPS-R), 130, 132, 137, 140–141, 386, 388, 391, 392, 393, 394
Ribgy, M., 388
Richardson, G., 270–271, 303–304, 389
Rigby, M., 84, 171–172
Rintala, D. H., 298, 388
Rivermead Behavioral Inattention Test (BIT), 54, 55
Rogers, C. S., 388
Rogers, J. C., 3, 4–5, 16–17, 238, 245, 388
Role Checklist, 282–283, 284, 386, 387, 388, 391, 393, 394, 395

role loss, 283
Romanow Report, 368
Rosenbaum, P., 331–332, 388
Rosenthal, M., 389
Roth, D. L., 240, 388
Rucks, V., 250–251

Sacco, J., 242, 388
Safety Assessment of Function and the Environment for Rehabilitation—Health Outcome Measurement and Evaluation (SAFER-HOME), 324–325, 385
Safety Assessment of Function and the Environment for Rehabilitation (SAFER Tool), 324–325
Scholastic Testing Service, Inc.
    Coping Inventory for Children, 98, 388
    Early Coping Inventory, 99, 388
School-Age Care Environment Rating Scale, 327
School Function Assessment (SFA), 25, 95, 96–97, 112–113, 349, 386, 388, 391, 392, 393, 394
school system, occupational therapists in, 371
Schulte, M., 388
Scott, R., 309, 388
self-actualization, 4
self-care measurement, 108, 181–182, 392
self-efficacy, 251
Self-Identified Goals Assessment (SIGA), 85
self-reports, 94, 230, 231
sensorimotor performance assessment, 56
Sensory Integration and Praxis Tests, 56
sensory processing, 56–57
Sensory Profile, 58–59
    Adult, 57, 61–62
        Infant Toddler, 63–64
        reliability and validity of, 59–60
Sensory Profile scale, 31
service systems, 347
Shapiro, M., 242, 388
Shear, E., 388
Shore, A., 213–214, 389
Short Blessed Test, 54, 55
Short Orientation-Memory-Concentration Test, 54
Sickness Impact Profile (SIP), 94
Simple Audition Test, 55
simultaneous occupational roles, 279
Singh, G., 208–210, 388
single-case research, 66
Skurla, E., 238, 388
Slosson Oral Reading Test—Revised, 54
Smith, N. R., 292–293, 388
snowballing, 72
social context measures, 93–103
social ecology approach, 287, 288–289
social environment, 309–310
social life measures, 395

social practices, 348

Social Problem Questionnaire, 281, 386, 387, 391, 393, 394

Social Security disability, 370

social support, 301–302, 306–309, 310

Social Support Inventory for People with Disabilities (SSIPD), 306–307, 308–309, 386, 388, 391, 393

societal needs, 377–378

sociocultural context, 6, 347–364

Spinal Function Sort, 175–176, 386, 387, 391, 392, 394

Spitzer, W. O., 302–303, 389

Stagnitti, K., 142–143, 389

standard score comparisons, 29

statistical tests, 25

Stratford, P., 219–220, 389

Structured Assessment of Independent Living Skills (SAILS), 233, 235, 236, 246, 386, 388, 391, 392, 393, 394, 395

Structured Observation and Report Technique (SORT), 288, 298, 386, 388, 391, 392, 393, 394, 395

subjective investigation, 69–70

Sunderland, T., 238, 388

Takata, N., 389

Talty, P., 269, 388

Task Analysis: An Individual and Population Approach, 156

Teri, L., 101–102, 389

Test of Environmental Supportiveness (TOES), 130, 132, 139, 146–147, 322, 386, 387

Test of Grocery Shopping Skills, 235, 239–241, 247, 386, 388, 391, 393, 394

Test of Playfulness (ToP), 130, 132, 322
    Version 4, 136–137, 386, 387, 391, 393
    testing, definition of, 15–16

Therapeutic Environment Screening Survey for Nursing Homes (TESS-NH), 327

Therapy Skill Builders, Pediatric Interest Profiles: Survey of Play for Children and Adolescents, 133, 264, 389
    Time Structure Questionnaire (TSQ), 288

time use measures, 288–298

top-down approach, 14–15, 49

Transdisciplinary Play-Based Assessment (TPBA), 2nd Ed., 130, 137, 144–145, 386, 388, 391, 392, 393, 394

transferability, 69

treatment planning, 70

triangulation, 69

Truax, P., 101–102, 389

trustworthiness, 69

Uniform Data System for Medical Rehabilitation, Functional Independence Measure (FIM) and WeeFIM, 204–207, 389

university databases, 30–31

Uomoto, J., 101–102, 389

Uttermohlen, D. M., 298, 388

validity, 69

Valpar Component Work Samples (VCWS), 161, 174, 386, 389, 391, 392, 393, 394, 395

Valpar International Corporation, 174, 389

values, enduring, 5

Velozo, C. A., 169–170, 389

Vineland Adaptive Behavior Scales (VABS), 100, 386, 387, 391, 392, 393, 394, 395

visual acuity
    corrected, 54
    diminished in older adults, 52–53

visual data, gathering, 73

visual impairment testing, 53–54

visual neglect, unilateral, 52, 54

Vitaliano, P. P., 101–102, 389

vocational rehabilitation, PEO factors in, 155

Walens, D., 84, 171–172, 388

Wandrei, K., 283, 389

Watts, J. H., 279–281, 292–293, 388, 389

Wechsler Intelligence Scales, 56

WeeFIM, 182, 204–207, 386, 389, 391, 392, 393

Weissinger, E., 253, 388

well-being, focus on, 377–378

Westaway, M., 219–220, 389

Westmead Home Safety Assessment, 326–327, 385, 387

White, E. T., 328, 388

Whiteneck, G., 270–271, 303–304, 389

Wilcock, A., 5, 6–7

Willer, B., 389

Williams, J. B. W., 283, 389

Williams, J. I., 302–303, 389

Wolenski, J., 85, 387

Wood-Dauphinee, S., 302–303, 389

Woodcock Johnson Psycho-Educational Battery, 56

Work Environment Impact Scale, 340–341

work environment measures, 157–158, 340–343, 385, 388

Work Environment Scale (WES), 158, 342–343, 386, 387

work performance
    assessment of
        common elements and variations in, 162–163
        functional capacity evaluation in, 160–165
        measuring environment in, 157–158
        measuring occupation in, 156–157
        measuring person in, 158–160
        occupational performance perspective on, 151–177
    context of, 151–152
    definition of, 152–154
    self-perception of, 160
    work simulation tasks, 161

Work-Site Analysis forms, 158

WorkCover New South Wales, guidelines of, 164

Worker Role Interview, 169–170, 386, 389, 391, 392, 394, 395

Workplace Environment: Work Environment Impact Scale, 385, 388

World Health Organization—Disability Schedule II (WHO-DAS II), 123, 386, 389, 391, 392, 393, 395

Wright, F. V., 213–214, 389

Yerxa, Elizabeth, 4

Young, N. L., 190–191

Zarit, S., 101–102, 389

Zimet, G. D., 335–336, 389

Zimet, S. G., 335–336, 389

Zung Self Rating Scale, 54

WAIT ...*There's More!*

SLACK Incorporated's Professional Book Division offers a wide selection of products in the field of Occupational Therapy. We are dedicated to providing important works that educate, inform and improve the knowledge of our customers. Don't miss out on our other informative titles that will enhance your collection.

Evidence-Based Reahbilitation: A Guide to Practice

Mary Law, PhD, OT Reg. (Ont.), FCAOT
384 pp., Soft Cover, 2002, ISBN 1-55642-453-1,
Order #44531, **$39.95**

While providing the most up-to-date information about evidence-based practice, this comprehensive and well-organized text focuses on building skills for understanding and using evidence, rather than simply doing research. By viewing evidence-based practice from a holistic perspective, this text also recognizes the need to include client preferences and therapists' clinical reasoning in the process.

Occupational Therapy: Performance, Participation, and Well-Being

Charles H. Christiansen, EdD, OTR, OT(C), FAOTA;
Carolyn M. Baum, PhD, OTR/L, FAOTA;
and Julie Bass Haugen, PhD, OTR/L, FAOTA
680 pp., Hard Cover, 2005, ISBN 1-55642-530-9,
Order #35309, **$67.95**

Highly valued by both therapists and educators, *Occupational Therapy: Performance, Participation, and Well-Being* has been integral to the evolution of occupational therapy services and functions. Incorporated within this impressive third edition are new features and topics that shape the modern era in occupational therapy practice.

Measuring Occupational Performance: Supporting Best Practice in Occupational Therapy, Second Edition

Mary Law, PhD, OT Reg. (Ont.), FCAOT; Carolyn M. Baum, PhD, OTR/L, FAOTA; and Winnie Dunn, PhD, OTR, FAOTA
432 pp., Hard Cover, 2005, ISBN 1-55642-683-6,
Order #36836, **$46.95**

Occupation-Based Practice: Fostering Performance and Participation

Mary Law, PhD, OT Reg. (Ont.), FCAOT; Carolyn M. Baum, PhD, OTR/L, FAOTA; and Sue Baptiste, MHSc, OT Reg. (Ont.), FCAOT
160 pp., Soft Cover, 2002, ISBN 1-55642-564-3,
Order #35643, **$38.95**

Best Practice Occupational Therapy: In Community Service with Children and Families

Winnie Dunn, PhD, OTR, FAOTA
400 pp., Soft Cover, 2000, ISBN 1-55642-456-6,
Order #34566, **$48.95**

Quick Reference Dictionary for Occupational Therapy, Fourth Edition

Karen Jacobs, EdD, OTR/L, CPE, FAOTA and Laela Jacobs, OTR
600 pp., Soft Cover, 2004, ISBN 1-55642-656-9,
Order #36569, **$26.95**

Client-Centered Occupational Therapy

Mary Law, PhD, OT Reg. (Ont.)
192 pp., Soft Cover, 1998, ISBN 1-55642-264-4,
Order #32644, **$34.95**

All About Outcomes: An Educational Program to Help You Understand, Evaluate, and Choose Adult Outcome Measures

Mary Law, PhD, OT Reg. (Ont.); Gillian King, PhD, OT Reg. (Ont.); Dianne Russell, MSc; Debra Stewart, MSc, OT(C); Patricia Hurley, BA (Hon); and Eric Bosch, BSc, Mmath
CD-ROM, 2000, ISBN 1-55642-727-1, Order #37271,
$49.95

All About Outcomes: An Educational Program to Help You Understand, Evaluate, and Choose Pediatric Outcome Measures

Mary Law, PhD, OT Reg. (Ont.); Gillian King, PhD, OT Reg. (Ont.); Dianne Russell, MSc; Debra Stewart, MSc, OT(C); Patricia Hurley, BA (Hon); and Eric Bosch, BSc, Mmath
CD-ROM, 1999, ISBN 1-55642-729-8, Order #37298,
$49.95

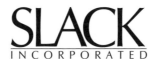